R TATE

D1349146

R TATE

# SPINE

# ORTHOPAEDIC SURGERY ESSENTIALS

# SPINE

## ORTHOPAEDIC SURGERY ESSENTIALS

**Spine**
Christopher M. Bono, MD
Steven R. Garfin, MD

**Pediatrics**
Kathryn E. Cramer, MD
Susan A. Scherl, MD

**Foot and Ankle**
David B. Thordarson, MD

**Sports and Medicine**
Anthony Schepsis, MD
Brian Busconi, MD

**Oncology and Basic Science**
Carol Morris, MD

**Adult Reconstruction**
Daniel J. Berry, MD

**Hand and Wrist**
James R. Doyle, MD

**Trauma**
Charles Court-Brown, MD
Margaret McQueen, MD
Paul Tornetta III, MD

# ORTHOPAEDIC SURGERY ESSENTIALS

# SPINE

**Series Editors**

**PAUL TORNETTA III, MD**
*Professor*
*Department of Orthopaedic Surgery*
*Boston University School of Medicine;*
*Director of Orthopaedic Trauma*
*Boston University Medical Center*
*Boston, Massachusetts*

**THOMAS A. EINHORN, MD**
*Professor and Chairman*
*Department of Orthopaedic Surgery*
*Boston University School of Medicine*
*Boston, Massachusetts*

**Book Editors**

**CHRISTOPHER M. BONO, MD**
*Assistant Professor*
*Department of Orthopaedic Surgery*
*Boston University School of Medicine*
*Boston University Medical Center*
*Boston, Massachusetts*

**STEVEN R. GARFIN, MD**
*Professor and Chairman*
*Department of Orthopaedic Surgery*
*University of California, San Diego*
*San Diego, California*

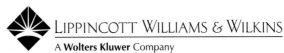

**LIPPINCOTT WILLIAMS & WILKINS**
A **Wolters Kluwer** Company
Philadelphia • Baltimore • New York • London
Buenos Aires • Hong Kong • Sydney • Tokyo

*Acquisitions Editor:* Robert Hurley
*Developmental Editor:* Lisa Consoli
*Production Editor:* Maryland Publishing Services
*Manufacturing Manager:* Colin Warnock
*Cover Designer:* Karen Quigley
*Compositor:* Maryland Composition
*Printer:* Quebecor World Kingsport

© 2004 by LIPPINCOTT WILLIAMS & WILKINS
530 Walnut Street
Philadelphia, PA 19106 USA
LWW.com

All rights reserved. This book is protected by copyright. No part of this book may be reproduced
in any form or by any means, including photocopying, or utilized by any information storage and
retrieval system without written permission from the copyright owner, except for brief quotations
embodied in critical articles and reviews. Materials appearing in this book prepared by
individuals as part of their official duties as U.S. government employees are not covered by the
above-mentioned copyright.

Printed in the USA

**Library of Congress Cataloging-in-Publication Data**

Spine / book editors, Christopher M. Bono, Steven R. Garfin.
    p. ; cm. — (Orthopaedic surgery essentials)
    Includes bibliographical references and index.
    ISBN 0-7817-4613-2
    1. Spine—Surgery. 2. Spine—Diseases—Treatment. 3. Orthopedics. I. Bono, Christopher
M. II. Garfin, Steven R. III. Series
    [DNLM: 1. Spine—surgery. 2. Orthopedi Procedures. 3. Spinal Diseases—surgery. WE
725 S75712 2004]
    RD768.S67232 2004
    617.5'6059—dc22                     2004046464

    Care has been taken to confirm the accuracy of the information presented and to describe
generally accepted practices. However, the authors, editors, and publisher are not responsible
for errors or omissions or for any consequences from application of the information in this
book and make no warranty, expressed or implied, with respect to the currency, completeness,
or accuracy of the contents of the publication. Application of this information in a particular
situation remains the professional responsibility of the practitioner.

    The authors, editors, and publisher have exerted every effort to ensure that drug selection
and dosage set forth in this text are in accordance with current recommendations and practice
at the time of publication. However, in view of ongoing research, changes in government
regulations, and the constant flow of information relating to drug therapy and drug reactions,
the reader is urged to check the package insert for each drug for any change in indications
and dosage and for added warnings and precautions. This is particularly important when the
recommended agent is a new or infrequently employed drug.

    Some drugs and medical devices presented in this publication have Food and Drug
Administration (FDA) clearance for limited use in restricted research settings. It is the
responsibility of the health care provider to ascertain the FDA status of each drug or device
planned for use in their clinical practice.

10 9 8 7 6 5 4 3 2 1

To my wife, Terri, and my parents, Ernest and Grace, who are the reasons
for any of my accomplishments
—CMB


This book is dedicated to the many fellows, of which Chris Bono, MD,
is a shining example, who have taught me and aided me
in much of what I know and do.
—SRG

# CONTENTS

## SECTION I: EXAMINATION AND DIAGNOSTICS

## SECTION II: TRAUMA

## SECTION III: INFECTION

# SECTION IV: TUMORS

# SECTION V: DEGENERATIVE DISORDERS

# SECTION VI: SPINAL DEFORMITY

# SECTION VII: METABOLIC AND INFLAMMATORY DISORDERS

# SECTION VIII: SURGERY

# SECTION IX: GENERAL KNOWLEDGE

# CONTRIBUTING AUTHORS

**Marc A. Agulnick, M.D.**
Assistant Clinical Instructor
Department of Orthopedic Surgery
SUNY at Stony Brook
Stony Brook, New York

**Todd J. Albert, M.D.**
Professor and Vice Chairman
Department of Orthopedics
Thomas Jefferson University Medical College
Philadelphia, Pennsylvania

**Rajesh George Arakal, M.D.**
Chief Resident
Department of Orthopaedics
New Jersey Medical School
Newark, New Jersey

**John M. Beiner, M.D.**
Clinical Instructor in Orthopaedics
Yale University School of Medicine
New Haven, Connecticut

**Carlo Bellabarba, M.D.**
Assistant Professor
Department of Orthopaedic Surgery and Sports Medicine
University of Washington
Seattle, Washington

**Scott D. Boden, M.D.**
Professor of Orthopaedic Surgery
Emory University School of Medicine
Atlanta, Georgia

**Christopher M. Bono, M.D.**
Assistant Professor
Department of Orthopaedic Surgery
Boston University School of Medicine
Boston, Massachusetts

**Gregory T. Brebach, M.D.**
Attending Orthopaedic Spine Surgeon
Department of Surgery
Good Samaritan Hospital
Barrington, Illinois

**Keith H. Bridwell, M.D.**
Asa C. and Dorothy Jones Professor
Department of Orthopaedic Surgery
Washington University School of Medicine
St. Louis, Missouri

**Eugene J. Carragee, M.D.**
Professor
Department of Orthopedic Surgery
Stanford University
Stanford, California

**Steven Caruso, M.E.**
Instructor, Orthopaedic Surgery
New York Medical College
Valhalla, New York

**Jens R. Chapman, M.D.**
Professor
Department of Orthopaedics and Sports Medicine
Joint Professor of Neurological Surgery
University of Washington
Seattle Washington

**Bradford L. Currier, M.D.**
Associate Professor
Department of Orthopedics
Mayo Graduate School of Medicine
Rochester, Minnesota

**Robert K. Eastlack, M.D.**
Orthopaedic Surgery
University of California, San Diego
San Diego, California

**Charles C. Edwards II, M.D.**
The Maryland Spine Center
Mercy Medical Center
Baltimore, Maryland

**Jeffrey S. Fischgrund, M.D.**
Spine Surgeon
Orthopaedics
William Beaumont Hospital
Royal Oak, Michigan

**Steven R. Garfin, M.D.**
Professor and Chairman
Department of Orthopaedic Surgery
University of California, San Diego
San Diego, California

**Jonathan N. Grauer, M.D.**
Assistant Professor
Department of Orthopaedics and Rehabilitation
Yale University School of Medicine
New Haven, Connecticut

**Mark G. Grossman, M.D.**
Attending Physician
Department of Orthopedics
Division of Sports Medicine
Winthrop University Hospital
Mineola, New York

**Thomas R. Haher, M.D.**
Professor of Orthopaedic Surgery
New York Medical College
Valhalla, New York
Chairman, Orthopaedic Surgery
Lutheran Medical Center
Brooklyn, New York

**Robert F. Heary, M.D.**
Associate Professor
Department of Neurological Surgery
UMDNJ–New Jersey Medical School
Newark, New Jersey

**Harry N. Herkowitz, M.D.**
Chairman
Department of Orthopaedic Surgery
William Beaumont Hospital
Royal Oak, Michigan

**Christopher P. Kauffman, M.D.**
Assistant Professor
Department of Orthopaedic Surgery
University of California, San Diego
San Diego, California

**Choll W. Kim, M.D., Ph.D.**
Assistant Professor
Department of Orthopaedic Surgery
University of California, San Diego
San Diego, California

**Brian K. Kwon, M.D.**
Vancouver Spine Program
Department of Orthopaedic Surgery
University of British Columbia
Vancouver Hospital and Health Sciences Center
Vancouver, BC, Canada

**Steven S. Lee, M.D.**
Orthopaedic Surgery
University of California, San Diego
San Diego, California

**Paul C. Liu, M.D.**
Department of Orthopaedic Surgery
Kaiser Hospital Fontana
Fontana, California

**John Louis-Ugbo, M.D.**
Instructor
Departments of Anatomy and Cell Biology and Orthopaedic Surgery
Emory University School of Medicine
Atlanta, Georgia

**Peter O. Newton, M.D.**
Associate Clinical Professor
Department of Orthopedic Surgery
University of California, San Diego
Children's Hospital
San Diego, California

**Mini Pathria, M.D.**
Professor
Department of Radiology
UCSD Medical Center
San Diego, California

**Bernard A. Pfeifer, M.D.**
Spine Surgery
Lahey Clinic
Burlington, Massachusetts

**Frank M. Phillips, M.D.**
Professor
Department of Orthopaedic Surgery
Rush University Medical Center
Chicago, Illinois

**Maya E. Pring, M.D.**
Clinical Assistant Professor
Department of Orthopedic Surgery
University of California, San Diego
San Diego, California

**John M. Rhee, M.D.**
Assistant Professor
Department of Orthopaedic Surgery
The Emory Spine Center
Atlanta, Georgia

**Dilip K. Sengupta. M.D., M.Ch. (Orth)**
Spine Fellow
Department of Orthopaedic Surgery
William Beaumont Hospital
Royal Oak, Michigan

**Gary Scott Shapiro, M.D.**
Northwestern University Medical School
Chicago, Illinois

**Edward D. Simmons, M.D., C.M., M.Sc., F.R.C.S.(C)**
Associate Clinical Professor
Department of Orthopaedic Surgery
State University of New York at Buffalo
Buffalo, New York

**Kern Singh, M.D.**
Chief Resident
Orthopedic Surgery
Rush University Medical Center
Chicago, Illinois

**Andrew V. Slucky, M.D.**
Chief
Spinal Surgery Service (Ortho)
Alta Bates Summit Medical Center
Oakland, California

**Mike H. Sun, M.D.**
Chief Resident
Orthopedic Surgery
University of Chicago
Chicago, Illinois

**Kenneth G. Swan, Jr., M.D.**
Orthopaedic Resident
University of Medicine and Dentistry of New Jersey
Newark, New Jersey

**Robert Talac, M.D., Ph.D**
Research Associate
Department of Orthopedic Surgery
Mayo Graduate School of Medicine
Rochester, Minnesota

**William Tontz, M.D.**
Professor
University of California, San Diego
San Diego, California

**Eeric Truumees, M.D.**
Attending Spine Surgeon
Department of Orthopedics
William Beaumont Hospital
Royal Oak, Michigan

**Alexander R. Vaccaro, M.D.**
Professor
Department of Orthopaedic Surgery
Thomas Jefferson University
Philadelphia, Pennsylvania

**Antonio Valdevit, M.Sc.**
Director, Research Engineering
Department of Surgery
Lutheran Medical Center
Brooklyn, New York

**Artem Y. Vaynman, M.D.**
Resident in Neurological Surgery
UMDNJ–New Jersey Medical School
Newark, New Jersey

**Michael J. Vives, M.D.**
Assistant Professor
Department of Orthopaedics
University of Medicine and Dentistry of New Jersey
Newark, New Jersey

**Matthew P. Walker, M.D.**
Department of Orthopaedic Surgery
Charleston Area Medical Center
Charleston, West Virginia

**Dennis R. Wenger, M.D.**
Clinical Professor of Orthopedic Surgery
University of California–San Diego
Children's Hospital
San Diego, California

**F. Todd Wetzel, M.D.**
Professor
Department of Orthopaedic Surgery and Neurosurgery
Temple University
Philadelphia, Pennsylvania

**Gregory C. Wiggins, M.D.**
Affiliate Assistant Professor
Neurological Surgery
University of Washington
Seattle, Washington

**Michael J. Yaszemski, M.D., Ph.D.**
Associate Professor of Orthopedic Surgery and
    Biomedical Engineering
Department of Orthopedic Surgery
Mayo Graduate School of Medicine
Rochester, Minnesota

**Hansen A. Yuan, M.D.**
Professor
Department of Orthopaedic and Neurological Surgery
SUNY, Upstate Medical University
Syracuse, New York

**Philip S. Yuan, M.D.**
Clinical Instructor
Department of Orthopaedic Surgery
Thomas Jefferson University
Philadelphia, Pennsylvania

**Yinggang Zheng, M.D.**
Research Fellow
Department of Orthopaedic Surgery
State University of New York at Buffalo
Buffalo, New York

# SERIES PREFACE

Most of the available resources in orthopaedic surgery are very good, but they either present information exhaustively—so the reader has to wade through too many details to find what he or she seeks—or assume too much knowledge, making the content difficult to understand. Moreover, as residency training has advanced, it has become more focused on the individual subspecialties. Our goal was to create a series at the basic level that residents could read completely during a subspecialty rotation to obtain the essential information necessary for a general understanding of the field. Once they have survived those trials, we hope that the *Orthopaedic Surgery Essentials* books will serve as a touchstone for future learning and review

Each volume is to be a manageable size that can be read during a resident's tour. As a series, they will have a consistent style and template, with the authors' voices heard throughout. Content will be presented more visu-

ally than in most books on orthopaedic surgery, with a liberal use of tables, boxes, bulleted lists, and algorithms to aid in quick review. Each topic will be covered by one or more authorities, and each volume will be edited by experts in the broader field.

But most importantly, each volume—*Pediatrics, Spine, Sports Medicine*, and so on—will focus on the requisite knowledge in orthopaedics. Having the essential information presented in one user-friendly source will provide the reader with easy access to the basic knowledge needed in the field, and mastering this content will give him or her an excellent foundation for additional information from comprehensive references, atlases, journals, and on-line resources.

We would like to thank the editors and contributors who have generously shared their knowledge. We hope that the reader will take the opportunity of telling us what works and does not work.

—Paul Tornetta III, MD

# PREFACE

As the field of spinal surgery advances, it has become increasingly difficult for the orthopaedic resident to collect, let alone master, necessary and pertinent knowledge and information. Notwithstanding, the resident is challenged further by the interdisciplinary nature of spinal surgery, with advances in knowledge being reported in various orthopaedic subspecialty and neurosurgical journals in addition to dedicated spine publications.

In accordance with the series' mission, the editors of *Orthopaedic Surgery Essentials: Spine* have attempted to collect, compile, and distill this information into one easily accessible and user-friendly source. The chapters have been written with one goal in mind—educating the resident. The chapters have been authored by established and upcoming leaders and pioneers in spinal surgery whose challenge it was, metaphorically, to fit an encyclopedia into a briefcase. After reading their splendid work, you will realize they have superbly succeeded!

# ACKNOWLEDGMENTS

For their outstanding work, which can be visibly appreciated between this book's covers, I thank all of the authors, who, regardless of how busy and renown, managed to find time for this project. For placing in my hands this opportunity, among so many others, I sincerely thank Paul Tornetta and Tom Einhorn. I pledge heartfelt gratitude to my mentor and coeditor, Steve Garfin, as this book represents yet another reinforcing bond to our already enduring friendship.

For their countless hours of dedication not otherwise visibly acknowledged in this book except in these words, I thank Bob Hurley and Lisa Consoli. Likewise, I thank all of the orthopaedic residents in Boston, San Diego, and Newark for teaching me how to be a teacher. Last, but most important, I acknowledge my patients who share with me the unending desire to make them well.

—Christopher M. Bono, MD

I particularly wish to thank my administrative staff and nurse practitioner, Elizabeth Stimson, FNP, who have given me the opportunities and time to work with residents and fellows. Their support has allowed efforts such as this book to be completed; with the help of many of the fellows we (as a team) have trained over the years.

—Steven R. Garfin, MD

# PHYSICAL EXAMINATION OF THE SPINE

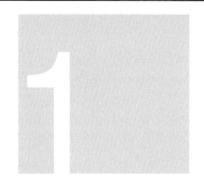

**STEVEN S. LEE**
**CHRISTOPHER M. BONO**

The physical examination remains the cornerstone of evaluation of spinal disorders. Despite great advances in imaging, such as computed tomography and magnetic resonance imaging, these modalities provide instantaneous images of continuously dynamic tissues. Clinical correlation of imaging findings with the physical examination provides the basis for treatment decision making. The development of a systematic physical examination is a fundamental skill for the spine surgeon. A routine approach improves the identification of subtle clinical findings and helps improve diagnostic accuracy.

A comprehensive physical examination can support a diagnosis that may have origins from spinal cord, root, or musculoskeletal pathology. Conversely, it can implicate disorders that mimic spinal pathology, such as lower extremity arterial insufficiency, which can feign neurogenic claudication. Only after a complete exam are diagnostic tests ordered to confirm a specific diagnosis. Ordering an array of diagnostic tests without a complete physical exam often adds costs unnecessarily and leads to confusion concerning the significance of incidental positive findings.

The surgeon first encounters the spine patient in one of two settings: the *emergency department* or the *outpatient clinic*. Patients may present to the emergency or trauma department with an acute spinal injury. This can range from spinal cord injury from a cervical fracture-dislocation after a diving injury to sudden-onset back and leg pain from lifting a heavy box. Initial examination is crucial to guide additional diagnostic evaluation and possible surgical intervention, with goals of preventing additional injury and restoring function.

Patients present to the outpatient clinic for evaluation of chronic and subacute problems. A thorough examination in the clinic is no less important than in the emergency setting. A greater emphasis is placed, however, on performing specific provocative tests in consideration of the patient's signs and symptoms.

This chapter presents an approach to a thorough and systematic spine examination. The patient's presentation in each of the two aforementioned settings results in emphasis on different aspects of physical examination. The fundamentals of examination remain the same, however.

## EXAMINATION IN THE EMERGENCY SETTING

The physical examination in the trauma setting requires the coordinated efforts of the spine surgeon, general trauma surgeon, and ancillary staff. Information regarding the accident scene can help estimate the mechanism of injury, severity, and approximate amount of energy that was imparted. This information can lead to a higher index of suspicion for some patients who present with minimal complaints in relation to the energy of the trauma. For example, significant front-end automobile damage may heighten the awareness of possible blunt intraabdominal injury, major vessel injury, or distracting ligamentous spinal injury from a sudden deceleration mechanism.

The initial evaluation of a trauma patient is guided by standard Advanced Traumatic Life Support protocol. The mnemonic *ABCDE* helps to remember the components: *Airway*, *Breathing*, and *Circulation* are mandatory in the initial evaluation of the patient. Proper oxygenation and perfusion of tissues helps to reduce further injury at the cellular level. This includes the possible prevention of further hypoxic injury after spinal cord injury. As the patient is hemodynamically stabilized, specific life-threatening injuries are addressed. After this, any *Deficits* are noted after proper *Exposure* of the patient; this can show posterior injuries or injuries concealed by clothing.

After adequate stabilization and resuscitation of the patient, it is imperative to perform a thorough and efficient examination of the spine. Full spine precautions are followed until injury is ruled out. The full exam must be completed despite detection of one spinal injury. The incidence of noncontiguous spinal injuries has been found in 15% of cases.

Spinal cord injury can occur with or without an obvious bony or ligamentous spinal injury. The determination of the type of spinal cord injury is important. An incomplete injury may have a good prognosis for some functional motor recovery, whereas complete injuries have a much poorer prognosis. An *incomplete spinal cord injury* is defined as the presence of some motor or sensory function more than three segments below the level of injury (American Spinal Injury

Association definition). A *complete spinal cord injury* is defined as the absence of motor or sensory function more than three segments below the level of injury.

## Inspection

Examination includes the following:

- Inspect the patient. Inspection requires adequate exposure of the entire patient and is mandatory to avoid missing injuries obscured by clothing or positioning.
- Assess the overall appearance and status of the patient. Unusual posturing, such as decerebrate or decorticate posturing, may signify a traumatic brain injury, which may limit detailed neurologic examination.
- Determine the need for mechanical ventilation. Patients with spinal cord injuries above the C4-5 level typically are unable to breathe independently because of denervation of the diaphragm and may require mechanical ventilation.
- Examine the head and skull to look for contusions, lacerations, or ecchymosis that can suggest a pattern or directional mechanism of cervical spine injury.
- Assess the chest wall and pelvis.
- Note any spontaneous movement of the extremities because in the intubated or obtunded patient this may represent the extent of the motor exam. The lack of spontaneous movement in uninjured extremities may signify a neurologic deficit.
- Look for subtle findings, such as shoulder or lap belt markings, which can raise the suspicion of thoracolumbar spinal injury.

## Palpation

Full spine precautions are followed during palpation of the neck and back (Table 1-1). Four people are required for the standard logroll maneuver used to examine the spine. One person stays at the head of the bed and coordinates the movements. Three people are positioned on the side of the patient to stabilize and turn the chest, pelvis, and limbs as a unit. As the head and neck are manually stabilized, the posterior portion of the cervical collar can be removed. Palpation begins at the base of the skull and proceeds caudally. No attempts at manipulation or range of motion testing of the cervical spine should be performed at this time.

The first region examined is the occiput. This represents the posterior base of the skull and marks the junction of the head with the cervical spine. Crepitus or ecchymosis can signify a basilar skull fracture. Palpation of the midline is performed next. The spinous processes of the upper cervical spine are difficult to palpate, but the overall sagittal and coronal alignment of the cervical spine can be assessed (Fig. 1-1). Any abnormal position of a spinous process, tenderness to direct palpation, associated paraspinal muscle spasm, torticollis, or neck malposition can signify an underlying injury. Common injuries encountered in the upper cervical spine are difficult to assess solely by physical examination. These injuries include dens fractures, atlantoaxial instability, and C1 ring fractures.

Next, palpation of the middle and lower spine is per-

### TABLE 1-1  GUIDELINES FOR SPINE PRECAUTIONS

| | |
|---|---|
| Principles | Protection of the full spine during management of the trauma patient |
| | Immobilization of the spine in neutral position on a firm surface |
| Prehospital | Use of semirigid cervical collar, side head supports, or bolsters |
| | Strapping of the head, shoulders/chest, and pelvis |
| | Full-length spine boards, scoop stretcher, or vacuum mattress for transport of the patient |
| In-hospital | Manual protection (cervical collar) replaced after examination or procedures (intubation) |
| | Four-person logroll for examination and rigid transfer slides for transferring the patient |
| | Minimization of the number of logrolls and transfers |

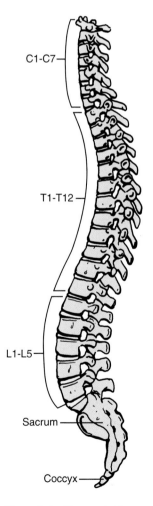

**Figure 1-1**  The axial alignment of the adult human spine as seen in the lateral view. Note the normal lordosis of the cervical and lumbar areas.

C1-C7

T1-T12

L1-L5

Sacrum

Coccyx

formed. The spinous processes here are easier to palpate, and sagittal and coronal alignment can be assessed more easily. Common injuries encountered in this region include fractures, subluxations, dislocations, and fracture-dislocations. The first large spinous process, or *vertebra prominens*, encountered is usually that of C7 or T1. This is a landmark for the cervicothoracic junction.

The spinous processes of the thoracic vertebrae are palpated easily. The ribs and associated costovertebral joints provide increased stability to the thoracic spine so that small amounts of displacement or step-off suggest high-energy injuries with a high rate of spinal cord injury. Systematic palpation along the thoracic spine is performed to note any point tenderness, malalignment, or interspinous widening. Rib fractures can be detected with tenderness to palpation.

The lumbar spine is palpated in continuity with the thoracic spine. The spinous processes are easily palpable. Alignment is noted along with tenderness or interspinous gaps. The tops of the iliac crests are usually at the level of the L4-5 interspace, which can be a useful surface landmark. Taking both hands on either side of the iliac crests and placing the thumbs toward the midline directs the examiner to the space between the L4 and L5 spinous processes.

Finally, palpation of the subcutaneous sacrum and coccyx is performed. This part of the exam is important because fractures of the sacrum frequently are missed initially. Missed, untreated sacral fractures can lead to persistent neurologic deficits, such as bowel, bladder, and sexual dysfunction from distal sacral root injuries. After palpation, the cervical collar is replaced, and the patient is gently and uniformly logrolled back to the supine position.

## Sensation

Sensation is evaluated by dermatomes according to respective nerve roots. The sensory dermatomes can overlap one another by one third of their width. Thoracic and lumbar nerve roots exit below the corresponding numbered vertebral body. Cervical roots exit above their corresponding numbered vertebrae, as there are eight cervical roots for seven cervical vertebrae. The C8 root exits below the C7 vertebral body (Fig. 1-2).

Comprehensive testing includes the following:

- Light touch
- Pinprick
- Vibration
- Proprioception
- Temperature
- Pain response

In the acute trauma setting, only the first two tests usually are feasible. Simple testing of light touch can entail the use of the examiner's fingertips or a cotton-tipped applicator against the skin. Testing is performed bilaterally to detect asymmetric innervation. This can delineate the general areas of sensory deficiency.

Pinprick testing can be performed to define further and demarcate specific dermatomes where sensory function may be diminished or absent. To perform pinprick testing, a cotton-tipped applicator or tongue depressor can be

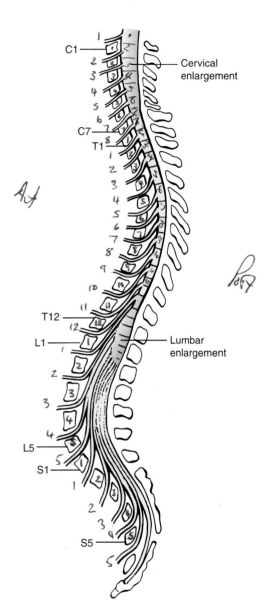

**Figure 1-2** The relationship of the spinal nerve roots to the vertebral bodies. The eighth cervical root exits below the C7 vertebra because there are eight cervical roots but only seven cervical bodies.

snapped in half and the pointed end used for testing. Alternatively, a manufactured device can be used if readily available. The affected areas or spinal cord level can be outlined with a skin marker for subsequent serial evaluations.

Cervical testing concentrates on the C5 to T1 nerve roots (Fig. 1-3). The C5 dermatome innervates the skin overlying lateral shoulder and deltoid muscle. C6 usually innervates the radial aspect of the forearm and the thumb. C7 usually innervates the middle finger distal to the metacarpophalangeal joint. C8 usually innervates the ulnar aspect of the forearm, including the ring and small fingers. T1 usually innervates the medial arm.

Discrete testing of the thoracic levels (T2-12) along the chest wall is difficult because of overlap among the roots.

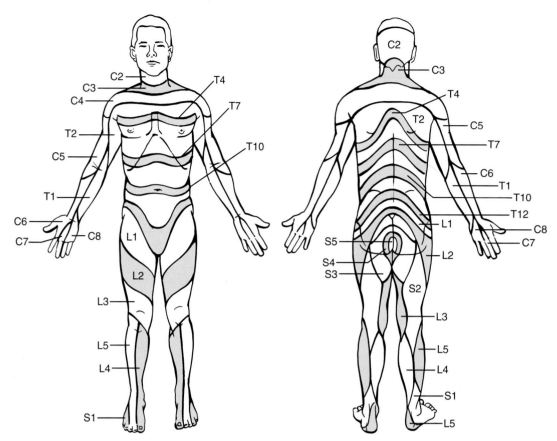

**Figure 1-3** Anterior and posterior sensory dermatomes. (From Browner BD, Jupiter JB, Levine AM, Trafton PG. Skeletal trauma, 2nd ed. Philadelphia: WB Saunders, 1998.)

Three regions can be used as landmarks, however, as follows:

- T4 dermatome usually innervates the chest wall at the level of the nipples.
- T7 usually innervates the chest wall at the level of the xiphoid process and the inferior border of the sternum.
- T10 usually innervates the skin along the abdominal wall at the level of the umbilicus.

Sensation in the upper chest (above the nipple line) can be supplied by distal cervical nerve roots, the so-called cervical cape. Sensation in this region should not be misinterpreted as thoracic level function because this can lead to inaccurate determination of the level or type of spinal cord injury.

The lumbar roots innervate the lower extremities. These levels correlate with skin patches that are oriented obliquely along the thighs and legs (see Fig. 1-3). The L2 dermatome corresponds to the anterior thigh. The L3 dermatome usually involves the anterior knee. The L4 to S1 dermatomes are tested in the foot. L4 innervates the medial foot; L5, the dorsal foot; and S1, the lateral foot.

The remainder of the sacral roots innervate the skin in the perineal region. They form concentric rings around the anus with S5 in the center (Fig. 1-4). Although the reflex examination is discussed in detail later, evaluation of rectal tone and the bulbocavernosus reflex is performed best in conjunction with perianal sensory testing. The "anal wink" is described as the contraction of the anal sphincter when the skin around the anus is stimulated. The *anal wink* is a normal response, and its absence can indicate spinal cord injury. Rectal tone is assessed and should be characterized as normal, decreased, or absent. The presence of rectal tone and perianal sensation can indicate sacral sparing and continued function of the sacral roots and their connections through the cord to the cerebral cortex. Sacral sparing may be the only indication of an incomplete cord injury during the initial trauma evaluation. Four common incomplete cord injury patterns are the central cord syndrome, anterior cord syndrome, posterior cord syndrome, and Brown-Séquard syndrome. These are described in further detail in Table 1-2.

In completing the rectal exam, the *bulbocavernosus reflex* is tested. This is elicited most easily by a gentle tug on a Foley catheter. During the digital rectal exam, this maneuver elicits a normal reflexive contraction of the anal sphincter. If a catheter has not been placed, the reflex can be elicited by a gentle squeeze of the glans penis in men or the clitoris in women. The absence of the bulbocavernosus reflex indicates spinal shock. *Spinal shock* is a state of flaccid paralysis, hypotonia, and areflexia that can occur immediately after a severe spinal cord injury. The reflex returns in most people after 24 hours, signifying the end of spinal shock. If there is no evidence of sacral sparing or spinal

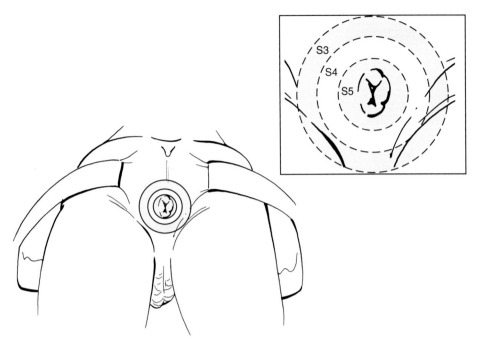

**Figure 1-4** The concentric rings of the dermatomes around the perineal area. (From Browner BD, Jupiter JB, Levine AM, Trafton PG. Skeletal trauma, 2nd ed. Philadelphia: WB Saunders,1998.)

cord function distal to the level of injury after the period of spinal shock is over, this is a complete cord injury and there is little chance for further recovery of function. No determination of the completeness of spinal cord injury can be made while the patient is in spinal shock.

## Motor

Associated extremity injuries may limit full evaluation of motor strength testing. Extremity injuries and associated pain should be noted in documenting strength testing.

Motor strength is graded by a 0-to-5 scale (Table 1-3). It is important to clarify a standard grading scale to optimize interexaminer and intraexaminer repeatability. Although some use a + or − to note slightly more or slightly less strength, this practice may create confusion. For example, subsequent examiners may not be able to differentiate between strength graded as 5− versus 4+.

Grading depends on the ability of the muscle to move a joint (see Table 1-3):

- *Grade* 5: Signifies full strength with the ability to move the joint against full resistance.

## TABLE 1-2 COMMON SPINAL CORD INJURY SYNDROMES

| Syndrome | Pathology | Frequency | Characteristics | Prognosis |
|---|---|---|---|---|
| Central | Age >50<br>Extension injury | Most common | Motor and sensory deficits<br>UE affected > LE | Fair |
| Anterior | Flexion/compression | Common | Motor deficit, some sensory loss<br>Deep pressure and proprioception preserved | Poor |
| Brown-Séquard | Penetrating trauma | Uncommon | Ipsilateral motor loss<br>Contralateral pain and temp loss | Good |
| Root | Foramina compression<br>HNP<br>Facet fracture | Common | Motor and sensory deficits in specific<br>neurologic level | Good |
| Complete | Burst fracture<br>Canal compression<br>Fracture-dislocation | Uncommon | No motor or sensory function below injury<br>level after spinal shock over | Poor |

HNP, herniated nucleus pulposus; LE, lower-extremity; UE, upper extremity.

## TABLE 1-3 MANUAL MOTOR TESTING GRADING SCALE

| | |
|---|---|
| 5 | Active movement against full resistance |
| 4 | Active movement against some resistance |
| 3 | Active movement against gravity |
| 2 | Active movement, gravity eliminated |
| 1 | Palpable or visible contraction |
| 0 | Paralysis, no visible contraction |

- *Grade 4:* Signifies the ability of the muscle to move the joint against some, but not full, resistance.
- *Grade 3:* Signifies movement against gravity alone without any added resistance.
- *Grade 2:* Signifies the ability to move the extremity or joint through a full range after gravity has been eliminated. Grade 2 biceps function means that the elbow can be flexed fully when the arc of motion is in a horizontal plane (e.g., the arm lying flat on the bed), but not when the arc of motion is in a vertical plane (Fig. 1-5).
- *Grade 1:* Signifies visible contraction of the muscle without the ability to move joint.
- *Grade 0:* Signifies no visible muscle contraction.

Similar to sensory innervation, most muscles are innervated by more than one root. Five major roots are evaluated in the upper extremity for cervical evaluation, C5 to T1, as follows:

- C5—evaluated by testing the deltoid with shoulder abduction
- C6—evaluated by testing the biceps and wrist extensors
- C7—evaluated by testing the triceps, wrist flexors, and finger extensors
- C8—evaluated by testing the finger flexors
- T1—evaluated by testing the intrinsic muscles of the hand through finger abduction and adduction

The intercostals and paraspinal muscles are not amenable to myotomal root level testing of thoracic spinal cord function. Although assessment of regional contraction in the thorax and abdomen can be performed, sensory testing of the dermatomes is used more accurately to determine the level of function.

Six major nerve roots are evaluated in the lower extremities, L1-S1, as follows:

- L1 and L2—evaluated by testing hip flexion
- L3—tested by knee extension, understanding that significant contributions to quadriceps innervation are made by L2 and L4
- L4—evaluated better alone by testing ankle dorsiflexion through the tibialis anterior
- L5—evaluated by testing great toe dorsiflexion through the extensor hallucis longus
- S1—evaluated by testing ankle plantar flexion through gastrocnemius complex

## Reflexes

Reflex testing is performed last to complete the initial spine trauma evaluation. The grading of reflexes also needs to

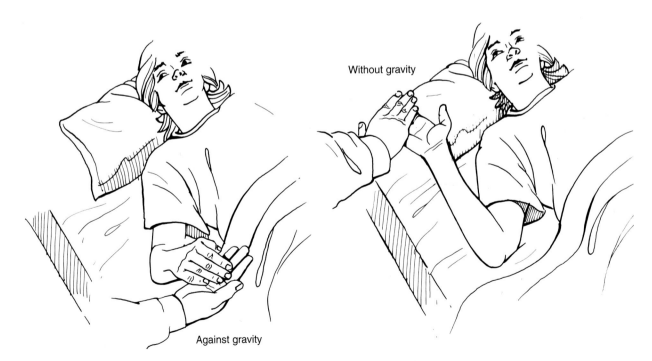

Without gravity

Against gravity

**Figure 1-5**   An example illustrating the difference between grade 2 versus grade 3 motor function of the biceps. If the elbow is able to be flexed without gravity, but unable to be flexed with gravity, the biceps is graded as having grade 2 strength.

be systematic and consistent to improve interexaminer and intraexaminer repeatability and reliability.

Reflexes are graded on a 0-to-3 scale, as follows:

- *Grade 3:* Hyperreflexia
- *Grade 2:* "Normal" response
- *Grade 1:* Hyporeflexia
- *Grade 0:* Absence of a reflex response

Testing reflexes should be performed with a standard reflex hammer to ensure an adequate response.

In the upper extremity, three major deep tendon reflexes are evaluated:

- C5 is tested by the biceps; C6, the brachioradialis; and C7, the triceps reflex. The reflexes are elicited at the musculotendinous junction near their insertion sites (Fig. 1-6).
- T7 to L1 levels can be tested by eliciting a superficial abdominal reflex. A light stroke of the skin along four quadrants centered on the umbilicus should result in contraction of the muscles to pull the umbilicus to that quadrant. T7-T10 is tested above the umbilicus, and T10-L1 is tested below the umbilicus. The bulbocavernosus and superficial anal reflexes were discussed earlier.

In the lower extremity, two major deep tendon reflexes can be tested (Fig. 1-7):

- L4 is tested by the patellar tendon reflex.
- S1 is tested by the Achilles tendon reflex.
- There is no reflex that can assess the L5 nerve root.

The presence of sustained clonus and a positive Babinski's sign indicate cranial or spinal upper motor neuron pathology. *Sustained clonus* is checked by quickly dorsiflexing the relaxed ankle joint. Greater than four beats of clonus is considered abnormal, with normal individuals usually exhibiting one to two beats. *Babinski's sign* (or *plantar reflex*) is checked by stroking the sole of the foot from the heel toward the toes with the handle end of a reflex hammer. It is considered positive with an up-going great toe. A normal response is flexion of the toes.

Reflexes may be absent if the patient is in spinal shock. This can last 24 to 48 hours. After spinal shock has ended, hyperreflexia, spasticity, and sustained clonus may be appreciated.

The initial trauma spine examination should enable determination of the following:

- Level of spinal cord injury
- Complete versus incomplete spinal cord injury
- Status of spinal shock and sacral sparing

# EXAMINATION IN THE OUTPATIENT CLINIC

Examination of the spine in the clinic usually is focused on areas pertaining to patient's complaints. A systematic exam is crucial, however, to avoid missing pathology and to make an accurate assessment. Principles of the examination are the same as that of the trauma exam, with more emphasis placed on the areas of symptoms and the use of provocative maneuvers. The goal of the exam is to determine if the patient's complaints arise from axial mechanical pathology, radiculopathy, myelopathy, or other pathology.

The combination of bilateral hyperreflexia, weakness or paralysis with little atrophy, Babinski's sign, clonus, and other pathologic reflexes suggests myelopathy and spinal cord compression. Other complaints related to an upper motor neuron lesion include the insidious onset of clumsiness in the hands and lower limbs, with increasing difficulty in maintaining balance.

Radiculopathy is suggested by pain, sensory, or motor dysfunction corresponding to a specific root level, usually in a unilateral distribution. Other signs of these lower motor neuron lesions include flaccid weakness of innervated muscles, marked muscle atrophy, and diminished or absent reflexes (Table 1-4).

## Inspection

Examination should include the following:

- Observe the overall patient, including affect, posture, and gait.
- Evaluate the patient's gait as he or she walks into the room or down the examination hallway. This aspect of the examination is often underappreciated and overlooked, but it can provide significant information. Although a comprehensive discussion of gait analysis is beyond the scope of this chapter, specific gait patterns should be noted that might be related to neural pathology:
  - □ Wide-based gait can signify instability related to myelopathy.
  - □ Locked knee can signify quadriceps weakness from L2-4 pathology.
  - □ Footdrop or steppage can signify loss of ankle dorsiflexion from weakness of tibialis anterior or extensor hallucis from L4-5.
  - □ Flatfoot or loss of push-off can signify loss of calf plantar flexion from weakness of the gastrocnemius-soleus from S1-2.
  - □ Abductor lurch most often is associated with hip pathology, but can be related to abductor weakness from L5 innervation of the gluteus medius.
- Assess the patient's posture, which can highlight areas of localized pain, muscle spasm, or deformity. Areas of splinting or awkward motion of the extremities can be appreciated.
- Evaluate the skin for any abnormalities and previous surgical scars.
- Evaluate the extremities for any muscle atrophy or cutaneous signs of diseases that may have spine-related pathology, such as rheumatoid arthritis or neurofibromatosis.
- With the patient standing upright, observe the coronal and sagittal alignment of the spine. Note exaggerated kyphosis, lordosis, or scoliosis in the spine with its orientation and location. Further curve analysis is done as the patient bends forward, noting differences in rib hump or paraspinal muscle prominence. Approximate rotation can be measured using a scoliometer at this time. As the

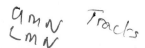
UMN  Tracts
LMN

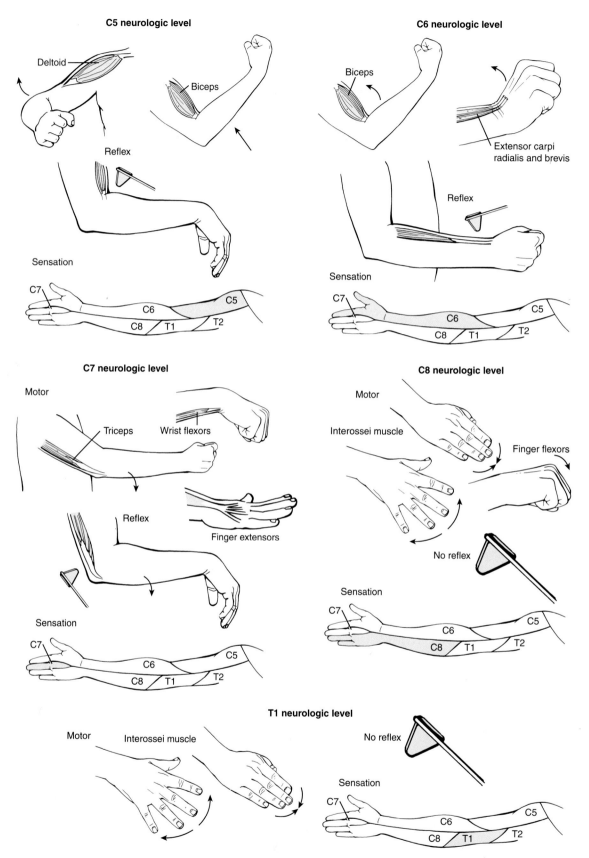

**Figure 1-6** Clinical testing of the C5-T1 nerve roots. (From Klein JD, Garfin SR: History and physical examination. In Weinstein JN, Rydevik BL, Sonntag VKG, eds. Essentials of the spine. New York: Raven Press,1995:71-95.)

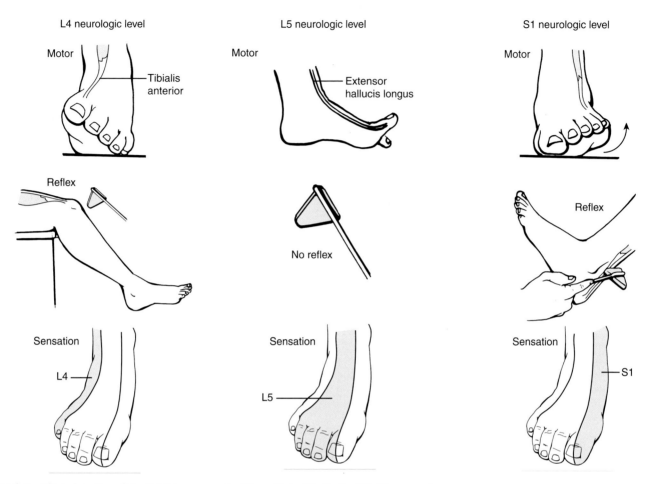

**Figure 1-7**   Clinical testing of the L4-S1 nerve roots. (From Klein JD, Garfin SR: History and physical examination. In Weinstein JN, Rydevik BL, Sonntag VKG, eds. Essentials of the spine. New York: Raven Press,1995:71-95.)

## TABLE 1-4  COMPARISON OF CLINICAL FINDINGS IN MYELOPATHY VERSUS RADICULOPATHY

|  | Myelopathy | Radiculopathy |
|---|---|---|
| Neurologic levels affected | >1 | Usually 1 |
| Bilateral symptoms | Common | Rare |
| Sensation | Variable | Decreased in dermatome distribution |
| Motor | Weakness with disuse atrophy | Weakness with marked atrophy of innervated muscles |
| Tone | Spastic | Flaccid |
| Reflexes | Hyperreflexic | Hyporeflexic |
| Gait | Wide based, poor balance | Depends on neurologic level affected (more related to specific muscle weakness, e.g., footdrop from L5 HNP) |
| Common finding(s) | Babinski sign, clonus<br>Presence of abnormal reflexes | Pain or dysesthesia in dermatome distribution |

HNP, herniated nucleus pulposus.

patient stands upright again, take care to note subtle curves in the thoracic and the lumbar portions of the spine. Normally the shoulders and pelvis should be level, and the head should be well balanced over the midline of the body. Note any pelvic or shoulder obliquity and trunk shift. The latter can be measured using a plumb line dropped from the base of the skull to determine amount of offset in centimeters from the center of the sacrum/coccyx.

■ Perform an active range of motion test for the cervical, thoracic, and lumbar spine. In the cervical spine, the distance from the chin to the chest is a measure of flexion and can be documented as the distance from the tip of the chin to the sternal notch. Full neck extension normally allows the patient to look straight up to the ceiling. Rotation and lateral bending are normally 70 and 40 degrees, respectively. The greatest amount of segmental flexion and extension occurs between the occiput and C1. The greatest amount of axial rotation (approximately 50%) occurs in the upper cervical spine, facilitated by the nearly flat orientation of the C1-2 facets.

There is limited motion in the thoracic spine owing to the stability provided by the ribs. In the lumbar spine, motion testing can be measured during the forward bending portion of inspection for curve deformities. Flexion can be measured by the distance of the fingertips to the toes. Extension is difficult to quantify accurately. Rotation and lateral bending can be measured in degrees from the orientation of the shoulders.

## Palpation

Palpation of the posterior spine as described for the trauma exam remains the same for the clinical examination. The anatomic landmarks can correlate areas of pain to specific vertebral levels. The paraspinal areas are checked for tenderness, muscle spasm, and masses. Lumbar strain is associated with paraspinal muscle spasm, tenderness to palpation, and pain with motion over several lumbar levels without radicular symptoms. Degenerative disc disease of a single level usually can be limited, however, to central tenderness to palpation with less paraspinal muscle spasm at a localized lumbar level, with or without radicular symptoms. The sacroiliac (SI) joints and the coccyx are evaluated for pain and tenderness.

Evaluation of the anterior spine begins at the neck. Structures to evaluate include the sternocleidomastoid muscle, carotid artery, and thyroid gland. If the patient reports mild difficulty swallowing, this may be caused by cervical bony abnormalities, osteophytes, or a mass that may be found by gentle palpation. The supraclavicular fossa also is evaluated for masses or a cervical rib. In the abdominal area, the umbilicus lies over the L3-4 levels near the aortic bifurcation. Deep palpation near this area may detect an aortic aneurysm, which can produce back pain.

The examination of peripheral pulses is performed at all extremities. Careful examination of pedal pulses is especially necessary to assess for possible peripheral vascular disease in patients with claudication symptoms.

## Sensory and Motor Testing

Sensory and motor function testing remain the same as for the trauma evaluation. Areas of pain or abnormal sensation are noted for dermatomal, peripheral nerve, stocking-glove, or nonanatomic distribution. Weakness of specific muscles or groups of muscles helps distinguish root versus peripheral nerve dysfunction. Additional attention should be paid to differentiating central nervous system from peripheral nerve function. Careful physical examination with a high index of suspicion can help differentiate between peripheral nerve versus spinal cord and root pathology. Detailed understanding of the brachial plexus and lumbosacral plexus is crucial.

## Reflexes

Reflex testing is the same as for the trauma evaluation. Generally, hyperreflexia, including clonus and positive Babinski's sign, indicates myelopathy. Hyporeflexia or areflexia usually indicates radiculopathy related to the specific root. Side-to-side differences are noted.

For the upper extremity, the patient rests the hands on the thighs. The examiner first can elicit the biceps reflex by palpating the tendon at the elbow crease with the thumb, then lightly tapping the reflex hammer against the thumb. Then the brachioradialis reflex is tested. Finally, the examiner takes the patient's relaxed arm and supports it at the side so that the elbow is hanging free. The triceps reflex is elicited at the tendinous portion of the triceps just proximal to the olecranon.

A few pathologic reflexes and signs (tests are described subsequently) that indicate myelopathy in the cervical area should be noted at this time. The scapulohumeral reflex suggests myelopathy of the upper cervical spine above the C4 neurologic level. This reflex is positive if the scapula elevates or the humerus abducts in response to tapping on the spine of the scapula or tip of the acromion with the patient seated. Myelopathy of the middle cervical levels is suggested by Hoffman's sign and inverted radial reflex. Hoffmann's sign is elicited by quickly flicking the middle finger into extension. A positive sign is noted when the thumb and other fingers flex in response to the maneuver. The inverted radial reflex also is noted when the thumb and fingers flex during testing of the brachioradialis reflex. Finally, myelopathy is suggested by two findings specific to hand dysfunction known as "myelopathy hand." The first is the finger-escape sign, which is seen when the ulnar digits drift into abduction and flexion when the patient is asked to extend the digits fully with the palm facing down. The second is the inability to perform a repeated grip and release maneuver rapidly with the fingers secondary to weakness and spasticity of the hand.

For the chest and trunk, the main normal reflex seen is the abdominal reflex. In the presence of myelopathy, this superficial reflex often is diminished or absent. The superficial reflexes require skin stimulation and are upper motor neuron reflexes. The two other superficial reflexes that can be tested are the cremasteric reflex and the anal reflex (anal wink).

For the lower extremity, the patient hangs the legs over

the examination table so that the feet are free to move and not resting on a step. The patellar tendon reflex is elicited easily with the examiner standing to the patient's side. The Achilles reflex is tested with the ankle in gentle dorsiflexion to "preload" the gastrocnemius-soleus. It is often difficult to obtain a good reflex response because many patients cannot relax fully and often try to "help" by keeping the ankle actively dorsiflexed. Pathologic reflexes indicating myelopathy in the lower extremities include the presence of clonus and Babinski's sign, which have been described earlier. A positive Oppenheim sign also is found in myelopathy when abnormal great toe extension with splaying of the great toes is elicited when running a finger firmly down the tibial crest.

## Special Tests and Provocative Maneuvers

The combination of the patient's history and initial exam lead to focused use of provocative maneuvers and special tests to help discern pathology related to spinal versus nonspinal pathology. An important consideration during provocative testing is to correlate the findings with the patient's reported symptoms. Pain can be produced during testing, but it may not be clinically significant unless it is concordant with the patient's symptoms of radiculopathy.

Simple axial compression and distraction of the cervical spine with the patient seated can reproduce and relieve symptoms related to cervical root compression. Reported pain in the head and neck areas should be noted because reliable patterns have been correlated to specific cervical levels with discography (Fig. 1-8). *Lhermitte's sign* is a shocklike sensation in the trunk or extremities associated with axial load combined with flexion or extension of the neck. The pain is believed to occur from a reduction in foraminal or spinal canal space during dynamic motion as a result of disc disease or herniation. Performing a Valsalva maneuver also can be associated with a sharp or shocklike pain in the neck or a dermatomal distribution from increased intrathecal pressure irritating a nerve root. The *Spurling maneuver* also can exacerbate symptoms of radiculopathy by the combination of lateral flexion and rotation of the neck to the affected side. This can help to differentiate radiculopathy from shoulder-related pain. *Adson's maneuver* can help distinguish pathology originating from compression of neurovascular structures from thoracic outlet syndrome or a cervical rib. This is suggested by noting a decreased radial pulse pressure at the wrist when the patient takes a deep breath; holds the arm in an abducted, extended, and externally rotated position; then rotates the head toward the arm being examined. The decreased pulse from compression of the subclavian artery can be associated with compression of the adjacent brachial plexus and not the nerve roots. Because shoulder problems often can mimic cervical radiculopathy (and vice versa), careful assessment of the shoulder, including rotator cuff testing, should be performed. Tests for peripheral nerve compression syndromes, such as Tinel's and Phalen's signs, may be performed because these syndromes can present with similar symptoms.

*Beevor's sign* may be the only way to test motor function of the thoracic roots. This is checked during a partial sit-up with the patient supine on the exam table. Normally the umbilicus should move proximally on the midline. Any weakness of the rectus muscle, which is innervated broadly by T5-12, would lead to deviation of the umbilicus away from the affected side. A positive test can be related to thoracic radiculopathy.

Symptoms of lumbar radiculopathy can be reproduced with provocative maneuvers of the lower extremities. The *femoral nerve stretch test* (L2-4) is performed by flexing the knee and passively hyperextending the hip while the patient is prone. The straight-leg test (SLR) for sciatica (L4-S1) can be performed while the patient is supine and while the patient is sitting. A positive test recreates symptoms of radiculopathy in the distribution of the affected nerve root (i.e., distal to the knee). Pain can be aggravated further with dorsiflexion of the ankle (*Lasègue's sign*). *Kernig's sign* is similar to the SLR test but with the addition of neck flexion during the maneuver to re-create sciatica. Reproduction of pain when a contralateral SLR is performed enhances specificity because it puts tension on the involved lumbar root from the opposite side. Tightness of the hamstring muscle is common in patients with associated mechanical low back pain. This can mimic sciatica during SLR testing but has the important distinction that pain usually does not extend distal to the knee.

A comprehensive evaluation includes a hip and knee exam to evaluate for range of motion and pain at these joints. Internal derangements in the knee or hip can mimic symptoms of spine pathology, such as radiculopathy. Pain originating from the SI joints also needs to be assessed. Manual compression of the iliac wings can elicit SI symptoms. The *FABER* (flexion, abduction, external rotation) figure-four position of the leg is performed to assess for pain originating from SI instability or pain. The final test for SI pathology is *Gaenslen's sign,* when the patient lies supine with both legs flexed to the chest similar to a fetal position with one buttock and leg over the edge of the table. Complaints of pain in the SI area when the leg is dropped and extended over the edge of the table suggest pathology in that area.

When a patient's symptoms and complaints are inconsistent with objective findings during the physical exam, a series of special tests may need to be performed to identify patients who may be exaggerating or magnifying pain symptoms. *Hoover's sign* is performed to detect if a patient is giving full effort for motor testing. In this test, both of the patient's ankles are cupped under the examiner's hands simultaneously. The patient is asked to perform an SLR with maximum effort. Usually the examiner feels downward pressure on the other hand as the opposite leg provides increased leverage for this strength test. If not, the patient simply is not attempting to move the leg. Also commonly seen is "giving way," or sudden lack of resistance during manual strength testing. Motor testing is graded against sustained resistance. Sudden giving way of the muscle group being tested is not a reliable indicator of objective weakness.

Waddell developed and validated a series of signs and tests, known as *Waddell's signs,* to identify patients who may respond poorly to treatment, including surgery or nonsurgical measures. These patients may be seeking secondary gain, malingering, or exhibiting nonorganic causes of pain.

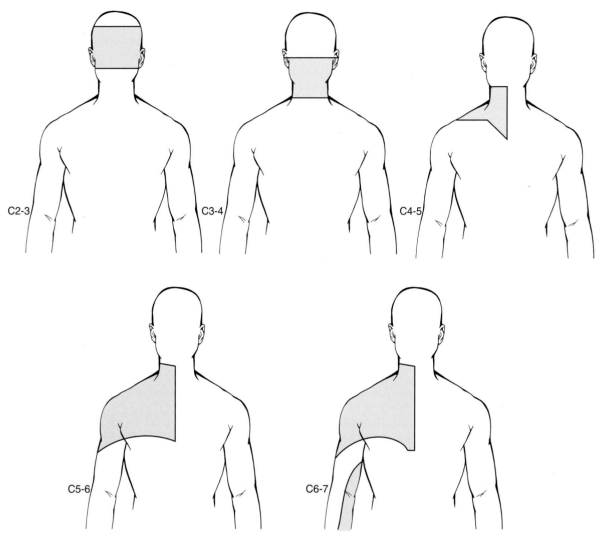

**Figure 1-8** Patterns of pain provoked by discography from the C2-3 to the C6-7 disc levels. (From Grubb SA, Kelly CK. Cervical discography: clinical implications from 12 years of experience. Spine 2000;25:1382-1389.)

Three patterns of abnormal pain behavior can be noted:

1. Pain in nonanatomic distributions
2. Pain out of proportion to stimulus
3. Exaggerated pain behavior

Four benign maneuvers that simulate a pain-provocative maneuver can be performed. These tests are insufficient to produce an organic pain response from spinal origin:

1. *Skin roll test* is performed by gently rolling the loose skin over the lower back while the patient is standing or prone and asking if radicular symptoms are produced. Radicular symptoms should not occur.
2. *Twist test* is performed by gently rotating the patient's torso at the hips as the patient is standing with the hands on the hips. This simulates spine motion, but all the rotation occurs through the knees and should not generate back pain.
3. *Head compression test* is performed by applying ap-

proximately 5 lb of axial load to the top of the head. This small amount of load is not sufficient to cause mechanical pain or instability. This is not to be confused with the Spurling maneuver.

4. *Flip test* is evaluation of the seated SLR test. Symptoms that are present during a supine SLR but not present during seated SLR indicate a positive test. Normally, if nerve root compression is present, radicular symptoms should be aggravated during the seated SLR with associated complaints of sciatic pain or physically leaning back to avoid the pain response.

Normal patients may have one or two positive Waddell's signs. The presence of more than three positive signs predicts poor treatment outcome, however.

## SUMMARY

A thorough and consistent spine examination is the cornerstone of the diagnosis of spine disease. The evaluations of the trauma patient and the clinic patient have some subtle differences and emphases but share most aspects of the exam. Each exam can be performed efficiently and reliably. The combination of patient history, physical examination, and radiographic evaluation leads to proper diagnosis and appropriate treatment plan.

# SUGGESTED READING

Albert TJ, Levine MJ, An HS, et al. Concomitant noncontiguous thoracolumbar and sacral fractures. Spine 1993;18:1285–1291.

Grubb SA, Kelly CK. Cervical discography: clinical implications from 12 years of experience. Spine 2000;25:1382–1389.

Henderson RL, Reid DC, Saboe LA. Multiple noncontiguous spine fractures. Spine 1991;16:128–131.

Klein JD, Garfin SR. History and physical examination. In: Weinstein JN, Rydevik BL, Sonntag VKG, eds. Essentials of spine. New York: Raven Press, 1995:71–95.

Rao R. Neck pain, cervical radiculopathy, and cervical myelopathy. J Bone Joint Surg Am 2002;84A:1872–1881.

Shimizu T, Shimada H, Shirakura K. Scapulohumeral reflex (Shimizu): its clinical significance and testing maneuver. Spine 1993;18:2182–2190.

Stauffer ES. Diagnosis and prognosis of acute cervical spinal cord injury. Clin Orthop 1975;112:9–15.

Vaccaro AR, An HS, Lin S, et al. Noncontiguous injuries of the spine. J Spinal Disord 1992;5:320–329.

Vroomen PC, de Krom MC, Knottnerus JA. Consistency of history taking and physical examination in patients with suspected lumbar nerve root involvement. Spine 2000;25:91–97.

Waddell G, McCulloch JA, Kummell E, Venner RM. Nonorganic physical signs in low back pain. Spine 1980;5:117–125.

# IMAGING

## WILLIAM TONTZ
## MINI PATHRIA

Diagnostic imaging plays an important role in the detection, preoperative management, surgical planning, and follow-up of orthopaedic spinal disorders. The use of routine radiography to identify fractures constituted the earliest application of imaging techniques for spinal pathology. Although fracture detection and follow-up remain common indications for spinal imaging, new imaging modalities, such as computed tomography (CT) and magnetic resonance imaging (MRI), allow accurate diagnosis of a broad range of osseous, articular, and soft tissue abnormalities in the spine. Currently, spinal imaging is used frequently for the evaluation of degenerative disorders of the spine. The appropriate use of these modalities is presented in relation to an accurate work-up of spinal trauma, neoplastic disease, infection, and degenerative conditions.

This chapter provides an overview of the role of radiography, MRI, CT, and myelography in the preoperative assessment of spinal disorders. Although imaging depicts the anatomy of the various disorders involving the spine, the importance of the physical examination for accurate diagnosis and surgical planning cannot be overstated. Although newer imaging modalities have high sensitivity for the detection of apparent pathology, their specificity is low in the absence of clinical symptoms at that particular level. Approximately 30% of asymptomatic individuals may display abnormal MRI changes consistent with disc degeneration in the absence of clinical symptoms. The findings from imaging studies must be used in conjunction with clinical and laboratory findings for accurate diagnosis and optimal patient management.

## QUALITY ASSURANCE

Before discussing advanced imaging of the spine, it is important to review the basic issues of quality assurance that apply to all imaging modalities. Imaging studies should be labeled appropriately with patient identification information and the date of the study. The examination should include the entire area of interest to the surgeon. For example, the lateral cervical spine radiograph should include C7-T1 for adequate assessment of a traumatized spine. The technical factors unique to the imaging exam should be optimized so that there is acceptable spatial resolution for fine ana-

tomic detail and adequate contrast resolution to differentiate anatomic structures. Correct patient positioning also is crucial for diagnostic imaging studies. These technical factors should be optimized for the best possible imaging quality without unnecessary patient discomfort or exposure of the patient to unwarranted high radiation doses.

## OVERVIEW OF IMAGING MODALITIES

Imaging modalities can be divided conveniently into two groups—modalities that employ ionizing radiation and modalities that do not. The modalities that employ ionizing radiation include radiography, tomography, and scintigraphy. MRI does not use ionizing radiation to form an image.

### Conventional Radiography

Conventional radiography is widely available and well suited to assess the osseous skeleton. Assessment of the soft tissues is limited, however, to identifying swelling, blurring, or displacement of fat stripes; visualizing focal masses; and identifying soft tissue gas or radiopaque foreign bodies. Despite their limited contrast resolution, radiographs typically are the initial imaging modality employed to assess spinal pathology. Bone lesions producing disruption or proliferation of the vertebral cortex are visualized relatively easily. Bone loss limited to trabecular bone from tumor, osteoporosis, or infection is seen less easily. It has been estimated that trabecular bone loss must be greater than 30% to 40% to be detected on conventional radiographs. Stress radiographs are x-rays obtained at the extremes of range of motion or during manual application of distraction or angular stress. These views may show instability or imply ligamentous injuries when no abnormalities are seen in the neutral position.

### Conventional (Plain Film) Tomography

Conventional tomography is a specialized radiographic technique that has been virtually replaced by CT. Synchronous motion of the radiographic film and x-ray tube produces blurring of objects outside the selected focal plane. This technique was used widely in the past for assessment of spinal injury and spinal fusion. Conventional tomography significantly increases radiation exposure to the patient and no longer is widely used or available.

## Computed Tomography

CT is a technique by which slicelike images of the body are obtained. CT is an important adjunct to x-rays, particularly in complex anatomic areas, such as the spine and pelvis. The contrast resolution for soft tissues is much better than with radiographs, although soft tissue contrast is still less than that achieved with MRI. CT is well suited to assess spinal trauma, particularly to identify retropulsed bone fragments narrowing the spinal canal and to identify posterior element fractures. Although conventional CT images are in the axial plane, manipulating the data can reconstruct serial axial images to create sagittal or coronal reconstructions. Reformatted three-dimensional images also can be generated, allowing the viewer to study the object from a variety of perspectives as the image is digitally rotated through space (Fig. 2-1). Metallic objects produce extensive artifact and limit the use of this technique.

## Scintigraphy

Bone scanning with technetium-99m-labeled phosphate or diphosphonate compounds plays an important role in orthopaedic imaging. For spinal imaging, scintigraphy is used most often to survey the skeleton for metastatic disease and to identify stress fractures and osteomyelitis. In contrast to CT and plain radiographs, which are purely anatomic, scintigraphy reflects bone metabolic activity. The spatial resolution of the exam is limited, and any lesion causing increased turnover of bone can produce abnormal uptake, resulting in low specificity. Single-photon emission computed tomography images provide improved image contrast and spatial resolution.

## Myelography

Previously considered the gold standard for spinal imaging, myelography now has been replaced largely by planar imaging techniques such as CT and MRI. Limitations of myelography include complications related to the procedure, reactions to contrast material, high radiation dose, indirect assessment of discal pathology, and relative insensitivity to pathology in the lateral spaces and epidural space in the lower lumbar spine. The two disorders for which myelography still is considered necessary for accurate diagnosis are arachnoiditis and traumatic nerve root avulsion. Currently, myelography rarely is used for presurgical planning, unless MRI is unavailable or contraindicated. When myelography is performed, it typically is combined with postmyelography CT to assess the spinal structures adequately (Fig. 2-2).

## Magnetic Resonance Imaging

MRI is playing an increasingly important role in the assessment of spinal disorders and is now the diagnostic imaging technique of choice for preoperative assessment. The major advantages of MRI are that the technique is noninvasive, is nonionizing, has multiplanar capability, and provides excellent contrast and spatial resolution. In contrast to CT, MRI can evaluate long segments of the spine, allowing visualization of a broad anatomic region in one image. The major disadvantages of MRI include relatively high cost (although cost has decreased considerably since the 1990s), long examination times requiring the patient to hold still, and limited availability. An important disadvantage of MRI for the surgeon is the extreme sensitivity of this technique to implanted metal, resulting in artifacts that often render

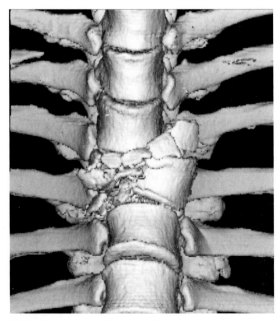

**Figure 2-1**   Three-dimensional reconstruction of a traumatic fracture-dislocation at the thoracic level.

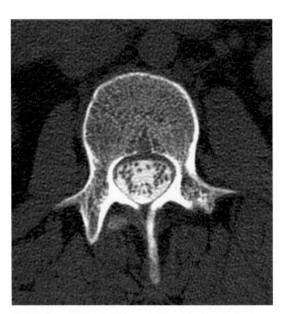

**Figure 2-2**   Normal CT myelogram shows excellent spatial resolution and detail.

the exam uninterpretable. Stainless steel instrumentation is ferromagnetic and leads to significant artifact (Fig. 2-3), whereas newer titanium devices do not cause any noticeable image degradation. Absolute contraindications for MRI include implanted pacemakers, cardiac valve replacement, implanted electrical devices, intraocular metallic bodies, and intracranial clips.

The soft tissue contrast resolution of MRI is superior to other modalities. Normal bone marrow in adults is of high signal intensity on T1-weighted and T2-weighted images owing to the predominance of fat. The intervertebral disc, which has a low signal on T1 images and increases to intermediate high signal on T2 images, is seen well and separated easily from adjacent tissues. Although mineralized bone is not as well seen as with CT, the adjacent medullary changes render MRI more sensitive than CT for bone trauma, osteomyelitis, and marrow replacement processes. MRI is an excellent technique to assess spinal tumors. Marrow replacement by tumor and soft tissue abnormalities are detected more accurately than with CT, and the multiplanar capabilities of MRI allow accurate anatomic staging of the lesion.

## SPECIFIC CONDITIONS

### Spinal Trauma

It is estimated that 10,000 patients each year in the United States sustain a spinal cord injury. The early identification, immobilization, and treatment of spinal cord injury and spinal trauma are paramount in preventing further morbid-

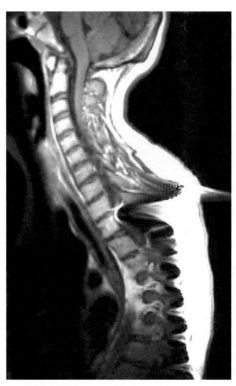

**Figure 2-3** Postsurgical MRI shows significant hardware artifact from ferromagnetic metallic implants.

ity or mortality. Spinal trauma is categorized by the location of the injury, its presumed mechanism, and the presence or absence of instability. The most common locations of injury include the lower cervical and thoracolumbar regions (Fig. 2-4). The most common mechanisms are flexion and axial loading.

Most fractures are readily apparent on good-quality radiographs. Advanced imaging often is required, however, for a complete assessment of injury to the intervertebral discs, interspinous ligaments, and direct cord injury (Fig. 2-5). Initial radiographic evaluation of the traumatized spine begins with conventional radiography, with the spine still protected by a cervical collar. A cervical spine series comprises a lateral view that includes the cervicothoracic junction, an anteroposterior view, and an odontoid view. If the lateral radiograph is inadequate secondary to body habitus or technique, a swimmer's view is obtained. Certain soft tissue "red flags" must be kept in mind. Greater than 5 mm of soft tissue swelling at the anteroinferior margin of C2 is considered abnormal. Greater than 14 mm of soft tissue swelling below the arytenoid cartilage level (C3-4 vertebral bodies) also is considered abnormal. The radiographs also are evaluated for spinal alignment, by assessing the normal "spinal lines" (Fig. 2-6) and adjacent segment angulation. The posterior vertebral margins and the spinolaminar lines are most useful in the overall assessment of spinal alignment. Findings indicating traumatic cervical spine instability include greater than 3 mm of anterior or posterior translation (Fig. 2-7), angulation greater than 11 degrees compared with other contiguous spinal segments, rotation or widening of facet joints, and focal widening of an interspinous process distance.

CT is useful to evaluate spinal bony injury and canal compromise and to assess the posterior arch of the spine. CT has been shown to be far more sensitive than conventional radiography for detection of spinal fractures. Several institutions now rely on CT for initial screening of the injured spine and use CT routinely in all cases of trauma. Other institutions use CT for evaluation of regions not seen adequately on the initial radiographs and to assess areas of suspected injury.

MRI also is useful to assess patients with spinal trauma, particularly patients with neurologic injury unexplained by CT. MRI is superior to CT in evaluating intervertebral discs, ligaments, and the spinal cord. The early detection of ligamentous and cord injuries is paramount in the polytrauma patient. Newer MRI techniques, such as short tau inversion recovery or fat saturation techniques, allow highly T2-weighted images to be obtained rapidly, increasing the sensitivity of MRI in detecting injuries about the spine.

### Cervical Spine Trauma

Occipitoatlantal dissociation is a rare injury that is almost always fatal at the time of impact. In the typical case, there is anterior and superior displacement of the occipital condyles with respect to the superior articular facets of C1. Radiographs show displacement of the anterior rim of the foramen magnum (basion) anterior to the dens and widening of the occipitoatlantal articulations, and Power's ratio (Fig. 2-8) is abnormal. Atlantoaxial rotary fixation may be due to

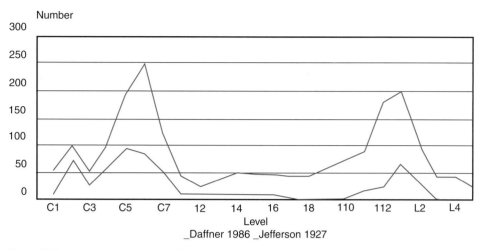

Number

_Daffner 1986 _Jefferson 1927

**Figure 2-4**   Bimodal distribution of frequency of spine fractures. The most common locations are the cervicothoracic and thoracolumbar junctions.

trauma or follow an upper respiratory tract infection. In this condition, the patient presents with a torticollis as C1 is fixed in rotation relative to C2. The anteroposterior odontoid view shows asymmetry in the sizes of the C1 lateral masses and in the distance between the dens and the lateral masses of C2. CT shows if the C1-2 axis is abnormally fixed in rotation.

Jefferson's fracture of C1 is an axial loading injury resulting in simultaneous anterior and posterior arch fractures. It may be unilateral or bilateral. The anteroposterior odontoid view shows lateral displacement of the lateral masses of C1 with respect to the articular pillars of C2. The fracture lines may not be seen directly on routine radiographs, although

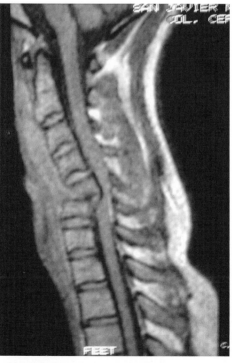

**Figure 2-5**   Cervical spine MRI shows gross disruption of the anterior longitudinal ligament after a displaced teardrop fracture. The posterior longitudinal ligament appears to be "peeled away" from the vertebral body, but it appears to be in continuity. Compression of the spinal cord is clearly visible.

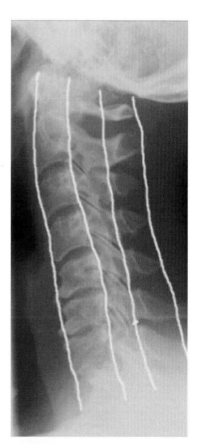

**Figure 2-6**   Diagram depicting cervical spine radiographic parameters of instability.

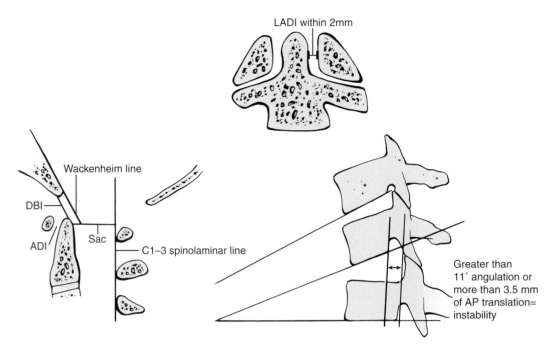

**Figure 2-7**   The spinolaminar junction and posterior vertebral body alignment lines. Note they are disrupted at the level of the injury (C5 dislocation). ADI, atlantodens interval; AP, anteroposterior; DBI, dens-basion interval; LADI, lateral atlantodens interval.

CT shows the fracture lines well. Odontoid fractures are overlooked easily, particularly if the fracture is undisplaced. The fracture line occurs obliquely in the upper dens in type 1 fractures, occurs at the base of the dens in type 2 fractures, and extends into the body of C2 in type 3 injuries. Anterior or posterior displacement results in malalignment

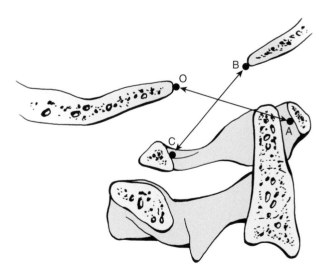

**Figure 2-8**   Power's ratio. A line is drawn from the basion (B) to the posterior arch of the atlas (C). Another line is drawn from the opisthion (O) to the anterior aspect of the atlas. Normally the ratio of BC is greater than AO. With atlantooccipital dissociation, BC increases while AO decreases. A ratio greater than 1 is diagnostic of atlantooccipital dissociation.

of the spinolaminar line at C1 and C2. Because the injury typically is transverse, routine axial CT may not show the fracture. The fracture is identified easily, however, on coronal and sagittal reconstructed images. Hangman's fracture, also known as traumatic spondylolisthesis of C2, is caused by hyperextension. The bilateral pars fractures of C2 occur just anterior to the inferior articular facets; 20% extend into the C2 vertebral body. Typically the fracture results in anterior displacement of C2 relative to C3, resulting in disruption of the C1-2 spinolaminar line and the C2-3 posterior vertebral body line.

Flexion instability is due to isolated rupture of the posterior ligaments. No fracture is seen, so the injury may be missed unless delayed flexion views are obtained. In severe injuries, the initial lateral film may suggest posterior ligament disruption by interspinous widening. CT is typically normal. The diagnosis of isolated ligament injury is made most effectively with MRI. The torn ligaments appear irregular and show high signal within their substance on T2-weighted images. The "clay shoveler's" fracture is an avulsion fracture limited to the spinous process of the vertebra. This injury is most common at T1 and C7, and the fractured spinous process typically is displaced inferiorly. Associated ligamentous tears may accompany this fracture, resulting in malalignment of the facet joint.

In the teardrop fracture, a triangular piece of bone arising from the anteroinferior vertebral body is avulsed, with malalignment of the spine. This unstable fracture is associated with posterior ligamentous tears and a high incidence of spinal cord injury. Serious injury to the spinal cord may occur if there is encroachment of the canal by displaced bone, disc fragments, or significant epidural hemorrhage.

Disruption of the facet capsule can result in the presence of a facet lock, which can occur unilaterally or bilaterally. Unilateral and bilateral facet lock are assessed best on the lateral view, which shows anterior displacement of the affected upper vertebra. Bilateral facet lock is due to flexion and is easy to recognize because the degree of displacement is large, averaging more than 50% of the vertebral body width. Unilateral facet lock is more difficult to appreciate, and careful analysis of the appearance of the facet joints is necessary to avoid missing this injury. CT shows a "naked" facet or shows the abnormal reversed position of the dislocated facet joint.

Hyperextension places the cord at high risk for neurologic deficit, particularly in the spondylitic or stenotic spine. Conventional radiographs may be normal after a hyperextension injury, even in the presence of profound neurologic deficit. MRI is the optimal method of assessing the spinal cord after a hyperextension injury and allows differentiation between a frank cord hematoma, which has a universally poor prognosis, and a cord contusion, which may resolve clinically.

### Upper Thoracic and Thoracolumbar Trauma

The upper thoracic spine is relatively rigid because of support provided by the rib cage and is injured infrequently. Injuries in this area, when they do occur, have a significant incidence of neurologic injury due to the small size of the spinal canal in this area. In young patients, upper thoracic injuries tend to be severe fracture-dislocations resulting in severe neurologic deficit. Although traumatic fractures are uncommon, osteoporotic compression fractures in this area occur with high frequency in the elderly.

Injuries at the thoracolumbar junction are classified according to the Denis classification system, which divides the spine into three columns:

- *Anterior column* consists of the anterior half of the vertebral body, the anterior longitudinal ligament, and the anterior half of the disc.
- *Middle column*, which is the most important for stability, includes the posterior half of the vertebral body, posterior half of the disc, and posterior longitudinal ligament.
- *Posterior column* includes all the osseous structures and ligaments from the pedicles posteriorly.

In the Denis classification, minor injuries include all fractures consisting of a single break limited to the posterior bony arch. Major injuries include compression fractures, burst fractures, seat belt–type injuries, and fracture-dislocations. On radiographs, burst fractures can be distinguished from simple compression fractures by loss of height of the posterior vertebral body, retropulsed bone fragments in the spinal canal, interpedicular widening, and posterior element fractures. CT is the best method for visualizing involvement of the posterior vertebral body column and assessing the extent of osseous retropulsion. Seat-belt injuries are due to flexion combined with distraction. They produce posterior element widening and horizontal vertebral fractures. Fracture-dislocations disrupt the entire spine, allowing large amounts of translation and displacement.

### Lower Lumbar Trauma

The lower lumbar spine is deep and protected by large overlying muscles and is injured rarely. The same types of injuries that occur at the thoracolumbar region also occur in the lumbar spine, although with decreased frequency. Transverse process fractures are stable injuries that are rarely significant clinically. In rare cases, they may be associated with injury to the genitourinary tract. Spondylolysis defects are a developmental abnormality that result in disruption of the pars interarticularis during early childhood. Most pars defects involve L5, with the upper levels involved in less than 5% of cases. The defects are seen best on oblique or lateral lumbar radiographs; on oblique views, they are shown as disruption of the collar of the "Scotty dog." On CT and MRI, the defects are seen as disruption of the posterior arch at the level of the basivertebral vein (Figs. 2-9 and 2-10). Spondylolysis may result in anterolisthesis of the vertebral body relative to the body below; this displacement also is termed *spondylolisthesis*. Spondylolisthesis accelerates degeneration of the intervening disc and can result in foraminal stenosis; this is depicted best on MRI.

## Infection

The combination of vertebral and disc infection commonly is referred to as *infectious spondylitis*. In infectious spondylitis, the initial site of infection is the anterior vertebral body, with subsequent erosion of the adjacent end plate and involvement of the adjacent disc. When the disc is infected, the organism can extend into the adjacent vertebral body.

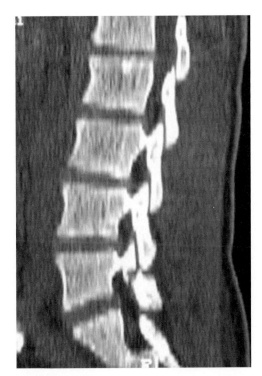

**Figure 2-9** Sagittal CT reconstructions can be useful in detecting and visualizing spondylolytic defects.

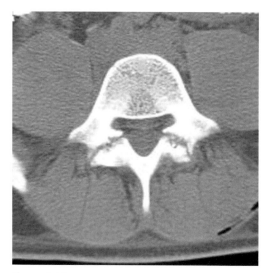

**Figure 2-10** On axial CT scans, bilateral spondylolytic defects might be mistaken for arthritic facet joints. This CT slice is at the level of the pedicles, however, which is above (or below) the level of the facet joints.

The radiographic findings of infectious spondylitis consist of disc space narrowing, adjacent end plate erosion, bone destruction, and soft tissue swelling. These radiographic findings are delayed, and definitive evidence of infection may not appear for several weeks after the onset of symptoms. MRI has replaced scintigraphy and CT as the definitive modality for the detection and evaluation of suspected spinal infection (Fig. 2-11). MRI is more sensitive than conventional radiography and CT for early infection and has been shown to provide equivalent sensitivity (96%), speci-

ficity (93%), and accuracy (94%) compared with gallium and with bone scans. MRI provides detailed anatomic information about the paraspinal and spinal tissues and the adjacent thecal sac. On T1-weighted MRI, there is decreased marrow signal in the affected vertebral bodies, with high signal intensity of the disc on T2 images. Enhancement is present after intravenous gadolinium administration, and the enhanced regions are more consistent with an abscess versus a phlegmon.

## Spinal Neuropathic and Inflammatory Disorders

Spinal neuropathic arthropathy or Charcot's spine is a relatively uncommon destructive process affecting the intervertebral disc space, adjacent vertebral bodies, and facet joints. The radiologic appearance may be similar to that of infection or other inflammatory processes. MRI shows great variability in the signal characteristics of these lesions. Findings suggesting spinal neuroarthropathy on CT and MRI include the presence of vacuum disc phenomenon, debris and disorganization of the involved areas, facet malalignment, spondylolisthesis, and rim enhancement of discs on gadolinium-enhanced MRI. Biopsy is frequently necessary for accurate differentiation from infection.

Rheumatoid arthritis shows inflammatory changes that predominate in the cervical spine, specifically the craniocervical junction. Synovial proliferation can cause pannus formation, erosions of the odontoid, vertebral bodies or facets, autofusion of facet joints, cranial settling, and atlantoaxial and subaxial subluxations. The most common radiographic pattern of spinal instability in these patients is widening of the atlantodens interval. Flexion-extension radiographs are essential to assess the atlantoaxial joint accurately because the instability frequently is manifested only

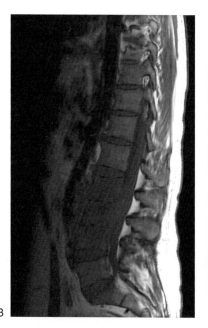
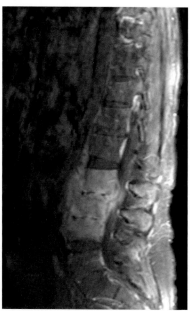
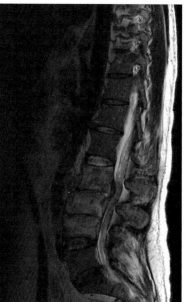

A,B  C

**Figure 2-11** T1-weighted (**A**), T2-weighted (**B**), and gadolinium-enhanced (**C**) images of a patient with lumbar osteomyelitis.

on the flexion examination. MRI can be helpful in identifying and characterizing the soft tissue pannus and assessing the degree of cord compression and canal compromise, which can be underestimated by plain radiographs. Some authors advocate the use of functional MRI of the cervical spine performed in varying degrees of flexion and extension to evaluate atlantoaxial instability and its effect on the spinal cord.

The seronegative spondyloarthropathies include ankylosing spondylitis, psoriatic arthritis, Reiter's syndrome, arthritis related to inflammatory bowel disease, and other much less common arthritides associated with the HLA-B27 antigen. The most common condition involving the spine is ankylosing spondylitis, which typically presents in young men. Symptoms usually are related to involvement of the spine and sacroiliac joints.

Early radiographic changes of ankylosing spondylitis include bilateral symmetric narrowing and erosion of the sacroiliac joints and later bone proliferation (syndesmophytes) and erosions ("shiny corners") at the thoracolumbar junction. CT and MRI are helpful in the detection and characterization of erosive changes at the sacroiliac joints. A major complication of ankylosing spondylitis is the development of a fracture and subsequent formation of a pseudarthrosis in the spine. On MRI, the pseudarthrosis can mimic infection, with signal changes surrounding the abnormal fractured disc. The detection of a horizontal fracture line through the posterior elements allows differentiation of a pseudarthrosis after traumatic fracture from discal infection (Fig. 2-12).

Crystal-induced arthritis of the spine is uncommon and frequently misdiagnosed. Deposition of urate crystals in the spine with advanced gout can cause erosions of the odontoid process and the end plates, disc space narrowing, and vertebral subluxation. Calcium pyrophosphate deposition disease is characterized by the presence of crystal deposition in the articular cartilage, menisci, synovium, and periarticular tissues. In the spine, calcium pyrophosphate deposition disease can cause destructive lesions of the vertebral bodies and disc spaces and calcification of the discs. Masslike deposits of calcium pyrophosphate deposition disease crystals have been described in the atlantoaxial region, and the cystic changes seen in the adjacent bone increase the risk of fracture of the dens significantly. Calcium hydroxyapatite crystal deposition disease more characteristically is associated with extraarticular tendinous calcific deposits. In the spine, hydroxyapatite crystal deposition disease is seen most frequently in the tendon of the longus colli muscle. A painful, inflammatory tendinitis is present with soft tissue swelling anterior to C2. The calcific deposit is seen best on CT. On MRI, prevertebral edema is seen in the upper cervical spine as thickening and signal alterations in the tendon.

Dialysis spondyloarthropathy can mimic infection radiographically. The etiology is thought to be amyloid deposition within the disc space. Slowly progressive end plate erosions, disc space narrowing, and vertebral destruction are seen typically in the cervical and lumbar regions. Multiple levels may be involved. In contrast to infection, the soft tissues remain normal in dialysis spondyloarthropathy. On MRI, the vertebral bodies also show normal marrow signal except for minimal alterations adjacent to the erosions. The T2-weighted image is particularly helpful because it shows no abnormal high signal in the affected region.

## Neoplastic Disease

The patient with a spinal neoplasm typically presents because of local pain, pathologic fracture, or neurologic deficit. Occasionally a spinal tumor is detected as an incidental finding in an asymptomatic patient; in this situation, the lesions are typically benign. MRI plays a complementary role with plain film radiography, CT, myelography, and scintigraphy for the assessment of spinal neoplasms.

### Metastatic Disease

The spine is a large reservoir of hematopoietic marrow and the most common site of metastasis to the skeleton. The vertebral body is involved with greater frequency than the posterior elements. Scintigraphy traditionally is used as the initial imaging test for the detection of metastatic disease in a patient with a known primary malignancy. Scintigraphy allows whole-body screening, which currently is not feasible by MRI. Scintigraphy is considerably less sensitive than MRI, however. The advantage of MRI is particularly evident for infiltrative neoplasms, such as multiple myeloma and lymphoma, which may have normal scintigrams in the presence of widespread disease. Another disadvantage of scintigraphy is that a positive exam provides no morphologic information about the spinal lesion. MRI can detect the presence of a fracture or soft tissue encroachment on the neural structures, which have an impact on therapy (Fig. 2-13).

Most patients with metastases have disseminated disease, with multiple noncontiguous sites of involvement. Metastases appear as areas of diminished signal loss within the bone marrow on T1-weighted images. The signal of metastatic disease on T2-weighted images is more variable, depending on the nature of the adjacent bony response. Lytic tumors are typically bright on T2-weighted images. Sclerotic lesions are highly variable and may appear hypointense, hyperintense, or isointense to normal bone marrow. Most metastases, with the exception of a few densely osteoblastic lesions, show enhancement after intravenous gadolinium. The use of fat suppression after gadolinium injection increases the ability to identify areas of enhancement.

### Primary Neoplasms

The accurate diagnosis of solitary primary tumors of the vertebra requires consideration of the patient's age, the location of the lesion, and the lesion's appearance. MRI is not particularly helpful for predicting the histologic type of neoplasm in many cases. Multiple myeloma is the most common primary osseous tumor, typically presenting with bone pain and osteopenia in an elderly individual. It may be in its solitary (plasmacytoma), disseminated (multiple plasmacytoma), or diffuse (multiple myeloma) form at the time of diagnosis. The MRI appearance of myeloma is variable and depends on the pattern and degree of infiltration. Mild disease, producing only subtle marrow inhomogeneity, is common and may be interpreted as within the normal

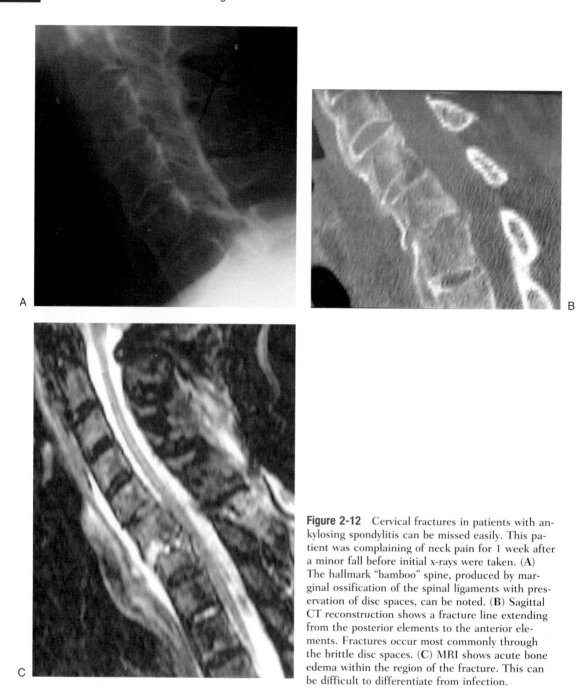

**Figure 2-12**  Cervical fractures in patients with ankylosing spondylitis can be missed easily. This patient was complaining of neck pain for 1 week after a minor fall before initial x-rays were taken. (**A**) The hallmark "bamboo" spine, produced by marginal ossification of the spinal ligaments with preservation of disc spaces, can be noted. (**B**) Sagittal CT reconstruction shows a fracture line extending from the posterior elements to the anterior elements. Fractures occur most commonly through the brittle disc spaces. (**C**) MRI shows acute bone edema within the region of the fracture. This can be difficult to differentiate from infection.

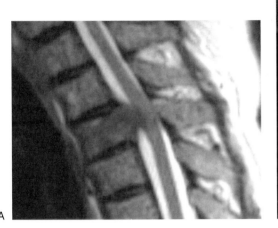

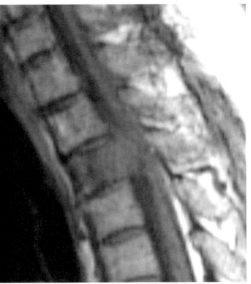

A                                                                                          B

**Figure 2-13**  T2-weighted (**A**) and T1-weighted (**B**) images of the upper thoracic spine of a patient who presented with bandlike chest pain at rest from activity. He had a history of lung cancer. Open biopsy confirmed the lesion to be metastatic adenocarcinoma. This is an example of direct tumoral expansion into the spinal canal without pathologic fracture.

range. Approximately 20% to 25% of cases of myeloma cannot be detected by MRI. Other common primary neoplasms of the skeleton include hemangioma, lymphoma, chordoma, and chondrosarcoma. Primary neoplasms typically do not involve the disc space and remain confined to the vertebral body or posterior arch (Fig. 2-14). Exceptions to this rule include chordoma, which frequently extends via the epidural space to involve the disc and adjacent vertebral body, and plasmacytoma, which frequently involves multiple contiguous vertebrae and the intervening disc spaces.

## Degenerative Diseases of the Spine

### Back Pain

Acute back pain is a common and expensive health care problem in society. Approximately 60% to 80% of all adults develop severe incapacitating low back pain sometime in their life. Approximately 2% of all adults visit a physician because of back pain each year. It is particularly common among middle-aged adults and accounts for 25% of missed workdays. Low back pain is also one of the leading causes of chronic work-related disability. The cause of back pain, the need for surgery, and the role of imaging in low back pain syndrome all are subjects of controversy (Fig. 2-15).

### Degenerative Disc Disease

In disc degeneration, an edema-like signal in the disc and adjacent end plates, mimicking infection, is seen in approximately 5% of patients. Modic et al classified the bone marrow changes according to the signal intensity on MRI. The described patterns include the following:

- *Modic type 1:* End plate changes are seen. Modic et al suggested this appearance is due to an inflammatory response to disc degeneration. Type 1 changes are hypointense on T1-weighted images and hyperintense on T2-weighted images (Fig. 2-16). Type 1 change routinely enhances with gadolinium and can simulate an osteomyelitis.
- *Modic type 2:* Marrow is converted to predominantly fat. This pattern has been shown to be stable over a 2- to 3-year period. Type 2 changes show a hyperintense signal on T1-weighted images and isointense-to-hypointense signal on T2-weighted images. Chronic disc disease leads to vertebral body end plate sclerosis, which is known as a type 3 change.
- *Modic type 3:* Hypointensity is displayed on T1-weighted images and T2-weighted images.

In contrast to infection, the soft tissues are normal, the marrow abnormalities are less extensive, the intranuclear cleft of the disc is preserved, and the end plates are not eroded and are preserved. Type 1 changes tend to resolve spontaneously over a few months. They can be difficult to differentiate from infection, and laboratory studies, such as C-reactive protein and sedimentation rate, are required.

### Scheuermann's Disease

Scheuermann's disease, also known as *juvenile kyphosis,* is a condition seen predominantly in adolescents and young adults. It is poorly understood, although many investigators think it is a postrepetitive stress osteochondrosis of the vertebral end plate, leading to secondary degenerative disc disease. The radiographic findings include end plate irregularity, multiple Schmorl's nodes, wedging of the bodies, and kyphosis. In most reported cases, MRI shows loss of disc

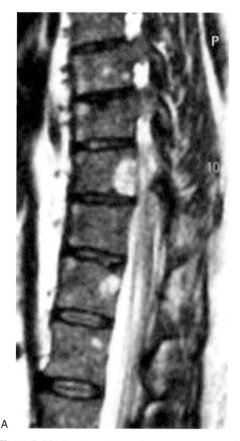

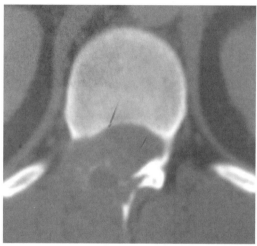

A                                                                                                    B

**Figure 2-14**   Benign primary bone tumors most often occur within the posterior vertebral body and posterior arch. (**A**) Sagittal MRI shows a benign hemangioma of the posterior vertebral body that extended into the pedicle (image not shown). (**B**) Axial CT scan of an aneurysmal bone cyst. The patient presented with pain and myelopathy.

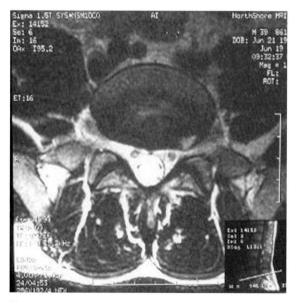

**Figure 2-15**   Small annular tears can be detected with MRI. They are thought to contribute to back pain.

height, disc dehydration, and variable herniation of nuclear material into the annulus fibrosus or vertebral end plates known as *Schmorl's nodes*. These herniations may incite an inflammatory response in the vertebra, which can be difficult to distinguish from focal osteomyelitis. On MRI, 10% of Schmorl's nodes may show vascularization and adjacent bone marrow edema. There is speculation that the degree of vascularity may reflect the age of the abnormality and the likelihood that it will be symptomatic. An inflammatory response to intrabody discal herniation also can be seen in adults, although it is much less common than in children. Hemispherical sclerosis results in a rounded area of sclerosis and mild bone marrow edema surrounding a Schmorl's node. This condition typically is seen in middle-aged women at L4.

The controversy regarding the role of imaging in patients with acute back pain is related to the high incidence of morphologic abnormalities in asymptomatic patients. Studies have shown that there is little difference between symptomatic and asymptomatic individuals in the frequency of spinal anatomic lesions, such as disc space narrowing, osteophyte formation, spondylolysis, and disc herniations. In 1994, Jensen et al published a landmark article regarding MRI findings in asymptomatic individuals. They performed

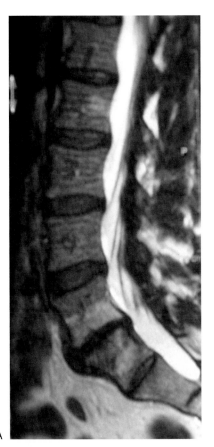
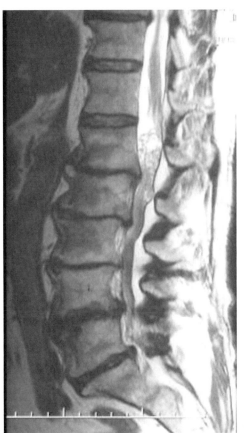

A                                                                                                          B

**Figure 2-16** Degenerative disc disease can manifest in many ways. (**A**) Sagittal MRI shows type 1 Modic changes within the adjacent end plates of the L5-S1 disc. Note the marked collapse of the disc space, with only minor bulging of the annulus. This has been referred to as the "flat-tire" syndrome. (**B**) Sagittal MRI of an elderly man who presented with neurogenic claudication. Type 2 and 3 Modic changes can be noted in multiple vertebral bodies. Of most interest, profound spinal stenosis is noted from L2-4. Nerve root clumping is evident above the level of stenosis (behind L1 vertebral body).

a prospective study of 98 people with no history of back pain or radiculopathy. In their study group, which was evaluated using the North American Spine Society (NASS) criteria, only 36% of persons had a totally normal examination. Of patients, 52% had at least one bulging disc, and 27% had at least one disc protrusion. Schmorl's nodes (19%), annular defects (14%), facet joint arthrosis (8%), and spondylolysis (7%) also were common. The only finding that was infrequent in asymptomatic individuals was the presence of disc extrusion. In their series, only one asymptomatic person showed a disc extrusion.

# SUGGESTED GUIDELINES FOR SPINAL IMAGING

Numerous guidelines for spinal imaging have been suggested. Although they differ in their details, all guidelines recommend conservative management of back pain for 4 to 7 weeks before any diagnostic imaging, unless the patient meets criteria for earlier radiographic evaluation. Suggested criteria for early imaging include the following:

- Neurologic deficit (myelopathy or radiculopathy or both) unexplained by plain films
- Suspected fracture (significant trauma, steroid use, severe osteoporosis)
- Suspected vertebral infection (immunocompromised, fever, or elevated laboratory values)
- Suspected metastatic disease (history of malignancy)
- Before radiation therapy
- Before spinal surgery
- New-onset or increasing postoperative back pain

## Terminology

Inconsistencies in terminology are widespread concerning degenerative disease of the spine. Perhaps the difficulties with the terminology are partly responsible for the poor correlation between imaging findings and symptoms. Terminology used by radiologists to describe degenerative diseases of the spine is highly variable. Terms such as *spondylosis deformans (annular degeneration), intervertebral osteochondrosis (nuclear degeneration), osteoarthrosis, osteoarthritis, diffuse skeletal hyperostosis, degenerative spondylosis, disc*

## BOX 2–1 NORTH AMERICAN SPINE SOCIETY (NASS) TERMINOLOGY FOR DISC HERNIATIONS.

**NASS Terminology**
- Disk dehydration
- Generalized bulge
- Annular fissure
- Disc protrusion
- Disc extrusion
- Sequestration

*desiccation, disc degeneration, annular fissure, annular tear,* and *disc herniation* commonly are used interchangeably when describing degenerative disease, often without precision or consistency. There is also considerable variability in the terminology used by spine surgeons in describing degenerative diseases of the spine. A study by the NASS found wide variation in description of common spinal degenerative conditions by eight highly experienced surgeons. The eight surgeons used almost 50 terms collectively to describe eight different imaging findings.

To lessen the problem, the NASS has recommended that consistent terminology be used for describing disc herniations (Box 2-1). This terminology was designed primarily to correlate MRI with surgical findings. It avoids use of the term *herniation,* which is confusing and medicolegally significant. The dehydrated disc shows loss of signal on T2-weighted sequences. A generalized bulge is due to weakening of annular fibers, allowing the disc to protrude greater than 2 mm circumferentially beyond the bone margin. A disc protrusion is broad based and is wider in the coronal

plane than in the sagittal plane. All of these findings are common in the asymptomatic population. A disc extrusion has a narrow pedunculated segment and is elongated in the sagittal plane. A sequestered disc has lost its attachment to the parent disc. Both of these findings are uncommon in the asymptomatic population. Although they can be missed with CT myelography, foraminal discs are detected readily on MRI (Fig. 2-17).

The natural history of disc "herniation" is not well known. In a series by Bozzao et al, 69 patients with disc herniation were followed longitudinally while undergoing nonsurgical, conservative therapy. Of patients, 63% showed spontaneous decrease in volume of the disc greater than 30%, and 48% showed decrease in volume of the disc greater than 70%. The most dramatic decrease in size was seen in the largest disc herniations. Perhaps some, or even most, of the decrease in size of the disc herniation apparent by MRI is due to resolution of the inflammation that surrounds the symptomatic herniated disc.

Clinical resolution of symptoms does not correlate with findings on postoperative imaging studies. In many patients, follow-up imaging studies show no improvement in the anatomic lesion thought to be responsible for symptoms, despite excellent response to the intervention.

Postoperative MRI is difficult to interpret. Ross et al and Boden et al reviewed MRI studies postoperatively in patients who were greatly improved or rendered completely asymptomatic after surgery. Both of these series showed no correlation between postoperative mass effect and patient outcome. In both studies, significant residual mass effect persisted in most patients after successful surgery. Persistent disc protrusion/extrusion was present in 69% of surgical responders. Imaging showed a slow, incomplete resolution of mass effect over 36 months, despite immediate clinical response.

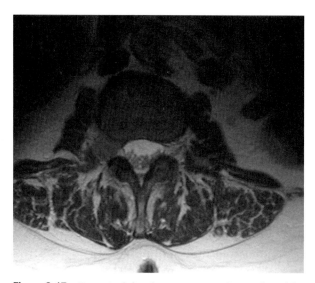

**Figure 2-17** Foraminal disc herniations are detected readily on MRI, whereas they may be missed by myelographic techniques. This is because the nerve root compression occurs beyond the point that the dura becomes confluent with the spinal nerve epineurium.

# SUGGESTED READING

## Spinal Trauma

Emery S, Pathria MN, Wilber RG, et al. MRI of posttraumatic spinal ligament injury. J Spinal Disord 1989;2:229–233.

Magid D, Fishman EK. Imaging of musculoskeletal trauma in three dimensions: an integrated two-dimensional/three-dimensional approach with computed tomography. Radiol Clin North Am 1989; 27:945–956.

Rockwood CG, DP. Rockwood and Green's fractures in adults. In: Bucholz RH, JD, eds. Vol. 1–2, 5th ed. Philadelphia: Lippincott Williams & Wilkins, 2001.

## Spinal Inflammatory Disorders

Bundschuh C, Modic MT, Kearney F, et al. Rheumatoid arthritis of the cervical spine: surface-coil MR imaging. AJR Am J Roentgenol 1988;151:181–187.

de Roos A, et al. MR imaging of marrow changes adjacent to end plates in degenerative lumbar disk disease. AJR Am J Roentgenol 1987; 149:531–534.

Freidman DP, Hills JR. Cervical epidural spinal infection: MR imaging characteristics. AJR Am J Roentgenol 1994;163:699–704.

Wagner SC, et al. Can imaging findings help differentiate spinal neuropathic arthropathy from disk space infection? Initial experience. Radiology 2000;214:693–699.

# Degenerative Spine

Bozzao A, Gallucci M, Masciocchi C, et al. Lumbar disk herniation: MR imaging assessment of natural history in patients treated without surgery. Radiology 1992;185:135–141.

Guinto, et al. AJNR Am J Neuroradiol 1984;5:632.

Stabler A, Bellan M, Weiss M, et al. MR imaging of enhancing intraosseous disk herniation (Schmorl's nodes). AJR Am J Roentgenol 1997;168:933–938.

Torgerson WR, Dotter WE. Comparative roentgenographic study of the asymptomatic and symptomatic lumbar spine. J Bone Joint Surg Am 1976;58:850–853.

# ELECTRO-MYOGRAPHY, LOCAL BLOCKS/ INJECTIONS, DISCOGRAMS

## EUGENE CARRAGEE

Most diagnoses in patients with spinal disorders can be made on the basis of clinical presentation. Fractures, dislocations, disc herniations, infections, and malignancies can be strongly suspected on clinical grounds and most often are confirmed with imaging studies. In the absence of clear pathologic findings (e.g., in patients with age-related degenerative changes), ancillary investigations using special diagnostic tests can be helpful. Some, such as electromyography (EMG) and nerve conduction studies (NCS), are objective and have established basic science in support of their use and findings. Others, such as provocative discography, are controversial and do not have clear basic science support in confirming a test-specific diagnosis.

## NEUROPHYSIOLOGIC STUDIES (ELECTROMYOGRAPHY, NERVE CONDUCTION STUDIES, SOMATOSENSORY EVOKED POTENTIAL)

Neurophysiologic studies sometimes are used in the evaluation of suspected spinal disorders that manifest neurologic symptoms. Usually spinal disorders with neurologic symptoms are not a diagnostic dilemma. The site of pathologic findings on imaging studies corresponds to the symptoms and signs on neurologic examination. In these cases, EMG and NCS rarely are indicated for diagnostic purposes. In patients with less clear relationships between pathoanatomic findings and clinical symptoms, EMG, NCS, or both may be appropriate.

Common indications for neurophysiologic testing include the following:

- To evaluate symptoms and signs of neurologic impairment without clear pathology
- To evaluate multiple anatomic (radiologic) levels of dis-

ease in the presence of focal neurologic signs (use to confirm the level)
- To distinguish radicular (nerve root) from peripheral neuropathy
- To distinguish spinal cord (myelopathy) from nerve root (radiculopathy) lesions
- To evaluate prognosis and estimate acute versus chronic injury

### Causes of Nerve Symptoms and Signs

Nerve injury with spinal disorders can occur at multiple levels and may be associated with or be confused by concomitant (extraspinal) neurologic dysfunction.

- The most common cause of neurologic symptoms in spinal disorders is irritation or compression of spinal nerve root.
- Spinal cord injury usually presents with different signs than root injury (spasticity versus pain/weakness); however, cord and root injuries can be present at the same time.
- Psychological issues are common in patients with back pain syndromes. It often is difficult to differentiate true neurologic weakness from lack of volitional effort to move.

Table 3-1 lists a practical set of neurologic presentations and common diagnoses. This is not an all-inclusive list but rather a reflection of the more common causes and important differential diagnoses in each group.

### Nerve Injury and Electromyography and Nerve Conduction Studies

Axonal loss with destruction of the axon and myelin sheath:

- Most frequently results in an abnormal EMG examination

## TABLE 3-1 PRACTICAL DIFFERENTIAL DIAGNOSIS OF NEUROLOGIC SYMPTOMS IN SPINAL DISORDERS

**Weakness and Pain**
Root injury/compression
Peripheral nerve injury/compression (mechanical injury, diabetic, or toxic neuropathy)
Intrinsic nerve disease (herpes zoster, nerve tumor)
Spinal cord injury (unusual)
Emotional/psychological disturbance (nonneurologic weakness)
Poor effort (pain or secondary gain issues)

**Painless Weakness**
Spinal cord injury or myelopathy
Brain injury (e.g., motor cortex, internal capsule)
Intrinsic nerve disease (polio, multiple sclerosis, amyotrophic lateral sclerosis)
Emotional disturbance ("hysterical paralysis," fear of injury)
Root or peripheral nerve injury (unusual)

**Predominantly Discoordination, Ataxia**
Brain injury
Spinal cord injury
Mild (inapparent) weakness
Vestibular disease
Psychological disturbance (flamboyant unsteadiness or collapse while under observation)

**Painless Sensory Changes without Weakness**
Peripheral neuropathy
Psychological disturbance (e.g., "conversion reaction")
Root injury (unusual)
Spinal cord injury or disease (e.g., posterior column disease, vitamin $B_{12}$ deficiency)
Brain injury

---

- Produces varying range of motor loss (mild to complete)
- Commonly results in muscle atrophy
- Has a guarded prognosis

Demyelination without axonal loss:

- Results in only mild or no muscle weakness
- Uncommonly results in atrophy
- Has a good prognosis with treatment (e.g., surgical decompression is better)
- Usually results in a normal EMG examination

Weakness from deconditioning, poor cooperation, and psychological factors do not influence nerve injury patterns on EMG or NCS.

- Severe paralysis attributable to root injury on physical examination cannot be normal on EMG.
- EMG and NCS data, when carefully acquired and interpreted, are objective and independent of patient effort.

## Common Electrodiagnostic Procedures

EMG, NCS, H-reflex, and somatosensory evoked potential (SSEP) are compared in Table 3-2.

### Electromyography

- EMG is the most useful test for radiculopathies.
- When positive, EMG can indicate injury distribution and level.
- Level of injury is estimated by usual innervation pattern of extremity muscles.
- Overlap and anatomic variation of innervation are common.
- Best estimation is to within one or two segments.
- Some findings have lag time after injury.
  - □ 1 week for most proximal muscles
  - □ 6 weeks for distal extremity muscles
  - □ Potential for false-negative results in early examination
  - □ *Spontaneous activity* refers to abnormal activity at rest, including fibrillations and fasciculations. These are indications of denervation of the tested muscle.
- Acute injury—fibrillation/fasciculation potentials
- Chronic injury—giant unit potentials

*Contraction activity* refers to the shape, amplitude, and duration of nerve firing and the number of phases of electrical potential compared with a normal muscle unit.

- Giant amplitude potentials indicate renervation.
- Some estimation of severity can be made (not very accurate).

### H-Reflex

- H-reflex is a monosynaptic spinal reflex specific for S1.
- H-reflex is abnormal immediately after injury.
- It is abnormal with S1 radiculopathy and corresponds to ankle reflex on physical exam.
- It also is abnormal in advanced age, tibial or sciatic nerve injuries (e.g., trauma, hip arthroplasty), and peripheral neuropathies (e.g., diabetic).
- H-reflex cannot differentiate acute from chronic injury.

### Nerve Conduction Studies

- NCS measure amplitude and speed of an applied signal traveling along a peripheral nerve.
- Velocity can be normal in radiculopathy proximal to the dorsal root ganglion.
- Amplitude should be normal, unless massive or multilevel axonal loss has occurred.
- When abnormal, it is usually due to peripheral neuropathy.

### Somatosensory Evoked Potential

- SSEP measures conduction between a large peripheral nerve and the cerebral cortex or the spinal cord.
- SSEP has poor detection of radiculopathy lesions.
- It is sensitive to certain spinal cord pathway lesions, including traumatic spinal cord injury or tumor, compressive myelopathy, and multiple sclerosis.
- Deficits in motor pathways may be missed.

## DIAGNOSTIC ANESTHETIC INJECTIONS

Diagnostic anesthetic injections are diagnostic procedures that rely on the premise that if pain is relieved by an anes-

**TABLE 3-2  COMPARISON OF BASIC FEATURES IN COMMON ELECTROPHYSIOLOGIC DIAGNOSTIC TEST**

|  | EMG | NCS | H-Reflex | SSEP |
|---|---|---|---|---|
| Root level specific | Moderate (1–2) | No | S1 only | No |
| Immediately positive after nerve injury | No | Yes | Yes | Yes |
| with spinal cord injury | No | No | No | Yes |
| with moderate radiculopathy | Yes | No | Yes | No |
| with massive or multiple root injury | Yes | Yes/no | Yes | Yes/no |
| in peripheral neuropathy | No | Yes | Yes | Yes/no |
| Different in acute versus chronic injury | Yes | No | No | No |

EMG, electromyography; NCS, nerve conduction study; SSEP, somatosensory evoked potential.

thetizing injection, that structure is a likely cause of the patient's pain. This method is used most commonly in the evaluation of nonspecific back pain. Local injections to the zygapophyseal (facet) joint, sacroiliac (SI) joint, spondylolytic defects, or selective nerve root blocks at the neural foramen are the most commonly used. Criteria for a positive result are arbitrary but can be estimated as the degree of subjective pain relief (e.g., 50%, 75%, 100%). In most cases, the predictive value of positive or negative blocks is not known because of the lack of an objective gold standard measure to confirm the result.

There are theoretical problems with anesthetic injections as a diagnostic technique, as follows:

▪ Injections proximal to a lesion may block afferent pathways. Pain from peroneal nerve entrapment may be relieved with a selective nerve root block of L5.
▪ Injections distal to a lesion (e.g., sciatic nerve anesthetic in root compression) also can give pain relief, albeit through an unclear mechanism. More worrisome is the overlap of segmental innervation of the spine from a single dorsal root ganglion. A single sensory afferent neuron may have branches that converge from two or more spinal segments (discs, bone, facets). Anesthetic injections to a painless site may modulate the input from a distant painful site, giving a misleading result.
▪ Placebo effects unrelated to presence or absence of a lesion may be 30% with spinal injections.

## Facet Joint Injections

Estimates of facet joint pain incidence in chronic low back pain (LBP) range from 15% to 40% based on diagnostic anesthetic blockage. These studies have no gold standard to confirm the diagnosis, however. Facet stimulation in normal subjects can induce pain in certain referred patterns with modest reproducibility, but this typical pattern has not been confirmed in symptomatic subjects. Experimental facet joint pain (distention with injection) can be blocked with simultaneous local anesthetic blockade of the *medial branches of the primary dorsal rami* above and below the stimulated facet.

There is a poor correlation between clinical symptoms, signs, or radiographic evidence of facet arthrosis and response to anesthetic facet blockade. The failure to identify

any reliable clinical syndrome or radiologic finding with facet block results may indicate the following:

▪ The painful lesion being locally anesthetized simply is not detectable by imaging studies and has a variable clinical presentation.
▪ The test does not identify a true clinical entity of any sort, and the response is related to secondary pain pathways or perception.

## Differential Anesthetic Blocks

Some authors suggest the use of sham injections or injections with short-acting and long-acting anesthetics as a means of increasing the specificity of diagnostic injection. Using this method, one group found ablation procedures relatively effective. These authors also reported, however, no difference in duration of pain relief when short-acting versus long-acting anesthetics were used in this trial (both about 4 to 5 hours). These findings reinforce the argument that diagnostic blocks are poorly understood pharmacologically and neurophysiologically.

## Sacroiliac Joint Injections

Diagnosis of SI joint problems usually is clear in cases of trauma (SI joint dislocation, Malgaigne's fracture), infection, or inflammatory disease; diagnostic injections usually are not needed or performed. With less clear presentation, SI joint injections are prompted by suggestive signs on physical exam. A positive response to provocative maneuvers (Faber and Galen tests) does not correlate, however, with a positive response to an SI joint anesthetic injection. In one small series, 20% to 30% of selected chronic LBP patients responded to a single or differential (short-acting versus long-acting agents) anesthetic block. The predictive value of SI joint blockade is unknown because of a lack of an objective gold standard test (i.e., pain resolution is subjective).

In summary:

▪ Patients who respond to SI joint injections do not always have a characteristic history or response to provocative maneuvers on physical exam.
▪ It is not clear whether patients who respond to SI injection with some pain relief represent only subjects with

"true" SI joint pathology, or whether they are a diverse group with various local, regional, or complex pain sites.

■ It has not been shown that a specific pathology found on imaging studies is seen only in subjects with response to SI joint anesthetic injections.

# PROVOCATIVE DISCOGRAPHY

Discography first was developed as a method to identify herniated discs in the lumbar spine. It coincidentally was noted that sometimes during injection of the contrast material into the disc the patient's usual sciatic symptoms were reproduced. With continued experience, it also was reported that familiar back pain could be reproduced during disc injection. The finding that disc injection in some patients seemed to *reproduce their usual and typical back pain* has led to use of discography as an evaluative maneuver in determining the cause of chronic LBP.

## Technique

Discography technique has evolved over time. Compared with original methods, injections use less irritating contrast dye, are directed by image guidance, and employ limited pressure. Discography is performed by injection of a water-soluble, radiopaque dye under fluoroscopic guidance into several intervertebral discs.

■ The central portion of the disc is penetrated percutaneously by a long fine-gauge needle through an introducer (large-gauge needle) in a "two-needle" technique. This can be done from a posterolateral approach in most cases. At L4-5 and L5-S1, the needle usually is bent into a gentle curve before introduction.

■ Discography should be performed with minimal sedation and local anesthetic at the skin puncture site. The patient needs to be comfortable but alert and able to describe the pain response to injections.

■ The dye is injected slowly into the nucleus of several lumbar discs with the patient blinded to the timing and site of injection.

■ The distribution and extravasation (if present) of the dye in the disc is noted, as is the patient's clinical response to injection.

■ Two key features of clinical response are noted:

  □ *Pain intensity*: The patient is asked whether each injection is painful and is asked to rate the pain against a standardized scale (e.g., 0 to 5, 0 to 10, "none" to "unbearable").

  □ *Concordancy*: The discomfort provoked by the injection, if any, is rated as similar (concordant) or dissimilar to the usual LBP. A patient with similar or exact pain reproduction usually is considered to have a concordant pain response.

## Criteria for a Positive Discogram

■ *Basic criteria*: A positive test includes "significant pain" with injection and a reproduction of usual pain.

■ *Walsh criteria*: Based on a study in 1990 by Walsh et al, a positive response is defined as 3/5 or 6/10 and patient describing the pain as bad or worse. These authors also

required that an observable pain reaction or pain behavior be present.

■ *Other criteria*: The following are used to limit the risk of false-positive injections:

  □ *Control disc injection*: Many discographers require at least one disc injection to be negative before an adjacent disc can be considered positive. It is not clear in the literature what a "negative" disc means (e.g., painless with injection, not "significantly painful," or not concordantly painful). This confusion has led most practitioners to include the disc above and below the suspected painful disc as a control levels.

  □ *Exact pain reproduction*: Some authors recommend that only "exact" pain reproduction be considered a positive response. Clinical and experimental studies have shown that patients with regional pain, not coming from the intervertebral disc, may confuse disc and regional pain and report both as exactly concordant with disc injections.

  □ *Annular disruption*: Some authors require the dye to reach the outer anulus. Morphologically normal discs or discs without fissuring to the outer anulus cannot be positive by this criteria.

  □ *Pressure-controlled injection*: Some authors propose that disc injections be limited to less than 80 to 100 psi and that positive responses to low-pressure injections (<15 to 20 psi) be differentiated from positive responses that occur only at higher pressures. This criterion was based on an observation of differential outcomes in a small cohort of low-pressure positive discs, which since have been termed *chemically sensitive* (rather than *mechanically sensitive*). Experimental studies in subjects without chronic LBP show less frequent positive injections at these low pressures, but still a false-positive injection rate at low pressures ranging from 10% to 30%.

## Specificity of Discography

The unresolved question remains: Does a positive injection of a disc, by whatever criteria, definitively identify the disc as a cause of chronic LBP? Because provocative discography relies entirely on the subjective reporting of pain perception, the pain intensity and concordancy are subject to the neurophysiologic modulation of pain pathways, which may amplify or downregulate nociceptive signals from the stimulated disc.

The concept of modulation of pain perception should be considered. Pain may begin at a local structure (e.g., disc, muscle, ligament), but the transmission of the nociceptive signal is modulated along the neural axis (i.e., local nerves, autonomic nerves, dorsal root ganglion, dorsal horn and ascending tracts, thalamic and associated processing areas of the cortical and higher/complex pain processing regions) (Figs. 3-1, 3-2, and 3-3).

## Discography in Asymptomatic Subjects

Walsh et al studied 10 healthy young men with little disc degeneration and no known psychological or chronic pain predisposing to pain amplification. One of 10 subjects had

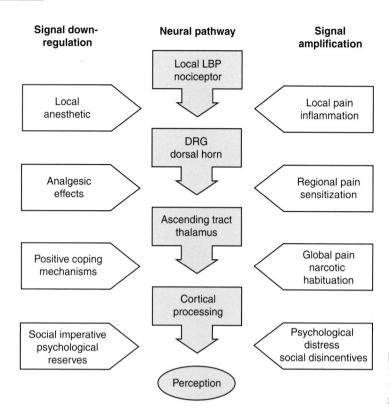

**Figure 3-1** Schematic of pain signal pathways for low back pain (LBP) with modulation from signal amplification factor and downregulators. DRG, dorsal root ganglion.

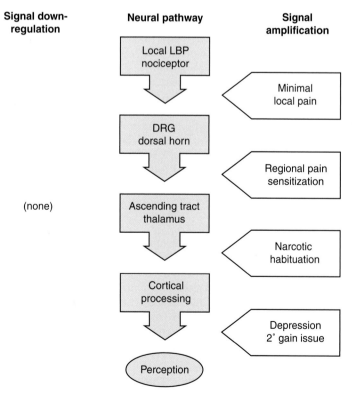

**Figure 3-2** Scenario of Pain Amplification Pathway: Low back pain (LBP) from minimal degenerative changes in a patient with multiple chronic pain syndromes, chronic narcotic habituation, depression, and workers' compensation claim (social disincentive). DRG, dorsal root ganglion.

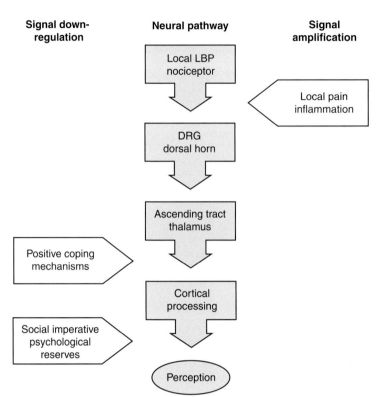

| Signal down-regulation | Neural pathway | Signal amplification |

**Figure 3-3** Scenario of down regulation pathway. Low back pain (LBP) from heavy physical training in well-motivated and conditioned soldiers. DRG, dorsal root ganglion.

pain at 6/10 level (10% significant pain) with disc injection (Fig. 3-4). Carragee et al studied 10 subjects asymptomatic for LBP with known degenerative disc disease and no chronic pain processes: 10% had significant pain with injection. In another study, Carragee et al studied 16 subjects asymptomatic for LBP but with distant chronic pain syndromes and increased psychological distress. Of subjects, 56% (9/16) had significant pain with injection.

Further studies of disc injections in subjects with no or minimal discogenic pain have shown the following risk factors for amplified pain response to disc injections:

- Increased psychological distress
- Nonlumbar chronic pain syndrome (concurrent)
- Disputed compensation claims
- Previous discectomy at the injected disc
- History of persistent clinically benign backache

All of these factors can increase the risk of false-positive injections if found in subjects with chronic LBP. These subjects may be at higher risk for a positive disc injection at levels that are not the primary cause of their chronic LBP.

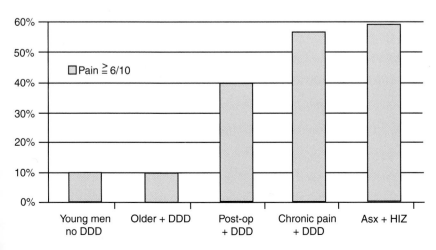

**Figure 3-4** Percent of asymptomatic subjects with pain (≥6/10) on disc injection in different subgroups. Note increasing risk factors for false-positive injections. Asx, asymptomatic; DDD, degenerative disc disease; HIZ, high intensity zone.

## Discography as Predictor of Clinical Outcomes

Calhoun et al, in an uncontrolled comparison of patients undergoing spinal fusion–based discography and imaging versus imaging studies alone, reported a moderate increase in success in the discography group. More recently, using a historical control design, adding discography to the preoperative evaluation was not found to improve outcomes.

## Summary

Provocative discography is an invasive method used to pressurize a suspected disc and elicit a pain response. The specificity of discography in determining the cause of LBP is unknown. False-positive rates seem to vary with psychological distress, chronic pain states, compensation issues, and certain morphologic changes (annular disruption). Studies are conflicting whether the use of this technique can improve clinical outcomes of various interventions in patients with chonic LBP (Table 3-3).

---

**TABLE 3-3 PRACTICAL GUIDE TO DISCOGRAPHY USE**

Best case utility
  Negative discogram to determine end of fusion in deformity or other clear pathology
  Positive, single-level disc in subject without risk factors for false-positive injection (e.g., normal psychological profile, no chronic pain behavior or history, no compensation issues)
Unclear utility
  Positive two-level discs, but no risk factors
  Postoperative discs, but otherwise no risk factors
  Intermediate (at risk) psychological profile, single level
Poor utility
  Spine with multilevel pathology
  Abnormal or very chronic pain behavior
  Abnormal psychometric findings
  Disputed compensation cases

# CERVICAL TRAUMA

**RAJESH G. ARAKAL**
**MICHAEL VIVES**

Traumatic injuries to the cervical spine are a common cause of morbidity and mortality throughout the world. Most patients with closed spinal column injury are young men, whose injury often results from motor vehicle accidents, falls, or sports injuries. A second peak in prevalence exists in adults age 50 and older. Injuries in this age group are related predominantly to falls. Categorizing these injuries has allowed spine care specialists to evaluate more adeptly and treat affected patients.

## ANATOMY

A thorough understanding of the complex anatomy of the cervical spine is essential for accurate injury identification and treatment planning. Although the anatomy of the subaxial cervical spine is largely consistent, the anatomy of the upper cervical spine is unique at each level. Bony restraints of the occipitocervical junction involve the convex occipital condyles articulating with the lateral masses of the atlas (C1). Children younger than 12 years old have more unrestricted motion and are predisposed to injury at the occipitocervical junction. The posterior arch of C1 provides a bony limit to occiput extension. Ligamentous restraints are formed primarily by the alar ligaments, which course from the superolateral aspect of the odontoid process to the medial occipital condyle. Motion at this segment approximates 21 degrees of extension, 3 degrees of flexion, 7 degrees of rotation to each side, and 5 degrees of lateral bending to each side.

The atlas is linked mechanically to the base of the skull and the axis. It relies on two lateral masses for weight bearing. Embryologically the caudal part of the C1 somite joins with the cranial C2 somite to form the odontoid process. By 3 to 6 years of age, the dens fuses with the body. In the absence of a disc between the occiput and C1, the anatomic relationship is maintained by ligamentous relationships. The atlantooccipital membrane attaches to a tubercle at the base of the skull and is confluent with the anterior longitudinal ligament. The apical ligament attaches the tip of the dens to the anterior edge of the foramen magnum. The posterior longitudinal ligament continues superiorly as the tectorial membrane. The most important ligamentous restraint to anterior translation of the C1-2 complex is the transverse ligament, which traverses posterior to the odontoid to attach to the C1 lateral masses. Secondary restraint comes from the alar ligaments, which arise along the medial aspect of the occipital condyles and lateral masses of C1 and insert onto the lateral aspect of the odontoid. Approximately 15 degrees of flexion/extension occurs at the occipitoatlantal junction. The muscular attachments to the cervical spine include the longus colli, which attach to the anterior and inferior portions of the arch of C1. The rectus capitis medialis and lateralis and the trapezius insert posteriorly.

Although the atlantoaxial joint (50%) and subaxial spine (50%) contribute equally to rotation, most of the flexion and extension in the cervical spine occurs from C3 to C7. At each motion segment of the subaxial spine, 17 degrees of sagittal plane motion can occur. Coronal motion ranges from 4 to 11 degrees per motion segment in this region. The anterior longitudinal ligament and anulus fibrosus act as a tension band limiting extension. Posteriorly the supraspinous and interspinous ligaments and the ligamentum flavum resist flexion. The cross-sectional area of the spinal canal is largest at C2 and smallest at C7. Anterior radicular arteries supply the anterior spinal artery (and the spinal cord) and posterior radicular arteries supply the posterior spinal arteries. In the cervical spine, the radicular artery originating from the deep cervical artery accompanying the left C6 spinal nerve root is the most significant.

## CLINICAL EVALUATION

All patients who present with traumatic injuries should have an initial evaluation according to standard advanced trauma and life support protocols. The patient should be logrolled carefully and the spine palpated for tenderness or step-off. A thorough neurologic exam should be performed, focusing on key motor groups as suggested by the American Spinal Injury Association classification. The Frankel scale (A through E) is part of spinal injury classification, with A representing complete motor and sensory function loss below the level of injury and E representing normal motor and sensory function.

## IMAGING

Standard plain radiographic evaluation involves anteroposterior, lateral, and open mouth views. The lateral view of the cervical spine shows 85% of injuries. The cervicothoracic junction should be visible. If the lateral view is not sufficient, a swimmer's view is obtained. If still unclear, a computed tomography (CT) scan of C7-T1 is obtained. In patients without significant clinical findings, there is a 3.1% incidence of occult cervical trauma at the cervicothoracic junction. Up to 16% of patients have noncontiguous spinal fractures. Frequently, fractures at C1-2 are associated with a remote subaxial fracture. The Power's ratio is useful to evaluate occipitocervical alignment (Fig. 4-1). The ratio of a line drawn from the basion to the posterior arch of the atlas over the line from the opisthion to the anterior arch of the atlas should be less than 1. A ratio greater than 1 suggests an anterior occipitoatlantal dislocation. Flexion/extension films normally should reveal less than 1 mm of translation between the occiput and C1. Greater than 1 mm indicates occipitoatlantal instability. The atlantodental interval (ADI) is used to determine the stability of the atlantoaxial segment. Values greater than 3 mm in an adult and 4 mm in a child suggest rupture of the transverse ligament. Soft tissue shadows often indicate undiagnosed cervical trauma. The normal prevertebral soft tissue shadow anterior to C1 should be less than 10 mm, less than 7 mm at C3, and less than 20 mm at C6 in the noninjured cervical spine.

The radiographic criteria for subaxial spinal stability continue to evolve. Angulation greater than 11 degrees compared with adjacent normal segments or translation greater than 3.5 mm are guidelines developed by serial sectioning studies in cadavers to simulate flexion injuries. Extension injuries can be subtle, necessitating evaluation for anterior disc space widening or increase in soft tissue density in the retropharyngeal space.

If the plain radiographs reveal osseous abnormalities, CT may help define the extent of bone damage. CT also is helpful when the lower cervical spine cannot be visualized adequately on plain radiographs.

Magnetic resonance imaging (MRI) may be indicated in:

- Patients with neurologic deficits, particularly when CT does not show a reason for the deficit.
- Patients with deteriorating neurologic status.
- Cases of suspected posterior ligamentous injury not evident by plain radiographs or CT reconstructions.

Davis et al showed that 50 of 130 patients with normal radiographs were found to have disc or soft tissue injuries by MRI. Controversy exists regarding the timing of obtaining these studies in the acute trauma setting. We favor early restoration of cervical alignment and protection, with traction, in an alert and cooperative patient before obtaining an advanced imaging work-up, which can result in delay or repeated transfers.

# CRANIOCERVICAL INJURIES AND THEIR TREATMENT

## Occipital Condyle Fractures

Injuries to the occipitocervical junction are becoming increasingly prevalent as improved trauma care has decreased acute mortality. Injuries occur primarily by three mechanisms: compression, distraction, and lateral rotation. Fractures are organized according to CT morphology and potential instability. Occipital condyle fractures may result from axial loading or distraction forces on the atlas as classified by Anderson and Montesano. A *type I injury* is a comminuted fracture due to impaction of the occipital condyle into the lateral mass of the atlas. It is usually stable. A *type II injury* is an occipital condyle fracture associated with a basilar skull fracture, usually from a direct blow. Stability is compromised when the entire condyle is separated from the occiput. Rotation or lateral bending may result in an avulsion fracture of the occipital condyle by the alar ligament; this is a *type III injury*. Any anteroposterior displacement or incongruent articulation may be an indication of underlying instability in type III patterns. Rigid collar immobilization for 6 to 8 weeks is recommended for type I and most type II injuries. Type III injuries are unstable and require posterior fusion.

A frequently used classification system for occipitocervical instability is based on the direction of displacement (Table 4-1):

- *Type I* injury involves anterior displacement of the occiput with respect to the atlas. Children, because of their

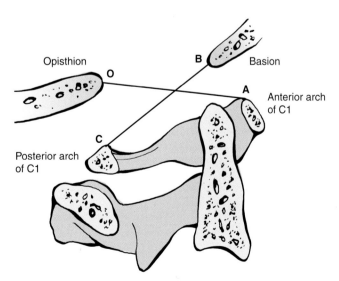

**Figure 4-1**   Power's ratio. The ratio of BC to AO normally equals 1. If the ratio is greater than 1, an anterior occipitoatlantal dislocation may exist.

Opisthion

Basion

Anterior arch of C1

Posterior arch of C1

| TABLE 4-1  CLASSIFICATION OF OCCIPITOCERVICAL INSTABILITY | |
| --- | --- |
| Type I | Anterior displacement between occipital condyles and atlas |
| Type IIa | Vertical displacement between occiput and atlas |
| Type IIb | Vertical displacement between atlas and axis |
| Type III | Posterior displacement between occipital condyles and atlas |

larger head size, are more prone to anterior displacement of the occiput.

- *Type II* injury is a distraction injury with vertical separation of the occiput from the atlas. These injuries should not be placed in traction because this may exacerbate the deformity and result in further neurologic compromise.
- *Type III* injury is a rare posterior displacement of the occiput with respect to the atlas.

Type I and III injuries may be treated with 5 lb of traction initially. If intubation is necessary, it should be nasotracheal. Halo vest immobilization usually is recommended for 3 months with subsequent flexion and extension radiographs to assess stability. Type II injuries usually require occipitoatlantal fusion.

Numerous methods of occipitocervical arthrodesis have been reported. Fusion can be achieved using posterior wiring from the outer table of the occiput to the atlas as described by Cone and Bohlman. Modifications include addition of a contoured rod and passage of sublaminar wires to achieve fixation. Occipitocervical plating with reconstruction plates also is an option with screw fixation of the occiput and transarticular C1-2 screw placement. C2 pedicle screws also may be placed as an alternative.

## Fractures of the Atlas

Fractures of the atlas represent 10% of all cervical spine fractures. Five distinct fracture patterns can be recognized, as follows:

- The most common injury is the posterior arch fracture, which usually occurs at the junction of the lateral masses.
- A second pattern involves fractures anterior to the lateral mass on one side and posterior on the contralateral side, creating a free-floating lateral mass.
- Simultaneous fractures of the anterior and posterior rings are characteristic of Jefferson's fracture, which tends to displace laterally.
- Horizontal fractures can occur through the anterior tubercle of C1.
- Transverse process fractures of C1 may be unilateral or bilateral.

Fractures of the posterior arch of C1 usually result from hyperextension. Associated injuries of C2, such as an anterior teardrop fracture and spondylisthesis of the axis, should be ruled out if this mechanism of injury is suspected. Lateral mass fractures are a result of combined axial loading and lateral bending. Associated fractures include lower cervical facet fractures. Combined displacement of the lateral masses (Jefferson's fracture) greater than 6.9 mm can be associated with failure of the transverse ligament. The alar and apical ligaments and the C1-2 capsule usually are spared, however. Severe hyperflexion movements disrupt the transverse, alar, and apical ligaments. Hyperextension results in an avulsion; this may be due to forceful contraction of the superior oblique portion of the longus colli. Transverse process fractures are usually from a forced lateral compressive (ipsilateral) injury with a contralateral avulsion fracture. This pattern may be associated with laminar fractures in the lower cervical spine as well.

Treatment of most C1 injuries is nonoperative and includes a cervical orthosis, Minerva cast, or halo fixator. If the transverse ligament is ruptured, early C1-2 arthrodesis may be considered. Surgery usually is indicated for the associated spine injuries. Commonly associated injuries are fractures of the dens and traumatic spondylolisthesis (hangman's fracture) of the axis. Fractures of the posterior arch of the atlas by themselves are stable injuries and amenable to closed treatment with a cervical orthosis. Lateral mass fractures with minimal displacement may be treated with rigid orthoses or halo immobilization. Displaced fractures with greater than 7 mm usually are associated with rupture of the transverse ligament. Some authors have recommended attempted reduction with axial traction through a halo ring as the initial step in treatment of this injury. This is followed by 1 to 2 weeks of bed rest with traction. Halo vest immobilization should be maintained for 3 months.

## Odontoid Fractures

Fractures of the odontoid constitute approximately 18% of cervical spine fractures. Motor vehicle accidents account for most injuries in patients age 16 to 34 years. Falls account for most injuries in patients older than age 55 and younger than age 15.

Anderson and D'Alonzo established the following classification system:

- *Type I* odontoid fractures involve the tip of the dens. This may result from a severe rotational or lateral bending force that causes an avulsion of bone through the alar and apical ligaments. Other distraction injuries must be ruled out.
- *Type II* fractures occur through the "waist" of the dens without involvement of the C2 body and have nonunion rates of 11% to 100%. Risk factors for nonunion are (1) age greater than 60, (2) more than 5 mm displacement and 9 degrees of angulation, and (3) smoking.
- *Type III* fractures are through the body of C2. In marked contrast, this has a union rate that may approach 100%, a consequence of larger surface areas and more vascular cancellous bone.

Type I injuries can be treated with a cervical orthosis, in the absence of occipitocervical instability. Type III fractures and type II fractures with less than 10 degrees of angulation and 5 mm of displacement can be treated with a halo fixator. Greater displacement should be treated with initial traction for a better reduction followed with early conversion to a halo vest. Displaced or significantly angulated type II fractures often are treated with posterior atlantoaxial arthrodesis using autogenous bone graft or osteosynthesis with an anterior odontoid screw, which theoretically preserves more motion.

## Transverse Ligament Insufficiency

Atlantoaxial instability may be caused by a disruption of the transverse ligament. This disruption can result from trauma and congenital, infectious, and inflammatory processes. The transverse ligament functions primarily as restraint against anterior subluxation of C1 on C2. Fielding reported that an intact transverse ligament allows a maximum of 3 mm of anterior translation of C1 on C2. Failure of the ligament is inferred with greater than a 3 mm ADI. High-resolution CT or MRI can be used to evaluate a midsubstance tear or avulsion fracture. Axial gradient-echo MRI is the best modality to visualize the transverse ligament. Treatment is aimed at restoring stability when the ADI measures more than 5 mm. Posterior C1-2 arthrodesis is preferred. Children may be managed with a trial of rigid halo fixation for 2 to 3 months. C1-2 arthrodesis is performed in the presence of persistent pain or an anterior ADI greater than 5 mm in flexion. The best healing rates with nonoperative treatments are with bony avulsion fractures.

## Traumatic Spondylolisthesis of the Axis (Hangman's Fracture)

The axis represents the transition between the upper and lower cervical spine. The superior articular facets of C2 lie anterior to the neural elements and in line with the C1-2 lateral masses, whereas the inferior facets are posterior to

the canal and are in line with the lower cervical lateral masses. The transitional nature of this vertebra places greater stresses on the pars interarticularis with loading. Injury occurs with a combination of extension, axial compression, and flexion. A fracture line results that propagates through the C2 pars interarticularis; this can result in anterolisthesis of the C2 body on C3. Patients rarely have neurologic deficit owing to the large size of the canal at this level. The fracture displacement tends to increase the effective canal size.

Classification of hangman's fractures currently is based on the degree of angulatory and translational deformity between C2-3 (Fig. 4-2):

- *Type I* fractures occur through the neural arch at the base of the pedicle and show less than 3 mm of translation and no angulation at the fracture site. They result from a hyperextension and axial load and do not include significant injury to the disc, longitudinal ligaments, or adjacent body of C3. *Type IA* injuries are less evident on lateral plain films because of the obliquity of the fracture line across the body of C2 (often through the foramen transversarium). There may be apparent elongation of

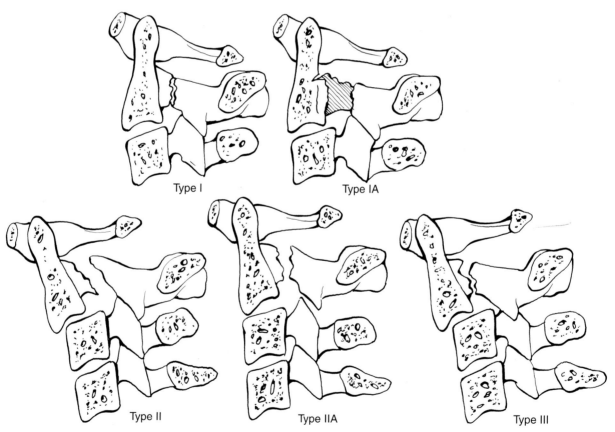

**Figure 4-2** Classification of hangman's fractures. Type I—minimal separation of the fragments, without significant angulation or translation. Type IA—oblique fracture through posterior portion of vertebral body may be difficult to visualize on lateral radiograph. There may be apparent elongation of the vertebral body and pars. Type II—relatively vertical fracture with separation of the fragments, angulation, and translation of C2 on C3. Type IIA—oblique fracture line by failure of pars in tension, no translation, but significant angulation of C2 on C3. Type III—combined injury, with type I fracture of pars and C2-3 facet dislocation.

C2 by 2 or 3 mm of translation of the anterior aspects of the C2 body with relative anatomic alignment of the posterior elements. A CT scan often is necessary to delineate this pattern. Type I and IA injuries (without neurologic deficit) can be treated with immobilization in a cervical orthosis.

- *Type II* injuries are characterized by translation greater than 3 mm and significant angulation at the fracture site. The anterosuperior portion of the C3 body can show some compression. The pars fracture line is usually vertical, close to the body-pedicle junction in the coronal plane. The anterior longitudinal ligament is stripped off the superior one third to one half of the front of the C3 body, but it is still in continuity. The mechanism of injury is one of an initial hyperextension and axial loading followed by hyperflexion. Disruption of the C2-3 disc often occurs. Traction reduction followed by halo immobilization is the usual treatment. *Type IIA* fractures have significant angular deformity but only minimal translation. Angulation can exceed 15 degrees, whereas translation rarely exceeds 2 or 3 mm. Type IIA injuries most commonly are a result of flexion/distraction injury resulting in failure of the neural arch in tension with rupture of the posterior aspects of the disc. Traction is contraindicated in this injury and would result in an increase in deformity and widening of the disc space. Type IIA injuries should be reduced with extension and compression. Image intensification may be helpful during halo positioning.
- *Type III* fractures have facet dislocations at C2-3 in addition to a displaced pars fracture. The mechanism of injury is flexion and distraction followed by hyperextension. They have a higher rate of neurologic injury. The distinguishing feature is the free-floating inferior facets of C2. It usually requires open reduction of the facet dislocation and posterior C2-3 fusion.

# SUBAXIAL CERVICAL INJURIES AND THEIR TREATMENT

Although a universally accepted classification system for fractures and dislocations of the lower cervical spine does not exist, classifications based on mechanism of injury generally have been found useful. Allen et al's classification is one of the most widely used. It is based on a retrospective evaluation of 165 cases. The authors proposed six categories, each named for the presumed position of the cervical spine at the moment of injury and the initial principal mechanism of load to failure. Categories include the following:

- Vertical compression
- Compressive flexion
- Distractive flexion
- Lateral flexion
- Compressive extension
- Distractive extension

The authors showed that the probability of neurologic injury could be predicted based on the type and severity of the fracture.

## Vertical Compression Injuries

Vertical compression injuries are commonly the result of motor vehicle accidents, diving injuries, and blows to the vertex of the skull. Vertical compression stage 1 injuries have central cupping of one vertebral end plate. Vertical compression stage 2 has disruption of both end plates. Stage 1 injuries often are treated with a rigid cervical or cervicothoracic orthosis. Vertical compression stage 2 injuries without neurologic injury can be treated with halo vest immobilization for 8 to 12 weeks. Vertical compression stage 3 injuries show fragmentation of the vertebral body with displacement of the fragments peripherally into the canal (burst fracture). In the setting of neurologic injury, most surgeons favor anterior corpectomy to decompress the spinal cord followed by strut fusion and instrumentation to reestablish anterior column integrity. Posterior instrumentation and fusion may be added.

## Compressive Flexion

Compressive flexion injuries comprise 20% of subaxial cervical spine fractures (Fig. 4-3). In this subtype, the force vector is anterior and inferior. The subtypes include the following:

- *Stage 1* consists of blunting at the anterosuperior margin of the vertebral body.
- *Stage 2* has further loss of anterior height, producing a beaklike appearance anteroinferiorly. Rigid collar immobilization is usually sufficient to allow healing and prevent development of late deformity.
- *Stage 3* results from greater force application, producing a fracture line passing from the anterior surface obliquely to the subchondral plate (the so-called "teardrop fragment"). These often can be managed successfully in a halo vest if minimally displaced or minimally kyphotic.
- *Stage 4* has a similar fracture pattern accompanied by less than 3 mm of displacement of the posterior body into the canal.
- *Stage 5* is characterized by more severe displacement and failure of the posterior ligamentous complex.

Some authors favor anterior decompression and fusion with instrumentation (with or without possible adjuvant posterior arthrodesis) (Fig. 4-4). Biomechanical studies of anterior plating (without structural bone graft) led to concern regarding the adequacy of anterior surgery alone for this injury. Clinical data of anterior structural grafting with a rigid plate have shown good results, however, even without postoperative halo immobilization.

## Distractive Flexion

Distractive flexion accounts for approximately 10% of subaxial cervical injuries. The distractive flexion stages include the following:

- *Stage 1* is a failure of the posterior ligamentous complex with facet subluxation only in flexion and divergence of the spinous processes. Radiographs often are negative.

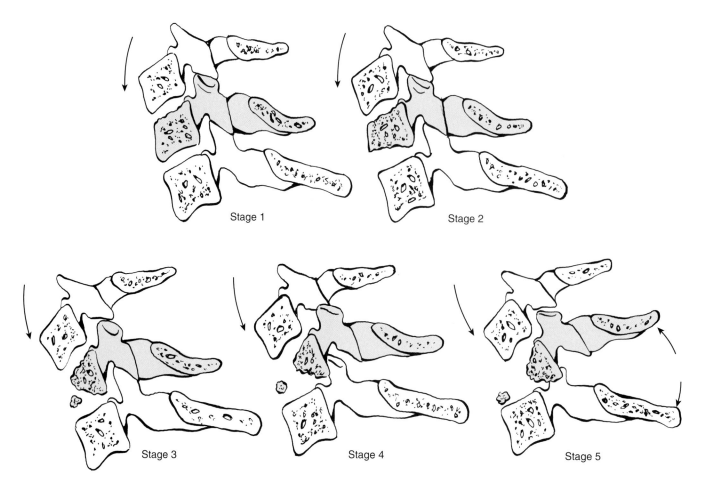

Stage 1

Stage 2

Stage 3

Stage 4

Stage 5

**Figure 4-3** Compressive flexion injuries. Stage 1—blunting of anterosuperior vertebral margin. Stage 2—additional loss of height, involvement of inferior end plate. Stage 3—oblique fracture from anterosuperior surface to subchondral plate. Stage 4—posterior displacement (<3 mm) into neural canal. Stage 5—further disruption of posterior ligamentous complex and posterior displacement of vertebral body (>3 mm).

Flexion/extension radiographs help identify these injuries and are best obtained in 2 to 3 weeks.

- *Stage 2* is a unilateral facet dislocation that may be associated with a fracture of the articular process or pedicle.
- *Stage 3* is a bilateral facet dislocation, which usually shows 50% anterior displacement.
- *Stage 4* is a bilateral facet dislocation with full width (100%) vertebral body displacement.

Unilateral facet dislocation can be distinguished from bilateral facet dislocation in that the former shows less than 25% translation of the vertebral body. The incidence of complete neurologic injury is more frequent with bilateral facet dislocation. Some authors recommend routine prereduction MRI to identify concomitant herniated nucleus pulposus because of the risk of disc fragment displacement during a reduction. The clearest indication for prereduction MRI is in the situation of an intubated and anesthetized patient; awake and cooperative patients have been reduced safely by closed means. Reduction usually is achieved by sequential addition of increasing weights to cervical tongs

until the facets are perched, followed by careful manipulation. Many times, the facets reduce spontaneously with sufficient weight. Definitive stabilization and fusion is required. Posterior instrumented fusion and anterior discectomy and interbody fusion with a plate may be successful for definitive treatment (Fig. 4-5).

## Compressive Extension

- *Stage 1* lesions involve a unilateral posterior arch fracture, usually accompanied by failure of the anterior portion of the disc in tension (Fig. 4-6). The posterior element fracture may consist of a linear fracture through the articular pillar, an ipsilateral pedicle and laminar fracture resulting in the "horizontal facet" appearance (Fig. 4-7), or a combination of an ipsilateral articular process and pedicle fracture (i.e., lateral mass fracture). Rotational instability around the contralateral intact lateral mass may result. Retrospective data on patients treated in either a hard collar or a halo brace have shown

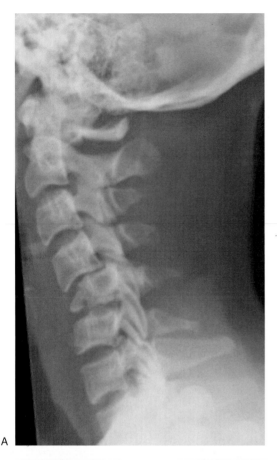

A

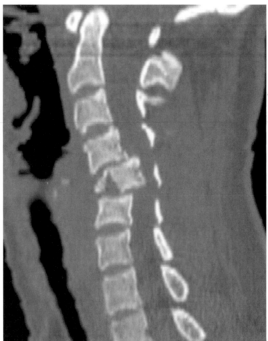

B

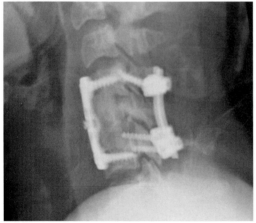

C

**Figure 4-4**   (**A**) Lateral radiograph of a patient with a compressive flexion injury involving C5. (**B**) Sagittal reconstruction showing posterior displacement of vertebral body into the neural canal, which resulted in spinal cord injury. (**C**) Lateral radiograph after anterior decompression and circumferential stabilization.

that such management was frequently unsuccessful. Posterior surgery traditionally has been advocated. Alternatively, anterior discectomy and plated interbody fusion also seems to be effective and may lead to better radiographic results (i.e., maintenance of kyphosis correction).

■ *Stage* 2 lesions involve bilaminar fractures without evidence of failure of anterior constraints. Multiple contiguous levels often are involved. Neurologic injuries are

unusual with this injury. Immobilization in a rigid cervical orthosis or halo vest usually is sufficient.

■ *Stages* 3, *4, and* 5 lesions involve progressively severe circumferential disruption, with stage 5 characterized by vertebral arch fractures and 100% anterior displacement of the vertebral body. These are true fracture-dislocations. Given the extreme disruption of both columns, combined anterior and posterior fusion with instrumentation is the best approach to surgical management.

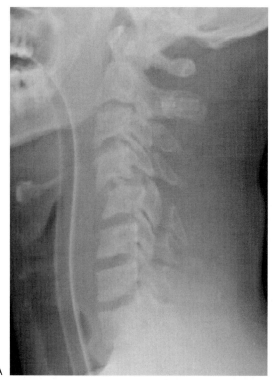

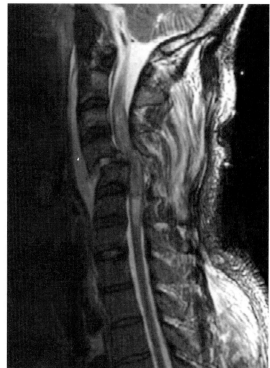

A

B

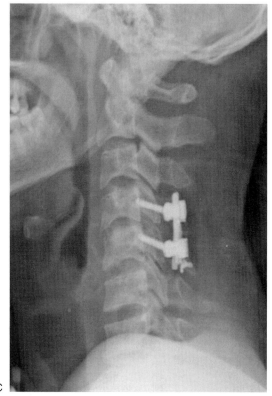

C

**Figure 4-5** (A) Lateral radiograph of a patient with a distractive flexion injury at C4-5. (B) MRI was per- -formed before reduction because the patient had a concomitant head injury with altered consciousness. (C) Lateral radiograph after posterior fusion.

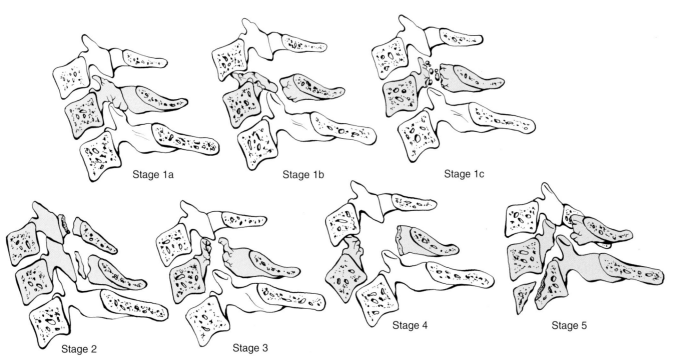

Stage 1a          Stage 1b          Stage 1c

Stage 2          Stage 3          Stage 4          Stage 5

**Figure 4-6** Compressive extension injuries. Stage 1 involves unilateral fracture through the articular process, pedicle, or lamina. Stage 2 involves bilaminar fracture, which often occurs at multiple contiguous levels. Stages 3 and 4 are hypothetical stages, not seen in Allen's initial observations. Stage 5 involves three contiguous levels, anterior displacement, and shear injury through the adjacent inferior centrum.

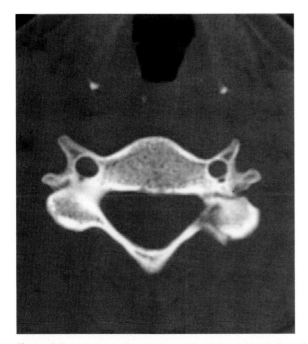

**Figure 4-7** CT scan of a patient with ipsilateral pedicle and lamina fracture resulting in a "floating facet."

## Distractive Extension

■ *Stage 1* lesions involve failure of the anterior ligamentous complex (anterior longitudinal ligament and intervertebral disc) or a transverse failure through the bony centrum. In the stage 1 lesion, there is no translation or posterior displacement. Lesions that involve largely bony injury may be managed best in a halo vest. Conversely, operative treatment and nonoperative treatment have been recommended for stage 1 lesions that involve only soft tissues. This category represents a spectrum of injuries that involve disruption of the anterior restraints from the anterior anulus and longitudinal ligament to the posterior anulus and posterior longitudinal ligament. If an initial nonsurgical route is chosen, immobilization in either a rigid orthosis or a halo should be accompanied by frequent serial radiographic follow-up. If surgical treatment is elected, either primarily or after failed nonoperative treatment, anterior reconstruction with a plate acting as a tension band can be effective.

■ *Stage 2* lesions, in addition to the features seen in stage 1, involve failure of the posterior ligamentous complex. The resultant instability may allow displacement of the upper vertebral body posteriorly into the spinal canal. Because these injuries involve disruption of the anterior and the posterior columns, circumferential stabilization procedures may ensure better long-term stability. Consideration may be given to approaching the spine posteriorly initially to align the spine in the sagittal plane adequately before anterior column reconstruction. Many of these injuries occur in patients with ankylosing spondylitis or diffuse idiopathic skeletal hyperostosis. The reduced capacity of the brittle spine to accommodate substantial distraction/extension force vectors may be responsible for this association.

### Lateral Flexion Injuries

Lateral flexion *stage 1* injuries comprise ipsilateral fractures of the centrum and posterior arch. Often CT scans are necessary to identify the posterior arch fracture, which may be in the pedicle, lamina, or articular processes. External immobilization may be adequate for most stage 1 injuries, if the articular process injury is not one that is predisposed to rotational instability (see under Compressive Extension). *Stage 2* injuries result in fracture of the vertebral body with contralateral bony or ligamentous failure in tension. These injuries usually require traction for reduction and operative stabilization.

## SUMMARY

Cervical trauma is a common cause of morbidity for patients in all age groups. Careful clinical evaluation and judicious use of imaging studies identify the spinal injury pattern and associated neurologic deficits. The upper cervical spine has a unique anatomy that leads to discrete injury patterns. Classifying subaxial cervical injuries by their mechanism of injury may be helpful in outlining operative and nonoperative treatment strategies.

## SUGGESTED READING

Aebi M, Mohler J, Zach G, Morscher E. Indication, surgical technique and results of 100 surgically treated fractures and fracture dislocations of the cervical spine. Clin Orthop 1986;203:244–257.

Beatson TR. Fractures and dislocations of the cervical spine. J Bone Joint Surg Br 1963;45:21–35.

Clark CR, Ingram CM, El-Khoury GY, et al. Radiographic evaluation of cervical spine injuries. Spine 1988;13:742–747.

Davis SJ, Teresi LLM, Bradley WG Jr, et al. Cervical spine hyperextension injuries: MR findings. Radiology 1991;180:245–251.

Esses S, Langer F, Gross A. Fracture of the atlas associated with fracture of the odontoid process. Injury 1981;12:310–312.

Fielding JW, Cochran GVB, Lawsing JF, et al. Tears of the transverse ligament of the atlas. J Bone Joint Surg Am1974;56:1683–1691.

Garvey TA, Eismont FJ, Roberti LJ. Anterior decompression, structural bone grafting, and Caspar stabilization for unstable cervical spine fractures and/or dislocations. Spine 1992;17(10 Suppl):S431–435.

Hecker P. Appareil ligomenteux occipito atloidoaxoidien: etude d'anatomie compare. Arch Anat Hist Embryol 1923;5:464–475.

Rorabeck CH, Rock MG, Hawkins AJ, Bourne RB. Unilateral facet dislocation of the cervical spine: an analysis of the results of treatment in 26 patients. Spine 1987;12:23–27.

Scaefer DM, Flanders AE, Osterholm J, et al. Prognostic significance of magnetic resonance imaging in the acute phase of cervical spine injury. J Neurosurg 1992;76:218–223.

Vaccaro AR, Klein GR, Thaller JB, et al. Distraction extension injuries of the cervical spine. J Spinal Disord 2001;14:193–200.

# THORACIC AND LUMBAR TRAUMA

## KERN SINGH
## ALEXANDER R. VACCARO

The thoracolumbar spine is the most common site of spinal injuries. Most of these injuries occur in males (15 to 29 years old) usually as the result of significant force impact, such as motor vehicle accidents. Most injuries (52%) occur between T11 and L1, followed by L1-5 (32%) and T1-10 (16%). Depending on the type of fracture, associated injuries occur in 50% of patients mainly as a result of a distraction force. Associated injuries include intraabdominal bleeding from liver and splenic injuries, vessel disruption, and pulmonary injuries (20% of patients). Contiguous and noncontiguous spine injuries are present in 6% to 15% of patients.

## THORACOLUMBAR ANATOMY

The thoracic spinal cord is protected from injury by the surrounding paraspinal musculature, the vertebral elements, and the thoracic rib cage. The sternum and the rib cage significantly limit motion in the thoracic spine. As a result of the significant amount of force necessary to disrupt the protective enclosure of the thoracic spinal cord, spinal injuries in this region are associated with a high incidence of neurologic injury. This high incidence also is a function of the decreased spinal canal diameter to spinal cord diameter ratio, particularly between T2 and T10. High-energy injuries in this area usually result in a 6:1 ratio of complete to incomplete neural deficits. The physiologic kyphosis of the thoracic spine may predispose it to flexion/axial load injuries.

The thoracolumbar junction is a transitional region between the less mobile thoracic spine and the more flexible lumbar spine. In this junctional region, the rib cage no longer provides protection and support to the vertebral column. Also, the thoracic vertebral bodies are not as large as the lumbar vertebral bodies; they are less able to resist deformity after specific load applications. These factors render the thoracolumbar junction more vulnerable to injury and make it the most common location for burst-type fractures.

## INITIAL TREATMENT AND EXAMINATION

Initial evaluation should begin with the ABCs (airway, breathing, circulation) of trauma care. A cervical collar should be placed and any extremity injuries splinted when the airway is secured. The patient now can be logrolled carefully, and the spine can be palpated for tenderness, step-offs, swelling, or visual deformities. Of patients with persistent localized tenderness after trauma to the thoracolumbar spine and absence of an obvious radiographic deformity, 30% may have an occult spinal fracture.

The detailed neurologic exam should include motor testing, dermatomal sensory testing, lumbar and sacral root motor evaluation, and examination of reflexes. *Spinal shock* refers to flaccid paralysis due to a physiologic disruption of all spinal cord function. The presence of the bulbocavernosus reflex heralds the end of spinal shock and allows for an accurate assessment of the patient's neurologic status typically 48 hours after the injury. The bulbocavernosus reflex is tested by squeezing the glans penis or clitoris and observing for reflex anal sphincter contracture. It also may be tested by tugging on an indwelling catheter and observing for an "anal wink."

A *complete* neurologic injury is marked by a total absence of sensory and motor function below the anatomic level of injury in the absence of spinal shock. In an *incomplete* lesion, residual spinal cord or nerve root function exists below the anatomic level of injury. An incomplete spinal cord lesion may manifest as one of four syndromes (Table 5-1).

Hypotension secondary to neurogenic or hemorrhagic shock must be reversed through fluid or blood replacement, with or without the use of vasopressors. Intravenous methylprednisolone is administered routinely within 8 hours of a spinal cord injury in the absence of specific contraindications (Table 5-2).

Deep venous thrombosis prophylaxis is paramount. The use of intermittent external pneumatic compression devices, static compression stockings, and, in select patients, subcutaneous (5000 U subcutaneously every 12 hours) or intravenous low-molecular-weight heparin helps to minimize potentially fatal pulmonary emboli.

## RADIOLOGIC EVALUATION

The radiographic evaluation begins with plain radiographs of the entire spine (anteroposterior and lateral views). The

45

## TABLE 5-1   SPINAL CORD INJURY SYNDROMES

| Syndrome | Characteristics | Prognosis |
|---|---|---|
| Central | Most common. UE > LE. Motor and sensory loss | Fair |
| Anterior | Loss of motor function with possible sparing of proprioception and pressure sensation | Poor |
| Posterior | Very rare. Loss of proprioception and pressure sensation. No motor loss | Good |
| Brown-Séquard | Ipsilateral motor loss and contralateral pain and temperature loss | Best |

LE, lower extremity; UE, upper extremity.

posterior vertebral body line should be assessed on the lateral radiograph. Disruption of this line may signal spinal canal compromise from a burst-type fracture. Other radiologic signs suggesting a compression spinal injury include buckling of the cortical margins, loss of vertebral body height, and an intravertebral vacuum sign. If the cervicothoracic junction (C7-T1) is difficult to visualize, a swimmer's view (lateral view with a maximally abducted arm) or an oblique view may help define the vertebral anatomy.

Vertebral alignment also should be assessed on the anteroposterior view. Vertebral body cortical disruption may suggest a lateral compression fracture. The spinous processes should be in the midline with a relatively consistent interpedicular distance. Displacement (i.e., spreading) may represent significant posterior element injury and spinal instability.

Further clarification of the degree of tissue disruption may require the use of computed tomography (CT) or magnetic resonance imaging (MRI). CT is useful in evaluating the integrity of the middle (posterior vertebral body) and posterior (posterior elements) columns of the vertebral body. On plain radiographs, approximately 25% of burst fractures may be misdiagnosed as stable compression fractures owing to lack of clear visualization of the vertebral bony anatomy. The greatest disadvantage of CT is its limited sensitivity in showing consistently specific soft tissue inju-

## TABLE 5-2   METHYLPREDNISOLONE DOSING

| Time from Injury (h) | Dose of Methylprednisolone (mg/kg/h) | Duration (h) |
|---|---|---|
| < 3 | 5.4 | 24 |
| 3–8 | 5.4 | 48 |
| > 8 | No treatment | No treatment |

ries (disc herniation, epidural hematoma, ligamentous disruption, or spinal cord injury) (Table 5-3).

MRI is useful when visualization of the nonbone structures of the spine is necessary. MRI is the definitive diagnostic modality in the evaluation of spinal cord injury. It is extremely useful in all cases with neurologic deficit to assess for intrinsic and extrinsic spinal cord pathology. MRI can help illustrate and elucidate the various spinal cord parenchymal findings, such as edema, hematoma, and physical transection of the neural elements.

Edema is seen as a fusiform enlargement of the spinal cord with increased signal intensity on T2-weighted images. Hematoma is characterized by decreased signal intensity on T2-weighted images acutely and often is surrounded by a halo of T2-weighted enhancement from adjacent edema. Edema extending more than two vertebral levels and the presence of hematoma within the spinal cord are considered poor prognostic signs for potential functional motor recovery.

MRI also can help define acute ligamentous disruption. A "black stripe sign" may indicate disruption of the posterior longitudinal ligament or supraspinous ligament. A bright signal within the substance of the interspinous space reliably represents ligamentous injury. MRI is helpful in the evaluation of acute traumatic disc disruptions, especially in the setting of a facet dislocation. MRI also may be useful in the postinjury period in cases of late development or worsening of a preexisting neurologic injury. In these situations, a treatable posttraumatic cyst or syrinx often can be diagnosed.

## CLASSIFICATION SCHEMES

The three-column theory of spinal instability by Denis is used commonly to define vertebral column injuries. The anatomic spine in this system is divided into three columns. Denis divided thoracic and lumbar spinal injuries into minor and major injuries. Fractures of the spinous and transverse processes, the pars interarticularis, and the facet articulations were categorized as minor injuries. Major spinal injuries were divided into compression fractures, burst fractures, flexion/distraction injuries, and fracture-dislocations (Figs. 5-1 to 5-4).

McAfee et al described a CT-based classification system. Their system included six fracture types based on the failure mode of the middle column: wedge-compression, stable burst, unstable burst, Chance, flexion/distraction, and translational fractures (Table 5-4).

Ferguson and Allen presented a mechanistic classification of thoracolumbar injuries. They described seven injury patterns: compressive-flexion, distractive-flexion, lateral-flexion, translational, vertical-compression, and distractive-extension injuries. This system categorizes injuries by the forces that create them and is useful in guiding nonoperative and operative treatment strategies (Table 5-5).

## SURGICAL DECISION MAKING

Surgical management of thoracolumbar injuries attempts to shorten hospitalization; maximize function; facilitate

## TABLE 5-3 DIAGNOSTIC IMAGING MODALITIES

| Imaging Modality | Advantages | Disadvantages |
| --- | --- | --- |
| Plain radiograph | Inexpensive, quick | Poor visualization of cervicothoracic junction and middle spinal column |
| CT | Excellent visualization of bony anatomy, particularly middle spinal column and cervicothoracic junction. Assesses spinal canal patency | Poor visualization of soft tissues |
| MRI | Excellent visualization of soft tissues, including ligaments, disc, and spinal cord | Poor visualization of detailed bony anatomy |

CT, computed tomography; MRI, magnetic resonance imaging.

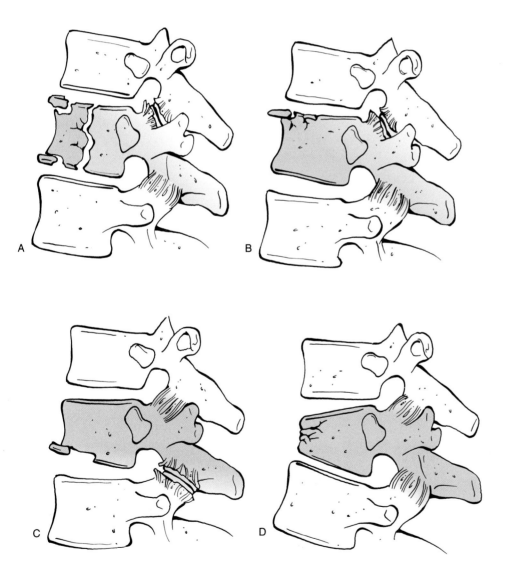

**Figure 5-1**   Denis's classification of thoracolumbar compression injuries. These fractures may involve both end plates, type A (**A**); the superior end plate only, type B (**B**); the inferior end plate only, type C (**C**); or a buckling of the anterior cortex with both end plates intact, type D (**D**).

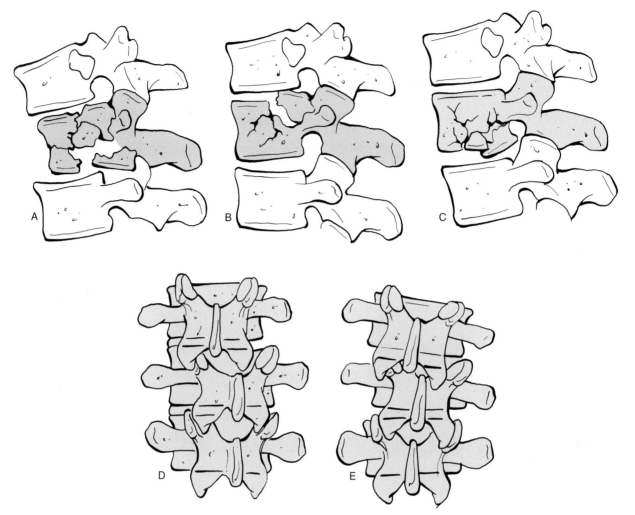

**Figure 5-2** Denis's classification of thoracolumbar burst fractures. Types A, B, and C represent fractures of both end plates (**A**), the superior end plate (**B**), and the inferior end plate (**C**). Type D fracture is a combination of a type A burst fracture with rotation (**D**), which is best appreciated on an anteroposterior radiograph. The superior or inferior end plate, or both, may be involved with this fracture. Type E fractures are burst fractures with lateral translation or flexion (**E**).

nursing care; and prevent deformity, instability, or pain. White and Panjabi defined clinical instability as the "loss of the ability of the spine under physiologic loads to maintain relationships between vertebrae in such a way that there is neither damage nor subsequent irritation to the spinal cord or nerve roots, and in addition, there is no development of incapacitating deformity or pain."

Surgical intervention often is determined by the assessment of the integrity of the posterior osteoligamentous complex. In a typical burst fracture, if there is marked widening of the posterior spinous processes with an obvious kyphotic malalignment, this would be considered an unstable fracture with the potential for deformity progression. Denis defined *instability* as a disruption of two or more of the three spinal columns and categorized instability into three groups: mechanical, neurologic, and combined. Mechanical instability included multiple column injuries in which the posterior elements were disrupted in distraction, and late kyphosis was a potential. Neurologic instability described a neurologic deficit in the setting of a spinal fracture. Combined instability described an unstable mechanical fracture in the setting of a neurologic deficit.

The optimal timing for medical or surgical intervention (decompression and stabilization) is unclear. A critical window of opportunity (possibly <3 hours) may exist in which the decompression of extrinsic pressure on the spinal cord and spinal stabilization may enhance functional neurologic outcome. Vaccaro et al reported the only controlled, prospective, randomized study on the timing of surgical intervention in cervical spinal cord injury. The authors found no significant difference in functional neural recovery when patients were operated on either early (<3 days) or late (>5 days). Progressive neurologic loss associated with an unstable fracture pattern with significant spinal cord compression is an indication for emergent surgical intervention.

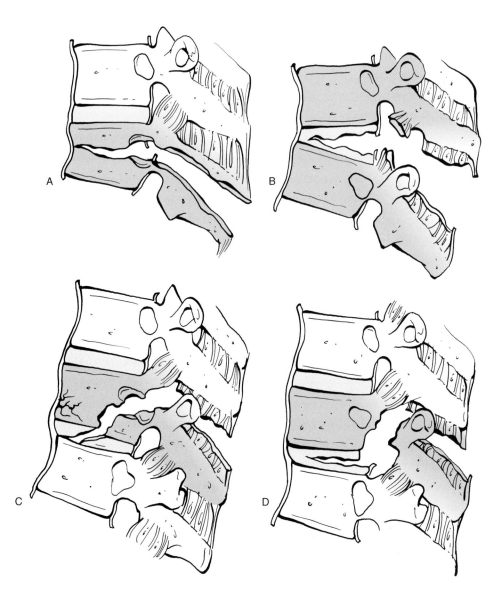

**Figure 5-3**  Denis's classification of flexion/distraction injuries. These may occur at one level through the bone (**A**), at one level through the ligaments and disc (**B**), at two levels with the middle column injured through the bone (**C**), or at two levels with the middle column injured through the ligament and disc (**D**).

# SURGICAL SPINAL DECOMPRESSION

The role of surgical decompression of thoracolumbar spinal injuries with symptomatic neural compression is unclear. Despite varied opinions, there is no direct correlation between the percentage of canal occlusion shown radiographically and the severity of neurologic deficit after burst fractures. Instead the initial force imparted to the spinal cord or the cauda equina, along with the associated hematoma, edema, and vascular ischemia perpetuated by various neurotrophic and vasoactive agents may be the underlying cause of neurologic injury.

Approximately 60% of patients with neurologic injury below T12 gain some return of neurologic function with nonoperative treatment. Neurologic recovery is more predict-able, however, following an anterior decompression in spinal cord compression. Late decompression, even several years after injury, may enhance neurologic recovery of the spinal cord, conus medullaris, and cauda equina.

The posterior approach is an indirect method of relieving canal compression via ligamentotaxis. This method is accomplished more efficiently if performed in the early peritrauma period. Several studies have shown that the spinal canal remodels or enlarges with time in nonoperatively treated and operatively treated fractures in a predictable fashion

The spinal level, degree and nature of canal compromise, and experience of the surgeon dictate the choice of surgical approach. Multiple variations on the approach to the thoracolumbar spine exist based on three methods to decompress the thecal sac: anterior, posterior, and posterolateral (Table 5-6).

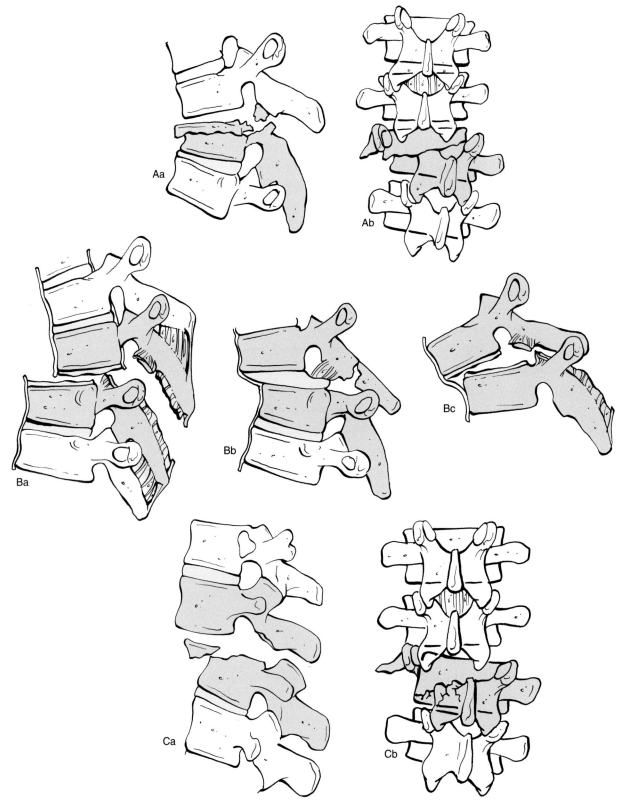

**Figure 5-4**  Denis's classification of fracture-dislocations. These injuries may occur at one level through the bone (**A**), at one level through the ligaments and disc (**B**), or at two levels with the middle column injured through the ligament and disc (**C**).

## TABLE 5-4  THE McAFEE CLASSIFICATION SYSTEM

| Type of Fracture | | | | Mechanism |
|---|---|---|---|---|
| Columns | Anterior | Middle | Posterior | |
| Wedge compression | Compression | None | None | Forward flexion |
| Stable burst | Compression | Compression | None | Compressive load |
| Unstable burst | Compression | Compression | Compression, lateral flexion, rotation | Compression, lateral flexion, rotation |
| Chance | Tension | Tension | Tension | Horizontal avulsion |
| Flexion distraction | Compression | Tension | Tension | Flexion distraction |
| Translational | Shear | Shear | Shear | Shear |

## TABLE 5-5  THE FERGUSON AND ALLEN CLASSIFICATION SYSTEM FOR SPINAL FRACTURES

| Type of Fracture | | | |
|---|---|---|---|
| Columns | Anterior | Middle | Posterior |
| Compressive flexion | | | |
|    Type I | Compression | None | None |
|    Type II | Compression | None | Tension |
|    Type III | Compression | "Blown out"* | Tension |
| Distractive flexion | Tension | Tension | Tension |
| Lateral flexion | | | |
|    Type I | Unilateral compression | Unilateral compression | None |
|    Type II | Unilateral compression | Unilateral compression | Ipsilateral compression/ contralateral tension |
| Translational | Shear | Shear | Shear |
| Torsional flexion | Compression/rotation | Disrupted | Tension/rotation |
| Vertical compression | Compression | Bony compression | Bony involvement |
| Distractive extension | Tension | | Compression |

* "Blown out"—evidence of middle column bone rotated into the neural canal between pedicles.

## TABLE 5-6  SURGICAL APPROACHES TO SPINAL DECOMPRESSION

| Approach | Advantages | Comments |
|---|---|---|
| Anterior | Easier access to retropulsed vertebral bone and discal material | Anterolateral approach—transthoracic T4-9, thoracoabdominal T10-L1, retroperitoneal T12-L5 |
| | Direct visualization of compressed neural tissue | Right-sided approach—above T10 to avoid great vessels |
| | Minimal manipulation of spinal cord | |
| Posterior | Effective when using distractive instrumentation to reduce retropulsed bone fragments | Posterior indirect reduction via ligamentotaxis is more efficient if done within 2–3 days of injury |
| Posterolateral | Instrumentation can be performed without the need for a second anterior staged procedure | One is able to access the thecal sac via the pedicle |
| | | Difficult anterior column reconstruction |
| | Advantageous in lower lumbar fractures and lateralized nerve root entrapment | Increased risk of neural injury secondary to neural manipulation |

# SPINAL INSTRUMENTATION

Since the introduction of Harrington rod internal fixation, there has been progressive development of various spinal fixation systems based on segmental fixation of the spine. The choice of spinal implant is determined by the nature, degree, or biomechanics of the existing instability; the quality (bone density) of the spinal elements; and the medical condition of the patient.

## Anterior Instrumentation

Approximately 80% of the axial load transmitted through the spine is through the intact anterior column. Direct restoration of the load-bearing function of the anterior spine is paramount in addressing spinal instability secondary to thoracolumbar trauma. Indications for anterior spinal surgery in patients with thoracolumbar injuries include unstable fractures requiring anterior column support, bony or discal compression of the thecal sac in the setting of a neurologic injury best addressed anteriorly, and unstable fractures (select burst injuries) that require stabilization best achieved through an anterior approach to preserve spinal motion segments (Fig. 5-5).

Interbody spacers inserted in an intracolumnar position act as a load-sharing device restoring axial stability until arthrodesis is obtained. With a deficient anterior column and no structural interbody spacer, a posterior spinal construct bears most of the axially applied loads leading to the potential for nonunion and instrument failure.

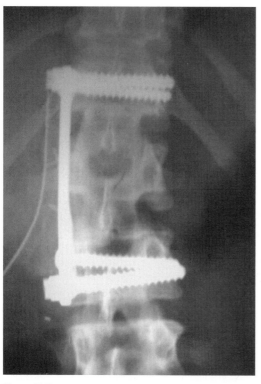

**Figure 5-5** Postoperative radiograph after completion of an anterior thoracolumbar decompression and stabilization procedure using autologous iliac crest bone graft and an anterior thoracolumbar plate and screws.

The most commonly used interbody spacer is an autologous tricortical iliac crest, although allograft sources, such as a tibial or femoral shaft or metallic mesh cages, are gaining popularity. Iliac crest interbody grafts allow for a faster rate of bony incorporation owing to their biocompatibility than do allograft strut grafts. Allograft strut grafts are able to withstand greater physiologic loads, however, in the erect spine in the early reconstruction and healing period. Several authors have reported successful results using anterior cortical allograft strut grafts in thoracolumbar fractures with fusion rates approaching greater than 90% at greater than 5-year follow-up with minimal graft subsidence and change in sagittal alignment.

A functional posterior osteoligamentous complex is crucial to the success of an anterior spinal construct. In the presence of posterior ligamentous injury, an anterior stand-alone procedure using a structural interbody graft followed by adjunctive internal fixation (i.e., a dual rod or plating fixation device) may be adequate in restoring enough stability until bone healing occurs. If significant posterior instability still exists, however, a staged posterior stabilization procedure should be done.

Anterior thoracolumbar decompression procedures followed by reconstruction are technically demanding procedures not without significant potential complications. Vascular complication rates of 5.8% have been reported, accompanied by a 2.4% rate of deep venous thrombosis and a 10% rate of dural laceration.

## Posterior Instrumentation

Posterior spinal approaches allow for efficient realignment of the spine, direct and indirect decompression of the neural elements, and protection against late deformity and instability through the application of spinal instrumentation and subsequent fusion. Posterior spinal instrumentation allows for application of specific vector forces to the spine to correct or improve spinal alignment. The most commonly applied vector forces are cantilever bending and distraction. With a prudent distraction force, restoration of vertebral body height and partial clearance of bone or discal fragments from within the spinal canal by ligamentotaxis can be achieved. Spinal canal clearance through ligamentotaxis optimally is achieved within the first 2 to 3 days after injury. Posterior distraction techniques may enlarge the compromised canal 40% to 75%.

Biomechanically, a longer applied longitudinal component (rod) reduces the risk of terminal implant cutout or dislodgment by increasing the distance from the fracture site, decreasing the forces on the hook. Especially with hook-based systems, this often requires the immobilization of five or six motion segments that may contribute to increased global spinal stiffness and subsequent junctional degeneration. Historically, in an attempt to preserve the motion of uninjured motion segments, the "rod long-fuse short" technique was introduced. With this method, only one level above and one level below the fracture were fused, and three levels above and below the injury were spanned by instrumentation, which was removed at 1 year after surgery. This technique eventually lost popularity as gross and histologic findings of osteoarthritis were noted along the unfused but instrumented spinal segments at the time of implant removal.

Shortcomings of distraction rod-hook techniques for fracture reduction and stabilization include hook dislodgment, late vertebral collapse, and progressive kyphosis after rod removal. Overdistraction with long rods may lead to iatrogenic loss of lumbar lordosis and the development of a painful flat back deformity. Various modifications of hook-rod constructs were initiated to address these issues. More square hooks, which prevented rod rotation, allowed for gentle contouring of the rod and as such decreased hook cutout. Edward sleeves, made of high-density polyethylene, which were placed along the rod, were developed to provide an anterior vector moment to the spine through three-point or four-point bending strategies.

The development of pedicle screw anchors provided an additional method of stabilizing an unstable three-column spinal injury through three-column bone fixation. Pedicle screw implants potentially, in nonosteoporotic patients, allow for shorter posterior fixation lengths, while conferring adequate spinal stability. Experimental data confirmed that short-segment pedicle screw constructs provide torsional, flexural, and compressive rigidity comparable to longer hook-rod constructs. Despite the increased rigidity of pedicle screw systems, posterior short-segment fixation of unstable thoracolumbar fractures has resulted in high failure rates.

The best candidates for posterior short-segment pedicle screw fixation (one level above and one level below the fracture level) seem to be patients with flexion/distraction injuries or lower lumbar burst fractures in which the weight-bearing line is posterior to the posterior vertebral body wall. Transpedicular intracorporeal grafting combined with short-segment instrumentation has been offered as an alternative to a staged anterior column reconstruction procedure. This technique has not been shown to decrease the incidence of loss of sagittal plane alignment or instrumentation failure, however, compared with nonintracorporeal grafted cases at long-term follow-up.

# FRACTURE SUBTYPES

Spinal injuries can be divided into several categories based on their biomechanical and anatomic characteristics and the patient's neurologic status (Table 5-7).

## Minor Injuries

Transverse process, spinous process, and articular process fractures resulting from direct trauma or severe muscular contractions may be treated symptomatically with or without a brace for comfort. The importance of assessing for spinal stability after an initial immobilization period, if deemed necessary, with flexion/extension plain radiographs cannot be overemphasized. Care must be taken to avoid undertreatment and missing a potentially unstable spinal injury. An acute isolated fracture of the pars interarticularis should be immobilized in a well-molded total contact thoracolumbosacral orthosis. If the fracture is below L3, a unilateral thigh extension usually is recommended.

## Compression Fractures

Surgical stabilization may be indicated in compression (wedge) fractures if there is greater than 20 to 30 degrees of initial kyphosis (significant posterior osteoligamentous disruption) and greater than 50% loss of anterior vertebral body height (Fig. 5-6). Ferguson-Allen type I compressive flexion injuries typically can be treated with an extension cast or orthosis and early ambulation. If the fracture is proximal to T7, a cervical extension to the brace or cast is recommended. Type II and type III compressive flexion injuries without a neurologic deficit generally are stabilized with posterior nonsegmental or segmental instrumentation. Ferguson-Allen type II compressive flexion injuries at the thoracolumbar junction often are treated with posterior compression instrumentation, with the intact middle column being used as a hinge to restore lordosis. Type III injuries (which are burst fractures) without significant canal compromise and evidence of significant posterior osteoligamentous disruption (i.e., kyphosis >20 to 30 degrees or anterior loss of vertebral body height >50% or both) may be treated with the use of distraction-lordosis instrumentation to restore anterior and middle column height. Care must be taken to avoid overdistraction in patients with posterior column. A tension force placed on the neural elements from overdistraction can result in significant neurologic injury. Often a posterior interspinous wire is placed at the level of the posterior ligamentous injury, preventing overdistraction, while accomplishing fracture realignment through subsequent spinal distraction. If short-segment fixation strategies are chosen, strict postoperative immobilization in a custom-molded hyperextension orthosis or body cast for a minimum of 3 months is recommended to decrease the potential for spinal deformity recurrence and internal fixation failure.

Many surgeons continue to use the time-honored procedure of segmental fixation using sublaminar wires (Luque rods [rectangle] and sublaminar wires). This procedure rarely is performed in the setting of an intact or incomplete neurologic examination. If this technique is chosen, the Luque rectangle is prebent in mild hyphokyphosis to reduce the segmental kyphosis at the level of injury. This technique generally incorporates three levels above and two to three levels below the level of injury.

More recently, the use of percutaneous cement augmentation in symptomatic osteoporotic compression fractures has been reported (vertebroplasty or kyphoplasty, which uses balloon elevation of the vertebral end plates before cement insertion). Currently the indications of these techniques for traumatic fractures of the thoracic and lumbar spine are unclear.

## Burst Fractures

Nonoperative treatment of burst fractures usually involves a period of bed rest until resolution of initial symptoms, followed by progressive ambulation in a full contact orthosis or cast for 12 to 24 weeks with or without a unilateral thigh extension for the initial 6 weeks of treatment. Several studies have evaluated back pain associated with burst fractures and nonoperative management. Most studies have con-

## TABLE 5-7  MANAGEMENT OF THORACOLUMBAR FRACTURES

| Type | Nonsurgical Management | Surgical Indications | Comments |
|---|---|---|---|
| Minor injuries | TLSO—fracture below L3 add unilateral thigh extension | Instability on flexion/extension plain x-rays | Minor injuries are transverse/spinous/articular process fractures |
| Compression fractures | Extension TLSO cast or orthosis Early ambulation If fracture proximal to T7, add a cervical extension to the brace or cast | >20–30 degrees of initial kyphosis (significant posterior osteoligamentous disruption) > 50% loss of anterior vertebral body height | Use nonsegmental hook-rod construct to apply distraction-lordosis force vectors for reduction Short-segment pedicle screw construct may be used if followed by immobilization in a custom-molded hyperextension orthosis or body cast for a minimum of 3 m |
| Burst fracture | Bed rest until resolution of constitutional symptoms Progressive ambulation in a full-contact orthosis or cast for 12–24 wk with or without a unilateral thigh extension (fracture L3 or lower) for the initial 6 wk of treatment | Neurologically intact Kyphosis >20 degrees Facet subluxation or spreading of the interspinous process distance >50% loss of anterior vertebral body height Neurologically compromised Surgical decompression with imaging documentation of significant neural compression | No definitive evidence that correlates the degree of neural impingement with the severity of neurologic deficit after thoracolumbar trauma Anterior approach affords best canal decompression, should be followed by anterior column reconstruction ± anterior and/or posterior instrumentation |
| Distraction/ flexion Injury | Rarely indicated in an adult patient owing to the unpredictable nature of healing of this injury subtype | A compression force vector is used to reduce the injury deformity. Care should be taken not to cause iatrogenic retropulsion of bone or discal material into the canal | ALL serves as a tension band with this injury Look for associated intraabdominal viscous injury with this injury mechanism |
| Fracture-dislocations | Rarely indicated owing to the significant degree of instability and deformity associated with this injury subtype | Posterior facet fracture-dislocation, rotational instability or a translational shear injury in the absence of a neurologic deficit requires an initial posterior segmental reduction and stabilization procedure before considering the need for an anterior decompressive and stabilization procedure | Awake intubation may minimize neurologic injury associated with positioning |
| Distraction/ extension injury | Consider an attempt to reproduce the preinjury sagittal profile of the patient regardless of neurologic status through bedding supplements or skeletal traction | Surgical stabilization with segmental internal fixation initially via a posterior approach Consider a staged anterior stabilization procedure if a significant anterior column defect is present | High association with metabolic bone disease and a preexisting spinal deformity, e.g., ankylosing spondylitis and diffuse idiopathic skeletal hyperostosis |

ALL, anterior longitudinal ligament; TLSO, thoracolumbosacral orthosis.

cluded that the back pain is due to progressive degenerative changes as a result of the initial injury. Residual symptomatic foraminal stenosis, segmental instability, or sagittal plane deformity is a rare late manifestation of a healed thoracolumbar burst fracture.

In a neurologically intact patient with significant disruption of the posterior osteoligamentous complex (i.e., initial kyphosis >20 degrees), the presence of facet subluxation or spreading of the interspinous process distance, or greater than 50% loss of anterior vertebral body height, surgical

stabilization may help to restore and maintain adequate spinal alignment. Surgical intervention also is performed in an acute burst fracture with imaging documentation of significant neural compression in the setting of an incomplete neurologic deficit. Neurologic improvement has been seen 2 years after an injury following a late decompression (Fig. 5-7)

From the literature, no conclusive evidence supports a direct relationship between preinjury canal size and the force imparted to the spine at the time of trauma and a

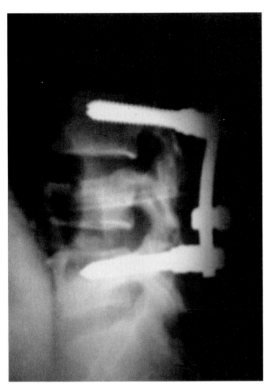

**Figure 5-6** Segmental pedicle screw construct used to treat a compression fracture that involved loss of greater than 50% of anterior vertebral height and disruption of the posterior interspinous ligaments.

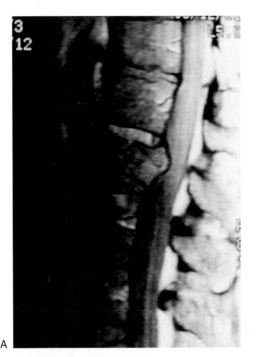

A

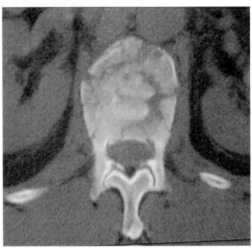

B

**Figure 5-7** (**A**) Sagittal MRI of a 34-year-old man who sustained a burst fracture to the T12 vertebral body. Note the retropulsion of the posterior vertebral body with compression of the anterior thecal sac. (**B**) Axial CT scan of the T12 burst fracture shows middle column failure with approximately 25% to 30% canal occlusion.

patient's resulting neurologic status. The degree of canal diameter and area is significantly more compromised at the time of trauma than that noted on postinjury MRI or CT evaluation.

## Distraction/Flexion Injuries

Distraction/flexion injuries with disruption of the interspinous ligaments and posterior longitudinal ligament (and possibly disc space) heal slowly and unpredictably and often benefit from surgical stabilization. Most posterior spinal implant techniques immobilize the vertebral level above and below the injury or at the vertebral level of injury and the level below if the injury is located anatomically below the pedicle of the cephalad vertebrae. Caution in the use of this reduction maneuver must be exercised if the middle column is comminuted for the fear of retropulsion of bone or disc material into the spinal canal or if the posterior facets are incompetent, which may prevent a controlled anatomic reduction. If the axis of rotation is posterior to the anterior spinal column and anterior column compression failure is present, a distraction maneuver may be applied at levels above and below the injury level when the posterior elements at the fracture site are stabilized to prevent posterior element distraction. The anterior longitudinal ligament in this case serves as a stabilizing tension band.

## Fracture-Dislocations

Any evidence of posterior facet fracture-dislocation, rotational instability, or a translational shear injury in the ab-

sence of a neurologic deficit requires an initial posterior segmental reduction and stabilization procedure before considering the need for an anterior decompressive and stabilization procedure. When reduction is complete, a neutralization spinal implant strategy may be employed to confer optimal stability and to prevent future fracture displacement (Fig. 5-8). An awake intubation followed by awake patient positioning is helpful in the absence of a complete spinal cord injury to help protect the neural elements from further injury due to voluntary patient splinting and afford real-time surveillance of the neurologic exam.

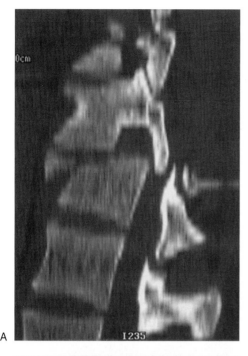

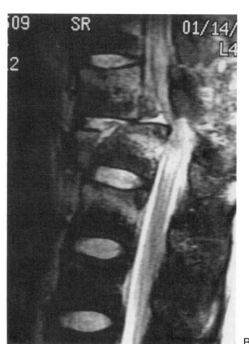

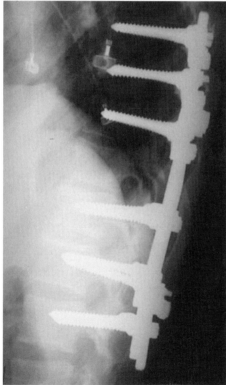

**Figure 5-8** (**A**) Sagittal CT reconstruction of a fracture-dislocation of the thoracolumbar spine shows marked vertebral body displacement and canal narrowing. (**B**) Sagittal MRI of the injury shows marked canal narrowing. Note the draping of the spinal cord over the posterosuperior edge of the caudal thoracic vertebrae. (**C**) Postoperative lateral radiograph shows reduction of the spinal deformity followed by a fusion and stabilization with segmental pedicle screw anchors spanning three levels above and below the level of injury.

## Distraction/Extension Injuries

Distraction/extension injuries are uncommon. Patients typically have an underlying metabolic bone disease and a preexisting spinal deformity (i.e., ankylosing spondylitis or diffuse idiopathic skeletal hyperostosis). Immobilization alone is inadequate because these are highly unstable injuries with a high likelihood of progression and neurologic worsening. Supine positioning may exacerbate the spinal deformity and cause neurologic decline due to the existence of a preinjury kyphotic spinal deformity. A principle of emergency management of this spinal injury is to attempt to reproduce the preinjury sagittal profile of the patient regardless of neurologic status through bedding supplements or skeletal traction. When

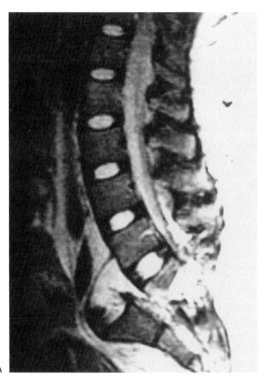
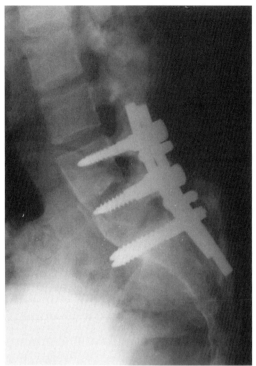

**Figure 5-9** (**A**) Sagittal T2-weighted MRI of a complete fracture-dislocation through the L5 vertebral body. (**B**) Lateral postoperative radiograph shows adequate reduction of the fracture-dislocation stabilized with pedicle screw instrumentation from L4-S1.

reduced, surgical stabilization with segmental internal fixation may be performed (Fig. 5-9).

## CONCLUSION

Despite advancements in spinal implants and radiographic imaging, controversy continues regarding the indications for surgical intervention, the timing of intervention, and the approach with which to correct any existing spinal deformity. Nevertheless, the basic tenets of trauma surgery should be strictly adhered to. When the patient is medically stabilized, a detailed neurologic exam and careful radiographic evaluation should be performed. The surgeon should be aware of the biomechanics of the thoracolumbar spine, the mechanism of injury, and the various implants available for treatment. Most thoracolumbar injuries, in the absence of a neurologic deficit, are stable and can be treated successfully nonoperatively. For the rare unstable spinal fracture, with or without a neurologic deficit, surgical treatment often is beneficial in improving patient mobilization and early functional return to society. The ultimate goals in managing thoracolumbar injuries are to maximize neurologic recovery and to stabilize the spine expeditiously for

early rehabilitation and an early return to a productive lifestyle.

## SUGGESTED READING

Abe E, Sato K, Shimada Y, et al. Thoracolumbar burst fracture with horizontal fracture of the posterior column. Spine 1997;22:83–87.

Bohlman HH, Kirkpatrick JS, Delamarter RB. Anterior decompression for late pain and paralysis after fractures of the thoracolumbar spine. Clin Orthop 1994;300:24–29.

Carlson GD, Minato Y, Okada A. Early time-dependent decompression for spinal cord injury: vascular mechanisms of recovery. J Neurotrauma 1997;14:951–962.

Ferguson Rl, Allen BL Jr. A mechanistic classification of thoracolumbar spine fractures. Clin Orthop 1983;189:817–831.

Gertzbein SD, Scoliosis Research Society: Multicenter spine fracture study. Spine 1992;17:528–540.

McAfee PC, Yuan HA, Fredrickson BE, Lubicky JP. The value of computed tomography in thoracolumbar fractures: an analysis of one hundred cases and a new classification. J Bone Joint Surg Am 1983; 65:461–473.

Oskouian RJ, Johnson JP. Vascular complications in anterior thoracolumbar spinal reconstruction. J Neurosurg 2002;96(1 Suppl):1–5.

Saboe LA, Reid DC, Davis LA, et al. Spine trauma and associated injuries. J Trauma 1991;31:43–48.

Vaccaro AR, Daugherty RJ, Sheehan TP. Neurologic outcome of early versus late surgery for cervical spinal cord injury. Spine 1997;22: 2609–2613.

Willen J, Lindahl S, Nordwall A. Unstable thoracolumbar fractures. Spine 1985;10:111–122.

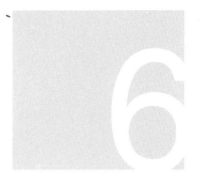

# SPINAL CORD INJURY AND PARALYSIS

**ROBERT F. HEARY**
**ARTEM Y. VAYNMAN**

## EPIDEMIOLOGY

Approximately 10,000 spinal cord injury (SCI) patients present to emergency departments annually in the United States. The immediate mortality of a complete cervical SCI is close to 50%. For survivors who make it to a hospital, the mortality is much lower (4% to 16%). The causes of SCI are divided according to age and gender. Of SCI patients, 80% to 85% are male, and 15% to 20% are female; at least 50% of patients are between 20 and 50 years old. The cervical spinal cord is the most common level of injury (50% to 60%). Thoracic, thoracolumbar, and lumbosacral spine regions represent 15% each in multiple series.

Fracture-dislocations and burst fractures are the most common mechanisms, constituting 70% of injuries that result in SCI. Compression fractures and isolated dislocations make up 10% and 5%, respectively. Since the advancements of magnetic resonance imaging (MRI) technology and the ready availability of MRI in most trauma centers, spinal cord injury without radiologic abnormality (SCIWORA) has become nearly obsolete. When imaged with MRI, SCIWORA shows signal changes in T2-weighted sagittal and axial sequences. The prognosis for patients with SCIWORA is good with cervical collar immobilization. Spinal cord injury without radiologic evidence of trauma (SCIWORET) also has been reviewed. High-resolution computed tomography (CT) and MRI usually show cervical spondylosis or congenital anomalies that predispose patients with minimal trauma to have profound deficits.

SCI is more common in patients with multiorgan injuries. A definite relationship exists between head injury and SCI, which makes an accurate physical exam more difficult and may lead to the diagnosis of SCI being delayed. Spinal shock resulting from SCI complicates the recognition and treatment of intraabdominal and chest injuries. Neurologic recovery of patients with SCI in the presence of multitrauma is reduced because of multiple factors that are discussed later.

## PATHOPHYSIOLOGY

The initial trauma to the spinal cord tissue can destroy a certain number of cells directly. It also sets in motion a multifactorial process that causes more cell death and damage. Disruption of the normal blood flow creates ischemia in the gray matter of the cord by either mechanical obstruction of feeding arteries or vasospasm of arterioles. This ischemia usually occurs within 2 to 3 hours after injury. Although the white matter blood supply may not diminish, vasospasm can affect the ascending and descending tracts as arterioles pass through the gray matter to reach these tracts. Vasoconstriction can increase progressively over the first 24 hours, and it is affected greatly by the release of histamine, prostaglandins, serotonin, and neurotransmitters such as norepinephrine. Thrombosis of injured arteries contributes to ischemia, which is tolerated poorly by central nervous system tissue, initiating a cascade of ion derangement, inflammation, and apoptotic cell death.

Injured cells release proinflammatory substances that attract neutrophils to the area within 24 to 48 hours; this causes an expansion of the damage in the rostral and the caudal directions. In 48 hours, macrophages and microglial cells migrate to the site and release reactive oxygen radicals that cause damage to the surrounding healthy tissue. Cellular membrane breakdown ensues with resultant ionic imbalance and nucleolysis. As the energy supply necessary for restoration of membrane potential is depleted, potassium ions move out of the cell, and sodium ions move into the cell. Additionally, calcium is released from storage granules, and it activates enzymes in the proteolytic pathway that destroy the cytoskeletons of cell bodies and axons. All of these events lead to demyelination and necrotic cell death.

The intrinsic suicide mechanism of cells, also known as *apoptosis,* is initiated by the release of excitatory neurotransmitters, such as glutamate, and by an increase in calcium concentration. Heat-shock proteins are synthesized and released. This release causes activation of a lytic cascade that results in apoptotic death of the oligodendrocytes. Because oligodendrocytes are responsible for the maintenance of myelinated pathways, demyelination of the ascending and descending tracts of the spinal cord, which were not injured by the initial trauma, causes further loss of function. All these events start 4 to 6 hours after SCI and can continue for 3 weeks.

At present, available scientific data suggest that acute

SCI is a complex phenomenon. Many interrelated events can lead to progressive, reversible and irreversible damage to spinal cord tissue. The primary damage, which occurs at the time of the SCI, is not correctable. Evidence from multiple investigators suggests, however, that inflammation and ionic disturbances initiate vicious cycles damaging tissue that was not injured by the initial trauma. This so-called secondary injury has been the focus of much research because this phase of the SCI cascade is potentially modifiable with effective treatments. Complex regeneration patterns also are being studied; however, further work is required before any definitive conclusions about the prevention of secondary injury or stimulation of regeneration can be made.

# CLASSIFICATION

At present, the American Spinal Injury Association (ASIA) scale, endorsed by the International Medical Society of Paraplegia (IMSOP) and published in 1992 in the *International Standards for Neurological and Functional Classification of Spinal Cord Injury,* is recommended for use by all physicians treating patients with acute SCIs. This system attempted to detail more accurately patients with incomplete neurologic deficits. Specifically, in the ASIA system, preserved sensation at the S4-5 level now is required for an incomplete classification to be made. A scoring method to describe sensation also has been added, with 0 = none, 1 = impaired, and 2 = intact. The previously used term *quadriplegia* has been replaced by *tetraplegia.* Another change is replacement of the term *zone of injury* with *zone of partial preservation,* which is defined as the number of levels below the neurologic level of injury that remain partially innervated. The motor exam consists of testing 10 bilateral muscle groups with assigned neurologic level of innervation and tabulating a score. All these data are entered into an ASIA card that can be used for statistical analysis.

# CLINICAL MANIFESTATIONS

Certain signs and symptoms, even in unconscious patients, can lead to a higher suspicion of SCI. Examples include the following:

- Flaccid paralysis
- Hemodynamic instability with bradycardia
- Priapism
- Lack of response to painful stimuli in the arms and legs
- Paradoxical respiration

Spinal shock occurs most frequently in cervical SCIs. It has a wide range of duration, but sensory and somatic motor symptoms usually resolve in 4 to 6 hours, whereas autonomic symptoms can persist for days or weeks.

Although complete SCI presents as a distinct entity, incomplete SCI has several well-described symptomatic patterns. Recognition of these patterns can help in determining the patient's prognosis.

## Cervicomedullary Syndrome

The cervicomedullary syndrome includes injuries from the lower medulla to the C4 region. It presents with the following:

- Respiratory difficulty
- Spinal shock
- Tetraplegia with the arms weaker than the legs
- Sensory level at C1-4
- Facial sensory loss (damage to the ascending tract of the spinal trigeminal nerve)

Examination of the face is important because the more lateral the facial sensory loss, the lower the lesion is. The prognosis is variable. The presence of significant motor deficits or spinal shock or both worsens the prognosis.

## Central Cord Syndrome

The presentation of the central cervical cord syndrome varies in its severity; the major diagnostic criteria include the following:

- Tetraparesis with arms, and in particular hands, weaker than legs
- Variable sensory loss that does not involve the face

Many patients with central cord syndrome show fast recovery and can be observed to plateau in 24 hours. This scenario occurs most commonly in elderly patients, with preexisting narrow spinal canals, who sustain an injury with an extension mechanism.

## Anterior Cord Syndrome

The anterior cord syndrome is due to a space-occupying lesion anterior to the cord, such as a disc, fragments of fractured vertebrae, or a hematoma. The presentation includes the following:

- Complete paralysis
- Preservation of vibration and touch sensations

In less severe cases, some motor function can be preserved through the lateral corticospinal pathways. Flexion mechanisms are the most common etiology, and the prognosis for neurologic recovery with these injuries is usually poor.

## Posterior Cord Syndrome

A distinct, although rare, entity, posterior cord syndrome is due to damage to the posterior tissue with some sparing of anterior cord.

- Tetraparesis is due to disruption of the lateral corticospinal tracts.
- Sensory loss is profound with the exception of pain and temperature.

## Brown-Séquard Syndrome

Brown-Séquard syndrome, initially described in patients with complete hemisection of the spinal cord, presents with the following:

- Ipsilateral paralysis
- Ipsilateral vibration and touch sensory loss
- Contralateral pain and temperature loss

Brown-Séquard syndrome also has been observed in combination with other types of incomplete injury, when different spinal levels are affected to varying degrees. It can present acutely or develop gradually over several days. Anal sphincter function can be preserved or recovered. This injury is seen most frequently in penetrating stab wounds.

## Conus Medullaris Syndrome

Compression or burst fractures of T12 or L1 can result in a loss of function involving only the sacral segments of the spinal cord, which are located in the conus medullaris. Paraparesis, loss of bowel and bladder function, and sensory loss in legs with perianal sparing can be observed. In severe injuries, progression to the development of a neurogenic bladder is inevitable.

## Cauda Equina Syndrome

Although it is included in the ASIA/IMSOP scale, cauda equina injury is strictly a peripheral nerve injury and carries a higher rate of recovery. It presents with varying degrees of motor and sensory loss, "saddle anesthesia," and bowel/bladder dysfunction. The better prognosis is believed to be due to the higher resistance of lower motor neurons to injury.

## Other Syndromes

Several well-described syndromes of SCI have variable degrees of functional loss and are transient in nature. "Burning hands syndrome" is seen most commonly among athletes and presents with paresthesias and dysesthesias of the hands, which usually disappear within several hours. It is thought to be due to a hyperextension injury. Spinal cord concussion also is common and presents with sudden onset of weakness and numbness with rapid improvement. This condition is associated frequently with congenitally narrowed spinal canals in athletes. The exact pathophysiology is unknown, but cellular-ionic and vascular mechanisms have been proposed.

SCI also can be observed in patients with cardiogenic shock or any other condition leading to prolonged hypotension. States of low blood flow or occlusion of major feeding arteries, such as vertebral arteries and radicular branches from the aorta, can lead to hypoperfusion of the spinal cord tissue and ischemia, resulting in spinal cord infarction. Infarction can occur even in the absence of cerebral ischemia and can be diagnosed by MRI.

# INITIAL MANAGEMENT

## Emergency Department Evaluation and Treatment

As previously mentioned, acute SCI is diagnosed most accurately in the presence of a high index of suspicion. Most often, either an abnormal physical exam or a history of symptoms and a mechanism of injury suggesting SCI are the clues to a correct diagnosis. All patients presenting to a hospital emergency department after a motor vehicle accident, fall, sports injury, multitrauma, or head injury and patients who are under influence of drugs, alcohol, or medication should be worked up for an acute SCI. If possible, a detailed motor exam of all groups of the upper and lower extremities should be completed. Additionally, a sensory exam of all dermatomes, including S4-5, should be performed. Deep tendon reflexes, rectal tone, and respiratory function should be evaluated at the same time. If a physical exam is unobtainable for medical or any other reasons, the spine should be assumed to be unstable. As such, the cervical spine should be immobilized with a rigid collar, and the rest of the spine should be immobilized with logroll precautions. Either plain anteroposterior and lateral radiographs of the cervical spine or a dedicated CT scan of the cervical spine with coronal and sagittal reconstructions should be obtained. If any destabilizing injury to the cervical spine is documented, and the physical exam is still unavailable, cervical traction with Gardner-Wells tongs should be considered. Data from animal studies support early decompression and realignment of the cervical spine, even in the absence of spinal canal compromise. We believe that relief of venous congestion and improvement of spinal cord blood flow may be obtained with cervical traction, and this may result in an improved outcome.

Any patient with an apparent SCI should undergo MRI of the cervical spine to rule out a traumatic disc herniation or a ligamentous injury or both. It is not advisable to manipulate the spine or get flexion/extension radiographs before the absence of such an injury has been documented. Because many patients with SCI present with other trauma and depressed mental status and cannot be examined reliably at the time of presentation, there is a risk of increased compression of the spinal cord during such manipulation. Specifically, flexion/extension radiographs should be avoided in patients with odontoid fractures, patients who are obtunded, and patients with central cord syndrome injuries because the motion can lead to an irreversible neurologic worsening.

Controversy exists over the timing of imaging studies in SCI patients. In our institution, patients who have spinal injuries who either are neurologically intact or have an incomplete neurologic deficit have MRI before any traction or surgery. In patients with a complete neurologic deficit and plain film evidence of bilateral facet subluxations, immediate traction with reduction is performed before any additional imaging studies. Although there is the theoretical risk of a herniated disc worsening the scenario, the time saved with these early reductions seems justified. Immediately after the emergent reduction, the patient is taken for advanced imaging studies.

## Medical Treatment of Spinal Cord Injury Patients

Since the 1990s, the medical treatment of SCI patients has received heightened attention. It now is apparent that allowing patients with acute cervical SCIs to remain hypotensive and bradycardic for the initial hours after injury is not ideal. The immediate treatment of acute SCI patients involves support with intravenous fluid administration and early use of vasopressors to combat hypotension. The goal is to get the mean arterial blood pressure to greater than 85 mm Hg immediately and keep it above this level for a minimum of 7 days. Likewise, it is essential to ensure the adequacy of oxygenation on initial evaluation and to supply supplemental oxygen, as necessary, to ensure that adequately oxygenated blood is perfusing the injured spinal cord.

Our practice, and that supported by the American Association of Neurological Surgeons/Congress of Neurological Surgeons Joint Section on Disorders of the Spine and Peripheral Nerves in the 2002 position statement, has been to maintain patients with cervical SCIs in an intensive care unit for a minimum of 7 days after the injury. Liberal use of vasopressors and judicious use of intravenous fluids to keep the mean arterial blood pressure greater than 85 mm Hg have proved to be rewarding in our institution. As in many aspects of the treatment of acute SCI, well-documented studies proving that this approach is optimal have not been completed.

## Pharmacologic Treatments

Many different pharmacologic agents have been used in the treatment of SCI patients. Although many experimental drugs have been tested, none has gained uniform acceptance. Based on existing basic science theories, three medications have undergone formal clinical testing in multicenter, prospective study formats. These pharmacologic agents include:

- Methylprednisolone
- Ganglioside GM$_1$
- Naloxone

One theory has been aimed at the prevention of oxidative phosphorylation as a method of treating SCI. This is the rationale behind the use of high-dose methylprednisolone in the treatment of SCIs. In the National Acute Spinal Cord Injury Study—Part II (NASCIS 2), published in 1990, a statistically significant benefit was found in SCI patients treated with high-dose methylprednisolone (30 mg/kg body weight bolus over 15 minutes, followed by a 45-minute delay, then 5.4 mg/kg/h for 23 hours) compared with patients treated with placebo. Used in this dosage regimen, methylprednisolone does not act by its glucocorticoid mechanism; rather, it functions as an antioxidant. It generally is held that the impact of methylprednisolone occurs in the gray matter of the spinal cord.

Criticisms of the NASCIS 2 study have centered on two main points. First, the benefits achieved were not of much functional benefit to the patients and may reflect merely a more rapid return of nerve root, rather than spinal cord, function. Second, in this high dose, methylprednisolone has side effects, including increased bleeding, increased infections, and detrimental effects on spinal fusions. None of these side effects were determined to have statistical significance in the NASCIS 2 study; however, with the questionable neurologic benefits achieved, the use of high-dose

methylprednisolone has not been embraced uniformly by spine surgeons. Additionally, in 1997, the NASCIS 3 protocol was published, which involved a minor alteration in the duration of methylprednisolone dosing.

There has been significant controversy over the use of methylprednisolone as recommended by NASCIS 2. A retrospective analysis of the raw data obtained in the NASCIS 2 study has shown that many confounding factors were omitted—accurate documentation of medical and surgical treatments at different centers, functional outcome, and medical complications. It has become clear that although steroids decrease inflammatory reaction within the injured spinal cord, the protocol recommended by NASCIS 2 does not offer a conclusive benefit over the risks of infection, bleeding, effects on subsequent fusions, pulmonary and endocrine complications, and difficulty with administration (there has been a national shortage of methylprednisolone). At present, our recommendations are as follows: There is no proven benefit that favors the administration of methylprednisolone for acute SCI, and because the risk-to-benefit ratio is not in favor of its use, we do not administer this drug routinely to SCI patients.

Further work is under way to develop drugs that would inhibit more specifically oxidative phosphorylation (antioxidants) without having the side effects of glucocorticoid agents. In a position statement of the American Association of Neurological Surgeons/Congress of Neurological Surgeons Joint Section of Disorders of the Spine and Peripheral Nerves published in 2002, the physician treating SCI patients is advised that methylprednisolone is an option that may be used in treatment with the understanding that the risks of this treatment outweigh its benefits.

An additional theory involves the use of GM$_1$ ganglioside. This agent is believed to exert its action at the white matter level in the spinal cord. A preliminary report published in 1991 was a cause for optimism with good results being reported on a few patients in a single center. A follow-up, multicenter, controlled study performed at 28 institutions failed to show benefit with the use of GM$_1$ ganglioside at 26-week or 52-week outcome analyses. As such, enthusiasm for this agent has waned.

One theory has emerged that attempts to explain the role of opiate receptors and opiate antagonists in SCIs. According to observations by different authors, naloxone, which is a μ-subtype antagonist, has a neuroprotective action. This action seems to be dose dependent and has such a multifactorial, multilayered activity that more studies are necessary to evaluate fully the possibility of naloxone use in treating acute SCI. In the doses used in the NASCIS 2 study, naloxone did not show a statistically significant beneficial effect in the treatment of acute SCIs.

## Selection of Surgical Candidates and Timing of Surgery

A large body of literature exists concerning the timing of surgery and candidate selection in the setting of an acute SCI. Until more recently, the prevailing opinion among spine surgeons was not to operate early after an injury, with "early" being defined as within 3 weeks. High morbidity and mortality from early intervention were documented in multiple studies. With advances in neurocritical care and neuroanesthesia, however, early surgical intervention after injury has become safer. It also is intuitive that the sooner the spinal cord and nerve roots are decompressed, the greater the potential is for recovery of function. In recent years, the definitions of "early" and "late" intervention have changed. We define "early surgery" as being done within 24 hours after injury and "delayed surgery" as being done after 24 hours. Although the NASCIS 2 study was not designed to evaluate the timing of surgery, an analysis of the raw data from this study did show an improved outcome from early surgical treatment. This outcome is equally true for most complete and incomplete injury syndromes, with the exclusion of central cord syndrome, in which injury usually is due to hyperextension with preexisting stenosis. In central cord syndrome patients, initial immobilization, with observation, and surgery at a later time is a common approach. Early intervention has other benefits in the cases of incomplete injuries. When the spine is stabilized, intensive physical therapy can be initiated so that other systemic complications of SCI can be reduced.

Other criteria used to select patients for early surgical
Author: Please verify drug doses.

intervention include associated systemic injuries and the general medical condition of the patient. Acute SCI, as previously mentioned, is associated with multiorgan trauma, plus SCI itself can cause systemic shock with hypotension, respiratory deterioration with pulmonary edema, and an increased risk for infection. When surgical decompression or stabilization of the spine is delayed, medical treatment of an acute SCI patient becomes essential in maximizing the neurologic outcome. At present, there is no consensus as to the timing of surgery for patients with SCI resulting from blunt trauma.

## SUGGESTED READING

Amar AP, Levy ML. Pathogenesis and pharmacological strategies for mitigating secondary damage in acute spinal cord injury. Neurosurgery 1999;44:1027–1040.

Benzel EC, Larson SJ. Functional recovery after decompressive spine operation for cervical spine fractures. Neurosurgery 1987;20:742–746.

Tator CH, Fehlings MG. Review of the secondary injury theory of acute spinal cord trauma with emphasis on vascular mechanisms. J Neurosurg 1991;75:15–26.

# SPINAL INJURIES IN SPORTS

**MARC A. AGULNICK**
**MARK G. GROSSMAN**

The spine is a concerning source of injuries in sports. Most acute injuries are related to participation in contact sports, such as football, wrestling, rugby, and hockey. Most injuries occur about the shoulder and neck and less commonly in the low back. Other conditions, such as thoracic outlet syndrome, effort-induced thrombosis, axillary artery occlusion, and peripheral nerve injuries, are infrequent but can present similarly to spinal disorders and should be considered in the differential diagnosis.

## CERVICAL ROOT AND BRACHIAL PLEXUS INJURIES

The brachial plexus is composed of the C5 through T1 nerve roots and is divided into roots, trunks, divisions, cords, and branches (Fig. 7-1). Usual mechanisms of injury are compression and traction. Traction usually is from forceful separation (i.e., lateral flexion of the neck) of the head from the shoulder. Arm position at the time of impact usually dictates the region of the plexus that is injured. If the arm is adducted, the upper roots are subjected to greater stress. If the arm is abducted, the lower roots are more susceptible to injury.

Compression injuries are usually the result of direct trauma or sustained external pressure to regions overlying the plexus, such as the supraclavicular fossa. A concomitant clavicular fracture frequently occurs. The nerve roots are compressed at the neural foramina with neck hyperextension or axial compression or both; neck hyperextension and axial compression are common in contact sports such as football.

### Diagnosis

Brachial plexus injuries usually are diagnosed clinically. Motor and sensory exams and reflexes should be documented for the upper and the lower extremities. A comprehensive vascular examination also should be performed. A thorough shoulder exam should rule out intrinsic shoulder pathology as the cause of symptoms.

Electrodiagnostic and advanced imaging studies can help confirm the diagnosis. Other diagnoses that may present similarly should be considered in the differential diagnosis, such as:

- "Dead arm" syndrome (from anterior instability of the shoulder)
- Occult fracture or developmental abnormality of the cervical spine
- Disc herniation
- Transient quadriplegia
- Acute brachial neuropathy (Parsonage-Turner syndrome)

### Provocative Maneuvers

Pain with range of motion or axial compression of the neck suggests a spine fracture. Spurling maneuver can reproduce radicular pain associated with disc herniation or foraminal stenosis (Fig. 7-2). Examination of the scapula should include forward elevation and wall push-off to detect medial scapular winging from serratus anterior palsy. Trapezius, levator scapulae, and rhomboid dysfunction can cause lateral winging.

Controlled separation of the athlete's head and shoulder can reproduce symptoms from a traction injury to the upper or lower trunk. Tinel's sign with percussion along the supraclavicular fossa may produce electric shock–like symptoms or pain into the extremity.

### Burners Syndrome

Burners syndrome is one of the most common injuries in contact sports. The "burner" or "stinger" was named after the pain, tingling, and burning experienced in the upper extremity of the athlete after contact. These injuries usually occur after the athlete strikes his or her head against another player, a wall, or a mat. After this event, the athlete experiences sudden pain, burning, and sometimes tingling that begins in the neck, radiates into the shoulder, and continues down the arm and into the hand. Symptoms do not follow a dermatomal pattern. Weakness of the supraspinatus, infraspinatus, deltoid, and biceps muscle often is noted, which usually presents hours to days after the injury.

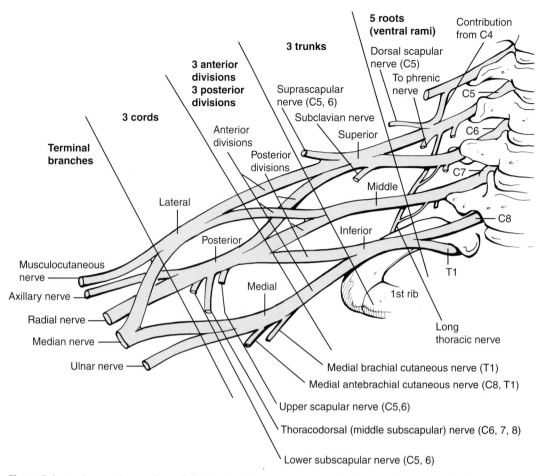

**Figure 7-1** A clear understanding of the brachial plexus is important in determining the level of the injury, which can influence prognosis.

Burners are a type of brachial plexus injury that usually result from traction to the brachial plexus or compression of the cervical root at the intervertebral foramen. Direct impact to the plexus within the supraclavicular region also has been reported. Traction injuries can occur with tackling. This causes sudden lateral deviation of the head away from the affected side and simultaneous depression of the ipsilateral shoulder. These injuries are more frequent in high school athletes, possibly because of less developed supportive neck musculature.

Cervical root compression occurs at the level of the intervertebral foramen. The foramen is dynamically narrowed during activities that cause cervical spinal extension, compression, and rotation toward the symptomatic side. These injuries are seen more commonly in collegiate or professional athletes. Patients present with more neck pain and diminished range of motion than do patients with traction injuries. Direct trauma to the supraclavicular region at Erb's point can produce a burners syndrome with upper trunk deficits predominating. Spurling maneuver is used to evaluate compression-type injuries, whereas the brachial plexus stretch test can be used to evaluate traction-type injuries.

Central cervical canal and foraminal stenoses are re-

ported as risk factors for recurrent burners. Logically, this association has been described for compression-type and extension-type injuries but not traction mechanisms. Athletes with a history of recurrent burners and associated degenerative disc disease or congenital stenosis should abstain from participation in contact sports.

The physician must determine whether symptoms are from cervical cord or root pathology. This important distinction often is made on the playing field. By definition, burners present with unilateral arm symptoms. Athletes who present with bilateral upper or any lower extremity symptoms are more likely to have had a more serious spinal cord injury. Focal neck tenderness or severe pain with motion should raise suspicion for a fracture or ligamentous injury to the cervical spine. In these cases, the spine should be immobilized using a collar and backboard, and the patient should be transported to a hospital for immediate imaging.

Burners are self-limited syndromes that usually do not cause permanent sequelae. Even with this favorable natural history, certain restrictions should be placed on athletes after sustaining these injuries to prevent more severe problems in the future.

Patients who are experiencing significant muscle weakness should rest the involved extremity until symptoms im-

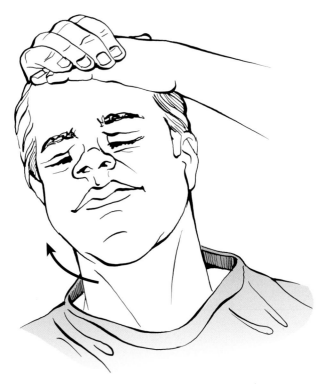

**Figure 7-2** Spurling maneuver—the patient turns head toward the symptomatic arm, while pressure is applied to the cranium. This applies load to the cervical spine and is positive if pain radiates to the affected upper extremity. Caution must be used because this test is nonspecific and must be taken in context with the entire history and physical exam.

prove. At that time, physical therapy can begin and be advanced as tolerated. Athletes also should be started on year-round trapezial strengthening programs. Theoretically, strengthening the neck musculature may increase the shock-absorbing capacity of the cervical spine. Athletes must fulfill particular criteria before they can return to play (Table 7-1).

Athletes who are prone to burners can use special equipment to help prevent injuries. Commonly used devices are thicker shoulder pads, neck rolls, springs, and the "cowboy collar" (Fig. 7-3). The devices must fit correctly and be used with properly fitting shoulder pads to be effective. Educat-

## TABLE 7-1 RETURN-TO-PLAY CRITERIA AFTER BURNERS SYNDROME*

1. Resolution of paresthesias
2. Full, painless range of motion
3. Negative Spurling maneuver and brachial plexus stretch test
4. Negative axial compression and resistive hand pressure tests
5. Normal strength to physical exam

*All must be satisfied.

ing participants about proper athletic technique also is important. Proper tackling and blocking techniques, with avoidance of spearing, should be taught to young football players as they first are learning the sport.

## CERVICAL SPINE INJURIES

Cervical spine injuries constitute a large percentage of spinal injuries in sports. Injuries range from cervical sprains to catastrophic complete spinal cord injuries (SCIs). An estimated 10% to 15% of football players experience an injury to the cervical spine. The overall incidence of SCI in the high school and college populations is around 1 in 100,000. Most are incomplete, with preservation of varying degrees of neurologic function.

### Mechanisms of Injury

Cervical spine injuries may occur by hyperflexion or hyperextension. A review by Torg et al of the data compiled by the National Football Head and Neck Injury Registry showed that axial loading of a slightly flexed head and neck is the most frequent contributing mechanism of injury. The slightly flexed posture reverses normal lordosis, potentiating axial load transmission down the straightened cervical spine. Preexisting spinal stenosis predisposes to SCI from these mechanisms. Athletes can sustain cord injury despite the absence of bone or ligamentous disruption. This phenomenon has been described by Penning. When the cervical spine is in hyperextension, the cord can be compressed between the posteroinferior margin of the superior vertebrae and the anterosuperior lamina of the subjacent vertebra. Infolding of the posterior longitudinal ligament and the ligamentum flavum contributes to central canal narrowing.

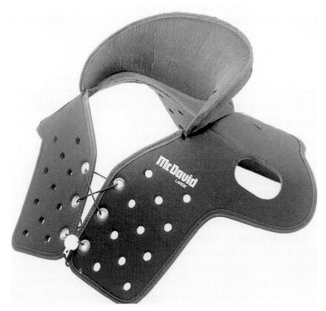

**Figure 7-3** The "cowboy collar" can be used for athletes who are prone to burners syndrome.

This transient compression can occur with energies not great enough to cause discoligamentous or bone disruption. SCI can occur without an "unstable" spinal injury. Some athletes experience multiple symptomatic episodes.

Contact sports, such as football, rugby, and wrestling, place patients at high risk for injury. Most cervical spine injuries in football players result from hyperflexion, but other mechanisms, including hyperextension, rotation, and lateral bending, have been reported. Gymnasts may sustain injuries after "missed" maneuvers that result in an uncontrolled fall. Wrestlers commonly exhibit neck hyperflexion, but also may endure rotational and horizontal shearing forces that place great stresses on the intervertebral discs, facet joints, and spinal ligaments. SCI also has been documented in noncontact sports, such as diving and surfing. These events usually result from the individual striking his or her head on the bottom of the pool or body of water, causing neck hyperflexion.

## Specific Conditions

### Cervical Stenosis

Narrowing or stenosis of the cervical spinal canal can predispose athletes to SCI. Two forms of cervical stenosis have been described in athletes: developmental and acquired.

- *Developmental*: Otherwise known as *congenital stenosis*, is present at birth, and is characterized by shortened pedicles causing an abnormally narrow canal, sometimes described as funnel-shaped.
- *Acquired*: The result of reactive bone thickening and ligamentous hypertrophy that can result from repeated collisions in sports over time. Other pathoanatomic features include disc bulges, spondylolysis, and osteophytes.

Methods for diagnosing and quantifying cervical stenosis have been suggested. Sagittal canal diameter is measured on a standard lateral cervical spine radiograph. The measurement is recorded as the anteroposterior distance between the posterior aspect of the vertebral body and the nearest point along on the spinolaminar junction. Wolf et al established normal parameters for this dimension. The average diameters at C1, C2, and C3-7 were 22 mm, 20 mm, and 17mm. Sagittal canal diameters of more than 15 mm were established as normal, and diameters of less than 13 mm were defined as stenotic. Evaluation of the sagittal canal diameter on a lateral cervical spine radiograph is limited by errors related to magnification, radiographic technique, and measurement variability.

Taking different vertebral sizes into account, Torg et al derived a ratio of the anteroposterior canal diameter and the anteroposterior vertebral body diameter. A value less than 0.8 was defined as spinal stenosis (Fig. 7-4). Herzog et al questioned the reliability of the Torg ratio, finding it to have a high sensitivity but a poor positive predictive value for detecting clinically significant cervical narrowing. Studies that have evaluated the cervical spines of clinically asymptomatic professional football players showed abnormal Torg ratios in 33% to 49%. The high incidence of these abnormally low ratios is due to the large vertebral body size in this population, with absolute dimensions of the spinal canal being adequately capacious for the spinal cord. Magnetic resonance imaging (MRI) evaluation of these players revealed adequate space available for the cord in the athletes and no true stenosis.

Presently, evaluation for functional spinal stenosis, with either MRI or computeed tomography (CT) myelogram, is becoming the new standard. Functional spinal stenosis is defined as obliteration of the cerebrospinal fluid cushion surrounding the cervical spinal cord. This method of evaluation is being used by many team physicians for decision making regarding athletes' return to play and treatment and activity modifications.

### Cervical Sprain and Strain

Neck pain, or the so-called jammed neck, is one of the most common complaints among athletes, especially football players. Patients can sustain an injury to the musculotendinous unit (sprain) or paraspinal muscle itself (strain): One sprains a tendon but strains a muscle. Typically an athlete presents with localized neck pain without radiation to the arms or back. Athletes may have decreased cervical range of motion secondary to pain. Sometimes the pain may be localized to one specific cervical level. There are no neurologic deficits.

Athletes presenting with acute cervical pain after a known contact event are placed in a cervical collar pending further work-up. Initially the radiographic evaluation includes anteroposterior, lateral, and odontoid views of the cervical spine. If these initial radiographs are normal, flexion and extension lateral radiographs are obtained after the pain and paraspinal muscle spasm have subsided. Instability based on Panjabi and White's criteria of displacement change of 3.5 mm or a change in angulation between two adjacent vertebral bodies of 11 degrees is assessed on plain lateral radiographs and preferably on flexion/extension views. Continuing symptoms and radicular pain may prompt further evaluation with MRI or bone scan.

Treatment is based on severity and etiology. Generally the use of a cervical collar and analgesic medications is continued until pain and spasm subside. After the collar is removed, range of motion exercises can begin. Return to athletic participation is delayed until painless full range of motion is achieved. Instability may necessitate surgical stabilization to prevent future neurologic injury.

### Intervertebral Disc Lesion

Acute disc herniation in contact sports is rare. Head-on collisions or other events leading to axial loading can result in increased intradiscal pressure. If large enough, cord compression can manifest as either transient or permanent quadriplegia or quadriparesis. Patients may present with acute paralysis of all four extremities and loss of pain and temperature sensation. Patients also may present with an anterior cord syndrome. Acute radicular symptoms can occur alone, however. MRI is the study of choice to detect a herniated disc. Patients with persistent clinical and radiologic evidence of spinal cord compression should be offered surgery, which may include anterior cervical discectomy and interbody fusion.

Radiographic evaluation of the cervical spine of football

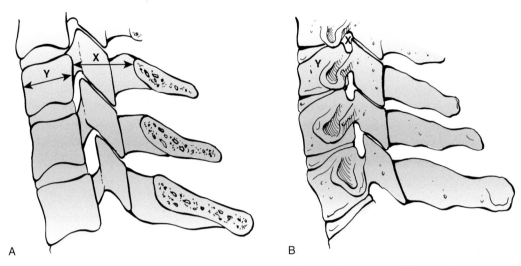

A          B

**Figure 7-4** (A, B) The Torg ratio is calculated by dividing the sagittal diameter of the vertebral canal (*x*) by the diameter of the vertebral body (*y*).

players can reveal asymptomatic cervical spondylosis. In one study, 7% of freshman college football players had abnormally narrowed disc spaces. Early degenerative changes have been attributed to years of repetitive loading from tackling. Severe degenerative changes, including foraminal stenosis, central canal stenosis resulting from posterior osteophytes, and loss of normal cervical lordosis, can result in the classic "spear tackler's spine."

### Transient Quadriplegia

*Neurapraxia of the cervical cord* with transient quadriplegia is fairly common in contact sports participants. Characteristics include:

- Bilateral burning pain
- Tingling
- Loss of sensation in the upper or lower extremities

An axial load with hyperextension or flexion of the cervical spine is thought to be the mechanism. A pincer mechanism that theoretically causes a brief compression of the cord is thought to play a role in the transient nature of the symptoms. Motor deficits can vary from mild weakness to total paralysis depending on the extent of insult to the spinal cord. By definition, symptoms are transient, and complete recovery usually occurs within 10 to 15 minutes, but it may take 48 hours.

Standard radiographic evaluation of the cervical spine usually is negative for fractures or dislocations. Incidental findings, such as congenital stenosis, spondylosis, Klippel-Feil syndrome, or evidence of intervetebral disc disease, may be present, however.

Patients may experience the "burning hands" syndrome originally described by Maroon. This is a variant of a central cord syndrome. It is characterized by burning dysesthesias and paresthesias that occur in a glovelike distribution. Symptoms usually last less than 24 hours. This syndrome has been documented after cervical spinal fractures and in athletes with no radiographic abnormality. Preexisting

cervical stenosis may be a predisposing factor. Reversible MRI spinal cord signal abnormalities have been documented.

### Permanent Neurologic Syndromes

SCI can be permanent. Permanent neurologic deficits are more common in association with fractures and dislocations, although permanent deficits may occur without such injuries.

Torg et al described spear tackler's spine, which occurs in athletes who employ improper tackling technique, using the top of their football helmet to hit an opposing player head on. This injury is associated with an increased risk for permanent neurologic damage. Affected athletes show the following:

- Narrowing of the cervical spinal canal
- Persistent straightening or reversal of the normal lordotic curve
- Concomitant preexisting posttraumatic radiographic abnormalities of the cervical spine

### Congenital Anomalies

Congenital anomalies of the cervical spine can predispose an athlete to spinal injuries by changing the mechanics and load-dissipating properties of the cervical spine. Congenital anomalies can occur by failure of formation or segmentation.

Klippel-Feil syndrome is secondary to failure of segmentation that may involve one or more motion segments. Torg and Glasgow classified Klippel-Feil syndrome into two types. Type I involves a long congenital fusion (more than two segments), whereas type II has one or two fused segments. As the number of fused segments increases, the ability of the cervical spine to dissipate loads decreases. More force is concentrated on the unfused motion segments, increasing the chance for injury in these regions with contact sports.

Failure of formation can manifest as odontoid agenesis, hypoplasia, or os odontoideum. These conditions can result in atlantoaxial instability, which places athletes participating in contact sports at great risk for SCI. In some instances, an athlete can have failure of formation of the atlantooccipital junction. These individuals are prone to experience compression of the posterior columns of the spinal cord at the posterior margin of the foramen magnum and should be restricted from contact sports.

Spina bifida occulta is another congenital anomaly. It is usually an incidental finding and asymptomatic. It usually does not hinder participation in athletics.

### Unstable Cervical Fractures and Dislocations

In an analysis of football players from 1977 to 1989, catastrophic SCIs were secondary to fracture-dislocations or anterior compression (burst) fractures in 33% and 22% of cases. In most cases, the cervical spine is straight on impact, which lessens its ability to dissipate the load. With increasing loads the spine fails in flexion, resulting in vertebral body comminution, subluxation, or facet joint dislocation. Experimentally, Maiman et al found the average axial load to failure to be less with a straightened versus a normal lordotic posture. The greatest force applied to the spine was found when the load was applied to the vertex of the skull. This force decreased as the load was moved forward on the skull.

Although axial loads combined with flexion cause most fracture-dislocations of the cervical spine, other mechanisms also can cause injuries. Rotation, extension, and shear forces alone or in combination have been implicated in various fracture patterns observed in the cervical spine. Although the multiple fractures experienced by athletes participating in contact sports such as football are beyond the scope of this chapter, they have led to the National Collegiate Athletic Association Football Rule Committee to outlaw the use of one's helmet to tackle an opponent.

### On-Field Evaluation and Initial Management of Suspected Spinal Cord Injury

Initial on-field management of athletes with suspected SCIs consists of the following measures:

- Remove the athlete from play.
- Institute immediate immobilization of the cervical spine.
- Perform a neurologic evaluation.
- Ensure proper airway control in unconscious patients.
- Remove the facemask (to allow airway access) without moving the cervical spine. Newer facemasks allow removal by cutting plastic attachment loops or unscrewing. Older facemasks may require removal with bolt cutters. As a rule, the chinstrap and helmet is left in place until arrival at a hospital, where a coordinated team can perform specialized removal maneuvers.

Athletes with a suspected SCI or altered mental status should be transported to a hospital for further evaluation. These patients should be immobilized on a spine board. Circumferential taping across the helmet, chest, torso, pelvis, and lower limbs is the most effective method of securing the athlete to the board (Fig. 7-5). All movements and transfers should use strict logroll precautions.

### Return-to-Play Decision Making

The decision to allow an athlete to return to play after an event dealing with the cervical spine is a difficult one to make. Many times the pressures placed on the physician or medical personnel by the athlete, coaches, and parents can cloud the decision. No definitive decisions should be made until a complete history and physical exam have been performed.

Players who have sustained a stinger may return to play after all neurologic symptoms have resolved and full strength and painless cervical range of motion are present. If this status cannot be achieved, the athlete is kept out of competition, and cervical immobilization should be maintained. Radiographic evaluation of patients with persisting symptoms is recommended.

A systematic approach using an algorithm may facilitate decision making after cervical injury (Algorithm 7-1). Patients with acute cervical strains are kept out of competition until painless full range of motion and full cervical strength are attained. If cervical spine plain films and flexion/extension films are normal, the athlete may return to play. It is essential that symptoms have resolved because reinjury rate in these patients is high.

Acute cervical disc herniations can have serious neurologic sequelae and can lead to decision-making dilemmas. Athletes with radiculopathy may return to play after symptoms have resolved. If the disc herniation is causing clinically symptomatic spinal cord compression, an anterior discectomy and fusion may be considered. Return to play may be considered if symptoms have resolved, definite radiographic fusion has been achieved, and full painless range of motion is restored. Although one-level or two-level fusions are not an absolute contraindication, many surgeons dissuade athletes from continuing contact sports.

Athletes with congenital or acquired stenosis of the cervical spine may be at higher risk for SCI. In these patients, the presence of instability, disc disease, degenerative changes, evidence of cord abnormalities on MRI, neurologic symptoms lasting more than 36 hours, and more than one recurrence of neurologic symptoms are contraindications to continued participation in contact sports. Athletes with radiographic evidence of spear tackler's spine should not be cleared for continued play. Torg et al deemed this condition to be an absolute contraindication to participation in football or other contact sports. In other cases, one episode of transient spinal cord neurapraxia is not a contraindication to returning to play after full resolution of symptoms. The presence of congenital spinal stenosis alone in an athlete is not an absolute contraindication to participation in contact sports. These patients and their families should be counseled adequately, however, as to the increased risks for SCI.

Congenital anomalies of the cervical spine are an absolute contraindication to participation in contact sports. All anomalies, even if found incidentally, should prompt removal from play. The only exceptions to this rule are Klippel-Feil type II deformities below C3. In these cases, there is a relative contraindication to participation in contact

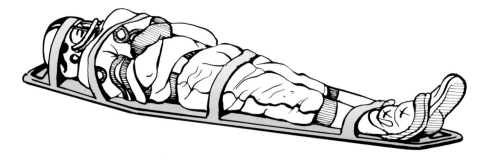

**Figure 7-5** Transfer of the athlete with a suspected cervical spine injury must be performed carefully. Optimally the helmet and body are secured to a rigid backboard using circumferential bands of tape.

sports. As always, decisions must be made on a case-by-case basis.

Bailes et al made specific recommendations concerning return to play by stratifying injuries into three types:

- *Type 1* denotes patients with a neurologic injury. These patients should not be allowed to return to sports.
- *Type 2* injuries consist of transient neurologic deficits without radiologic evidence of abnormalities. These athletes are allowed to return to activity unless they have sustained repetitive injuries or had particular risk factors, such as congenital stenosis.
- *Type 3* injuries that have radiographic abnormalities. This group represents a wide spectrum of disorders with

varying recommendations. Athletes who sustain fractures in the presence of congenital cervical stenosis should not be cleared for return to contact sports.

In the study by Bailes et al, other radiographic abnormalities, such as congenital fusion, disc herniations, and degenerative cervical spinal disease, were evaluated on a case-by-case basis.

## LUMBAR SPINE

Low back pain usually affects an athlete at some point. This pain can be from an overuse syndrome or acute trauma.

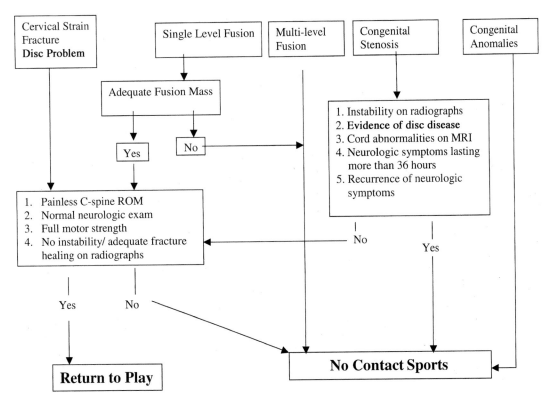

**Algorithm 7-1** Return-to-play criteria after cervical spine injury.

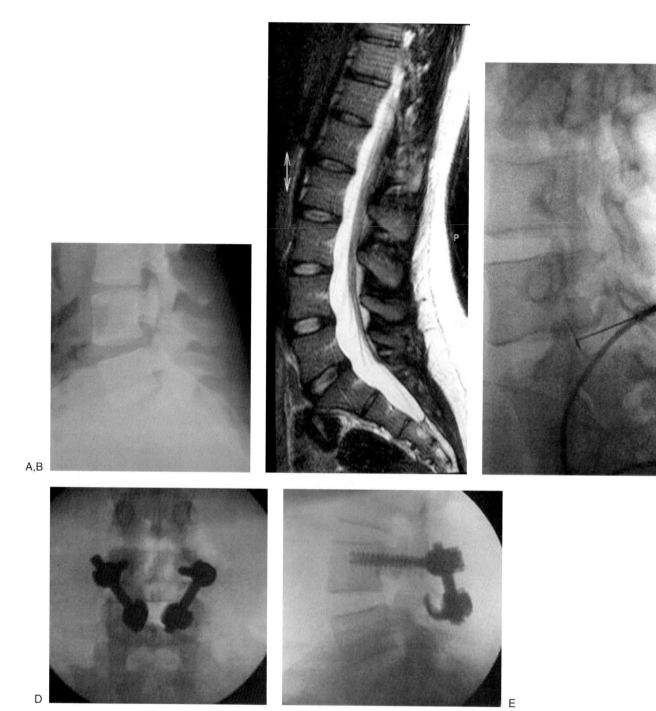

A,B

C

D

E

**Figure 7-6** In athletes with painful spondylolysis that is recalcitrant to nonoperative care, a pars repair may be performed. (**A**) Preoperative lateral radiographs of a 20-year-old college baseball player show a spondylolytic defect of the L4 pars. There is no evidence of spondylolisthesis. (**B**) For best results, there should be no or minimal disc degeneration. (**C**) A preoperative pars defect injection temporarily alleviated most or all of the patient's pain. Although various techniques for pars repair exist, common to all is autograft interposition in and around the defect to encourage healing. Translaminar screws, tension wiring, or pedicle screw-hook constructs provided rigid fixation. In this patient, screws were inserted into the L4 pedicle, and up-going hooks were placed beneath the L4 lamina. (**D, E**) A short rod was used to connect the two, enabling compression across the grafted defect. (Courtesy of Christopher M. Bono, MD, Boston University Medical Center, Boston, MA.)

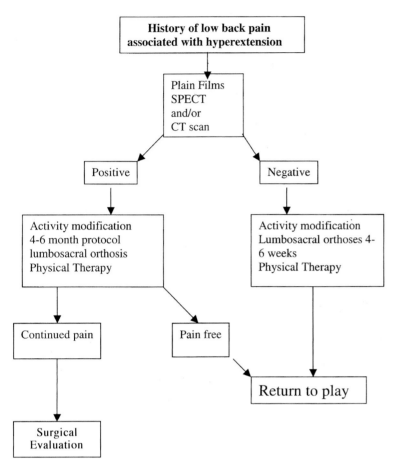

**Algorithm 7-2**  An algorithmic approach to the diagnosis, return-to-play decision making, and treatment of spondylolysis can be useful.

Complaints may range from mild to severe pain after a game or practice. Some injuries are characteristic of certain sports: lumbar herniated discs in weightlifters, sacral stress fractures in runners, and spondylolysis in football players and gymnasts. Position, hours, and number of years played can indicate overuse. Predominantly axial low back pain suggests internal disc disruption from degenerative disc disease. Predominantly leg symptoms suggest radiculopathy from a herniated disc. Infections, tumors, and inflammatory arthritis more typically are suggested by nonmechanical back pain. Other red flags are night pain, pain at rest, fever, or weight loss.

Radiographs should be obtained to evaluate low back pain that occurs after acute trauma during a sporting event. Chronic pain should be assessed according to protocols used for nonathletes for the specific suspected diagnosis, such as disc herniation, spinal stenosis, or axial back pain. An adolescent athlete with substantial back pain lasting longer than 3 weeks should be evaluated with plain lumbar radiographs and a bone scan or single photon emission computed tomography (SPECT). A retrospective study comparing 100 adolescent athletes and 100 adults with acute low back pain showed that 47% of the adolescent athletes had spondylolysis compared with only 5% of the adult subjects. The presence and grade of spondylolysis/spondylolisthesis can influence the decision to allow return to play.

Nonsurgical treatment of mechanical low back pain in athletes includes rest and pain control. Rest should be limited to no more than 48 hours to avoid deconditioning. Medications include nonsteroidal antiinflammatory drugs and a brief course of mild narcotics or muscle relaxants. Physical therapy may decrease recurrences, although no particular regimen is superior. Spinal orthoses may be used for short-term relief of mechanical symptoms from spondylolysis or low-grade spondylolisthesis.

For most conditions, athletes can return to sports after 8 weeks if they are pain-free, show a full range of motion, and are neurologically intact. Surgical treatment is specific for the diagnosis. Among other postoperative considerations, such as solid fusion, athletes may return to play after lumbar surgery after normal strength, endurance, and power have been regained. Because spondylolysis is so commonly encountered, an algorithm for its treatment is presented (Algorithm 7-2). Although a single-level fusion is the current standard in recalcitrant cases, a pars defect repair may be considered in some cases (Fig. 7-6).

## SUGGESTED READING

Albright JP, Moses JM, Feldick HG, et al. Nonfatal cervical spine injuries in interscholastic football. JAMA 1976;236:1243–1245.

Bailes JE, Hadley MN, Quigley MR, et al. Management of athletic injuries of the cervical spine and spinal cord. Neurosurgery 1991; 29:491–497.

d'Hemecourt P, Zurakowski D, Kriemler S, Micheli LJ. Spondylolysis: returning the athlete to sports participation with brace treatment. Orthopedics 2002;25:653–657.

Hershman EB. Brachial plexus injuries. Clin Sports Med 1990;9: 311–329.

Koffler KM, Kelly JD: Neurovascular trauma in athletes. Orthop Clin N Am 2002;33:523–534.

Meyer SA, Callaghan JJ, Albright JP, et al. Cervical spinal stenosis and stingers in collegiate football players. Am J Sports Med 1994;22: 158–166.

Penning L. Some aspects of plain radiography of the cervical spine in chronic myelopathy. Neurology 1962;12:513–519.

Reilly PJ, Torg JS. Athletic injury to the cervical nerve root and brachial plexus. Operative Techniques in Sports Medicine 1993;1:231– 235.

Torg JS, Das M. Trampoline-related quadriplegia: review of the literature and reflections on the American Academy of Pediatrics' Position Statement. Pediatrics 1984;74: 804–812.

Vegso JJ, Lehman RC. Field evaluation and management of head and neck injuries. Clin Sports Med 1987;6:1–15.

Wu WQ, Lewis RC. Injuries of the cervical spine in high school wrestling. Surg Neurol 1985;23:143–147.

# PYOGENIC INFECTIONS

**ROBERT K. EASTLACK**
**CHRISTOPHER P. KAUFFMAN**

Infections of the spine are relatively rare compared with musculoskeletal infections in general. The potential long-term consequences of these infections can have much more serious repercussions for affected patients, however, including neurologic compromise and death. Infection of the spine is usually an indolent process and often can be well tolerated if diagnosed early. Commonly, patients have vague back pain that is not evaluated fully until weeks or months after it began. The profound consequences and the indistinct clinical presentations of spinal infections highlight the importance of maintaining a reasonable index of suspicion. Occasionally, precipitous deterioration occurs, causing patients to present with sepsis, pathologic fracture, and neurologic compromise. The incidence of spinal infections is increasing, likely owing to an increase in spinal procedures, more immunocompromised patients, and escalating numbers of invasive procedures.

## PATHOGENESIS

### Etiology

Spinal infections of this type generally are categorized as discitis, pyogenic osteomyelitis, or epidural abscess. Pyogenic spinal infections usually arise through hematogenous or contiguous (direct) spread. Hematogenous spread, the most common pathway, involves seeding of the spinal elements through bacteremia from unrelated infections. Examples of distant sources include urologic, respiratory, and skin infections. Direct or contiguous spread may occur through posttraumatic inoculation, overlying decubitus ulcers, or adjacent infections (i.e., retropharyngeal or retroperitoneal abscesses), among others.

Despite the pathways taken by pathogens, there are a variety of potential sources. Iatrogenic causes represent a substantial portion of the problem. Potential liabilities include indwelling catheters; invasive spinal procedures, such as surgery or injections; and pharmacologic immunosuppression. Urologic procedures have a well-known association with bacteremia and subsequent seeding of the spinal elements.

### Epidemiology

The age distribution of spinal infections typically is bimodal, with a small peak between 10 and 20 years of age and a large peak in the elderly population (>50 years old). More recently, a new peak has been developing in the young adult group, possibly corresponding to increased rates of infection with human immunodeficiency virus (HIV) and intravenous drug abuse. Males are affected more commonly than females in all age groups, comprising 60% to 80% of the infected population. Other important risk factors include (see also Table 8-1):

- Diabetes
- Alcohol abuse
- Organ transplantation

Discitis most commonly affects children and is responsible for most spinal infections in the younger age group. There is no indication that discitis is more or less prevalent currently. In developed countries, vertebral osteomyelitis constitutes 2% to 8% of all cases of osteomyelitis, ranking it a distant third behind femoral and tibial infections. Epidural

## TABLE 8-1 RISK FACTORS FOR PYOGENIC SPINAL INFECTIONS

Alcohol abuse
Diabetes
Distant infections (genitourinary, respiratory, skin)
HIV (AIDS)
Iatrogenic immunosuppression
Indwelling catheters
Intravenous drug abuse
Male sex
Malignancy
Malnutrition
Morbid obesity
Previous spinal procedures
Renal disease
Rheumatoid arthritis
Skin infections
Smoking
Trauma (penetrating or nonpenetrating)

AIDS, acquired immunodeficiency syndrome; HIV, human immunodeficiency virus.

abscesses tend to occur in elderly patients after spinal injections and other invasive procedures.

It has been suggested that the incidence of spinal infections in general is increasing, likely due to an enlarging elderly population, more immunocompromised patients, and intravenous drug abuse. Although there has been a presumed increased incidence in more recent years, no definitive evidence supporting this conclusion exists in the literature. The true dynamics are obscured further by a considerable improvement in detecting infections.

Pathogens associated with pyogenic spinal infections are numerous and include, but are not limited to, the following (Table 8-2):

- *Staphylococcus aureus* is the most common and traditionally almost always the cause of spinal infections, but with changes in risk factor dynamics it now is isolated in only 50% to 60% of cases.
- *Pseudomonas* more commonly is associated with intravenous drug abusers than other patient subgroups.
- Other gram-negative organisms, such as *Escherichia coli, Klebsiella,* and *Proteus,* usually occur through genitourinary pathways.
- Patients with sickle cell disease are more susceptible to *Salmonella.*
- Vertebral osteomyelitis in children can develop from *Bartonella henselae* infection (cat-scratch disease).
- Postoperative infections associated with instrumentation often involve coagulase-negative *Staphylococcus* (S. *epidermidis*) or other normal skin flora.
- Other reported organisms include *Streptococcus* and *Acinetobacter* species. In the presence of hardware, even traditionally benign organisms are thought to be pathologic.

Approximately half of all infections occur in the lumbar spine. Most remaining infections occur in the thoracic spine, and only about 7% involve the cervical spine. The thoracolumbar and lumbosacral junctions each comprise approximately 5% of spinal infections.

## TABLE 8-2  ORGANISMS: PYOGENIC SPINAL INFECTIONS

*Staphylococcus aureus*
*Streptococcus* species
*Staphylococcus epidermidis*
*Escherichia coli*
*Klebsiella pneumoniae*
*Proteus* species
*Pseudomonas aeruginosa*
*Enterobacter* species
*Salmonella* species
*Serratia marcescens*
*Brucella* species
*Acinetobacter* species

Data from Sapico FL, Montgomerie JZ. Vertebral osteomyelitis. J Bone Joint Surg Am 1997;79:874–880; and Carragee EJ. Pyogenic vertebral osteomyelitis. Infect Dis Clin North Am 1990;4:539–550.

Postoperative infection rates vary with the length and complexity of the index surgery. Studies of discectomies and laminectomies consistently have shown infection rates of less than 1%. Instrumented posterior lumbar fusions generate an approximately 6% rate of postoperative infection. Cervical spine surgeries show similar statistics, with infection rates after instrumented posterior arthrodesis around 4%. Some specific additional risk factors associated with postoperative infections are revision surgery, instrumentation, allogeneic blood transfusion/higher blood loss, longer surgery time, posterior approach to spine, and congenital deformity.

## Pathophysiology

The pathophysiology of spinal infections has not been elucidated clearly. Because most infections are thought to be hematogenous, current theories are based mainly on vascularity. Early in life, there is a fairly rich blood supply to the nucleus pulposus. This blood flows from the adjacent end plates and anulus fibrosus into this central disc region. Through the aging process, vascularity into the nucleus pulposus diminishes significantly. As an adult, blood flow is limited mainly to the end plates and minimally at the peripheral anulus fibrosus. Nutrition is delivered to the adult disc via diffusion.

This vascular physiology seems to play a major role in the development of infection. Seeding of the disc via hematogenous spread of bacteria can result in discitis, which tends to be more prevalent in children. As blood flow to the central disc decreases with age, pyogenic infections tend to originate within the vertebral bodies.

Postoperative infections spread through hematogenous and direct means. When the organisms have involved the deeper wound, instrumentation may be seeded. Formation of a glycocalyx allows adherence to metal that often can protect the pathogen from otherwise bactericidal levels of antibiotics. Implants may have a variable propensity for this bacterial self-preservation. In a study comparing metal implants and wound infections after bacterial inoculation, rabbits showed a much higher infection rate in the stainless steel group (75%) than in the titanium group (35%). This finding has been correlated with a higher rate of bacterial adherence to stainless steel than to titanium.

## Classification

As discussed previously, there are three major regions of focus for infection around the spine. Involvement of the disc alone commonly has been referred to as *discitis.* Vertebral osteomyelitis denotes infection limited to the vertebral body, which eventually may cross the end plate to involve the disc, then adjacent segments (Fig. 8-1). This combination of involvement has been termed *spondylodiscitis.* Infections localized to the epidural space traditionally have been called *epidural abscesses.* Frequently, radiographic work-ups occur late in the process and can show diffuse involvement of one or more of these regions.

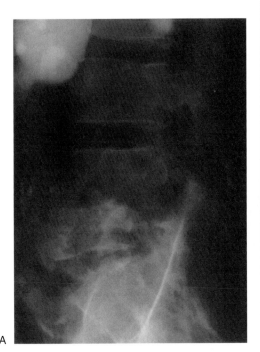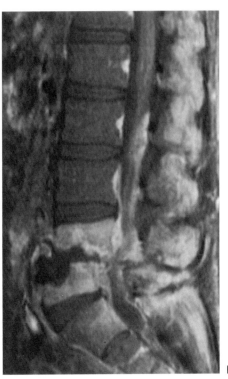

A                                                                                                    B

**Figure 8-1**   Plain radiograph (**A**) and MRI (**B**) of spondylodiscitis with adjacent vertebral bodies and the intervening disc involved in the infection.

# DIAGNOSIS

## Clinical Features

The most common presenting complaint for adult patients with spinal infection is back pain. The vague nature of this complaint contributes greatly to the frequent delay in diagnosis. Although the back pain may occur acutely, it usually has an insidious onset. Of patients, 50% to 70% have symptoms longer than 3 months before diagnosis.

Quality of the back pain has been described as constant with worsening at night, but it also can heighten with activity. Frequently, pain is accompanied by fever, night sweats, chills, weight loss, or other constitutional symptoms. Persistent and worsening back pain in the presence of one or more of these constitutional symptoms helps differentiate it from typical mechanical low back pain. In addition, there is often paraspinal muscle spasm with limited back range of motion due to pain. Involvement of the adjacent psoas muscles can result in painful hip flexion and extension.

Radicular complaints are relatively rare, but neurologic findings have been reported in about 10% of patients. Epidural abscesses and late, complicated infections tend to be more responsible for these findings. Neurologic compromise is associated more frequently with thoracic and cervical spinal infections.

Children show a unique pattern of presenting symptoms that varies with age. Irritability is common in infants and toddlers, with occasional difficulty and eventual refusal to walk. Older children may complain of abdominal or back pain and have spinal rigidity or localized tenderness on exam. High temperatures are the exception rather than the rule, with an average temperature of 37.6°C in one series.

Postoperative infections of the spine most commonly present with wound discharge and fever. These findings usually become apparent 1 to 2 weeks after surgery. Postoperative infections have presented nearly 2 years after surgery, however, and may show no more clinical symptoms than chronic or worsening pain.

## Laboratory Features

Laboratory evaluation is an important component to the work-up of patients suspected of having a spinal infection. White blood cell (WBC) count generally provides little help because the WBCs are abnormally elevated in only one third of patients. Epidural abscesses can cause substantial elevations, however, with an average WBC count of approximately 22,000 cells/mm$^3$. Epidural abscesses also have been associated with thrombocytopenia.

Erythrocyte sedimentation rate (ESR) is a general marker for systemic inflammatory response and is the most sensitive laboratory test for spinal infection. The ESR is elevated in 90% to 100% of children with discitis and approximately 90% of patients with vertebral osteomyelitis. Normal ESR values range from 0 to 20 mm/h, but some normal conditions can cause mild elevations. Most series of spinal infections and associated ESR testing report values greater than 40 mm/h. The ESR normalizes slowly after surgery (≥4 to 6 weeks) and is less useful when evaluating for postoperative infections.

A more useful laboratory test in the postoperative period

is the C-reactive protein (CRP) level. CRP is an acute-phase reactant that accumulates rapidly during infectious or injurious processes. In contrast to the ESR, the CRP level generally normalizes by 6 to 10 days after surgery. This characteristic makes it more valuable when evaluating for infections postoperatively. Additionally, because the CRP level normalizes relatively quickly, it is used frequently for longitudinal appraisal of successful treatment. The CRP level is highly sensitive, and it tends to be more specific than the ESR.

Blood cultures should be drawn during temperature spikes on all patients suspected of spinal infection. Although they are positive in only one third to three quarters of patients with documented infection, isolation of the responsible microbes is an important step in long-term management. Microbial identification yield also may be improved by culturing other potentially infective sources, such as sputum or urine.

Biopsy specimens often can be obtained percutaneously, usually with computed tomography (CT) or fluoroscopic guidance. Percutaneous biopsy is successful 60% to 96% of the time. Antimicrobials should be withheld before attempting to obtain biopsy specimens.

## Radiologic Features

The plain radiograph is the frontline imaging modality (Table 8-3). Despite this universal approach, plain x-rays usually are negative early on in the infectious process and may take 12 weeks to show notable changes. An exception occurs in children with discitis. By several weeks after the onset of symptoms, childhood discitis usually causes disc space narrowing seen on radiographs (Fig. 8-2). Vertebral disc height can return to normal (more often in younger children), but usually takes several months to a year.

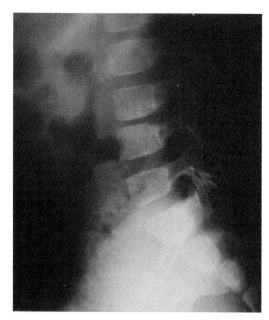

**Figure 8-2** Plain radiograph of discitis in a child. Note the classic disc space narrowing at L3-4 and the more subtle loss of lordosis.

Vertebral osteomyelitis also can present with radiographic narrowing of the disc space, but this follows osseous destruction of the adjacent end plates as shown in Figure 8-3. This distinguishes the process from most malignancies, which usually are confined to the vertebral body and do not cross the disc space. Vertebral body destruction and compression occur later in the process. Epidural abscesses alone rarely show significant abnormalities on plain radiographs.

Magnetic resonance imaging (MRI) is the diagnostic imaging modality of choice. MRI displays abnormalities in the disc, epidural space, and paraspinal anatomy, and its sensitivity for detecting infection reportedly is 99%. With infection of the vertebral body or disc, T1 signal intensity is decreased owing to inflammation and edema. Such a relative increase in water content causes the T2 signal intensity to increase. The use of contrast agents (i.e., gadolinium) allows even greater accuracy in identifying spinal infections with MRI (Fig. 8-4). It is useful in detecting epidural abscesses.

CT can be used to evaluate bone infection within the spine, with findings of osteolysis more clearly visible than on plain radiographs. The general quality of bone can be assessed best with this modality. CT scans often can be extremely valuable when planning surgical treatment and guiding biopsy procedures around the spine.

Scintigraphy (nuclear medicine studies) may be obtained if MRI is contraindicated (e.g., pacemaker) or not possible (e.g., stainless steel implants, claustrophobia). Nuclear medicine studies include three-phase technetium-99m, gallium, and indium-labeled WBC scans. A combined technetium and gallium scan provides the best sensitivity and specificity. Although indium-labeled WBC scans are highly specific, a high rate of false-negative results limits its role in the detection of spinal infection.

---

### TABLE 8-3  RADIOGRAPHIC IMAGING OF PYOGENIC SPINAL INFECTIONS

Plain radiographs
   Discitis: narrowing of intervertebral disc space
Vertebral osteomyelitis: end plate destruction, osteolysis, collapse, disc-space narrowing (late)
MRI
   $T_1$: Low intensity
   $T_2$: High intensity
   Gadolinium: ring-enhanced area of low intensity
CT scan (with/without contrast)
   Discitis: hypodensity in disc
   Vertebral osteomyelitis: osteolysis
   Evaluate bony anatomy (extent of true destruction) and use in guided biopsies
Nuclear medicine scans
   Technetium-99 diphosphonate
   Gallium-67 citrate
   Indium-111–labeled WBCs: high false-negative rate—use in combination

CT, computed tomography; MRI, magnetic resonance imaging; WBC, white blood cells.

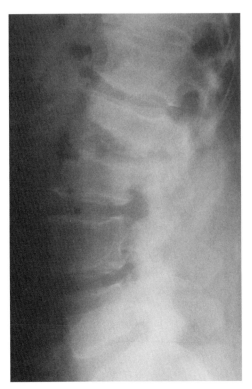

**Figure 8-3** Plain radiograph of infectious end plate rarefaction and narrowing with probable involvement of the intervertebral disc.

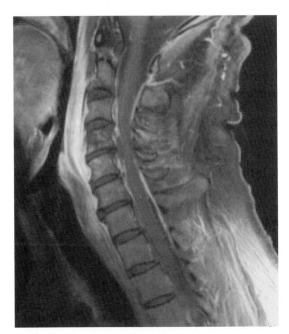

**Figure 8-4** T1-weighted MRI with gadolinium contrast enhancement elucidates a cervical epidural abscess within the anterior canal. Note the surrounding contrast halo, which is a classic finding with these infections.

### Diagnostic Work-up Algorithm

Diagnostic work-up includes the following:

- A thorough history and physical examination are done first.
- Plain radiographs are obtained.
- Screening laboratory tests always include WBC count, ESR, and CRP.
- Other initial laboratory studies can be directed by history specifics (e.g., exposure to *Mycobacterium tuberculosis*).
- Blood cultures should be obtained initially if the index of suspicion is high.
- MRI is the next radiographic study of choice, although nuclear medicine studies or CT can be performed when MRI is not feasible.
- When radiographic and laboratory work-up has revealed a likely infectious process, a biopsy specimen should be obtained through percutaneous or open means or directly at the time of surgery (if indicated).

## TREATMENT

### Nonoperative Treatment

Nonoperative treatment can be attempted initially with primary infections, although this treatment should be reserved for younger and more immunocompetent patients. In one series of 111 patients with vertebral osteomyelitis, the one third who failed nonoperative treatment tended to be older and immunodeficient. It is important to obtain the offending microbe via blood cultures or guided biopsy before beginning antibiotic treatment. Antibiotic regimens should be selected based on the organism's sensitivity profile and should be begun parenterally with an eventual switch to oral regimens in some cases.

Treatment of discitis in childhood typically begins with intravenous antibiotics empirically, even with negative blood cultures (guided biopsy rarely is indicated). A short (1 to 2 days) period of bed rest may be beneficial, but further activity restrictions should not be imposed. While awaiting clinical and laboratory (CRP) responses, an oral antibiotic regimen is begun. If this trend in improvement continues on the appropriate oral antibiotics, they are continued for 4 to 6 weeks. Occasionally, use of a brace may be indicated if symptoms persist. Children almost universally respond to these treatments and rarely require subsequent surgical intervention.

Vertebral osteomyelitis and discitis in adults must be approached slightly differently. Spinal immobilization plays a larger role in this population, but early ambulation should be encouraged. High-dose parenteral antibiotics should be administered for at least 4 to 6 weeks before any switch to oral agents. Infectious disease specialists can be helpful with optimizing drug regimens, especially when dealing with virulent or resistant species that may require a multidrug approach. Elimination of spine pain may occur in nearly 75% of patients, and spontaneous fusion often occurs.

Because epidural abscesses often cause neurologic compromise, nonoperative treatment rarely is indicated. Nonoperative treatment should be reserved for young, immunocompetent patients with minimal radiographic abnormalities and no neurologic changes. Immobilization and parenteral antibiotics should be used as in vertebral osteomyelitis, with little hesitancy for surgical intervention should neurologic changes develop.

Postoperative discitis that is uncomplicated by epidural abscess or osteomyelitis can be treated nonoperatively. A biopsy specimen should be obtained, if possible, to isolate the offending organism and direct the appropriate intravenous antibiotics for approximately 6 weeks. Orthoses can be considered for pain control, and close monitoring should be done to detect development of an epidural abscess or instability (deformity).

## Operative Treatment

Indications for surgical intervention include the following (Table 8-4):

- Failure of nonoperative treatment
- Need for open biopsy
- Presence of spinal abscess
- Sepsis
- Progressive spinal deformity
- Refractory spine pain
- Spinal instability
- Neurologic compromise

Advanced age (>60 years old) and the presence of immunodeficiency are relative indications for surgery before a trial of medical treatment alone. Progressive neurologic deficits usually necessitate urgent operative intervention. Postoperative spinal infections after fusion procedures also usually warrant surgical débridement.

The key surgical principles for treating spinal infections are adequate débridement, neural element decompression (if necessary), and rigid stabilization. Anterior infections, including vertebral osteomyelitis and discitis, should be approached with an anterior decompression and débridement. This procedure commonly is followed by anterior structural bone grafting and a concomitant or staged posterior instrumentation (Fig. 8-5). Choices for anterior structural support are numerous, but current recommendations are for autogenous structural bone graft (e.g., fibula, rib, tricortical iliac crest). Cortical allograft and vascularized bone graft

also are used, but allografts may harbor residual microbes more readily. Anterior instrumentation, in addition to bone grafting, has been successful in the cervical spine when treating infection and may obviate the need for posterior instrumentation (Fig. 8-6). Some surgeons now are using metal cages successfully for anterior reconstruction in the thoracic and lumbar spine without increasing the risk of recurrent infection. In a preliminary study, titanium cages were associated with a 58% reduction in hospital time, a decrease in brace time, an improvement in sagittal alignment, and an 18% reduction in postoperative complications compared with other methods. Widespread use of anterior instrumentation has been limited, however, by concerns over the potential for pathogen incubation on metal implants. Examples of anterior instrumentation include plates, rods, and metal cage devices (Fig. 8-7). The addition of posterior instrumentation allows more rigid spinal fixation, which may lead to earlier mobilization and diminished pain.

Posterior approaches alone rarely are indicated for decompression alone except when directed at posteriorly located epidural abscesses without anterior spinal involvement. In general, results have been poor when attempting posterior decompression without fusion in other circumstances.

Although not as common as the combined anterior/posterior approach, some surgeons advocate posterior decompression and fusion alone. Decompression of anterior elements and placement of a strut graft through a posterior approach is more technically demanding, but results have

## TABLE 8-4  SURGICAL INDICATIONS FOR PYOGENIC SPINE INFECTIONS

Failure of nonoperative treatment
Neurologic compromise (static or progressive)
Sepsis
Spinal instability
Progressive or advanced spinal deformity
Refractory pain
Need for pathogen identification
Relative indications:
    Incompetent immune system
    Age >60

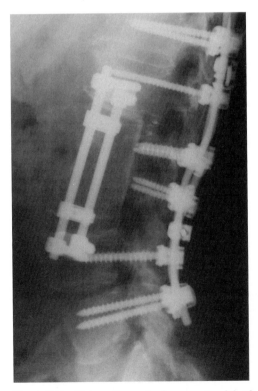

**Figure 8-5**  Plain radiograph after anterior débridement, anterior strut grafting (femoral allograft) with instrumentation, and posterior fusion with instrumentation. This treatment was performed for multisegmental pyogenic osteomyelitis.

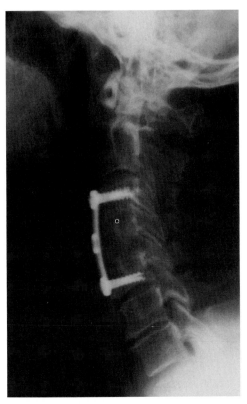

**Figure 8-6** Plain radiograph after anterior cervical débridement and fusion with anterior instrumentation only. This was performed for the infection seen in Figure 8-4.

been encouraging in several series. If the posterior spinal elements and epidural space are free of infection, some surgeons advocate immediate (rather than delayed) placement of posterior instrumentation.

# POSTOPERATIVE MANAGEMENT

Postoperative antibiotic courses should be similar to the drug regimens discussed in the nonoperative treatment section. After decompression of an epidural abscess without bone involvement, parenteral antibiotics may be administered for only 2 weeks after surgery. The proper postoperative antibiotic regimens should be based on isolation and sensitivity results and sequential laboratory markers (ESR and CRP). Patients with a history of intravenous drug abuse should be covered empirically for gram-negative infection.

Rehabilitation after operative treatment depends on the specific surgical management. Patients who undergo anterior decompression and fusion without instrumentation should be protected with 3 months of external stabilization, whereas patients with combined anterior/posterior procedures may not require long-term bracing or casting. Despite these general guidelines, surgeon preference is the rule when determining postoperative immobilization parameters. Despite these differences, most surgeons recommend early and progressive mobilization to prevent bed rest-associated morbidity.

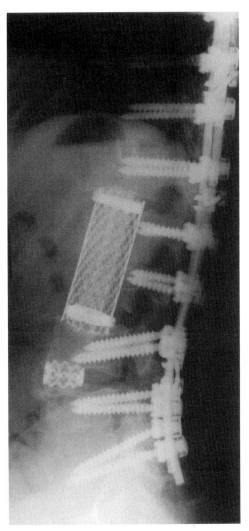

**Figure 8-7** Postoperative radiograph shows the use of metal cage instrumentation anteriorly after débridement of infection in these areas. Autograft or allograft bone can be used to fill and supplement the cages.

Postoperative infections after fusion or large decompression procedures should be thoroughly débrided and irrigated. Hardware most often is left in place, but exchanging metal rods or loose screws can be done. Suction drains should be placed or the wound should be packed open. Serial débridements may be necessary for appropriate treatment, and occasionally tissue flaps or tissue expanders are employed for adequate hardware and wound coverage.

# SUGGESTED READING

Arens S, Schlegel U, Printzen G, et al. Influence of materials for fixation implants on local infection: an experimental study of steel versus titanium DCP in rabbits. J Bone Joint Surg Br 1996;19: 109–116.

Bender CE, Berquist TH, Wold LE. Imaging-assisted percutaneous biopsy of the thoracic spine. Mayo Clin Proc 1986;61:942–950.

Cahill DW, Love LC, Rechtine GR. Pyogenic osteomyelitis of the spine in the elderly. J Neurosurg 1991;74:878–886.

Digby JM, Kersley JB. Pyogenic non-tuberculous spinal infection: an analysis of thirty cases. J Bone Joint Surg Br 1979;61:47–55.

Eismont F, Bohlman H, Soni P, et al. Pyogenic and fungal vertebral osteomyelitis with paralysis. J Bone Joint Surg Am 1983;65:19–29.

Fehlings MF, Cooper PR, Errico TJ. Posterior plates in the management of cervical instability: long term results in 44 patients. J Neurosurg 1994;81:341–349.

Garcia A, Grantham SA. Hematogenous pyogenic vertebral osteomyelitis. J Bone Joint Surg Am 1960;42:429–436.

Ratcliffe JF. Anatomic basis for the pathogenesis and radiologic features of vertebral osteomyelitis and its differentiation from childhood discitis. Acta Radiol Diag 1985;26:137–143.

Sampath P, Rigamonti D. Spinal epidural abscesses: a review of epidemiology, diagnosis, and treatment. J Spinal Disord 1999;12:89–93.

Tang HJ, Lin HJ, Liu YC, et al. Spinal epidural abscess—experience with 46 patients and evaluation of prognostic factors. J Infect 2002;45:76–81.

# ATYPICAL SPINE INFECTIONS

**ROBERT K. EASTLACK**
**CHRISTOPHER P. KAUFFMAN**

Atypical spine infections are fungal and granulomatous processes that are most often tuberculous in nature. In addition to *Mycobacterium tuberculosis*, however, there are a wide variety of other offending agents. Tuberculosis is of particular concern owing to its high worldwide prevalence, with approximately one third of the world's population infected. Immigration, drug resistance, and immunoincompetency have resulted in a reemergence of tuberculosis within the United States, necessitating a new focus on its complications and treatments. Immunosuppression and immunodeficiency resulting from various conditions also have led to an increased incidence of nontuberculous granulomatous infections.

## PATHOGENESIS

### Etiology

Most atypical spine infections involve *M. tuberculosis* (also called *Pott's disease*) so that much of the causal discussion becomes skewed by its particular population dynamics. An overall increase in incidence of all atypical infections within the United States can be attributed to immunocompromised states. Iatrogenic immunosuppression and human immunodeficiency virus (HIV)-related immunodeficiency are the primary contributors to this immune system dysfunction. In particular regard to *M. tuberculosis*, the resurgence is due to several other factors as well. There is an ever-increasing immigration of infected individuals into the United States from Asia and Central America. In addition, poor compliance to antimicrobial treatment regimens has generated multidrug resistance within strains of the organism. Finally, elderly and homeless populations continue to grow, with an accompanying increase in nursing home and shelter inhabitants.

Fungal osteomyelitis also has become more prevalent owing to increased immunosuppression, but it has been associated with greater use of hyperalimentation and chronic disease states. Inoculation of the spine is almost universally through hematogenous or lymphatic spread with atypical infections, generally after infestation through other portals

to the body (e.g., respiratory, genitourinary, indwelling blood vessel catheters).

## Epidemiology

Nearly one third of the world's population is infected with *M. tuberculosis*, and approximately 10% to 15% of infections disseminate to extrapulmonary sites. Only about 5% of these patients have spinal involvement (approximately 0.5% of the world's population, or 30 million people). Approximately 50% of extrapulmonary bone involvement is found in the spine. In the United States, the incidence was at 17 per 100,000 in 1991, with that level trending upward over the last several decades.

As with pyogenic infections, atypical spine infections have a predilection for elderly patients. Immigrants, homeless individuals, alcoholics, intravenous drug abusers, and other immunocompromised individuals (iatrogenic or HIV-related) compose the bulk of people at highest risk in the United States. Children are the most commonly affected in underdeveloped nations. Approximately one third of patients with active tuberculosis of the spine develop neurologic impairment. Although most cases of tuberculosis are caused by *M. tuberculosis*, *M. africanum* and *M. bovis* infection also may result in "tuberculosis," as we know it.

*Aspergillus* species are ubiquitous in the environment and rarely cause serious disease in healthy individuals. Other atypical organisms have particular geographic proclivities. Brucellosis is found more commonly in areas that do not pasteurize milk. *Mycobacterium avium-intracellulare* also is associated with poorly processed milk. Blastomycosis has a regional distribution in the southeastern and midwestern United States, whereas coccidiodomycosis exists in the southwestern United States, Central America, and South America. Histoplasmosis has a large endemic focus within the central eastern United States. *Cryptococcus neoformans* is found in the excreta of birds, such as pigeons and chickens.

Additional organisms include *Actinomyces israelii*, *Cryptococcus*, *Histoplasma*, and *Treponema pallidum* (syphilis) (Table 9-1). Compared with *M. tuberculosis*, the other atypical infections are exceedingly rare, but a broad differential

## TABLE 9-1 ORGANISMS CAUSING ATYPICAL SPINE INFECTIONS

Atypical bacteria
   *Mycobacterium tuberculosis* (most common)
   *Mycobacterium bovis*
   *Mycobacterium africanum*
   *Mycobacterium avium-intracellulare*
   *Brucella abortus*
   *Bartonella henselae*
   *Actinomyces israelii*
   *Nocardia asteroides*
   *Sporothrix schenckii*
Spirochetes
   *Treponema pallidum*
Fungi
   *Coccidioides immitis*
   *Histoplasma capsulatum*
   *Aspergillus* species
   *Cryptococcus neoformans*
   *Candida* species
Yeast
   *Blastomyces dermatitidis*

diagnosis should be considered when taking the history and ordering laboratory studies.

## Pathophysiology

Many fungal and granulomatous organisms are contracted through inhalation; however, other avenues are possible.

Most atypical spine pathogens infect the vertebral column through hematogenous spread. Another less common conduit is the lymphatic system, which frequently can be accessed by mycobacteria via lung or pleural drainage. Spinal involvement rarely occurs via direct spread.

*M. tuberculosis* is highly contagious through inhalation of aerosolized organisms. After primary pulmonary involvement, many individuals develop secondary or disseminated disease, in which extrapulmonary metastasis occurs. Involvement of the vertebral body begins with deposition of bacilli in the vertebral body, then accumulation of monocytes, epithelioid cells, and Langerhans' cells as part of a delayed-type hypersensitivity reaction. The continued host immune response of the human body generates the enlarging masses and subsequent damage to surrounding tissues. Expansion occurs within the vertebral body and progresses outward along the longitudinal ligaments or into the spinal canal, but usually spares the intervertebral disc space (Fig. 9-1). Granulomas of the vertebral body may originate in the metaphyseal area near the subchondral end plates, anteriorly or centrally, and typically cause collapse and deformity (Table 9-2). Tuberculosis of the spine almost always occurs in the anterior elements, although it has been identified rarely in the posterior elements (vertebral arch) or primarily in neural tissue.

Much less is known about the precise pathophysiology of other atypical pathogens, but it is thought to be similar in most cases. Granulomatous reactions are elicited by most of these organisms, and indolent clinical courses tend to be the rule, rather than the exception. Syphilis has shown an ability to involve the neural elements directly, causing tabes dorsalis and bone structures by gumma formation. Gummas

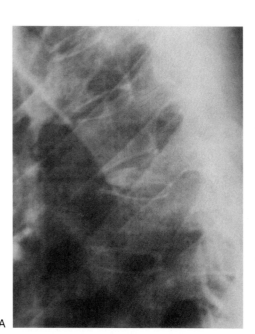
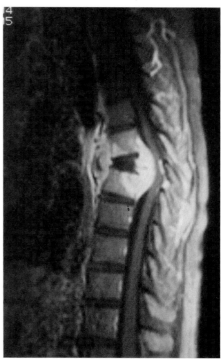

**Figure 9-1** Plain radiograph (**A**) and T1-weighted MRI (**B**) of a patient with tuberculous infection of the thoracic spine. Note the kyphotic gibbous deformity at the site of collapse.

## TABLE 9-2 TUBERCULOSIS: SITES OF VERTEBRAL ORIGIN

Vertebral body
Anterior
   Associated with migration along longitudinal ligament
   Produces "scalloping" of anterior spine on radiographs
Central
   Usually restricted to one segment
   Collapse and deformity common
Paradiscal/peridiscal
   Associated with end plate deposition of organisms
   > 50% of cases
Posterior elements
   Rare
   Neurologic deficits common

are granulomatous lesions with large central zones of acellular necrosis.

# DIAGNOSIS

## Clinical Features

In contrast to pyogenic infections, back pain usually presents late in the disease with atypical spine infections. There is wide variability in initial clinical presentation due to the insidious nature of these infections. A thorough history often elicits reports of constitutional symptoms, such as weakness, night sweats, chills, weight loss, and fever. In the presence of HIV or other chronic disease states, it can be difficult to make immediate assumptions based on such symptoms, however. Pain often begins with vertebral collapse or spinal deformity and tends to occur more frequently with thoracic involvement.

A thorough neurologic examination should be performed. Paraplegia is the most common neurologic deficit with tuberculosis of the spine. Deficits usually are associated with cervical or thoracic involvement, with a 40% incidence of cord compression when found in the cervical spine. Physical examination sometimes may reveal draining sinus tracts. Truncal rigidity and muscle spasm can be present.

## Laboratory Features

Laboratory tests may show the following:

- Anemia
- Albumin and total protein depletion
- Lymphocytosis
- Mild elevations in white blood cell count and erythrocyte sedimentation rate

Indicators of systemic inflammatory response (erythrocyte sedimentation rate and C-reactive protein) are less elevated than with pyogenic infections.

Purified protein derivative (PPD) skin testing and an anergy panel should be performed on all patients suspected of having tuberculosis. Sputum samples or biopsy specimens should be sent for acid-fast stains and cultures. Identification by culture can take 8 weeks, but polymerase chain reaction and other serologic testing can accelerate the identification process.

Brucellosis can be associated with an elevated D-arabinitol-to-L-arabinitol ratio, whereas Fontana-Masson stain should be ordered if cryptococcosis is the suspected pathogen. Aspergillosis, as with many other fungi, can be detected with potassium hydroxide preparations of affected tissues.

## Radiologic Features

The radiographic work-up should be similar to the work-up for pyogenic infections. The insidious nature of atypical spine infections causes plain film abnormalities to develop more slowly. Bone changes often are advanced on initial radiographs owing to the delayed presentation of many patients. These include the following:

- Collapse of affected segments that may lead to kyphotic gibbous deformities (Fig. 9-2)
- Paravertebral encroachment, which may be seen more readily on x-rays of atypical infections, as the granulomatous mass spreads outward, along the longitudinal ligaments

A chest x-ray should be ordered on all patients suspected of having tuberculosis.

Magnetic resonance imaging (MRI) is the preferred modality for confirming spinal involvement and can help differentiate infection from metastatic disease. Although pyogenic infection can be differentiated from neoplastic disease by the former involving (crossing) the disc space, this distinction may not be useful in evaluating tuberculosis of the spine. Tuberculous infections often spare the disc space. With advanced disease, large anterior soft masses eventually can involve two or more vertebral bodies, however, "crossing" disc spaces. Use of gadolinium may help define the margins of active disease when performing an MRI. Computed tomography scans can be used for diagnostic imaging, if MRI is unavailable, and may serve as an important tool for surgical decision making. Nuclear medicine studies have roles similar to their roles in pyogenic infections.

## Diagnostic Work-up Algorithm

The reader is referred to the pyogenic infection work-up in Chapter 8 because it is similar at the outset. Based on history of a more indolent process, and a higher suspicion of atypical pathogens, unique laboratory studies (e.g., serologic testing, PPD) may be warranted initially. Public health agencies also may need to be contacted early in the process.

# TREATMENT

## Nonoperative Treatment

Infectious disease consultation should be considered when dealing with any atypical spine infection. In the United States, tuberculosis infection confirmation activates a cas-

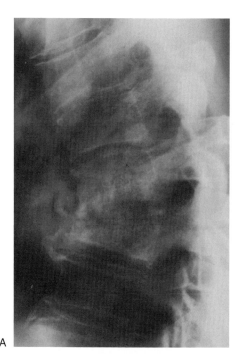
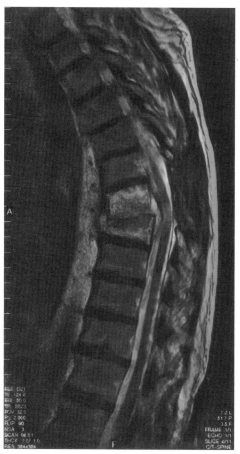

**Figure 9-2** Thoracic brucellosis infection shows adjacent segment involvement and kyphotic collapse on plain film (**A**) and T1-weighted MRI (**B**).

cade of public health events. Pharmacotherapy is the primary modality of treatment for patients with tuberculosis of the spine. Because of progressively worsening drug resistance, treatment regimens almost always consist of at least two medications. A standard empirical regimen comprises isoniazid, rifampin, pyrazinamide, and streptomycin (or ethambutol). Withdrawal of one or more medications may be prudent when cultures and sensitivities are complete. Treatment duration recommendations range from 6 to 12 months and can vary based on clinical response. Vitamin $B_6$ should be given with isoniazid to prevent peripheral neuritis. Other medications used to treat tuberculosis include aminosalicylic acid, capreomycin, cycloserine, ethionamide, kanamycin, thioacetazone, and viomycin. These medications may be employed in the case of multidrug resistance, immunodeficiency, or inability to tolerate standard regimens.

Early brucellosis can be treated with amphotericin B and 5-fluocytosine, but advanced disease usually requires surgical intervention. Aspergillosis most often can be treated with amphotericin B and rifampin initially. Amphotericin B and ketoconazole combined are effective for coccidioidomycosis and blastomycosis.

Bracing during medical treatment plays a similar role as in pyogenic infections. Reduction of pain, stabilization for improved healing of infection, and prevention or slowing of deformity all are theoretical advantages.

## Operative Treatment

Surgical indications include the following (Table 9-3):

- Neurologic compromise
- Failure of nonoperative treatment
- Spinal instability
- Progressive spinal deformity
- Need for tissue biopsy
- Advanced disease
- Recurrence of infection

Because of the insidious nature of most atypical infections, urgent surgical intervention usually is required only in the presence of progressive neurologic deficit. Surgical decompression has shown significantly better results for neurologic recovery than pharmacotherapy alone, even when done late in the disease course.

Surgical approach varies according to the site of infection. Most commonly, the anterior spine is affected and requires anterior débridement. Rarely, posterior elements are the focus of infection, and in these unique circumstances, a posterior approach and débridement can be employed. Although there have been reported series of anterior débridements alone, progression of kyphosis has been significant in nearly one fifth of these patients. For this reason, current recommendations are for anterior reconstruction

## TABLE 9-3  SURGICAL INDICATIONS FOR ATYPICAL SPINE INFECTIONS

Failure of nonoperative treatment
Neurologic deficit
Spinal instability
Progressive spinal deformity (usually kyphotic)
Advanced disease
Need for open biopsy (unidentified pathogen)
Recurrence of infection

via strut graft. There are many different strut graft options, including autograft and allograft bone, to be used for anterior reconstruction. Anterior instrumentation can be added for reinforcement without significant concern for persistent infection from hardware seeding, as is the case with pyogenic infections. It also may reduce the chances of progressive kyphotic deformity. Options for anterior instrumentation are evolving, but currently they include plates, rods, and metal cages.

Posterior instrumentation should be considered with unstable anterior constructs or when multilevel corpectomies are performed. Because of the increased likelihood of growth-related deformity, some authors have advocated posterior instrumentation in all immature spines after anterior débridement. In addition, any posterior débridements that destabilize the spinal column necessitate posterior instrumentation for definitive treatment. Posterior fusion alone, in the presence of anterior disease, does not protect adequately against progressive kyphotic deformity. In the presence of advanced kyphosis, posterior closing wedge or pedicle-subtraction osteotomy variants may be considered

for deformity correction. These are technically demanding procedures with increased neurologic risks.

Postoperatively, all patients should be treated adequately with proper pharmacotherapy. External support with bracing or other methods of immobilization should be chosen based on fixation quality and surgeon preference.

Complications are common with surgical intervention, but with current treatments consisting of surgery and medications, the cure rate is high. Fusion success with the recommended approaches exceeds 90%.

## SUGGESTED READING

Babhulkar SS, Tayade WB, Babhulkar SK. Atypical spinal tuberculosis. J Bone Joint Surg Br 1984;66:239–242.

Bass JB Jr, Farer LS, Hopewell PC, et al. Treatment of tuberculosis and tuberculosis infection in adults and children. Am J Respir Crit Care Med 1994;149:1359–1374.

Bloom BR, Murray CJ. Tuberculosis: commentary on a reemergent killer. Science 1992;257:1055–1064.

Currier BL, Eismont FJ. Infections of the spine. In: Herkowitz HN, Garfin SR, Balderston RA, et al, eds. The spine, 4th ed. Philadelphia: WB Saunders, 1999:1207–1258.

Davidson PT. Treating tuberculosis: what drugs, for how long? Ann Intern Med 1990;112:393–395.

Freilich D, Swash M. Diagnosis and management of tuberculous paraplegia with special reference to tuberculous radiculomyelitis. J Neurol Neurosurg Psychiatry 1979;42:12–18.

Halpern AA, Rinsky LA, Fountain S, et al. Coccidiomycosis of the spine: unusual roentgenographic presentations. Clin Orthop 1979; 140:78–79.

Konstam PG, Besovsky A. The ambulatory treatment of spinal tuberculosis. Br J Surg 1962;50:26–38.

Medical Research Council Working Party on Tuberculosis of the Spine. A 15-year assessment of controlled trials of the management of tuberculosis of the spine in Korea and Hong Kong. J Bone Joint Surg Br 1998;80:456–462.

Moon MS. Tuberculosis of the spine: controversies and a new challenge. Spine 1997;22:1791–1797.

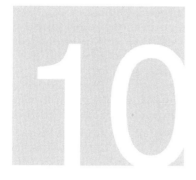

# PRIMARY BENIGN TUMORS

PHILIP S. YUAN
CHOLL W. KIM
MICHAEL J. YASZEMSKI
BRADFORD L. CURRIER

Patients with spinal tumors constitute only a small percentage of patients who seek medical attention for symptoms originating in the spine. Delays in diagnosis can occur if a physician is not aware of the features that distinguish spinal tumors from nonneoplastic spinal disorders. Advances in imaging techniques allow earlier diagnosis and more sophisticated preoperative evaluation and staging of spinal tumors. Advances in systemic therapy, surgical implants, biomaterials, and surgical procedures have improved greatly short-term and long-term outcomes in tumor patients. The principles of orthopaedic oncology that apply to the extremities may not always be applicable to the spine.

Primary tumors of the spine represent less than 10% of all bone tumors and are much less common than metastatic lesions. Benign primary lesions affecting the spinal column are far less common than malignant primary tumors. Diagnosing primary benign tumors of the spine requires a high index of suspicion. Spinal tumors occur in patients of all ages and at any level of the spine. Primary spinal tumors in children and adolescents are usually benign. Benign tumors are rare in elderly patients. In one series of patients with primary spinal tumors, nearly 70% of patients age 18 years or younger had benign spinal lesions. Of tumors in patients older than age 18 years, only 20% were benign. The mean age at diagnosis was 20.9 years for patients with benign tumors.

Benign primary spinal tumors involve the vertebral body and posterior elements of the spine, with a slight overall predilection for the posterior elements. Location of the lesion is an important factor in determining the type of tumor. Osteoid osteoma and osteoblastoma have a tendency to affect the posterior elements, whereas eosinophilic granuloma (EG) and hemangioma tend to involve the vertebral body.

## DIAGNOSIS

### History and Physical Examination

Pain is the most consistent complaint among patients presenting with primary benign spinal tumors. In one series,

pain was the chief complaint in nearly 85% of patients with spinal tumors. Pain usually is localized to the site of the lesion in the neck or back, but radicular pain is not atypical. The pain is characterized classically as progressive, gradual in onset, worse at night, and often unrelated to activity. Occasionally, patients may associate the onset of symptoms with a traumatic episode, which may be the case when fracture occurs in an already compromised vertebra. Pathologic fracture also should be considered, however, when patients report the acute onset of pain in the absence of severe trauma. In the case of nerve root compression by tumor or as the result of vertebral collapse, patients may present with radicular symptoms. Less commonly, patients may have weakness; bowel or bladder incontinence; palpable mass; or constitutional symptoms such as fevers, chills, night sweats, weight loss, and anorexia. Spinal deformity also may result from spinal tumors. Focal kyphosis can result from any tumor that causes vertebral body collapse. Scoliosis is a common presentation of osteoid osteoma and osteoblastoma in younger patients.

A careful physical examination is important in diagnosing primary spinal tumors. Focal tenderness is more common with spinal tumors than in nonneoplastic disease. Thorough inspection of the entire spine, including the forward bending test, is essential to look for any curvature of the neck or back. Torticollis or scoliosis, especially when associated with pain, can be attributed to spinal tumors. Although a tumor rarely presents with a palpable mass, it is important to palpate along the spinous processes from occiput to sacrum and the paraspinous areas. Subtle findings, such as a stiff neck or back, may be the only clues to recognizing a benign spinal tumor.

### Laboratory Evaluation

Laboratory work-up is recommended but may not be helpful in establishing a diagnosis. Complete blood cell count, erythrocyte sedimentation rate, and C-reactive protein level usually are obtained. In most patients with benign primary spinal tumors, the results of laboratory studies are normal.

## Imaging Studies

Routine radiography is relatively insensitive in identifying benign spinal tumors. Before a bone lesion can be detected by plain radiography, at least 30% to 50% bone loss must be present. If scoliosis is evident radiographically, spinal tumor must be included in the differential diagnosis. Technetium bone scanning is much more sensitive than biplanar radiography because it measures bone activity and can identify small lesions before extensive bone loss. Computed tomography (CT) has become a valuable imaging tool, particularly in evaluating bone anatomy and determining the amount of canal compromise after pathologic fracture of the spine. CT is not the best screening tool, however, because it does not image the entire spine. Magnetic resonance imaging (MRI) has become the criterion standard in the diagnosis of primary benign spinal tumors. MRI can detect the presence of a bone lesion, identify the presence of neural compression, and determine the involvement of the surrounding soft tissue. This information is crucial for treatment planning.

The most common benign lesions of the spine are:

■ Osteochondroma
■ Osteoid osteoma
■ Osteoblastoma
■ Hemangioma
■ Aneurysmal bone cyst (ABC)
■ EG and giant cell tumor (GCT)

Each has distinct features in terms of clinical presentation, location, imaging characteristics, and treatment. Each tumor type is discussed individually, with the exception of osteoid osteoma and osteoblastoma, which are differentiated primarily by size.

# OSTEOID OSTEOMA AND OSTEOBLASTOMA

In any young patient with axial pain, painful scoliosis, or radicular or referred-type pain into the extremities, osteoid osteoma and osteoblastoma should be included in the differential diagnosis. Osteoid osteoma and osteoblastoma are identical histologically and have similar clinical presentations. Pain usually is the first and only complaint of patients with these lesions. The pain associated with osteoid osteoma classically is relieved with aspirin when it involves the extremities, but this finding is not as consistent when the spine is involved. The only physical examination findings that may be present are spinal stiffness and spinal curvature in the form of scoliosis or torticollis. A few features distinguish between these two benign lesions (Table 10-1).

Idiopathic scoliosis is rarely painful, and another cause for the deformity needs to be sought when pain is an associated complaint. Benign osteoid osteoma and osteoblastoma may be the most common causes of scoliosis provoked by pain. These tumors, which often are difficult to view radiographically, tend to involve the cancellous lamina and pedicle of the vertebra but have been found in rib heads adjacent to thoracic vertebrae (Fig. 10-1).

**TABLE 10-1  DISTINGUISHING FEATURES OF OSTEOID OSTEOMA AND OSTEOBLASTOMA**

| Feature | Osteoid Osteoma | Osteoblastoma |
|---|---|---|
| Typical age at presentation (yr) | 10–20 | Early 20s |
| Size of lesion (cm) | <1.5 | 2 |
| Histologic characteristics | Osteoid nidus surrounded by sclerotic bone | Less sclerotic, more expansile mass |

Osteoid osteoma and osteoblastoma are believed to produce pain even before they are visible radiographically. Technetium bone scanning is nearly 100% accurate in locating these lesions, even when plain radiographs are negative, by showing a nonspecific but intense focal uptake of activity (Fig. 10-2). When these tumors are evident radiographically, they classically are located on the concavity of the deformity and near the apex. The painful lesion leads to muscle spasm on the ipsilateral side of the spine and increases pressure on the vertebral epiphyseal growth plate. The resulting growth retardation coupled with the continued growth of the contralateral vertebral epiphysis may result in true rotatory scoliosis.

The goals of treatment for osteoid osteoma and osteoblastoma of the spine are:

■ Early diagnosis
■ Complete excision
■ Relief of pain
■ Correction of deformity

The key to early diagnosis is having a high index of suspicion. Despite the fact that the natural course of osteoid osteoma may lead to spontaneous remission, a lesion should be removed when it is diagnosed because the time interval

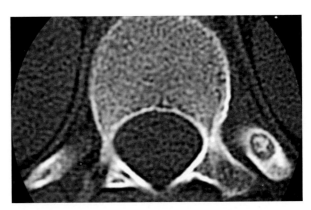

**Figure 10-1**  Axial CT scan shows osteoid osteoma in the rib head of the 12th thoracic vertebra. The patient was a 12-year-old boy with a 1-year history of back pain and mild spinal asymmetry. He was treated with en bloc excision.

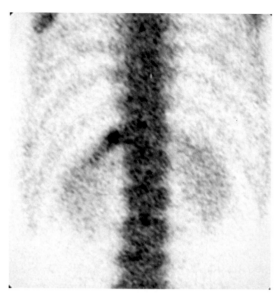

**Figure 10-2**    Technetium bone scan shows focal uptake in T12 rib head.

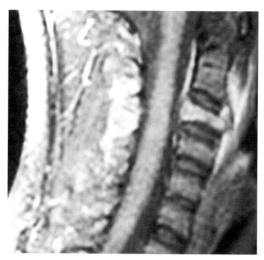

**Figure 10-3**    Sagittal MRI shows collapse of C3 vertebral body consistent with vertebra plana in a 10-year-old boy with a 3-week history of neck pain and torticollis.

before remission can range from 2 to 8 years, and the scoliosis can become structural during that time. Complete surgical resection via a posterior approach usually is curative. Patients often note immediate relief. Resolution of scoliosis also has been reported extensively in the literature. In patients who develop symptoms at or around skeletal maturity, complete resolution of scoliosis after excision is the norm. In skeletally mature individuals, the deformity is thought to be merely a postural response to the painful stimulus. Because these patients have no vertebral rotation, the deformity resolves instantaneously after the lesion is excised. In a growing child, the interrelationships of the age of onset of symptoms, duration of symptoms, severity of deformity, and time interval to skeletal maturity have a direct bearing on whether scoliosis resolves after removal of the painful stimulus. The crucial time span between the onset of symptoms and surgical excision has been reported to be 12 to 15 months. Complete or almost complete resolution of the spinal deformity occurred in nearly every patient treated before or within the crucial period. When diagnosis was delayed beyond 18 months, permanent deformity was the rule. Early diagnosis and complete excision of osteoid osteomas and osteoblastomas of the spine can reduce the duration of pain and may reverse associated deformity.

## EOSINOPHILIC GRANULOMA

Solitary EG has been described in nearly every bone of the body. The spine is one of the more common locations for these lesions, with only the skull and pelvis being involved more frequently. EG, a granulomatous process of unknown cause, destroys focal areas of bone. The disease occurs more frequently in young people than in adults.

The typical patient is a child with neck or back pain and without a history of serious trauma. In contrast to most benign tumors, the onset of pain usually is relatively sudden. Cervical lesions often present with associated torticollis. Neurologic deficits as a result of EG of the spine have been reported but are not common. The radiographic appearance is variable when EG involves the spine. Changes range from early cavitation and destruction of the body or neural arch to partial collapse, producing wedge-shaped deformities, and finally to uniform and complete collapse of a vertebral body. This uniform collapse is called *vertebra plana* (Fig. 10-3). Vertebra plana also can be attributed to other lesions, but it classically is associated with EG. EG always must be considered in the differential diagnosis of a lytic vertebral lesion, especially in children.

Confirming the diagnosis of EG requires biopsy and tissue analysis. Needle biopsy seldom is used today because of the tendency for negative results or inadequate amounts of recovered tissue. Open biopsy is preferred to establish the diagnosis of EG. Reports in the literature have shown satisfactory healing of these lesions with simple biopsy or even immobilization.

Treatment of EG involving the spine is controversial. EG is a self-limited disease, and simple biopsy and curettage alone frequently are sufficient to stimulate regression of the lesion. Radiotherapy also has been successful in treating this disease, even with associated neural deficit. Surgical decompression is rarely necessary. Spinal stabilization sometimes is necessary when open biopsy destabilizes a vertebral segment.

## ANEURYSMAL BONE CYST

ABCs are rare in the spine. First described in 1942, ABCs are neither aneurysms nor cysts, but the name has remained. Similar to EGs, ABCs are found in nearly every bone in the body, with a slight predilection for the spine.

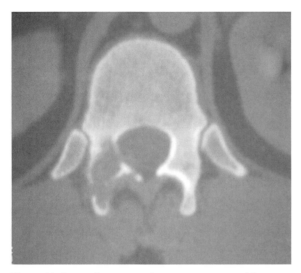

**Figure 10-4** Axial CT scan shows an aneurysmal bone cyst involving the posterior elements. The lesion is lytic and expansile with blown-out, thinned cortex. This 35-year-old patient presented with a 6-week history of sudden-onset back pain.

The cause of this condition also is unknown. These lesions tend to affect adolescents and have a slightly higher incidence in females.

Ill-defined somatic pain and stiffness are the clinical features associated with a typical ABC. Depending on the size of the lesion, the complete spectrum of neurologic signs also has been seen in patients with an ABC of the spine. Because of their tendency to expand, ABCs are associated more frequently with neural deficits than any of the aforementioned benign spinal tumors. They also may invade adjacent vertebrae. These lesions are identified easily on radiographs.

The typical ABC of the spine involves the neural arch and is an expansile, osteolytic cavity that often contains fine strands of bone surrounded by an eggshell of blown-out cortex (Fig. 10-4). Approximately 60% of ABCs involve the posterior elements, and the remainder involve the vertebral body. They are most common in the lumbar spine. Destruction of a vertebral body leading to vertebra plana has been observed in patients with ABC.

Needle biopsy is futile in most cases, and neurologic deterioration has been reported as a result of hemorrhage from the needle tract. Open biopsy is recommended to establish a diagnosis, usually at the same setting as definitive treatment. Complete excision at the time of biopsy reduces the risk of recurrence. A quarter of ABCs recur with incomplete resection. ABC is a benign condition in which disappearance has occurred spontaneously and with simple biopsy, making treatment controversial. If neurologic deficits are present, surgical decompression with excision of the tumor is recommended. Surgical instrumentation and fusion is indicated only when instability develops either from the extent of the lesion or from the surgical debulking. The prognosis tends to be excellent overall in the treatment of ABC of the spine.

# HEMANGIOMA

In contrast to other primary benign tumors, vertebral hemangioma is relatively common. Autopsy studies have shown an overall incidence of 10% of the population. Most cases are asymptomatic and undiagnosed. Pain and neural deficit have been reported in association with hemangioma of the spine but not typically. Less than 1% of vertebral hemangiomas are believed to be symptomatic. The thoracic spine is the usual location for these lesions, and multiple-level involvement is common. The diagnosis of hemangioma frequently can be made on the basis of plain radiographs.

Classically, prominent vertical striations are visible on anteroposterior and lateral views of the spine because of the thickened trabeculae of the affected vertebral body. Pathologic compression fractures also can occur in patients with hemangiomas. CT provides further information about cord impingement or pathologic fracture. MRI also can be helpful for surgical planning. Vertebral hemangioma can present as a cold defect on bone scintigraphy.

Treatment rarely is necessary for spinal hemangioma because most lesions are asymptomatic, incidental radiographic findings. Radiotherapy is the most common treatment for symptomatic lesions and has an antiinflammatory effect on these benign, slow-growing tumors. Radiotherapy is easy to use and is a highly effective analgesic treatment modality. In the rare patient who requires surgical decompression, it should be preceded by angiography, and preoperative embolization should be done whenever possible. Surgical excision may be difficult because of the vascularity of the tumor. Radiotherapy often is used to supplement the surgery in cases of subtotal resection.

# OSTEOCHONDROMA

Osteochondromas are benign cartilaginous tumors of bone that arise from any zone of endochondral bone formation. They develop by progressive endochondral ossification in anomalous foci of metaplastic cartilage in the periosteum. They make up almost 10% of all bone tumors and 40% of all benign tumors. Osteochondromas are common in the appendicular skeleton but occur rarely in the spine (<5%). These lesions can be solitary or multiple when they occur as part of the genetic disorder called *hereditary multiple exostoses*.

Solitary osteochondroma has a predilection for the cervical spine; the C2 vertebra is the most common location. OCs also originate in the thoracic and lumbar spine but rarely in the sacrum. In the case of multiple exostoses, the incidence of lesions occurring in the thoracic region increases.

Osteochondroma usually is located eccentrically in the neural arch of the vertebra. Vertebral body involvement is uncommon. Slow growth of the tumor can result in protrusion into the neuroforamen or spinal canal. The plain radiograph of osteochondroma is characteristic: a sessile or pedunculated osteoblastic mass adjacent to the marrow and the cortex of the bone from which it arises. When the spine is involved, the mass may be difficult to discern because of obstruction by the surrounding bone column. CT and MRI can be used to locate the lesion.

The clinical presentation is usually one of local pain. Neurologic symptoms also occur frequently in vertebral osteochondroma, as a consequence of the tendency for expansile growth into the spinal foramen. Occasionally a palpable mass can be detected on physical examination of the spine. There also is a case report in the literature of scoliosis resulting from a thoracic osteochondroma.

Treatment of symptomatic spinal osteochondroma usually consists of:

- Surgical decompression, when indicated
- Complete resection of the tumor

Total excision prevents the progression of neurologic deficits and eliminates the potential risk of sarcomatous degeneration, which reportedly occurs in 1% of the solitary lesions and in 5% to 15% of multiple osteochondromas.

# GIANT CELL TUMOR

GCT is the most aggressive of all benign spinal tumors. GCT constitutes 2% to 8% of all primary bone tumors but accounts for less than 1% of all vertebral tumors. GCT is found more commonly in the sacrum and less frequently in the anterior portion of the spinal column. Patients with GCT of the spine usually present with focal pain and neurologic deficit caused by the locally aggressive nature of the lesion. Pathologic compression fractures also are common and can result in relatively acute onset of pain. Patients often have symptoms for several months, however, before presenting to a physician.

Detection of sacral GCT can be difficult on plain radiographs, but spinal GCT usually presents as an osteolytic lesion involving the vertebral body. Although the radiographic appearance may be similar to ABC and metastatic disease, the diagnosis usually can be made if all information is taken into consideration. Although ABC and GCT appear as expansile osteolytic lesions, ABC tends to present in the posterior elements, and GCT almost always is situated anteriorly. The age at diagnosis in patients with GCT is usually 15 to 30 years, and metastatic tumors generally present later in life. CT scans define the bony anatomy more clearly and show osteolysis and possibly soft tissue extension. CT is especially important in the preoperative evaluation of these tumors because complete resection is crucial to eradication of local disease.

GCT of the spine has the worst prognosis of all benign tumors. Some authors believe that GCT is moderately malignant in nature. Despite its benign histologic appearance, transformation to malignancy or recurrence after high-dose irradiation was reported in the early 1970s. More recent studies indicate that radiotherapy can be used safely and effectively to treat GCT, especially as a supplement to surgical excision. Optimal treatment of GCT of the spine is controversial.

The treatment of choice for GCT is complete surgical excision; however, this is not always possible in the spine. The proximity of the spinal lesion to vital structures makes en bloc resection difficult. Intralesional excision may be

necessary, and adjuvant therapy is recommended. The options for adjuvant treatment include:

- Cement implantation
- Using a high-speed bur around the periphery of the lesion
- Irradiation

Prolonged disease-free survivals have been reported after resection or curettage and radiotherapy, although additional procedures were required in some patients because of local recurrence. With more aggressive surgical excision, radiotherapy is unnecessary, and good disease-free intervals have been obtained.

# SUMMARY

Benign primary tumors are uncommon in the spine. These tumors tend to occur in young patients and are diagnosed less commonly in adults. A high index of suspicion is essential for early diagnosis and improved overall patient satisfaction. The interval between the onset of symptoms and eventual diagnosis and treatment has prognostic importance. The clinical presentation usually provides clues to alert the physician to suspect spinal neoplasm. Although benign spinal tumors may remain asymptomatic for extended periods, when symptoms develop, they usually are a consequence of one or more of the following:

- Expansion of the cortex by tumor mass
- Compression of the spinal cord or nerve roots
- Pathologic fracture
- Spinal instability

Surgical treatment is recommended in most benign tumors of the spine and usually is curative. In planning the surgical approach, the anatomic extent of the lesion must be understood, and the need for stabilization or reconstruction must be anticipated. Improved imaging techniques have assisted greatly in this process. In general, vertebral body lesions should be approached anteriorly, and posterior tumors should be approached from behind.

Each type of benign tumor that involves the spine has features that distinguish it from the others and assist in making the correct diagnosis. When the diagnosis is made, the appropriate treatment can be applied. With advances in imaging techniques, equipment, biomaterials, and surgical procedures, prognosis and outcomes have improved greatly in the management of these lesions.

# SUGGESTED READING

Akbarnia BA, Rooholamini SA. Scoliosis caused by benign osteoblastoma of the thoracic or lumbar spine. J Bone Joint Surg 1981; 63A:146–155.

Bandiera S, Gasbarrini A, De Iure F, et al. Symptomatic vertebral hemangioma: the treatment of 23 cases and a review of the literature. Chir Organi Mov 2002;87:1–15.

Fowles JV, Bobechko WP. Solitary eosinophilic granuloma in bone. J Bone Joint Surg 1970;52B:238–243.

Graham GN, Browne H. Primary bony tumors of the pediatric spine. Yale J Biol Med 2001;74:1–8.

Hay MC, Paterson D, Taylor TK. Aneurysmal bone cysts of the spine. J Bone Joint Surg 1978;60B:406–411.

Jackson A, Hughes D, St. Clair Forbes W, et al. A case of osteochondroma of the cervical spine. Skeletal Radiol 1995;24:235–237.

Keim HA, Reina EG. Osteoid-osteoma as a cause of scoliosis. J Bone Joint Surg Am 1975;57:159–163.

Malawski SK. The results of surgical treatment of primary spinal tumors. Clin Orthop 1991;272:50–57.

Ransford AO, Pozo JL, Hutton PA, et al. The behaviour pattern of the scoliosis associated with osteoid osteoma or osteoblastoma of the spine. J Bone Joint Surg 1984;66B:16–20.

Sherk HH, Nicholson JT, Nixon JE. Vertebra plana and eosinophilic granuloma of the cervical spine in children. Spine 1978;3:116–121.

Yan SC, Xu QM, Lin JR. Diagnosis and treatment of giant cell tumor in the thoracic spine. J Surg Oncol 1989;40:128–131.

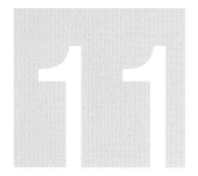

# 11 PRIMARY MALIGNANT TUMORS

**CHOLL W. KIM**
**PHILIP S. YUAN**
**MICHAEL J. YASZEMSKI**
**BRADFORD L. CURRIER**

Primary malignant tumors of the spine are extremely rare. Most spinal tumors are caused by metastatic spread from another primary source. Of the 2000 primary bone sarcomas and 6000 soft tissue sarcomas diagnosed annually in the United States, only about 10% arise from the spine. Primary tumors of the spinal column are difficult to classify as one clinical entity. The complex neuromusculoskeletal development of the spine may account for a spectrum of malignant tumors with distinct biologic behaviors. Because of biologic heterogeneity, these tumors have variable sensitivity to radiotherapy and chemotherapy. Characterization of the tumor type is essential for devising an appropriate therapeutic strategy.

## DIAGNOSIS

### History and Physical Examination

The most common presenting symptom is back pain. Approximately 85% of patients with spinal tumors have back pain as the initial complaint. Diagnosis often is delayed because this presentation resembles degenerative disc disease. Useful clues to an underlying neoplasm include slow, gradual onset of pain in the absence of a clear traumatic event; gradual progression of pain; persistent pain at night; and symptoms unrelated to mechanical stressors. Although uncommon, systemic signs may occur, such as weight loss, loss of appetite, fevers, night sweats, and generalized malaise. Only 10% of patients have a severe neurologic deficit, but many have radicular pain. Patients with spinal tumors are more likely to have a specific site of focal tenderness compared with patients with degenerative disc disease, particularly if they also have a pathologic compression fracture of the involved vertebrae. In younger patients, primary malignant tumors usually are osteosarcoma or Ewing's sarcoma (Table 11-1). In older adults, the most common primary malignant spinal tumors are multiple myeloma (the most common primary tumor of the spine), chordoma, chondrosarcoma, and malignant fibrous histiocytoma. Sacral tumors often are diagnosed late in the disease process because

the mass is difficult to appreciate on general musculoskeletal examination. More than half of all patients with a sacral chordoma have a palpable mass on rectal examination, however, at the time of presentation.

### Imaging Studies

Primary bone tumors, such as chondrosarcoma or osteosarcoma, often have an associated soft tissue mass extending beyond the vertebral body and evident on plain radiographs. Bone destruction, increased sclerosis, and deformity also may be appreciated on plain radiographs. Magnetic resonance imaging (MRI) is the study of choice after plain radiography. With the addition of gadolinium, MRI can be used to evaluate surrounding soft tissue, neural elements, and disc involvement and to distinguish between extradural, intradural, extramedullary, and intramedullary tumors (Fig. 11-1A, B). Pathologic lesions that involve the posterior elements, especially in patients younger than age 30 years, are more likely to be benign than malignant. Diffusion-weighted MRI of the bone marrow helps to differentiate benign from pathologic vertebral compression fractures. Malignant pathologic vertebral compression fractures are hyperintense. In contrast, benign compression fractures are isointense or hypointense on diffusion-weighted images. Infections usually start in the disc space and spread to adjacent vertebral bodies above and below the disc space, whereas neoplasms start in the vertebral body, and the disc inhibits their spread (see Fig. 11-1A).

Additional imaging modalities often are used to obtain further information. Bone scintigraphy allows the entire skeleton to be screened. Bone scintigraphy can identify lesions 2 to 12 months before they can be seen on plain radiography. Certain tumors, particularly multiple myeloma, may not be seen on this study, however. A solitary lesion in the spine raises the possibility of a primary bone sarcoma. Computed tomography (CT) with intrathecal contrast is a useful alternative when MRI is unavailable or cannot be tolerated. Cerebrospinal fluid can be obtained for additional testing. CT is better than MRI for determining the degree

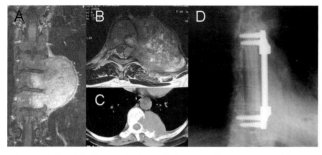

**Figure 11-1** (**A**) Coronal MRI of thoracic fibrosarcoma. Tumor invades bone readily but is inhibited by the disc space. (**B**) Axial T2-weighted image shows canal invasion and spinal compression. (**C**) Axial CT scan shows bone destruction, but contralateral pedicle is free of destruction. (**D**) Radiograph after resection and reconstruction. Anterior column support is provided by a strut allograft, fixed with anterior instrumentation.

of bone involvement (Fig. 11-1C). Positron emission tomography and single-photon emission computed tomography are newer techniques that may be used in lieu of bone scintigraphy, but they are not widely used to date.

## Biopsy

Before formulation of a treatment plan, a tissue diagnosis must be established. Techniques for obtaining tissue for pathologic evaluation include fine-needle aspiration, percutaneous core needle biopsy, and open biopsy. The choice of technique depends on the location and extent of the tumor. Fine-needle aspiration is useful when the tissue component is large and only a small sample is required. CT guidance is the most common localization technique. Percutaneous core needle biopsy is useful when bone tissue is needed. A common approach is transpedicular with multiplanar fluoroscopy. The diagnostic yield of needle aspiration and core biopsy of tumors is relatively high (75% to 85%) but lower for infections (50% to 60%). In all cases, the biopsy tract should be placed to allow its excision during future procedures. The surgeon who would perform any resection procedure should participate in the initial patient evaluation and biopsy.

## STAGING

### Enneking Classification

The Enneking system for classification of benign and malignant tumors has been used for more than 20 years. Malignant tumors are staged according to histologic grade, compartmental location, and presence of metastases. Stage I tumors are low grade, and stage II tumors are high grade. Stage III tumors are tumors of any grade with regional or distant metastases. Each stage is subdivided further into *A* for intracompartmental tumors and *B* for extracompartmental tumors. A high-grade osteosarcoma with extension into the paravertebral soft tissues is Enneking stage IIB. The

Enneking staging system was designed for pelvic and extremity tumors. In the spine, differentiating extension of tumor into the spinal canal and the anterior paraspinal soft tissue is crucial for surgical treatment. This key characteristic is not reflected, however, in the Enneking staging system.

### Weinstein-Boriani-Biagnini Classification

The Weinstein-Boriani-Biagnini staging system was designed specifically for the spine. This system divides the vertebra into 12 sectors in a clock-face arrangement (Fig. 11-2). Tumor location is defined further by involvement in six areas:

- *A*, extraosseous soft tissues
- *B*, intraosseous (superficial)
- *C*, intraosseous (deep)
- *D*, extraosseous (extradural)
- *E*, extraosseous (intradural)
- *M*, metastasis.

Detailed staging and surgical planning can be accomplished with this system.

## TREATMENT

Treatment is tailored individually according to tumor type, location, and size and the patient's neurologic status and overall health. Treatment modalities include (see Table 11-1):

- Chemotherapy
- Radiotherapy
- Surgery.

### Chemotherapy and Radiotherapy

Chemotherapy is used most commonly to treat osteosarcoma, Ewing's sarcoma, and multiple myeloma. For Ewing's sarcoma and osteosarcoma, multiagent chemotherapy achieves 90% tumor kill; subsequent surgical resection leads to 75% to 85% 5-year survival. For osteosarcoma, tumor kill of less than 90% with preoperative chemotherapy has a 25% 5-year survival. Postoperative radiotherapy is instituted if margins are positive after surgical resection. Chordomas and chondrosarcomas are not well treated with chemotherapy or radiotherapy. Treatment is mainly marginal or wide en bloc resection. Multiple myeloma is treated best initially with radiotherapy. If systemic involvement is widespread, chemotherapy may be added. Solitary plasmacytoma is an isolated form of multiple myeloma. Although it occurs rarely as a true solitary lesion, the 5-year survival is significantly better than for disseminated multiple myeloma (see Table 11-1).

### Surgery

Surgical treatment focuses on several goals:

- The neural elements are protected from further injury caused by compression.

A. Extraosseous
   soft tissues
B. Intraosseous
   (superficial)
C. Intraosseous
   (Deep)
D. Extraosseous
   (Extradural)
E. Extraosseous
   (Intradural)

M. Metastasis

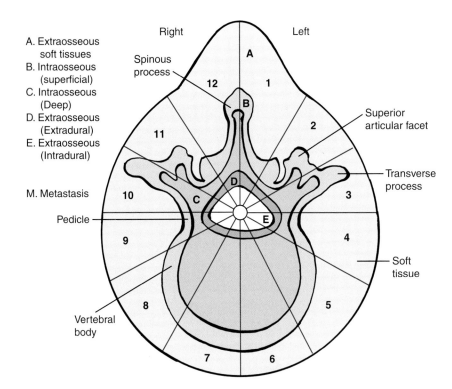

**Figure 11-2** Weinstein-Boriani-Biagini staging system for spine tumors. On the transverse plane, the vertebra is divided into 12 radiating zones (numbered clockwise 1 to 12) and into five layers (A to E from prevertebral to dural involvement). The longitudinal extent of the tumor is recorded. Each tumor is identified by the numbers of the sectors occupied, the letters of the layers involved, and the vertebrae of occurrence. (From Boriani S, Chevalley F, Weinstein JN, et al. Chordoma of the spine above the sacrum: treatment and outcome in 21 cases. Spine 1996;21:1569–1577.

## TABLE 11-1  PRIMARY MALIGNANT TUMORS OF THE SPINE

| Disease | Age at Presentation (yr) | Chemotherapy Sensitive | Radiation Sensitive | 5-yr Survival (%) | Unique Characteristics |
|---|---|---|---|---|---|
| Multiple myeloma | 60 | Yes | Yes | 18 | Radiation and chemotherapy are treatments of choice |
| Solitary plasmacytoma (spine) | 50–60 | Yes | Yes | 60 | Single myeloma lesion in the spine. Rare |
| Osteosarcoma | 10–20 | Yes | Unclear in spine | 25–85 | Only 2% occur in spine. Survival depends on tumor kill with chemotherapy. >90% tumor kill with preoperative chemotherapy leads to 85% 5-yr survival. <90% tumor kill leads to 25% 5-yr survival |
| Secondary osteosarcoma | 40–60 | Poor response | No | 5–17 | Usually arises from Paget's or irradiated bone. 30% of all osteosarcomas of spine |
| Ewing's sarcoma | Children, young adults | Yes | Yes | 75 | 3.5% occur in spine. Good 5–7 yr survival with multimodality treatment |
| Chondrosarcoma | 50–60 | No | No | 20–75 | 2–10% occur in spine. Prognosis greatly improved with en bloc excision with negative margins |
| Chordoma | 40–60 | No | No | 50 | Usually reaches large size before metastasizing. Arises from notochord. Half of all sacral tumors |

- Spinal stability is maintained.
- Resection is performed to achieve a cure.

The Musculoskeletal Tumor Society has recommended a uniform system to describe surgical margins. Surgical procedures are defined as intralesional, marginal, wide, or radical.

In intralesional procedures, the tumor is entered during the resection. The tumor can be entered intentionally, when a curettage technique is used, or inadvertently, when access to normal tissue around the tumor mass is limited. In a marginal resection, the plane of dissection is through the reactive zone of the tumor. A wide resection requires that a cuff of normal tissue completely surround the tumor mass. At no place should the tumor be encountered in either marginal or wide resection. Within the canal, the dura must be excised in most cases to achieve a wide tumor margin. A radical resection is not possible in the spine because this requires that the entire compartment be resected. Even if the patient were willing to sacrifice the spinal cord or cauda equina, the spinal canal causes the compartment to extend the entire length of the spine, making radical resection impossible. En bloc resections in the spine have marginal or wide margins.

Wide resections can be performed for low sacral lesions, with only minor neurologic sequelae (Fig. 11-3). Most patients maintain relatively normal bowel and bladder function if the resection spares one S3 nerve root and both S1 and S2 nerve roots (Table 11-2). Preserving all the nerve roots on one side (unilateral S1-5), while resecting the entire contralateral side, also enables most patients to maintain normal bowel and bladder function.

When a malignant tumor resides in the mobile spine, marginal or wide resections can be performed by anterior and posterior approaches (Fig. 11-4). To remain outside the tumor, a portion of the canal ring, such as one of the pedicles, must be free of tumor. Remaining outside the tumor is important because local recurrence correlates highly with poor clinical outcome. The likelihood of recurrence is two to five times higher if the surgical margin contains tumor cells, whether it is microscopically or macroscopically evident. The method of tumor resection also may be important. A piecemeal resection, even though negative margins in the

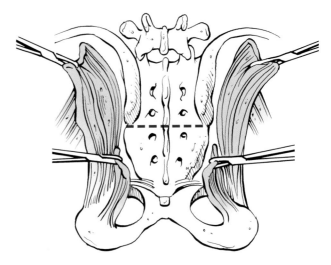

**Figure 11-3** Technique of low sacral resection of a chordoma or other primary tumor distal to S3. (From Levine AM, Crandall DG. The textbook of spinal surgery, 2nd ed. New York: Lippincott-Raven, 1997:1983–2006.

tumor bed are achieved, leads to a higher recurrence rate than en bloc resection.

After tumor resection, the spine generally requires stabilization. In most cases, anterior column support is established with a strut graft or cage. Instrumentation provides fixation until arthrodesis is achieved (see Fig. 11-1D). Stable fixation, which is imperative after resection, may require anterior and posterior fixation with long constructs.

## Outcomes

The overall outcome of combined medical and surgical treatment varies, depending on tumor type, size, location, and overall patient health (see Table 11-1). Most authors agree that persons with life expectancies greater than 3 months should be offered surgical treatment, even if palliative, to treat pain caused by spinal instability and neurologic dysfunction attributable to neural compression.

## TABLE 11-2 BOWEL AND BLADDER FUNCTION AFTER SACRAL RESECTION

| Resection | Spared Level | Normal Bowel No. (%) | Normal Bladder No. (%) |
|---|---|---|---|
| Bilateral S2–5 | Both S1 | 0/10 (0) | 0/10 (0) |
| Bilateral S3–5 | Both S2 | 2/5 (40) | 3/12 (25) |
| Bilateral S4–5 | Both S3 | 4/4 (100) | 9/13 (69) |
| Variable | Unilateral S3 | 2/3 (67) | 3/5 (60) |
| Unilateral S1–5 | Contralateral S1–5 | 7/8 (87) | 8/9 (89) |

From Todd LT Jr, Yaszemski MJ, Currier BL, et al. Bowel and bladder function after major sacral resection. Clin Orthop 2002; 397: 36–39.

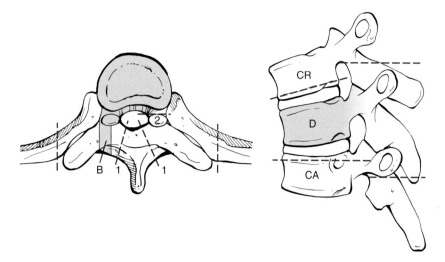

**Figure 11-4** Method of resection of tumor involving almost the entire vertebral body. When one portion of the canal ring is intact, such as a pedicle, a two-stage resection can be performed with negative margins. The laminae initially are removed along dashed lines *1*. The uninvolved transverse process and posterior part of the pedicle are removed up to dashed line *2*. *B* is the site of a previous transpedicular biopsy. *D* is the involved vertebra. If more than one vertebra is involved, *D* is the most cranial involved vertebra. *CR* is the adjacent uninvolved cranial vertebra. *CA* is the adjacent caudal uninvolved vertebra.

## SUMMARY

Evaluation and treatment of primary malignant tumors of the spine are challenging. A unique feature of musculoskeletal tumors of the spine, compared with tumors in the extremities and pelvis, is the proximity of the neural elements. En bloc resection with negative margins is difficult to achieve without injuring the spinal cord and nerve roots. Successful treatment relies on prompt diagnosis based on clinical history and physical examination findings, advanced imaging, and carefully planned biopsy. Multidisciplinary treatment regimens are applied according to tumor cell type, location, and size and overall patient health. Surgical treatment must consider not only the tumor itself, but also the status of the surrounding neural elements and the overall biomechanical stability of the spine.

## SUGGESTED READING

Bergh P, Gunterberg B, Meis-Kindblom JM, et al. Prognostic factors and outcome of pelvic, sacral, and spinal chondrosarcomas: a center-based study of 69 cases. Cancer 2001;91:1201–1212.

Boriani S, Biagini R, De Iure F, et al. Lumbar vertebrectomy for the treatment of bone tumors: surgical technique. Chir Organi Mov 1994;79:163–173.

Boriani S, Chevalley F, Weinstein JN, et al. Chordoma of the spine above the sacrum: treatment and outcome in 21 cases. Spine 1996; 21:1569–1577.

Boriani S, Weinstein JN, Biagnini R. Primary bone tumors of the spine: terminology and surgical staging. Spine 1997;22:1036–1044.

Cheng EY, Ozerdemoglu RA, Transfeldt EE, et al. Lumbosacral chordoma: prognostic factors and treatment. Spine 1999;24: 1639–1645.

Fidler MW. Radical resection of vertebral body tumours: a surgical technique used in ten cases. J Bone Joint Surg 1994;76B:765–772.

Oliverio PJ, Davis BT. Imaging of malignant and benign lesions of the vertebral column. Semin Spine Surg 2000;12:2–16.

Sundaresan N, Steinberger AA, Moore F, et al. Indications and results of combined anterior-posterior approaches for spine tumor surgery. J Neurosurg 1996;85:438–446.

Talac R, Yaszemski MJ, Currier BL, et al. Relationship between surgical margins and local recurrence in sarcomas of the spine. Clin Orthop 2002;127–132.

Todd LT Jr, Yaszemski MJ, Currier BL, et al. Bowel and bladder function after major sacral resection. Clin Orthop 2002;36–39.

Weinstein JN, McLain RF. Primary tumors of the spine. Spine 1987; 12:843–851.

York JE, Berk RH, Fuller GN, et al. Chondrosarcoma of the spine: 1954 to 1997. J Neurosurg 1999;90:73–78.

# METASTATIC TUMORS

**MATTHEW P. WALKER**
**MICHAEL J. YASZEMSKI**
**CHOLL W. KIM**
**ROBERT M. TALAC**
**BRADFORD L. CURRIER**

The management of metastatic disease of the spine is a challenging problem for spinal surgeons. Advances in imaging and spinal instrumentation have enhanced the surgeon's ability to perform complex decompression and stabilization procedures. The lack of a validated set of criteria to predict bone instability and neurologic compromise has made it difficult, however, for the surgeon to decide whether aggressive surgical intervention or nonoperative care is best for the individual patient. This chapter presents current information on the evaluation and treatment of metastatic disease of the spine.

## PATHOGENESIS

The spine is the most common site of skeletal metastases. In North America, approximately 18,000 new patients annually present with spinal cord compression from metastatic diseases. After a review of nearly 2800 cases from various clinical series, Mclain and Weinstein reported that nearly 60% of all metastases to the spine were secondary to breast, lung, or prostate carcinomas; myeloma; or lymphoma (Table 12-1). The high frequency of metastatic involvement of the spine is not completely understood. Batson's paravertebral venous plexus may play an important role. This plexus of thin-walled, valveless vessels most likely accounts for the predilection of metastatic lesions for specific areas of the spine. Metastases from breast and lung carcinomas more commonly occur in the thoracic spine, and prostate carcinoma metastases are more common in the lumbar spine.

## DIAGNOSIS

### History

Pain is the most common presenting complaint for patients with metastatic disease of the spine. The pain is gradual in onset, but progressive. It often is unrelenting, nonmechanical pain that worsens at night. Early in the disease course, the pain is usually axial. As the disease progresses, neural compression can lead to complaints of radicular pain.

Neurologic symptoms usually occur late in the disease process, and they frequently prompt patients to seek medical attention. Motor weakness has been reported as the presenting symptom in 76% of patients, including 17% who were paralyzed; 50% of the patients noted numbness or paresthesias. Radicular pain often accurately localized the tumor to within one or two vertebral levels. Isolated bowel and bladder dysfunction are uncommon presenting complaints but, when present, must be assessed with magnetic resonance imaging (MRI) or computed tomography (CT)-myelography to determine if neurologic compression is the cause. Patients who present with progressive neurologic signs or symptoms must undergo urgent evaluation. Severe deficits or rapidly progressive deficits portend a much poorer prognosis.

Other important historical items are unintentional weight loss, anorexia, fatigue, hemoptysis, hematuria, hematochezia, hematemesis, and tobacco use. The presence of a mass in the neck, axilla, breast, abdomen, or groin and a previous personal or family history of malignancy should be sought.

### Physical Examination

A general physical examination, including a rectal examination, should be performed on all patients suspected of having metastatic disease of the spine. The examination should focus on areas in which most primary tumors occur, including the breasts, chest, prostate, abdomen, and lymphatic system. A detailed neurologic examination also must be performed and documented for future comparison if neurologic deterioration occurs. Localized spinal tenderness often is present over the area involved with tumor. Multilevel tenderness may represent multilevel disease.

### Radiography

The imaging modalities most useful in the assessment of metastatic disease of the spine include plain radiography, bone scan, CT, CT-myelography, and MRI. Each modality has advantages and limitations. Plain radiography is helpful in assessing overall spinal alignment and spinal instability.

## TABLE 12-1 PRIMARY TUMOR IN SPINAL METASTASES

| Primary Tumor | Spinal Metastases (%) |
| --- | --- |
| Breast | 21 |
| Lung | 14 |
| Myeloma | 9 |
| Prostate | 7.5 |
| Lymphoma | 6.5 |
| Kidney | 5.5 |
| Gastrointestinal | 5 |
| Thyroid | 2.5 |
| Miscellaneous | 29 |

Small metastatic lesions may be overlooked, however, because 30% to 50% of the trabecular bone must be destroyed before radiographic evidence of bone destruction is apparent. A technetium-99m bone scan is a useful test for identifying metastatic lesions with an osteoblastic response. False-negative scans do occur, however, most commonly with tumors having a minimal osteoblastic response, such as multiple myeloma. CT is helpful in defining bony integrity, which aids in the assessment of impending spinal instability and preoperative planning. CT-myelography is useful for patients who cannot undergo MRI for evaluation of neural element compression. Limitations of this technique include possible rapid neurologic deterioration caused by cerebrospinal fluid pressure shifts and the potential to miss additional sites of neural compression in the presence of a complete block.

MRI is the imaging modality of choice for evaluation of metastatic disease of the spine. Bone involvement, soft tissue extension, and neural element compression can be assessed in the same study. A sensitivity of 93% and a specificity of 97% for MRI have been reported in the assessment of metastatic disease. Gadolinium-enhanced MRI is not helpful in most cases of vertebral metastases.

Studies reviewing the usefulness of MRI in differentiating benign versus malignant compression fractures have shown mixed results. Complete bone marrow replacement by tumor, resulting in a low T1-weighted signal, has been described in 88% of metastatic fractures. In 77% of benign fractures, normal marrow elements were preserved on T1-weighted images. These findings helped to delineate benign versus malignant fractures. In contrast, other studies have shown a high false-positive rate when MRI was used to detect malignant compression fractures. Early in fracture healing, the presence of fracture hematoma, marrow signal changes, and paraspinal mass effect can lead to the misinterpretation of benign lesions as malignant. On the basis of this information, a reasonable approach for a neurologically intact patient presenting with an acute compression fracture is to provide symptomatic relief with bracing and analgesics, then regular follow-up. Patients with benign compression fractures usually improve markedly in 2 to 3 months. Patients with malignant compression fractures

have progressive symptoms and should undergo work-up at that time.

### Biopsy

Before treatment for metastatic disease of the spine can be initiated, the diagnosis must be confirmed. This is accomplished most readily by confirming the presence of a primary lesion through a metastatic work-up. This work-up includes CT scan of the chest, abdomen, and pelvis; chest radiograph; bone scan; and appropriate laboratory studies, including serum protein electrophoresis. When a primary lesion is identified, the presence of a metastatic lesion can be confirmed via needle or open biopsy. In the case of multifocal lesions, a biopsy specimen of the most accessible lesion should be obtained. When the diagnosis of metastatic disease has been confirmed, it is not necessary to obtain more biopsy specimens of the spine for subsequent lesions if the imaging studies and time interval are consistent with metastasis.

## TREATMENT

Treatment for metastatic disease of the spine is palliative, not curative. The goal of treatment is to maximize the patient's quality of life by providing pain relief and maintaining or restoring neurologic function. In most cases, this goal is reached through nonoperative means, primarily by chemotherapy and radiotherapy. For patients who do not respond to nonoperative treatment and are appropriate candidates, surgical intervention offers an opportunity to maintain or restore quality of life.

### Classification Systems

Several classification schemes have been proposed to guide treatment of patients with metastatic disease. The Harrington scheme divided patients with spinal metastases into five categories based on the extent of neurologic compromise and bone destruction:

- *Class I*: Patients have minimal neurologic involvement.
- *Class II*: Patients have involvement of bone without collapse or instability and minimal neurologic involvement.
- *Class III*: Patients have major neurologic impairment without spinal instability.
- *Class IV*: Patients have vertebral collapse with pain attributable to mechanical causes or instability but without severe neurologic compromise.
- *Class V*: Patients have vertebral collapse or instability with major neurologic impairment.

Class I and II patients generally obtain pain relief with chemotherapy or hormonal manipulation. If these modalities are unsuccessful, local radiotherapy is recommended. Class III patients usually respond to radiotherapy alone. If neurologic compromise is acute, the addition of corticosteroid treatment should be considered. Surgery is reserved for radioresistant tumors and progressive tumors after radiotherapy. Surgical treatment is recommended for class IV and V patients.

The Tokuhashi scheme is an assessment system to determine the prognosis and life expectancy of patients with metastatic spinal tumors. This system assigns a point value to six characteristics, and the total determines a prognostic score. Treatment recommendations are based on this prognostic score. The six characteristics are:

- General health condition (poor, 0 points; moderate, 1 point; good, 2 points)
- Number of extraspinal bone metastases ($\geq 3$, 0 points; 1 to 2, 1 point; 0, 2 points)
- Number of vertebral metastases ($\geq 3$, 0 points; 2, 1 point; 1, 2 points)
- Metastases to the major internal organs (unremovable, 0 points; removable, 1 point; no metastases, 2 points)
- Primary site of cancer (lung, stomach, 0 points; kidney, liver, uterus, others, unidentified, 1 point; thyroid, prostate, breast, rectum, 2 points)
- Spinal cord palsy (complete, 0 points; incomplete, 1 point; none, 2 points)

The Tokuhashi system was applied to 64 patients, and patients with a total score of 9 or higher survived an average of 12 months or longer, patients with a score of 8 or lower survived 12 months or less, and patients with a score of 5 or lower survived 3 months or less. On the basis of this information, it was recommended that patients with a score of 9 or higher undergo an excisional procedure, and a palliative operation was indicated for patients with scores of 5 points or less.

A similar prognostic scoring system proposed by Tomita provides a treatment strategy for patients with spinal metastases (Fig. 12-1). An appropriate surgical procedure is selected on the basis of a score derived by assessing three prognostic factors:

- Grade of malignancy (slow growth, 1 point; moderate growth, 2 points; rapid growth, 4 points)

- Visceral metastases (no metastasis, 0 points; treatable, 2 points; untreatable, 4 points)
- Bone metastases (solitary or isolated, 1 point; multiple, 2 points)

Summation of these three factors gives a prognostic score between 2 and 10. For patients with a score of 2 or 3 points, the treatment goal is long-term local control, and a wide or marginal excision is recommended. For patients with a score of 4 or 5 points, marginal or intralesional excision is recommended for medium-term local control. For patients with a score of 6 or 7 points, the treatment goal is short-term palliation, and palliative surgery is recommended. A score of 8 to 10 points indicates nonoperative supportive care. In a series of 61 patients, successful local control was achieved in 43 (83%) of 52 surgically treated patients.

Our general approach to evaluation and treatment of patients with metastatic disease of the spine is shown in Algorithm 12-1. For patients with an acceptable prognosis for survival (>3 to 6 months) and satisfactory medical status, surgical indications include progressive neurologic deficit secondary to neurologic compression from a radioresistant tumor; spinal instability; severe intractable pain unrelieved by nonoperative measures; radioresistant tumor that is enlarging, causing intractable pain or impending instability; and the need for a definitive histologic diagnosis. Patients with inadequate bone stock, multiple areas of epidural compression, or life expectancy less than 3 months generally are not considered for operative treatment.

## Criteria for Spinal Stability

To make appropriate treatment decisions, the presence of spinal instability in patients with metastatic disease of the spine must be determined. No validated system exists for

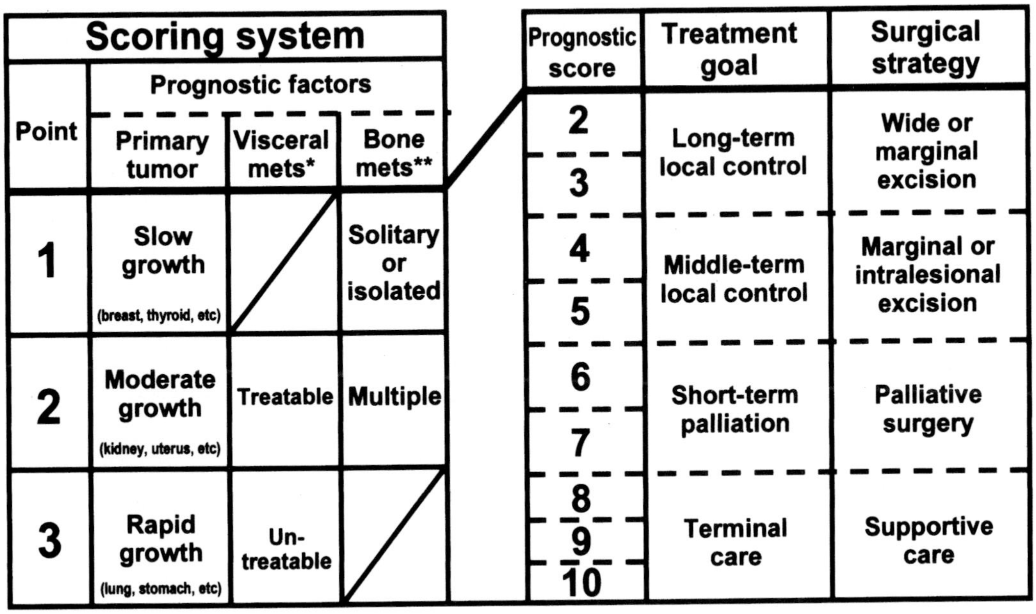

| Scoring system | | | | Prognostic score | Treatment goal | Surgical strategy |
|---|---|---|---|---|---|---|
| **Point** | **Prognostic factors** | | | | | |
| | **Primary tumor** | **Visceral mets\*** | **Bone mets\*\*** | | | |
| **1** | **Slow growth** (breast, thyroid, etc) | | **Solitary or isolated** | **2** | **Long-term local control** | **Wide or marginal excision** |
| | | | | **3** | | |
| **2** | **Moderate growth** (kidney, uterus, etc) | **Treatable** | **Multiple** | **4** | **Middle-term local control** | **Marginal or intralesional excision** |
| | | | | **5** | | |
| **3** | **Rapid growth** (lung, stomach, etc) | **Un-treatable** | | **6** | **Short-term palliation** | **Palliative surgery** |
| | | | | **7** | | |
| | | | | **8** | **Terminal care** | **Supportive care** |
| | | | | **9** | | |
| | | | | **10** | | |

**Figure 12-1**  Surgical strategy for spinal metastases (mets). (From Tomita et al.)

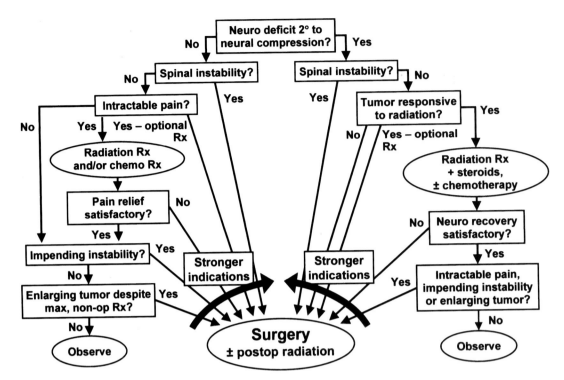

**Algorithm 12-1** Treatment algorithm for metastatic tumors of the spine.

making this determination, however. Nevertheless, multiple criteria have been proposed to determine the presence of spinal instability.

There are several classification systems for the assessment of spinal instability as it relates to spinal trauma. White and Panjabi defined stability as "the ability of the spine, under physiologic loads, to prevent initial or additional neurologic damage, severe intractable pain, and gross deformity." Radiographic criteria are used widely in the form of checklists for the diagnosis of spinal instability after cervical spine trauma. These criteria have not been validated for instability caused by neoplasms.

For thoracolumbar spinal trauma, the most widely used classification scheme is the three-column system of Denis:

- *Anterior column*—includes the anterior longitudinal ligament and the anterior half of the vertebral body, disk, and annulus
- *Middle column*—includes the posterior half of the vertebral body, disk, and annulus and the posterior longitudinal ligament
- *Posterior column*—includes the posterior elements and their associated ligaments and facet capsules

The spine is considered unstable if two of the three columns are disrupted.

Because these criteria were devised for the assessment of spinal stability after trauma, their usefulness in patients with metastatic disease of the spine has been questioned.

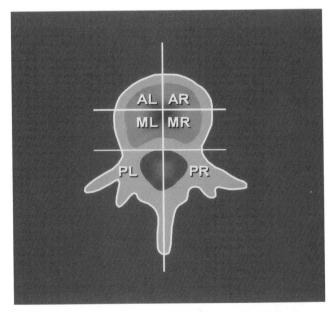

**Figure 12-2** Six-column system for evaluation of stability in spine tumors. (From Kostuik JP, Errico JN. Differential diagnosis and surgical treatment of metastatic spine tumors. In: Frymoyer JW, ed. The adult spine: principles and practice. Vol 1. New York: Raven Press, 1991:861–888.)

In an attempt to design a set of criteria specific for instability in spinal tumors, Kostuik and Errico proposed a six-column system (Fig. 12-2). The spine is divided into three columns as just described, then subdivided further into left and right halves. The spine is considered unstable if at least three of the six columns are destroyed or if more than 20 degrees of angulation is present.

In 1990, a classification system was developed by Asdourian et al to describe the stages of vertebral deformity in metastatic vertebral breast cancer. This information was used to define spinal instability and impending instability (Fig. 12-3). Four stages of vertebral deformity were recognized:

■ *Stage I*: A portion (IA), or all (IB), of the vertebral body marrow is replaced by tumor.
■ *Stage II*: Vertebral body collapse may occur at either one end plate (IIA) or both end plates (IIB). With progressive collapse, a bone fragment from the posterior vertebral body, termed the *delta sign*, may cause spinal canal encroachment.
■ *Stage III*: With end-stage collapse, resulting in either a kyphotic deformity (IIIA) or symmetric collapse (IIIB), the delta sign is consistently present.
■ *Stage IV*: Subluxation creates a translational deformity.

Type IA or type IB deformity is said to represent impending axial instability, and type II or type III deformity indicates axial instability. Impending translational instability is defined by type II or type III vertebral deformity with accompanying metastatic involvement of the posterior elements. Translational instability is present with type IV vertebral deformity. Treatment guidelines for metastatic vertebral breast cancer were proposed on the basis of these data. For impending axial instability, radiotherapy, chemotherapy, or hormonal manipulation was recommended. If spinal canal compromise was present, surgical decompression was considered if the tumor was radioresistant. When axial instability was present, with or without spinal canal compromise,

surgical stabilization was recommended. An anterior approach was advised for single-level involvement and a posterior approach for multilevel involvement. Impending translational instability, with or without canal compromise, was thought to indicate surgery with either an anterior-alone or a combined anterior-posterior approach. For translational instability, a posterior approach was recommended for stabilization, and a posterolateral or anterior approach was added for decompression.

To determine risk factors for vertebral collapse and to establish criteria for impending spinal instability, 100 thoracic and lumbar vertebrae with osteolytic lesions were analyzed radiologically by Taneichi et al. The data yielded a set of criteria to determine impending vertebral collapse in metastatic disease. For the thoracic spine (T1-10), the criteria are 50% to 60% involvement of the vertebral body with no destruction of other structures or 25% to 30% body involvement with costovertebral joint destruction. In the thoracolumbar and lumbar spine (T10-L5), the criteria are 35% to 40% involvement of the vertebral body or 20% to 25% body involvement with posterior element destruction.

In attempting to determine the presence of spinal instability in patients with metastatic disease, all of the available classification systems should be considered. None of these systems has been validated for use in metastatic disease, however, and all have limitations. These systems aid in guiding treatment, but other factors also should be considered when trying to determine the appropriate treatment option, including the biology of the specific tumor type, the radiosensitivity of the tumor, the response of the bone (blastic versus lytic metastasis), the patient's ability to withstand an operative procedure, the severity of pain, the quality of the host bone, and, above all, the wishes of the individual patient.

## Surgical Approach and Technique

The Weinstein, Boriani, and Biagnini surgical staging system for primary neoplasms also can be applied to metastatic lesions. In this system, the vertebral body is divided into zones of involvement to determine the optimal surgical approach. The tumor is classified by dividing each vertebra into 12 triangular zones (numbered 1 to 12 in clockwise order) and into five layers from the paravertebral extraosseous region to the intrathecal region (Fig. 12-4). The longitudinal extent of tumor involvement is obtained by recording the spinal segments involved. This system has been used to characterize primary bone tumors. The principles of the classification system, describing the anatomic location and providing information for surgical planning and communication, are applicable to metastatic spinal disease.

The percentage of satisfactory outcomes of the major clinical series of patients treated surgically for cord compression due to metastatic tumors has been tabulated by Mclain and Weinstein. The overall trend indicated improved results with anterior decompression, but the location of epidural compression should dictate the approach for decompression. After tumor excision, the spine must be reconstructed. In patients who have a limited life expectancy or in whom postoperative radiotherapy is planned, methyl methacrylate is a good choice for anterior recon-

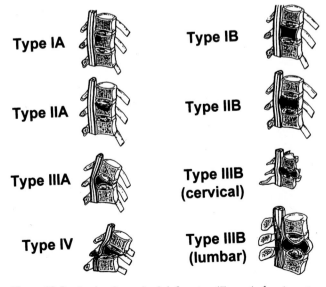

**Figure 12-3** Stage of vertebral deformity. (From Asdourian et al.)

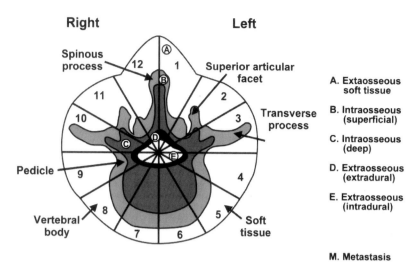

**Right**    **Left**

Spinous process

Superior articular facet

Transverse process

Pedicle

Vertebral body

Soft tissue

A. Extaosseous soft tissue

B. Intraosseous (superficial)

C. Intraosseous (deep)

D. Extraosseous (extradural)

E. Extraosseous (intradural)

M. Metastasis

**Figure 12-4**   Weinstein, Boriani, and Biagnini surgical staging system.

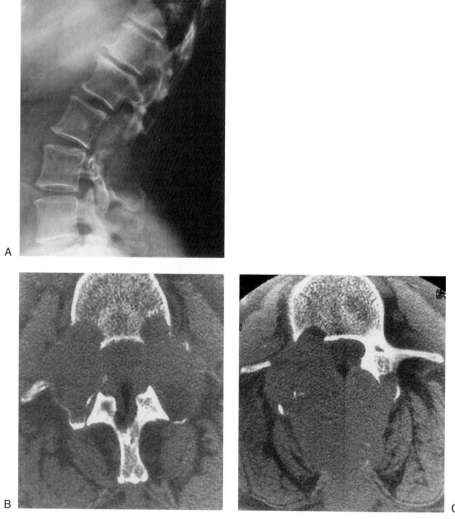

**Figure 12-5**   (**A**) Lateral radiograph of the lumbar spine shows lytic destruction of the posterior elements of L2 and L3. (**B**) CT scan shows bilateral pedicular involvement at L2. (**C**) CT scan shows right pedicular involvment at L3.

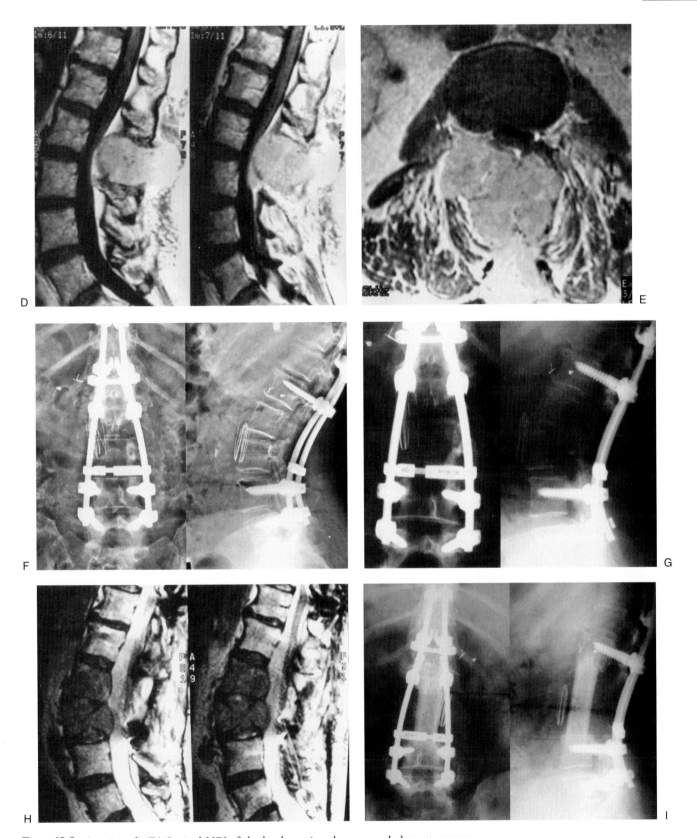

**Figure 12-5** (continued) (**D**) Sagittal MRI of the lumbar spine shows neural element compression. (**E**) Axial MRI shows spinal canal encroachment by metastatic lesion. (**F**) Posteroanterior and lateral radiographs after decompression and stabilization. (**G**) Posteroanterior and lateral radiographs show lytic destruction of L2 and L3 vertebral bodies. (**H**) Sagittal MRI shows tumor involvement of L2 and L3 vertebral bodies with neural compression. (**I**) Posteroanterior and lateral radiographs after L2 and L3 corpectomy and strut grafting.

struction because of its excellent resistance to compressive loads and immediate stabilizing effect. Posterior reconstruction with methyl methacrylate is discouraged because of its poor ability to resist tensile forces. When patient life expectancy is expected to be measured in years, the use of allograft or autograft bone is preferred because, without the support of a bony arthrodesis, methyl methacrylate is likely to fail with time.

## CASE EXAMPLE

In December 1997, a 64-year-old woman sought medical attention for back pain with an associated midline mass in the upper lumbar spine. Her history revealed a recent 15-lb weight loss and worsening back pain over the last month with no previous malignancy. Physical examination confirmed posterior midline tenderness over the mass and mild right-sided iliopsoas weakness. Radiographic evaluation of the spinal lesion was performed; the lateral plain film, CT, and MRI images are shown in Figure 12-5A through E. A work-up to identify a primary malignancy revealed a right kidney mass. Biopsy of the posterior spinal mass confirmed the diagnosis of metastatic renal cell carcinoma. Further metastatic work-up revealed no other lesions. The treatment decision at this time was to proceed with radiotherapy in an attempt to decrease tumor size and improve pain control. Despite maximal radiotherapy, the patient's symptoms progressed. Operative decompression and stabilization were planned. Before surgery, the patient developed a lower extremity deep venous thrombosis requiring filter placement.

In February 1998, the patient underwent preoperative embolization followed by L2-3 decompression with intralesional tumor excision and posterior spinal fusion from T10-L5 with instrumentation (Fig. 12-5F). The postoperative course was complicated by wound dehiscence that responded to operative débridement and dressing changes. She otherwise did well postoperatively with considerable improvement in pain.

One year later, the patient noticed a severe increase in back pain. Radiography and MRI revealed progression of disease into the L2 and L3 vertebral bodies (Fig. 12-5G, H). Because radiotherapy was maximized previously, treatment options were limited and consisted of either permanent bracing or surgery. The patient chose to proceed with operative intervention, and in March 1999, she underwent an L2 and L3 corpectomy with strut grafting after preoperative embolization (Fig. 12-5I). She did well postoperatively, with considerable improvement in back pain until her death 1.5 years later.

This case highlights several principles in the management of spinal metastasis. Initially the patient was thought to be in Harrington's class III, and radiotherapy was administered. Because renal cell cancer is not sensitive to radiotherapy, it would have been reasonable to perform surgery before radiotherapy. She did not respond to radiotherapy, and her symptoms progressed. Her Tokuhashi score showed that she was an acceptable candidate for surgery, and she underwent a posterior decompression and fusion. The results of anterior decompression and fusion are better than posterior procedures, but the surgery must be done from the side that is involved. Preoperative embolization is required in cases of renal cell metastasis to decrease intraoperative bleeding. A wound infection developed postoperatively. This complication occurs in approximately 35% of cases in which a posterior procedure is done after radiotherapy and is one of the reasons to consider early surgery in selected cases before radiation.

After treatment of her infection, the patient did well for 1 year until the disease spread into the anterior aspect of the spine and caused compression of the cauda equina. Her Tokuhashi score was still acceptable, and after another embolization, she underwent a decompression and stabilization procedure. This time the surgery was performed from the front because the disease was located anteriorly. She did well for another 1.5 years until she died. One could argue that when she initially presented to us, her Tomita score was only 3, and because the tumor type is not radiosensitive, we should have considered an en bloc spondylectomy to decrease the risk of local recurrence. In her case, however, the CT scan in Figure 12-5B shows that it would not have been possible to perform an en bloc spondylectomy with clear margins because of the extent of the tumor. The surgical classification schemes are helpful in determining the appropriate approach and likelihood of success when an aggressive treatment option is considered.

## SUMMARY

The treatment of patients with metastatic disease of the spine is a multidisciplinary effort that should follow a logical, orderly protocol such as the one proposed in Algorithm 12-1. The goal should be clearly defined. Patients considered for possible surgical intervention should have a reasonable life expectancy and have failed to attain treatment goals through nonoperative measures. If surgical intervention is chosen, the approach should be based on the location of epidural compression, presence of instability, or both. Stabilization can be achieved with methyl methacrylate, bone graft, and instrumentation, either alone or in combination. Above all, treatment should be tailored to the individual patient, always adhering to the goal of maximizing the patient's overall quality of life.

## SUGGESTED READING

Abdu WA, Provencher MT, Weinstein JN. Classification of spinal metastases. In: Heiner JP, Kinsella TJ, Zdeblick TA, eds. Management of metastatic disease to the musculoskeletal system. St. Louis: Quality Medical Publishing, 2002:371.

Barcena A, Lobato RD, Rivas JJ, et al. Spinal metastatic disease: analysis of factors determining functional prognosis and the choice of treatment. Neurosurgery 1984;15:820–827.

Edelstyn GA, Gillespie PJ, Grebbell ES. The radiologic demonstration of osseous metastases: experimental observations. Clin Radiol 1967;18:158–162.

Gilbert RW, Kim JH, Posner JB. Epidural spinal cord compression from metastatic tumor: diagnosis and treatment. Ann Neurol 1978; 3:40–51.

Harrington KD. Anterior decompression and stabilization of the spine as a treatment for vertebral collapse and spinal cord compression from metastatic malignancy. Clin Orthop 1988;233:177–197.

Kostuik JP, Errico JN. Differential diagnosis and surgical treatment of metastastic spine tumors. In: Frymoyer JW, ed. The adult spine: principles and practice. Vol 1. New York: Raven Press, 1991: 861–888.

Li KC, Poon PY. Sensitivity and specificity of MRI in detecting malignant spinal cord compression and in distinguishing malignant from benign compression fractures of vertebrae. Magn Res Imaging 1988;6:547–556.

Riley LH, Frassica DA, Kostuik JP, Frassica FJ. Metastatic disease to the spine: diagnosis and treatment. Instr Course Lect 2000;49: 471–477.

Tokuhashi Y, Matsuzaki H, Toriyama S, et al. Scoring system for the preoperative evaluation of metastatic spine tumor prognosis. Spine 1990;15:1110–1113.

# CERVICAL SPONDYLOSIS AND STENOSIS

**GREGORY T. BREBACH**
**JEFFREY S. FISCHGRUND**
**HARRY N. HERKOWITZ**

Cervical spondylosis is ubiquitous; it occurs as a person ages and manifests as degenerative changes in the cervical spine, including disc degeneration, facet arthropathy, osteophyte formation, ligamentous thickening, and straightening of cervical lordosis. When the spondylotic changes progress, they may cause narrowing of the cervical canal, leading to spinal stenosis. This condition can cause symptoms and signs consistent with radiculopathy, myelopathy, or a combination of both. *Spinal stenosis* is defined as a decreased space for the spinal cord. Spondylosis often is thought of as a progressive and dynamic process, with most patients with radiographic findings compatible with spondylosis remaining asymptomatic.

## PATHOGENESIS

### Epidemiology

Spondylosis is analogous to aging of the spine, with its associated clinical complaints of neck pain, referred scapular pain, and possibly nerve root or cord compression or both. Radiographic changes are seen in 95% of patients older than age 65 years. Men are affected more than women, and the changes that occur in men often are more severe. There are identifiable risk factors, including frequent lifting, cigarette smoking, driving, and a congenitally narrow spinal canal. Congenital spinal stenosis predisposes a patient to myelopathy when spondylosis develops.

### Pathophysiology and Anatomy

Much of the relevant clinical anatomy is reviewed in Chapter 14, but a few salient points are reviewed here. The cervical spine comprises seven cervical vertebrae, of which C3, C4, C5, and C6 are considered typical vertebrae. The typical sagittal alignment of the cervical spine is 20 degrees of lordosis. Vertebral discs compose 22% of the height of the cervical spine, allow motion between segments, and distribute weight evenly over the surface of the vertebral bodies.

A *motion segment* is defined as an intervertebral disc and the vertebrae above and below. Each motion segment has five articulations. These articulations include the intervertebral disc anteriorly, two facet joints posteriorly, and two neurocentral (uncovertebral) joints that lie along the posterolateral border of each typical vertebral body. With aging, these joints become arthritic and hypertrophied. Disc degeneration often is the instigating factor in spondylosis. With aging, the water content of the nucleus decreases, as does the concentration of glycosaminoglycans, and there is a resultant loss of disc height. There is a marked increase in the glycosaminoglycan keratin sulfate and decrease in chondroitin sulfate in the nucleus. Loss of intervertebral height and possible segmental instability interfere with the normal hydrostatic load-bearing function of the disc.

With degeneration, the border between the anulus and the nucleus becomes less well defined. Desiccation of the disc results from increased strain on the anulus, which fibrillates and weakens, contributing to decreased disc height. Segmental instability may occur at either a micro or a macro level. With the loss of disc height, the spine may lose its lordotic posture, and kyphosis may result. Kyphosis due to spondylotic changes leads to an abnormal strain on the posterior facet joints, also called the *zygapophyseal joints*. These true diarthrodial joints, with synovial membranes and fibrous capsules, may form osteophytes, which decrease the space available for the spinal cord. In addition, the neurocentral joints (the joints of Luschka) hypertrophy and may encroach on the spinal canal. Spondylytic change also affects the foramina, resulting in restricted motion and possible nerve root compression. Osteophytes also may form at the anterior and posterior aspects of the vertebral bodies. The posterior osteophytes may impinge further on the neural space.

### Etiology

Neck pain often is related to inflammation and neurologic compression secondary to a mechanical etiology. Spondylosis is most common at C5-6 followed by C6-7; these are the individual motion segments with the most mobility in the lower cervical spine. Disc function is the first to be affected, often by the 20s. When discs degenerate, discogenic pain may be the result. This symptom complex leads to axial neck and referred pain. Men present commonly with shoulder and lower neck pain, and women present with midline pain. Typically, axial pain increases with activity and decreases with rest. The pain often is insidious, without a clear inciting event, and may wax and wane over time. The exact anatomic location of the pain generator is difficult to identify.

## Pathophysiology

Radiculopathy can develop from either a soft disc or a hard disc. *Soft discs* are defined as herniations of the nucleus pulposus, and *hard discs* are defined as the osteophytes or bone spurs that result from spondylosis. Lower motor neuron signs predominate in patients with radiculopathy and include the following:

▓ Numbness
▓ Paresthesia
▓ Weakness
▓ Decreased deep tendon reflexes

Lateral disc herniations are intraforaminal and compress the exiting nerve root (i.e. at C3-C4, the C4 nerve root). Herniations of the nucleus most commonly are posterolateral, however, between the posterior edge of the uncinate process and the lateral border of the posterior longitudinal ligament. Here the exiting nerve root is compressed along with the spinal cord if the herniation is large. When the cord is compressed, myelopathic syndromes can develop. Central disc herniations compress the cord directly and can manifest as myelopathy or myeloradiculopathy.

## Classifications

Stenosis is classified into three types:

▓ Central stenosis
▓ Lateral recess stenosis
▓ Foraminal stenosis

It is classified further as follows:

▓ Congenital stenosis
▓ Acquired (degenerative) stenosis

Degenerative spinal stenosis is part of the aging process and becomes significant if the patient is symptomatic. Degenerative changes consisting of loss of disc height (with buckling of the ligamentum flavum posteriorly), osteophytic change in the uncovertebral joints and facets, and bulging or herniated discs all contribute to stenosis. Lateral recess stenosis is a result of osteophyte formation on the superior facet and ligamentum flavum hypertrophy. Foraminal stenosis is a narrowing of the foramen secondary to spondylosis of the superior facet. Congenital stenosis is primarily responsible for causing central stenosis and may exist primarily or in combination with degenerative stenosis. Congenital stenosis often predisposes the patient to myelopathy, leaving less space available for the cord to compensate for spondylotic changes.

Ossification of the posterior longitudinal ligament (OPLL) is a hereditary disease found primarily in Asians.

OPLL is a pathologic condition found in 2% of the Asian population. OPLL stenosis is a dynamic condition, wherein the compression of the cord becomes more profound in extension of the neck. It has been shown in biomechanical studies that the volume of the neural canal decreases in extension and increases in flexion. Additionally the diameter of the cord increases in flexion. OPLL may present with insidious progression of myelopathy or myeloradiculopathy, with the ossified ligament often compressing several levels of the spinal cord within the cervical canal.

## Natural History

Myelopathy does not have a readily definable natural history. There have been several retrospective studies with varying outlooks on this condition. Epstein et al reported a series of nonoperatively treated patients; 36% of patients improved, and 63% did not. Of the group that did not improve, 26% deteriorated, with decreasing neurologic function over time. Clark, in a similar study, showed that 75% of patients did not improve, with 67% of these deteriorating, some more rapidly than others. Symon published a series in which 67% of patients displayed relentless, linear progression of symptoms. There is a proportion of patients who do improve without operative intervention, but currently there are no clinical or radiographic signs that allow the physician to determine who would benefit from conservative therapy and who would not. It is necessary to follow these patients closely clinically and radiographically. Patients who do deteriorate may decompensate steadily or may follow a more rapid course. The best results from operative decompression are in patients who are not yet severely myelopathic, because their spinal cord has not yet been altered irreversibly pathologically by the compressing lesion. Congenital stenosis often predisposes the patient to myelopathy, leaving less residual space available for the cord to compensate for spondylotic change. Most cases of myelopathy develop slowly, in a stepwise fashion; however, with vascular insufficiency, the onset is acute and the results are devastating, with irreversible ischemic changes occurring within the cord.

## CLINICAL SYNDROMES

Spinal cord compression syndromes can be associated with stenosis and spondylosis. These syndromes require a thorough history and physical examination; they often occur in elderly patients with preexisting spondylosis or congenital stenosis or both. Older patients are especially susceptible to traumatic injury to the cord, especially hyperextension injuries. These syndromes are by definition incomplete, with some neurologic function below the level of the lesion.

Anterior cord syndrome resembles amyotrophic lateral sclerosis with localized dysfunction of the corticospinal tract. The corticospinal tract contains efferent nerve impulses that control voluntary motor function. These fibers decussate at the level of the medulla to the contralateral corticospinal fascicles. Anterior cord syndrome results from compression of the anterior spinal artery, which provides blood flow to the corticospinal tract. Motor function is affected severely, with paralysis below the level of the lesion. Pain, temperature, and light touch also are impaired with the involvement of the spinothalamic tract. Partial sensory function is intact, however, with the posterior columns (tactile discrimination, proprioception, and vibration) remaining viable. In anterior cord syndrome, the upper and lower extremities are affected equally. This syndrome has a poor prognosis for functional recovery.

Central cord syndrome spares the most lateral tracts in the corticospinal fasciculus, where the tracts for the upper extremities are medial to the tracts for the lower extremities; therefore, motor function often is retained in the lower extremities. In the upper extremities, there is decreased motor and sensory function, often with profound hand weakness. Central cord syndrome also is characterized by sacral sparing. The mechanism of injury is usually a hyperextension cervical injury that occurs in older patients with preexisting cervical spondylosis. Some functional recovery can be anticipated in 75% of these patients, in a specific pattern: first recovery of the lower extremities, then bowel and bladder control, then finally, and least predictably, hand function.

Brown-Séquard syndrome is uncommon and is characterized by injury to the lateral half of the spinal cord, with ipsilateral motor and proprioception loss and contralateral pain and temperature loss. This presentation is due to the spinothalamic tract decussating two to three levels above a lesion. The prognosis for recovery is good for these patients, with greater than 90% regaining some function.

# HISTORY AND PHYSICAL EXAMINATION

In diagnosing myelopathy, a thorough history is crucial. The duration of symptoms before clinical diagnosis ranges widely. Changes in the patient's activities may be subtle and not readily associated by the patient with an ongoing problem. Neck and arm pain are common presenting symptoms. A combined radicular and myelopathic syndrome is the most common presentation of cervical spondylotic myelopathy. Patients typically have compression of one or more roots, leading to lower motor neuron findings of radiculopathy in the upper extremity. Below the lesion, the spinal cord is compressed, manifesting as upper motor neuron involvement. Upper motor neuron signs predominate in myelopathy. Below the offending lesion, hyperreflexia (87% according to Lundsford), spasticity, and clonus in lower extremity are typical. Large central disc herniations also are implicated in myelopathy. Radicular pain with or without neurologic deficit, bowel or bladder dysfunction, gait disturbances, and long tract signs often are found together at presentation, creating a myeloradiculopathy. In central disc herniations, the corticospinal tracts are compressed anteriorly and are the first tracts to be affected, with patients presenting with diffuse lower extremity weakness. The posterior column is affected in more severe stenosis. An impairment in proprioception leads to a wide-based gait and ataxia.

Myelopathy also can be caused by vascular insufficiency, which is known as *indirect compression*. Compression of the anterior spinal artery is a cause of sudden-onset myelopathy.

Lower motor lesions, similar to the lesions of radiculopa-thy, also may be found at the level of the lesion and include areflexia, atrophy, and fasciculations. Bilateral or unilateral upper extremity (lower motor neuron compression) and bilateral lower extremities (spinal cord compression and upper motor neuron compression) may be affected. Weakness, clumsiness, and fatigability often are present. Most commonly, there is a decreased ability to ambulate, with a jerky, broad-based gait and an uneven cadence. Patients may report an unsteady feeling on their feet, difficulty walking, and an inability to maintain their balance. There is often a loss of fine motor function in the upper extremities, leading to difficulty holding a pen, combing one's hair, or opening bottles or jars, secondary to diminished dexterity.

The physical examination consists of observing the patient's gait to identify the telltale broad-based, jerky gait. This gait may be the presenting symptom and mimics a parkinsonian gait. The neck should be palpated for painful muscle spasms. Range of motion should be assessed, noting any decreased motion and noting maneuvers that may exacerbate the patient's symptoms. Extension maneuvers, which effectively decrease the amount of space available for the cord in the spinal canal, often elicit an increase in symptoms. A complete, root-specific neuromuscular exam follows. Pain and paresthesia in a radicular pattern are common presenting symptoms (34% to 39%), with variable presentations due to the involvement of multiple roots. Lower extremity weakness and spasticity (58%) are early presenting symptoms. Patients often notice decreased dexterity in their hands, often noting that they are becoming clumsy. A "myelopathy hand" can be caused by a lesion at or above C6-7 and manifests as a loss of power grip and subtle loss of proprioception and vibratory sense in the hand. Spasticity and hyperreflexia (50%) are found in the lower extremities and are signs of an upper motor neuron lesion. Bladder abnormalities present as retention and incontinence, with retention (50%) being more common. In extreme cases, the anal sphincter loses its tone, resulting in cases of fecal incontinence.

The physician must be familiar with several clinical signs that are associated with myelopathy. Lhermitte's sign is a shocklike feeling that progresses down the spine to the extremities when the neck is flexed and compressed. The scapulohumeral reflex, occurring with C1-3 myelopathy, consists of tapping on the acromion, with resultant abduction of the humerus and elevation of the scapula. Hoffmann's sign consists of flicking the nail of the long finger of a relaxed hand with resultant thumb or index finger flexion at the distal interphalangeal joint (13%). A myelopathic hand also can present with the "finger escape sign": The small finger cannot be adducted back to the palm, signaling an upper motor nerve lesion to nerves supplying the intrinsic musculature of the hand (C8 and T1). The inverted radial reflex is elicited with a reflex hammer tap to the brachioradialis, resulting in a diminished brachioradialis reflex accompanied by finger flexion. Clonus, which often is present in the lower extremities, is a rhythmic, repetitive oscillation of the foot at the ankle in response to dorsiflexion of the foot and stretch of the Achilles tendon. Babinski's reflex often is seen in conjunction with hyperreflexia. A positive Babinski's (50%) reflex is manifested by up-going toes when

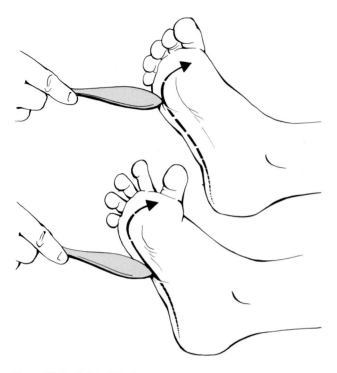

**Figure 13-1**  Babinski's sign.

the sole of the foot is stimulated with the handle of a reflex hammer (Fig. 13-1).

## Classification of Myelopathy

Nurick developed the following classification, which focuses on gait, to stratify disability in spondylotic myelopathy:

- *Grade 0*—root signs and symptoms without cord involvement
- *Grade I*—signs of cord involvement with a normal gait
- *Grade II*—mild gait abnormality; patient remains employable
- *Grade III*—gait abnormality prevents employment
- *Grade IV*—able to ambulate only with assistance
- *Grade V*—chair bound or bedridden.

This clinical classification is relevant because the clinical examination is prognostic of recovery, with lower grade patients predictably responding more favorably to operative and nonoperative treatment. Additional factors associated with an optimistic prognosis for recovery include duration less than 1 year, unilateral motor deficit, and younger age. The presence of Lhermitte's sign also has been shown to have a positive predictive value for recovery.

## Radiographic Features

Radiographic imaging is essential to establishing a causal relationship between the patient's presenting symptoms and structural changes of and around the spinal column. Radiographs are the initial studies to be obtained for acute symp-

toms. Clinical correlation is poor in patients older than 40 years old, with a high percentage of asymptomatic patients showing radiographic evidence of spondylosis. It is crucial to correlate the patient's symptoms to the radiographic findings and not to treat the radiograph reflexively.

Initial radiographs should include anteroposterior, lateral, and oblique views. In advanced spondylosis, these studies reveal narrowing of the intervertebral space, degenerative changes in the facets and neurocentral joints, loss of cervical lordosis, osteophyte formation, and foraminal encroachment (Fig. 13-2). Instability of the cervical spine can be determined radiographically by White's criteria. An unstable segment is diagnosed by noting a translation of one vertebra on another of 3.5 mm or an angulation of the end plates of two adjacent vertebrae of 11 degrees more than a normal adjacent segment.

A decreasing canal size suggests a risk of myelopathy, which is not determined easily with radiographs. Measurements are determined best with either computed tomography (CT) or magnetic resonance imaging (MRI). CT is excellent for evaluating canal diameter, as long as the gantry of the CT machine is aligned properly parallel to the disc spaces. MRI has been shown to overestimate the amount of canal stenosis by overstating the contribution of soft tissues. Each modality provides enough information, however, to evaluate spinal canal diameter. A normal canal diameter in the subaxial cervical spine is 17 mm. A measurement of less than 13 mm is defined as relative stenosis, and a measurement of 10 mm is absolute stenosis. The proportion of patients who present with myelopathy is related directly to

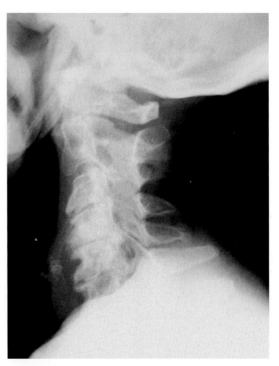

**Figure 13-2**  Lateral radiograph shows severe spondylosis. Note the loss of disc height and osteophyte formation at the anterior and posterior margins of the end plates. There also is a loss of physiologic lordosis.

lower measurements of canal diameter. Ratios also can be measured to determine stenosis. The Torg ratio divides the canal diameter by the length of the vertebral body as measured on a lateral radiograph. A ratio of less than 0.8 is considered stenotic. The cord compression ratio is the sagittal diameter of the cord divided by the transverse diameter on MRI; a ratio of less than 0.40 represents a significant amount of cord compression.

MRI is the first choice for advanced imaging of cervical disc disease and is useful for identifying intradural lesions and tumors. It is noninvasive, but a high-resolution machine is required with a powerful magnet of at least 0.5 Tesla and preferably 1.5. This high resolution affords a high degree of sensitivity of identification of compressive lesions of the cervical spine (Figs. 13-3 and 13-4). There is a high incidence of abnormalities in asymptomatic patients, with a low specificity due to a high false-positive rate. In one study, MRI was interpreted as abnormal in 19% of asymptomatic patients. When stratified by age, the false-positive rate was 28% in patients older than 40 years old and 14% in patients younger than 40. The clinician must be cautious in recommending operative treatment based on diagnostic tests alone; findings must match clinical signs and symptoms.

MRI largely has supplanted CT-myelography, but this study still has indications. CT-myelography is better than CT alone in patients with spondylosis, allowing direct visualization of compression. An ideal indication for this study would be a patient who has undergone previous instrumentation. In this case, the artifact associated with the ferromagnetic metal implants likely would not allow an accurate reading of an MRI study. The myelogram may reveal nonfilling of the proximal nerve root sleeves, flattening of the spinal cord, obstruction of contrast flow, or multiple indentations anteriorly (disc) or posteriorly (ligamentum flavum).

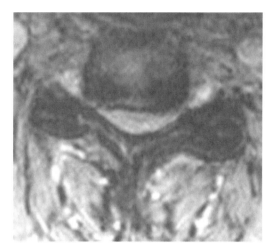

**Figure 13-4**    Axial cut T2-weighted MRI in a myelopathic patient. Note the central stenosis with decreased room available for the cord, facet hypertrophy, and foraminal stenosis.

CT-myelography allows direct visualization of compression. Its disadvantages are the difficulty in differentiating soft disc from hard disc protrusions, the difficulty in determining the extent of intradural lesions, and the possibility that distal pathology may be missed if a myelographic block is present.

Electrodiagnostic studies are adjuncts to the clinical and radiologic examinations and are not useful by themselves. They are not required for diagnosis of radiculopathy or myelopathy. Electrodiagnostic studies are used effectively to confirm a diagnosis of myelopathy or to rule out neurologic disorders, such as amyotrophic lateral sclerosis, multiple sclerosis, or peripheral nerve entrapment syndromes. Electromyography reveals fibrillations and sharp waves in a positive test done 3 to 6 weeks after radicular symptoms develop, and nerve conduction velocity exams reveal decreased amplitudes and velocities.

## Differential Diagnosis

The diagnosis of myelopathy is based on the history and physical exam and is supported by radiographic studies. Radiographs must correlate with clinical findings because more than 70% of patients older than age 70 have degenerative changes on radiographs. The differential diagnosis for myelopathy is vast. Patients with tumors or infections can present with myelopathic symptoms. Nonmechanical pain; night pain; and systemic signs, such as weight loss, night sweats, fever, and chills, all should be red flags for the evaluating physician. The pain associated with tumor and infection is often constant in nature and may escalate over time, occasionally with a rapid increase in pain. Multiple sclerosis may present with fatigue and focal deficits similar to myelopathy. Multiple sclerosis is associated with visual changes and upper motor neuron lesions that wax and wane over time. MRI may reveal focal plaques within the brain or spinal cord consistent with multiple sclerosis. Serum and cerebrospinal fluid with increased oligoclonal bands and immunoglobulins help to confirm this diagnosis. Amyotro-

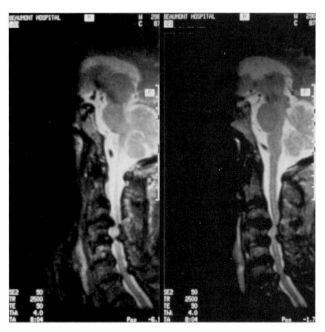

**Figure 13-3**    Multiple-level cervical spondylosis with loss of disc space, facet hypertrophy, buckling of the ligamentum flavum, and resultant cervical stenosis.

phic lateral sclerosis often presents in people in their 50s through 70s with painless weakness beginning about the shoulder girdle and progressing to complete motor loss without sensory involvement. Peripheral neuropathies can mimic cervical pathology and can be ruled out with a thorough physical exam and electromyography or nerve conduction velocity test.

# TREATMENT

## Nonoperative Treatment

Nonoperative treatment is the standard of care for discogenic and axial neck pain without accompanying myelopathy or radiculopathy. Axial neck pain tends to resolve on its own, but less frequently completely in patients with spondylosis (79% improved, 43% pain-free). Treatment regimens include nonsteroidal antiinflammatory drugs, moist heat, isometric and aerobic exercises, and occasionally a soft cervical collar. Surgery for discogenic neck pain is less rewarding than surgery for cases of radiculopathy or myelopathy.

Mild cases of myelopathy, involving only mild hand and arm symptoms, may respond to nonoperative treatment. Epidural injections may be of short-term benefit to a patient with radiculopathy, but there is no long-term research proving their efficacy. Myelopathy rarely resolves completely.

## Surgical Treatment

### Indications

The surgical management of myelopathy should address the pathophysiology of the disease by directly decompressing the cord. Candidates for surgery include patients who have difficulty using their arms, hands, or legs in activities of daily living; patients who rely on ambulatory aids for walking; and patients who are confined to a bed or chair. Radiculopathy commonly is present in myelopathic patients, and radiculopathy with persistent or disabling pain is an indication for surgery. The greatest predictor of postoperative recovery is the extent of preoperative involvement, as outlined by Nurick's classification, with age, sex, and duration of symptoms having less of an effect on outcome.

### Approaches

The anterior approach allows direct decompression of the offending discs and osteophytes. The procedure can be used for single-level and multilevel disease (Fig. 13-5). An anterior cervical discectomy and fusion is the procedure of choice for removing a single central disc herniation. A subtotal corpectomy and strut graft is a successful procedure for multilevel disease, providing 80% of patients with pain relief and 90% with some neurologic improvement (Fig. 13-6). In this operation, most of the vertebral body is removed, leaving only the lateral walls behind. A 3-mm margin on each side of the corpectomy leaves a safety zone between the surgeon's bur (used for removing the vertebral body) and the vertebral arteries, which course just lateral to the lateral margins of the vertebral body. Either structural allograft or autograft can be used to fill the corpectomy defect. If autograft is chosen, the iliac crest and the fibula are fre-

quent choices. Harvesting is associated with some morbidity, including hematomas, infection, and nerve damage. For these reasons, many surgeons prefer to use allograft—graft taken from a cadaver donor. The graft is placed while the anesthesiologist distracts the head. Plating has been shown to improve the fusion rates.

The anterior approach offers several advantages, including direct removal of compressive pathology, stabilization of the cervical spine with an arthrodesis, ability to correct a kyphotic deformity, and excellent relief of axial neck pain. The disadvantages are that the procedure is technically demanding and may require postoperative bracing. Additionally, graft extrusion or collapse is worrisome owing to the proximity of the graft to the neural structures posteriorly and the esophagus anteriorly. The graft should be well placed in the midline between the vertebral end plates. The end plates should be well prepared with a posterior lip to help prevent posterior dislodgment.

Posterior decompressive procedures also can be used to treat cervical myelopathy. Laminoplasty is a canal-expanding procedure that maintains cervical stability by leaving an intact hinge on the posterior elements (see Fig. 13-6). This procedure is most effective for unilateral radiculopathy at multiple levels with accompanying stenosis, especially for patients with OPLL. Laminoplasty is contraindicated in a patient who has lost physiologic lordosis on the lateral radio-

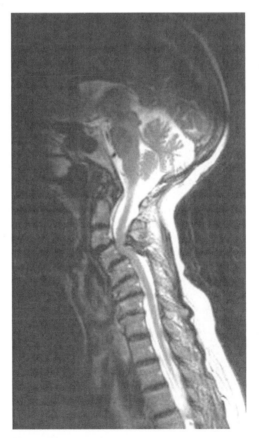

**Figure 13-5**  Sagittal T2-weighted MRI in a myelopathic patient. Note the decreased room available for the cord and loss of lordosis resulting from severe spondylosis.

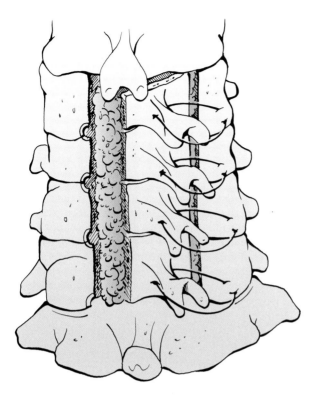

**Figure 13-6**   Laminoplasty: open door technique with sutures from the lateral mass to the spinous process to anchor the laminoplasty open.

graph, or has preoperative instability. Advantages of laminoplasty over wide laminectomy include retention of the osseous protection of the spinal cord and maintenance of soft tissue stabilizers.

Laminectomies are an alternative for multiple-level compression. It is a less technically demanding procedure than either the anterior approach or laminoplasty. The spine should be stable, with preservation of lordosis. If excessive motion does exist (as defined on flexion/extension radiographs), the laminectomy should be followed by posterior instrumentation and fusion to avoid subsequent postlaminectomy kyphosis. Laminectomies are used most commonly after failed laminoplasties or in patients with bony ankylosis of the anterior cervical spine. Advantages associated with the posterior approach include a minimal loss of motion (compared with the anterior approach) and a less technically demanding procedure. Disadvantages include the understanding that this is an indirect decompression, expanding the canal volume, but not directly addressing the anterior pathology. Kyphosis resulting from instability is an often cited complication of laminectomies in which an excessive amount of the facets have been removed; posterior instrumentation and stabilization may be recommended in patients with preoperative instability or patients who require excessive facet resection for decompression (Fig. 13-7).

### Complications

Myelopathic patients are susceptible to neurologic injury during surgery owing to the compromised state of the cord.

There is a higher incidence of neurologic injury with posterior procedures, especially laminectomies. Canal stenosis creates an environment of cord vulnerability. Postoperatively, 5.5% of myelopathic surgical patients may experience neurologic deterioration. The postoperative deficit may be secondary to surgical manipulation, such as a surgical instrument's being introduced into the spinal canal, but it is more commonly due to late kyphotic deformity or hematoma formation. Nerve root irritation most commonly is related to graft complications, either displacement or collapse of the graft. The C5 nerve root most commonly is involved, leading to deltoid weakness. Postoperative C5 nerve root dysfunction may be due to the following:

- C5 is often at the center of the decompression in myelopathic patients and is subject to more stretch from being tethered to the spinal cord.
- C5 root is shorter than other roots.

Autograft harvest site complications are the most commonly cited and include pain, hematoma, infection, abdominal herniation, and injury to the lateral femoral cutaneous nerve (meralgia paresthetica, with anterior harvest) or the superior cluneal nerves (with posterior harvest). Postoperative pain from iliac crest bone harvest has been reported, with 12% to 14% of patients having severe, but temporary pain. One study by DePalma noted 36% of patients had severe persistent pain.

Infections at the cervical site are uncommon, especially anteriorly (0.7% to 2.8%); this may be due to the abundant blood supply of the neck and the relatively atraumatic tissue dissection involved in the exposure. Prophylactic antibiotics, usually a first-generation cephalosporin, given 1 hour before surgery, have proved to be invaluable in preventing infection. Conditions associated with an increased risk of infection include diabetes, malnutrition, immunocompromised status, rheumatoid arthritis, malignancy, alcoholism, and poor dentition.

Iatrogenic nerve root injuries are uncommon, occurring in less than 2% of all anterior cervical procedures. Hoarseness may develop postoperatively secondary to excessive traction or, more seriously, transection of the recurrent laryngeal nerve. The recurrent laryngeal nerve on the right side courses transversely across the field at the C6-7 level, exposing it to injury with sharp dissection or retraction. For this reason, many surgeons prefer the left-sided approach. The recurrent laryngeal nerve courses in the tracheoesophageal groove and is protected by the trachea and esophagus. Transient sore throat and difficulty swallowing commonly are seen in the immediate postoperative period. Esophageal laceration is a rare but potentially lethal injury if not addressed intraoperatively. Postoperative tears may be evident by saliva or food in the wound, dysphagia, or neck pain; this can progress quickly to systemic sepsis. Esophageal perforation can be diagnosed with an esophogram. A positive exam shows water-soluble contrast material extravasating into the operated region. Treatment includes placement of a nasogastric tube, and the patient usually is taken back immediately to the operating room. Late perforations are related to prominent hardware (i.e., plates and screws) that are too proud on the anterior vertebral bodies. Finally, the thoracic duct of the lymphatic system enters the subclavian vein on

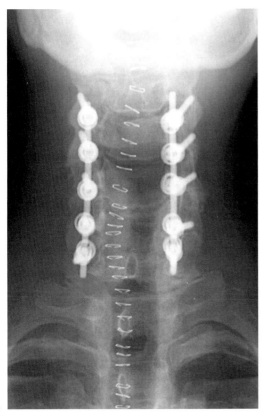 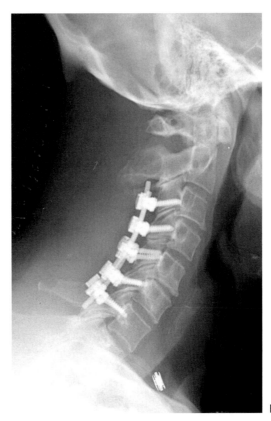

A                                                                                                          B

**Figure 13-7**   Postoperative anteroposterior (**A**) and lateral (**B**) radiographs after wide decompressive laminectomy and the use of posterior instrumentation to prevent postoperative kyphosis from developing.

the left side. Low, lateral approaches on the left potentially can injure the duct. If the thoracic duct is damaged, it should be double ligated.

Grafts always should be harvested with a power saw to avoid microfactures in the graft, which can occur when osteotomes are employed in the harvest. The graft should be well placed in the midline between the vertebral end plates. The end plates should be well prepared with a posterior lip to help prevent posterior dislodgment. Grafts that are too thick may lead to collapse, and grafts that are too thin may predispose to pseudarthrosis.

Pseudarthrosis, the failure of fusion of the interbody graft, is not always clinically significant, but it is related to a poorer clinical outcome. Pseudarthrosis is related directly to the number of levels fused. One-level fusion has a pseudarthrosis rate of 5% to 10%; two-level, 10% to 15%; and three-level, 20% to 30%. Rates also are increased with smoking and the use of allograft. Pseudarthrosis may be diagnosed in a patient experiencing continued mechanical cervical pain after 6 to 9 months. Motion on flexion/extension lateral films confirms the diagnosis. An asymptomatic pseudarthrosis can be observed. With graft resorption and resultant kyphosis, a partial anterior corpectomy with bone graft and plating would be the recommended revision surgery through an anterior approach. In partial fusions in which lordosis is maintained, a posterior fusion with for-

aminotomy (if radicular symptoms persist) stabilizes the construct.

## SUGGESTED READING

Boden SD, McCowin PR, Davis DO, et al. Abnormal MRI scans of the cervical spine in asymptomatic subjects: a prospective investigation. J Bone Joint Surg 1990;72A:1178–1184.

Epstein JA, Carras R, Epstein BS, Lavine LS. Cervical myelopathy caused by developmental stenosis of the spinal canal. J Neurosurg 1979;51:362.

Ferguson RJ, Kaplan LR. Cervical spondylitic myelopathy. Neurol Clin 1985;3:373–382.

Garfin SR, Herkowitz H, Mirkovic S. Spinal stenosis. Instr Course Lect 2000;361–376.

Herkowitz H. The surgical management of cervical spondylotic radiculopathy and myelopathy. Clin Orthop 1989;239:94–108.

Kimura I, Oh-Hama M, Shingu H, Yonago K. Cervical myelopathy treated by canal expansive laminoplasty. J Bone Joint Surg 1984; 66A:914–920.

Lees F, Aldren Turner J. Natural history and prognosis of cervical spondylosis. BMJ 1963;2:1607–1610.

Nurick S. The natural history and the results of surgical treatment of spinal cord disorder associated with cervical spondylosis. Brain 1972;95:101–108.

Poggi JJ, Martinez S, Hardaker WT, Richardson WJ. Cervical spondylolyis. J Spine Dis 1992;5:349–356.

Truumees E, Herkowitz H. Cervical spondylotic myelopathy and radiculopathy. Instr Course Lect 2000;339–360.

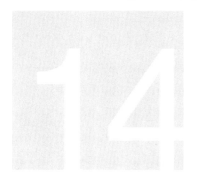

# CERVICAL RADICULOPATHY

**GREGORY T. BREBACH**
**HARRY N. HERKOWITZ**

Cervical disc disease is commonly manifested by nerve root dysfunction. Abnormalities in motor, sensory, or reflex function of a specific nerve root often are attributable to the herniation of disc fragments from the intervertebral disc and resultant compression of the nerve root by this fragment. The diagnosis begins with a thorough history and physical examination. Accurate diagnosis depends on an understanding of the differential diagnosis, which includes peripheral nerve entrapment syndromes and primary diseases of the neuromuscular system. The physician also should be familiar with the natural history of cervical radiculopathy, because most patients with radiculopathy improve with nonoperative treatment. For patients not responding to nonoperative therapies, several surgical options are described in this chapter, along with indications, results, and complications.

## PATHOGENESIS

### Epidemiology

Herniated cervical intervertebral discs occur most commonly in men 30 to 50 years old; age is the most significant risk factor. Other risk factors include frequent lifting, driving, working overhead (i.e., painting a ceiling), and smoking. Genetics also plays a role, with individuals predisposed to cervical radiculopathy presenting at an earlier age. Radiculopathy most commonly occurs without antecedent trauma, but trauma may aggravate an asymptomatic "abnormal" disc.

### Pathophysiology

A review of anatomy is essential to understanding the pathogenesis of cervical radiculopathy. There are seven cervical vertebrae, which can be divided into the upper and lower cervical spine. The upper cervical spine consists of the atlas, or C1, and the axis, C2. These two levels rarely are involved in producing radiculopathy. Radiculopathy of the cervical spine occurs most frequently in the lower cervical spine, defined as the intervertebral space of C2-3 to the intervertebral space of C7-T1. The C5-6 level is the most common site of compression, followed by C6-7. The five vertebral bodies of the lower cervical spine are similar in their anatomy. Each motion segment (a motion segment consists of a single intervertebral disc and the vertebra above and below) consists of five articulations. These articulations include the intervertebral disc anteriorly, the two facet joints posteriorly, and the two neurocentral joints, which lie along the posterolateral border of the vertebral body. The neurocentral joints also are called the *joints of Luschka* (or uncovertebral joints) and are osseous projections directed upward from the superior aspect of the inferior vertebral body and articulate with the uncinate process. These articulations are not true joints because they lack an articular capsule, but they can become arthritic. Because of their interposition between the disc and the intervertebral foramen, the neurocentral joints can cause impingement via mechanical compression of nerve roots as they exit the neural canal. The facet joints are oriented at 45 degrees in the sagittal plane and neutral in the coronal plane. The facet joints are true diarthrodial joints complete with a synovial membrane, articular cartilage, and fibrous capsule.

It is important to consider the location of the facet joints in relation to the intervertebral foramina. The intervertebral foramen comprises the vertebral body, intervertebral disc, and neurocentral joint anteriorly and the facets posteriorly. The superior and inferior pedicles constitute the superior and inferior borders of the foramina. As the nerve root enters the foramen medially, it lies at the level of the superior articular facet of the inferior vertebrae. The nerve courses inferiorly and laterally and forms the dorsal root ganglion within the lateral aspect of the neural foramen. With an understanding of this anatomy, it becomes clear how a disc herniation or arthritic hypertrophy of either the joints of Luschka or the facet joints may impinge mechanically on an exiting nerve root to cause radiculopathy. The process of degenerative change of these joints is called *spondylosis*, which is discussed more thoroughly in Chapter 13.

The anatomy of the intervertebral disc also has been well studied. The structural components of the disc include the nucleus pulposus and the anulus fibrosus, surrounded on the superior and inferior sides by cartilaginous end plates. The nucleus pulposus is a centrally located structure, occupying approximately 30% to 60% of the volume of the entire disc. It consists of a loose array of type II collagen arranged in an irregular meshwork. An extracellular matrix of proteoglycans gives the nucleus an elastic quality that accommodates compressive forces. The proteoglycans, primarily chondroitin sulfate and dermatan sulfate, are hydrophilic and maintain a high water content (70% to 90%) within the disc. As a person ages, the character of the nucleus pulposus changes. The ratio of proteoglycans changes, with a decrease in chondroitin sulfate, and an increase in dermatan sulfate and subsequent loss of water content. The nuclear composition undergoes age-related changes and no longer optimally can transmit, modify, and distribute forces evenly.

The biomechanics of the anulus is crucial to normal disc function, resisting tensile stresses of motion and transmitted forces from the nucleus. The anulus consists of type I collagen fibers peripherally and some type II fibers centrally. The anulus is formatted in concentric laminated bands of these collagen fibers, which attach to the vertebral body end plates and insert into the anterior longitudinal ligament and posterior longitudinal ligaments. The anulus' water content remains steady throughout life, but it, too, undergoes degeneration. Circumferential tears in the anulus begin to present around the 20s and progress to fraying and splitting of the collagen fibers. With the progression of degeneration, there is continued loss of the fluid properties of the nucleus, which undergoes a gradual replacement with fibrous tissue. This process occurs from the 30s to the 50s. By the 60s, there is advanced degeneration of the intervertebral disc, and the disc loses its ability to attenuate shock and vibration and to distribute loads evenly. Some environmental factors contribute to disc degeneration, such as driving, lifting, and smoking.

## Etiology

Herniated nucleus pulposus often results in mechanical deformation of the dorsal root ganglion or nerve root. This mechanical deformation—be it compression or stretch of the involved nerve root—causes release of substance P, phospholipase 2, and vasoactive intestinal polypeptide from the cells of the nucleus pulposus, which act to inflame the affected nerve root. These chemical mediators lead to paresthesia and sensory or motor deficit.

## Classification

When the nucleus herniates through the degenerated anulus, it can be classified into one of three forms:

- *First,* the nucleus pulposus may be a protrusion, with a radial tear in the anulus allowing for the nuclear material to force the outer annular fibers to bulge out and encroach on neural elements.
- *Second,* there is an extruded disc. In this scenario, nuclear elements have herniated through the anulus but are restrained by the posterior longitudinal ligament.
- *Third,* there is the sequestered disc, wherein nuclear material is directly compressing the neural elements, having herniated through the outer annular fibers and the posterior longitudinal ligament (Fig. 14-1).

Soft disc herniations typically cause acute radiculopathies, with chronic radiculopathy caused by hard discs re-

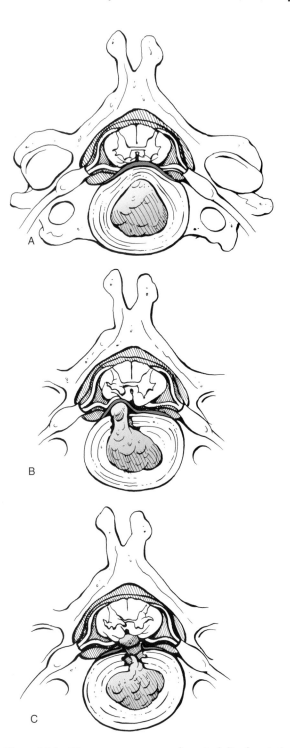

**Figure 14-1**  Three common types of cervical disc herniation. (**A**) Central protrusion, with the outer anulus remaining intact. (**B**) Posterolateral extrusion, with the anulus having a tear and the nucleus being restrained by fibers of the posterior longitudinal ligament. (**C**) Central sequestered fragment, lying posterior to the posterior longitudinal ligament. (From Jenis L, An H. Cervical disc disease. In: Chapman MW, ed. Chapman's orthopaedic surgery, 3rd ed. Philadelphia: Lippincott Williams & Wilkins, 2001:3749.)

sulting from the degenerative changes of spondylosis. *Hard discs* are posterior or posterolateral osteophytes that commonly cause spinal stenosis and radiculopathy in patients older than 55 years of age. The acute *soft disc* herniation is most common in men age 30 to 50. Disc herniations are categorized by their location relative to the neural canal—foraminal, posterolateral, and midline herniations—with posterolateral herniations being the most common cervical disc herniation.

Knowledge of neuroanatomy is essential to identify the specific symptoms and signs. The neuroanatomy of the cervical spine is unique in that the nerve roots exit above the pedicle of the same number, with the exception of C8, which exits below the pedicle of the same level. C5 exits above the pedicle of C5 in the C4-5 interspace. Compare this with the thoracic and lumbar spines, where the nerve root exits below the pedicle of the same number: The L4 nerve root exits below the L4 pedicle at the L4-5 interspace. The location of the herniation determines the presenting symptoms. Intraforaminal or lateral herniations most commonly manifest as pure radicular pain (pain in a dermatomal or radicular distribution). Posterolateral herniations, between the posterior edge of the uncinate process and the lateral border of the posterior longitudinal ligament, often present with motor deficits in the affected myotome. Midline herniations often are responsible for myelopathy, compressing directly on the cord itself.

# DIAGNOSIS

## History and Physical Examination

### Clinical Features

The patient's history is paramount in evaluating a suspected radiculopathy because there is an extensive differential diagnosis to be considered. Symptoms of cervical radiculopathy may develop acutely, with an initial episode of neck pain followed by radiation of pain in a dermatomal pattern or weakness in the affected extremity. Referred trapezial and periscapular pain often accompanies the radicular component. The patient may describe positions that alleviate symptoms, such as rotating the head away from the affected side, effectively enlarging the intervertebral foramina of the involved side, and the abducted shoulder sign, in which the patient describes pain relief with the affected shoulder abducted and the hand resting on top of the head.

The initial part of the physical exam includes observation of the patient, noting the position of the head and neck contours. Next the painful area of the neck is identified by palpation, checking for muscle spasm. In assessing range of motion, cervical flexion may alleviate symptoms, whereas extension may exacerbate the patient's symptoms. The range of motion in a normal patient involves the following:

- *Flexion*—chin to chest
- *Extension*—looking directly at the ceiling
- *Rotation*—chin in line with the shoulder
- *Lateral bending*—45 degrees to each side

There are helpful tests and signs in pursuing the diagnosis of cervical radiculopathy and differentiating the diagnosis from shoulder pathology, peripheral nerve entrapment syndromes, vascular syndromes, and lesions above the foramen magnum. The Spurling maneuver involves turning the patient's head toward the affected side, then applying axial compression, recreating symptoms of radiculopathy. The shoulder abduction sign often is observed as the patient enters the physician's office, with the affected arm abducted fully at the shoulder and the hand placed squarely on the head. The jaw jerk reflex is a tap on the temporomandibular joint, which, if hyperactive, indicates pathology above the foramen magnum.

A detailed and documented neurologic exam follows. The presentation of radiculopathy is nerve root specific, so a review of individual nerve root findings follows.

- Radiculopathy is rare above C2 and presents with occipital headaches and jaw pain without any neurologic deficit.
- C3 radiculopathy most commonly involves the C2-3 disc and presents with pain and numbness in the back of the neck around the mastoid process and the pinna of the ear. No weakness or reflex change is readily detectable. The pain often is accompanied by an occipital headache and must be differentiated from a tension headache.
- Compression of the C4 nerve root typically involves the C3-4 disc. There is more motion at this level than C2-3 and is more often involved. Pain and numbness at the base of the neck at the trapezium muscle predominates. Although the phrenic nerve is innervated by C3-5, involvement of the diaphragm is unusual secondary to bilateral denervation. There are no readily detectable weaknesses or reflex changes, with the exception of some weakness in neck extension with involvement of the levator scapula muscle.
- Disc herniations at C4-5 impinge on the C5 nerve root. This impingement typically presents with pain or numbness radiating down the side of the neck to the top of the shoulder to the lateral aspect of the deltoid muscle. The difficulty with C5 radiculopathy is differentiating it from intrinsic shoulder pathology, so a complete shoulder examination is mandatory. In a rotator cuff tear, there is weakness of the supraspinatus, infraspinatus, teres minor, or subscapularis. A shoulder examination shows weakness in abduction with external rotation, adduction with external rotation, or a posterior push-off test in a tear of one of the rotator cuff muscles. In a C5 radiculopathy, there is often weakness of the deltoid without involvement of the rotator cuff muscles. In advanced cases of C5 compression, the deltoid can become markedly atrophied. Although the biceps reflex frequently is associated with C5, findings of decreased reflexes here are unreliable findings.
- Radiculopathy at C6 involves the C5-6 disc and is the most common site of herniation in the cervical spine. It presents as pain radiating down the lateral side of the arm and forearm to the tip of the thumb and index finger. There is weakness of the biceps muscle, which often is subtle in its presentation. The examining physician should check not only elbow flexion, but also supination of the forearm. There also is a weakness of wrist extension. With C6 radiculopathy, there often is a diminished

brachioradialis reflex and possibly a decreased response of the biceps reflex.

■ C7 is the second most common site of cervical radiculopathy. The offending disc is at C6-7. Pain or numbness or both radiate down the middle of the forearm to the middle finger, with possible involvement of the index and ring fingers. There is a weakness in the triceps muscle and a loss of wrist flexion strength. Patients also may have decreased push-off strength. The triceps reflex is diminished.

■ Disc protrusions affecting C8 originate from the C7-T1 interspace. This relatively uncommon herniation is associated with numbness on the medial aspect of the forearm to the ring and small fingers. Pain is an infrequent complaint at this level. The intrinsic muscles of the hand, the lumbricals and the interossei muscles, weaken and atrophy, affecting finger flexion, abduction, and adduction. Weakness of grip strength results. No reflex changes are associated with this level.

## Radiographic Features

Radiographs are obtained usually after 6 weeks of symptoms. Exceptions to this practice are red flag cases, and include patients with progressive weakness, intractable pain, trauma, suspected infection, or tumor. A review of the patient's symptoms always should include a history of fever, chills, weight loss, and past malignancy. Plain radiographs often reveal the age-related changes of spondylosis, which are ubiquitous in patients older than age 40. Greater than 70% of radiographs show spondylotic or degenerative change in patients by age 70. Plain films may not be helpful in securing the diagnosis. When indicated, anteroposterior, lateral, and right and left oblique views should be ordered. Plain radiographs help to rule out tumor, infection, or fracture. Radiographs also show sagittal alignment. The oblique views are useful in evaluating the foramina; a narrowed foramen has a figure-of-eight appearance. Flexion/extension films may be helpful if trauma is involved or if instability due to severe facet degeneration is present.

Magnetic resonance imaging (MRI) is the preoperative imaging study of choice for cervical radiculopathy. A 1.5 Tesla magnet or higher is preferred. The test is noninvasive and is useful for diagnostic confirmation and preoperative planning. T1-weighted and T2-weighted images should be obtained. T1-weighted images show herniated discs and bone spurs as hypointense, making it more difficult to discern these structures from bone and ligament. T2-weighted images often are more revealing, creating a myelographic picture of the spinal cord and roots (Figs. 14-2 and 14-3). MRI tends to overestimate stenosis and, similar to radiographs, should be used with strict clinical correlation. Asymptomatic disc degeneration and herniation commonly are encountered in individuals older than 30 years.

Computed tomography (CT)-myelography is used in patients who are claustrophobic or when MRI is contraindicated or nondiagnostic. In an acute disc herniation, CT-myelography reveals extradural filling defects, cord flattening, and obstruction of flow to affected nerve roots in an axial plane (Fig. 14-4). Disadvantages include inability to differentiate between hard and soft disc protrusions, inabil-

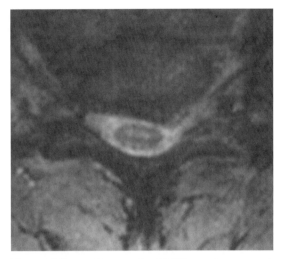

**Figure 14-2**   Axial T2 weighted MRI reveals a posterolateral soft disc herniation. The disc is impinging on the left nerve root (the right side of the MRI image) and effectively reducing the foraminal area.

ity to assess pathology below a complete myelographic block, and invasiveness.

Electrodiagnostic studies are used to rule out nonradicular pathology. Electromyography (EMG) and nerve conduction velocity studies detect motor changes secondary to compression. Demyelination must be present for nerve conduction tests to show decreased amplitude. This rarely occurs in radiculopathy; it occurs more commonly in peripheral nerve entrapment syndromes. Nerve conduction studies evaluate peripheral nerves and their responses to surface electrodes. The amplitude and the latency (time between the stimulus and response) are measured and compared against normal controls. EMG uses intramuscular needle electrodes to evaluate muscle function. A peripheral neuropathy, such as carpal tunnel or cubital tunnel syn-

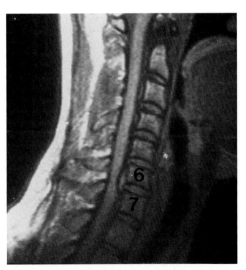

**Figure 14-3**   T2-weighted MRI reveals soft disc herniations at C4-5, C5-6, and C6-7.

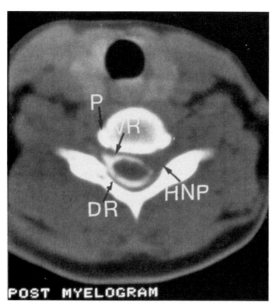

**Figure 14-4**   CT-myelogram shows a herniated nucleus pulposus (HNP). Note the loss of contrast material in the left nerve root, representing compression of the exiting nerve root. DR, dorsal root; VR, ventral root; P, uncinate process of the vertebral body.

drome, would present with fibrillations and sharp waves on EMG. EMG is not useful until 4 weeks after injury; normal (latent) responses are obtained before 4 weeks. These tests may be ordered in patients with unusual presentations, diabetes, suspected neurologic syndromes, or suspected peripheral nerve entrapment syndromes.

### Differential Diagnosis

A history of night pain or unrelenting symptoms should alert the physician to the possibility of a tumor or infection. Systemic signs of weight loss, night sweats, lack of energy, fever, and chills also are strong indicators of possible tumor or infection.

Peripheral nerve entrapment syndromes can affect any of the branches of the brachial plexus. Ulnar, median, posterior, and anterior interosseous nerve compressions can mimic radiculopathy. Pronator syndrome, involving the median nerve, may present similar to a C6-7 radiculopathy. Specific EMG and nerve conduction velocity studies are helpful in ruling out these entities, showing a change in potential, 3 weeks after injury.

Symptoms from shoulder disorders often are difficult to distinguish from radiculopathy. Rotator cuff tears, impingement syndromes, bursitis, tendinitis, arthritis, and shoulder instabilities can present with nonspecific shoulder and arm pain. A detailed shoulder examination is necessary to clarify the diagnosis.

Thoracic outlet syndrome involves compression of the lower cervical roots by a cervical rib or vascular compression of C8 and T1. Bruits in the lower cervical spine and a cervical rib on radiographs are clues to the diagnosis. Syringomyelia is a cystic dilation within the spinal cord itself often resulting from trauma or secondary to Chiari malformations and tumor. A syrinx typically presents with weakness and atrophy of the hands with a loss of pain and temperature sensation and sparing of light touch. A headache often precedes neurologic findings. The presence of syringomyelia can be confirmed with MRI.

Multiple sclerosis may present with fatigue and focal deficits similar to myelopathy. Multiple sclerosis is associated with visual changes and upper motor neuron lesions that wax and wane over time. MRI may reveal focal plaques consistent with multiple sclerosis. Serum and cerebrospinal fluid with increased oligoclonal bands and immunoglobulins help to confirm this diagnosis. Amyotrophic lateral sclerosis often presents in people in their 50s through 70s with painless weakness beginning about the shoulder girdle and progressing to complete motor loss without sensory involvement. Lesions above the foramen magnum, such as cerebrovascular insults or brain tumors, also may present with deficits that must be differentiated from cervical radiculopathy.

## TREATMENT

The goals of treatment are to reduce pain, improve function, provide stability, and resolve neurologic deficits. Understanding the natural history of cervical radiculopathy is important in formulating a treatment plan. Lees and Turner found, that 45% of cases of radiculopathy occurred as single episodes, 30% recurred with intermittent episodes, and 25% had persistent radiculopathy. DePalma and Rothman reported that 29% of patients had complete relief of symptoms, 49% had partial relief, and 22% had no relief. Gore's retrospective review showed that 32% of patients had persistent pain.

### Nonoperative Treatment

Nonoperative treatment begins with restricting activity and advising the patient to avoid lifting and extension movements about the neck. Soft cervical collars may be used for 1 to 2 weeks. These braces do not stop cervical motion effectively, but they serve more effectively as reminders to the patient that a problem exists. Medications are employed effectively to relieve inflammation, including aspirin, nonsteroidal antiinflammatory drugs, short-term oral steroids, and epidural steroid injections. Epidural steroids have been shown to provide short-term symptom relief, but currently there is no evidence of long-term symptomatic relief. Physical therapy plays an active role in conservative treatment. Isometric muscle strengthening and stretching and modalities such as heat, traction, ultrasound, and massage are helpful. Traction usually provides some relief of radicular pain and accompanying spasms. Active exercise that is limited by the patient's symptoms serves to keep the neck from becoming deconditioned. Chiropractic care may be considered in patients without significant spondylosis at the initial onset of symptoms.

### Surgical Treatment
#### Indications

Indications for surgery include persistent or recurrent arm pain with or without weakness, not responsive to 3 months of nonoperative treatment. A progressive neurologic deficit with confirmatory imaging studies consistent with the clinical picture is an absolute operative indication. The results of operative intervention for axial neck pain are inferior to the results for radiculopathy, with operative results for radiculopathy being 70% to greater than 90% good to excellent. Mitigating factors that should be considered include workers' compensation cases, mental health issues such as depression, and substance abuse. These factors have a negative impact on treatment, with surgical results for these patients lagging behind results of other patients.

## Approaches

There are two common approaches to the cervical spine—anterior and posterior—and there are several factors to consider in selecting one over the other. Single-level or double-level involvement is addressed best with an anterior approach, whereas multiple-level involvement may be addressed better by a posterior approach. The location of the impingement and the contour of the spine also are important to consider. Central herniations place the cord at risk if approached posteriorly, so an anterior approach is recommended. A unilateral soft intraforaminal disc may be approached posteriorly with a laminofacetectomy and foraminotomy. Laminoplasty, wherein the posterior elements are hinged open like a door, employs a right-sided or left-sided osteotomy at the intersection of the lamina and the lateral mass. This approach is most effective for unilateral radiculopathy at multiple levels with accompanying stenosis. Laminoplasty is contraindicated in patients who have lost physiologic lordotic contour of the cervical spine. Laminectomies are an alternative for multiple-level radiculopathies but are employed more commonly in myelopathic patients with central stenosis. If instability is present, laminectomy should be followed by posterolateral fusion to avoid subsequent kyphotic collapse. The anterior approach is the most common surgical approach for cervical radiculopathy. A transverse incision is used for one-level to two-level discectomies, and a longitudinal incision is used for three or more levels. A left-sided approach is preferred because of the predictability of the recurrent laryngeal nerve on this side. The nerve courses between the esophagus and the trachea and is protected. The thoracic duct of the lymphatic system inserts at the confluence of the jugular and subclavian veins on the left side and must be avoided in low-level discectomies. When approaching from the left, the level of the incision is determined by palpating anatomic landmarks: The hyoid bone is at the C3 level, the thyroid cartilage is at C4-5, and the cricoid cartilage is at C6 (Fig. 14-5).

## Results

An anterior cervical discectomy and fusion produces 70% to 90% satisfactory results. Tricortical autograft harvested from the patient's iliac crest remains the gold standard, providing stability, osteoinductivity, and osteoconductivity. Allograft, usually patella or fibula, has shown to be as effective in single-level fusions as autograft, without the morbidity associated with graft harvest. Tricortical grafts:

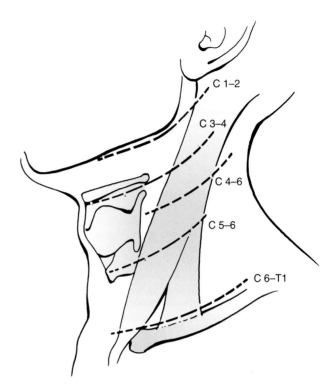

**Figure 14-5** Landmarks for the incision of the Smith-Robinson approach for anterior cervical discectomy and fusion. C1-2 is at the level of the mandible. C3 is at the level of the hyoid. C4-5 is at the level of the superior and inferior borders of the thyroid cartilage. C6 is at the level of the cricoid cartilage. C7-T1 exposure is just above the clavicle. (From Fischgrund J, Herkowitz H. In: Bradford DS, ed. Master techniques in orthopaedic surgery: spine. Philadelphia: JB Lippincott, 1997:92.)

- Offer some immediate stability to the motion segment
- Eventually lead to interbody fusion (which may arrest or reverse spur formation). Posterior osteophytes often resorb after solid fusion.
- Can increase the dimension of the neuroforamina by distraction (Figs. 14-6 and 14-7).

Anterior plating improves the fusion rate of multiple-level discectomies but does not improve the fusion rate in single-level anterior cervical discectomy and fusions. Plating should be used for multiple-level interbody fusions, single-level fusions in smokers, single-level fusions in which allograft is employed, and pseudarthrosis repair. In practice, plating allows for a more aggressive rehabilitation and decreased duration of immobilization (Fig. 14-8). Postoperative immobilization consists of a cervical orthosis for 6 weeks if plating is not used and less than 2 weeks if plating is employed. If an anterior plating system is placed, an orthosis is used for 1 week.

## Complications

Complications of cervical surgery are infrequent but well defined. They range from graft harvest complications to permanent neurologic injury, with an overall complication rate of 6.7%. Autograft harvest site complications are the most

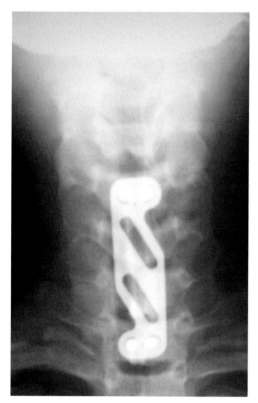

**Figure 14-6** Anteroposterior radiograph after a three-level anterior cervical discectomy and fusion with tricortical grafts for multiple-level herniations. The anterior plate assists with stability and improves fusion rates, especially in multiple-level operations.

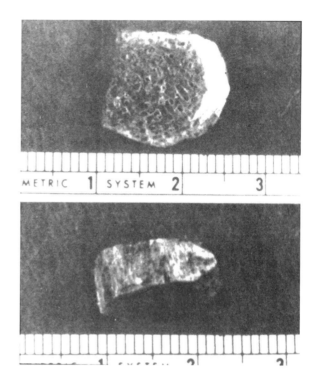

**Figure 14-7** Tricortical bone graft. Autograft tricortical graft is harvested from the iliac crest. Allograft tricortical graft often is taken from donor fibula or patella. Typical dimensions for a man would be 8 mm high × 14 mm deep × 14 mm wide.

commonly cited and include pain, hematoma, infection, abdominal herniation, and injury to the lateral femoral cutaneous nerve (meralgia paresthetica).

Infections at the cervical site are uncommon, especially anteriorly (0.7% to 2.8%); this may be due to the abundant blood supply of the neck and the relatively atraumatic tissue dissection involved in the Smith-Robinson exposure. Prophylactic antibiotics, usually a first-generation cephalosporin, given 1 hour before surgery reduce the risk of infection. Conditions associated with an increased risk of infection include diabetes, malnutrition, immunocompromised status, rheumatoid arthritis, malignancy, alcoholism, and poor dentition.

Iatrogenic nerve injuries are uncommon events; they occur in less than 2% of all anterior cervical discectomies. Hoarseness may be encountered secondary to excessive traction or, more seriously, division of the recurrent laryngeal nerve. The recurrent laryngeal nerve on the right side courses transversely across the spine at the C6-7 level, exposing it to injury with sharp dissection or retraction. For this reason, we recommend the left-sided approach, in which the recurrent laryngeal nerve courses in the tracheoesophageal groove and is protected by the trachea and esophagus. Transient sore throat and difficulty swallowing commonly are seen in the immediate postoperative period and usually resolve within 1 to 2 weeks. Esophageal injury is a rare but potentially lethal injury. Injury may be evidenced by saliva or food in the wound, dysphagia, and increasing neck pain. A perforated esophagus is diagnosed with an esophagogram. Late perforations may be related to prominent hardware. Finally, the thoracic duct of the lymphatic system enters the subclavian vein on the left side. Low, lateral approaches on the left potentially can injure the duct. If the thoracic duct is damaged, it should be double ligated. Clinically this injury presents with an expanding mass similar to that of a hematoma. Surgical exploration may be necessary to address the lymphatic drainage.

Graft extrusion occurs in 2% to 8% of cases. It is important to seat the graft properly. Graft collapse can be avoided by harvesting with a power saw to avoid microfactures that can occur when osteotomes are used. Grafts that are too thick may lead to collapse; grafts that are too thin may predispose to pseudarthrosis. Grafts should be 2 mm greater than the intervertebral space. If the graft collapses or migrates, revision surgery is advised. Neurologic injury, dysphagia, kyphosis, and respiratory distress all are possible complications of graft extrusion.

Persistent neurologic symptoms may be a result of irreparable damage done to the neural structures before surgery, wrong level of surgery, or an inadequate decompression. The level of surgery always should be checked with an intraoperative radiograph. Neurologic injury can occur during or shortly after surgery. Implant malposition or displacement should be considered and evaluated with radiographs and CT-myelography in patients with postoperative neurologic deficit.

Pseudarthrosis, the failure of fusion of the interbody

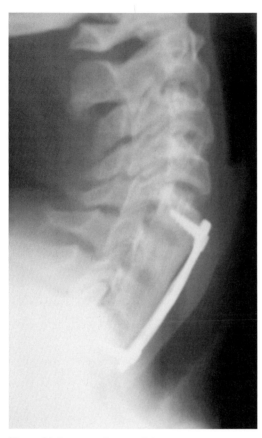

**Figure 14-8** Lateral view of the same patient as in Figure 14-7, 6 months postoperatively. Note the beginning of a fusion anteriorly.

graft, is related directly to the number of levels fused. One-level fusion has a pseudarthrosis rate of 5% to 10%; two-level, 10% to 15%; and three-level, 20% to 30%. Rates also are increased with smoking and the use of allograft. Pseudarthrosis may be diagnosed in a patient experiencing continued mechanical cervical pain. Motion at the graft segment seen on flexion/extension lateral films and a lack of bony trabeculae across the end plates confirm the diagnosis. Pseudarthrosis can be asymptomatic; surgical indications are based on the degree of instability and its attendant risk of injury to the spinal cord.

## SUMMARY

The diagnosis and treatment of cervical radiculopathy rely on the physician's knowledge of cervical anatomy and understanding of the differential diagnoses that may mimic its signs and symptoms. When cervical radiculopathy is diagnosed, nonoperative therapies should begin, including physical therapy and short-term use of a soft cervical collar. Plain radiographs show the degree of degeneration and the sagittal alignment and help to rule out neoplastic and infectious conditions. MRI and CT-myelography help confirm the diagnosis and detect the source of compression. Surgery is indicated in patients with progressive neurologic deficits or intractable, persistent pain for more than 3 months. The surgical results in patients with cervical radiculopathy are 70% to 90% good to excellent.

## SUGGESTED READING

Ahlgren BD, Garfin SR. Cervical radiculopathy. Orthop Clin North Am 1996;27:253–263.

Albert TJ, Murrell SE. Surgical management of cervical radiculopathy. J Am Acad Orthop Surg 1999;7:368–376.

Boden SD, McCowin PR, Davis DO, et al. Abnormal magnetic-resonance scans of the cervical spine in asymptomatic subjects: a prospective investigation. J Bone Joint Surg 1990;72A:1178–1184.

Dvorak J. Epidemiology, physical examination, and neurodiagnostics. Spine 1998;23:2663–2673.

Epstein NE. A review of laminoforaminotomy for the management of lateral and foraminal cervical disc herniations or spurs. Surg Neurol 2002;57:226–234.

Fager CA. Identification and management of radiculopathy. Neurosurg Clin N Am 1993;4:1–12.

Herkowitz HN. Cervical laminaplasty: its role in the treatment of cervical radiculopathy. J Spinal Disord 1988;1:179–188.

Levine MJ, Albert TJ, Smith MD. Cervical radiculopathy: diagnosis and nonoperative management. J Am Acad Orthop Surg 1996;4:305–316.

McCormack BM, Weinstein PR. Cervical spondylosis: an update. West J Med 1996;165:43–51.

# THORACIC SPONDYLOSIS, STENOSIS, AND DISC HERNIATIONS

## CHRISTOPHER M. BONO

Thoracic disc disease can manifest in many ways. Back pain can be associated with *disc degeneration* or herniation. Advanced degeneration may result in bone changes called *spondylosis*. Neurologic compression can occur from *disc herniation* or spondylosis (facets, ligaments, osteophytes). The latter is called *thoracic stenosis* and, as with a disc herniation, may result in myelopathy, radiculopathy, or both. Symptomatic thoracic disc disease is relatively rare. Thoracic disc herniations represent less than 2% of all disc operations, and less than 4% of symptomatic discs. Compared with cervical and lumbar stenosis, thoracic stenosis represents a small percentage of surgically treated cases.

## ANATOMY

Thoracic vertebrae have several distinct features. The spinous processes are long with considerable "overlap" between levels. In the upper thoracic spine, the facets resemble cervical articulations. Progressing toward the middle thoracic region, the joint surfaces are nearly coronal, and in the lower thoracic region, they are sagittal. The ribs articulate with the vertebrae in two areas:

■ At the anterior aspect of the transverse process
■ At the posterolateral aspect of the vertebral body

Each rib head articulates with two vertebrae (Fig. 15-1). The spinal canal in the thoracic spine is smaller in relation to the lumbar or cervical spine, resulting in a high rate of paraplegia with traumatic injuries. Because of the stabilizing contribution of the rib cage, more energy is needed to cause the initial injury. The borders of the neural foramina are the pedicles superiorly and inferiorly, the vertebral body and disc anteriorly, and the facet joint posteriorly. The inferolateral edge of the inferior articular process at its junction with the transverse process is the approximate entry point for a thoracic pedicle screw (Fig. 15-2).

## PATHOGENESIS

### Etiology

#### Axial Pain

The etiology of thoracic disc disease is most likely degenerative. The degenerative process has been described more extensively in the lumbar spine, which is discussed in subsequent chapters. Briefly summarized, initial disruption of the integrity of the intervertebral disc, including delamination, fibrillation, and annular tears, leads to a change in the disc's ability to withstand force. At each motion segment (two vertebrae = one motion segment or functional spinal unit), multiple joints interact. In the thoracic spine, these are the intervertebral disc, the facet joints, and the costovertebral junctions. In contrast to the cervical and lumbar regions, the interaction of the ribs gives a substantial amount of additional support. With a compromised disc, greater than normal demands are placed on the other joints. These joints can undergo subsequent articular surface breakdown with corresponding changes, such as hypertrophy and osteophyte formation.

How does the degenerative process produce symptoms? The most common complaint is pain. Pain can be axial (central, nonradiating) or radicular (follows dermatomal distribution). Axial pain is thought to be generated from the degenerated disc or facets or both. Both structures are innervated by nociceptive nerve endings. In the lumbar and thoracic spine, the facet is innervated by medial branches of the dorsal root ganglion. These branches arise from the two nerve roots *below* the joint. The T3-4 facet joint is innervated by branches from the T4 and T5 nerve roots. The posterior anulus of the disc is innervated by branches of the sinuvertebral nerve, which itself is a branch from the rami communicantes between the dorsal root ganglion and the autonomic ganglion. Dysfunction, instability, or degeneration may transmit pain through these nerves.

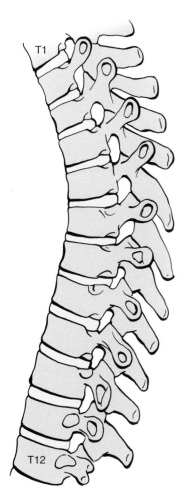

**Figure 15-1**  The rib head articulates with the anterior aspect of the transverse process and the posterolateral aspect of suprajacent and infrajacent vertebral bodies. This "bridging" between vertebral bodies provides additional stability to the thoracic spine.

Advanced degeneration is evidenced by pronounced spondylotic (not spondy*litic*) changes, including osteophytes protruding from the anterior, posterior, or lateral aspects of the vertebral bodies adjacent to the disc spaces. These changes are age dependent and are most often clinically asymptomatic. Facet joint hypertrophy also is characteristic.

## Myelopathy and Radiculopathy

The exact mechanism of neural dysfunction with thoracic disc disease is unclear. Most authors believe that mechanical compression is a key factor. Stenosis, whether central or foraminal, is a radiologic/pathoanatomic finding. Thoracic stenosis can be detected by imaging studies, such as computed tomography (CT) or magnetic resonance imaging (MRI), and represents narrowing of the spinal canal or space for the exiting nerve roots. Not all patients with these findings have neurologic signs or symptoms. Additional mechanisms are likely, such as neural vascular insuffi-

ciency, but they cannot be detected by presently available imaging techniques. Myelopathy and radiculopathy are clinical diagnoses and should not be based solely on imaging studies that may show evidence of neural compression. The actual etiology is probably multifactorial and remains to be elucidated clearly.

By default, detecting and addressing areas of neural compression remains the focus of surgical treatment of thoracic disc disease. Osteophytes, overgrown facets, or infolded ligamenta flava can compress the spinal cord or nerve roots. Disc herniations may protrude into the spinal canal or foramina as well, causing a similar clinical picture. Recognizing the cause and nature of the offending elements is crucial to effective treatment.

Compression of a thoracic nerve root (T2-11) usually does not result in clinically apparent sensory or motor deficits. It would be difficult to show isolated weakness of the right T9-10 intercostal muscles. Radicular pain is a more common complaint, presenting as a bandlike sensation wrapping around the chest. Patients can mistake this for the pain associated with a heart attack. In animal studies, pure compression of a nerve root, although it produces anesthesia, is not enough to cause pain (dysesthesia). Exposure to chemical factors from an injured disc might potentiate nerve root irritation. This "irascible" nerve root is more susceptible to symptomatic compression. Often, removal of small discs with little evidence of root compression relieves pain. Myelopathy itself is not painful but frequently presents with concomitant radicular or axial pain symptoms.

The spinal canal can be compromised by other structures. Hypertrophy of the facets or infolding of the ligamenta flava can encroach on the posterior aspect of the spinal canal. Ossification of the posterior longitudinal ligament, albeit rare, has been documented as a cause of thoracic myelopathy. Synovial cysts, which may be related to the degenerative process, also have been reported. Kyphotic deformity can be a predisposing factor. Case reports of cord compression in patients with Scheuermann's disease have been documented. Scheuermann's kyphosis can be associated with disc herniations that protrude into the vertebral bodies or the neural elements.

### Trauma

In rare cases, an acute traumatic event can lead to thoracic disc herniation with or without neural dysfunction. About 30% of affected patients relate a traumatic episode with the onset of pain or neurologic dysfunction or both. In most cases, the disc likely had been degenerated to some extent before the incident. Torsion and bending may risk injury to the thoracic disc more than other movements.

## Epidemiology

Radiologic studies indicate that thoracic disc abnormalities can be detected in 73% of asymptomatic patients. The estimated incidence of symptomatic discs is about 1 in 1 million. Symptomatic individuals usually are between 30 and 50 years old; men and women are affected equally. In a two-part natural history study of asymptomatic patients, about 58% of people had an annular tear, 37% had a her-

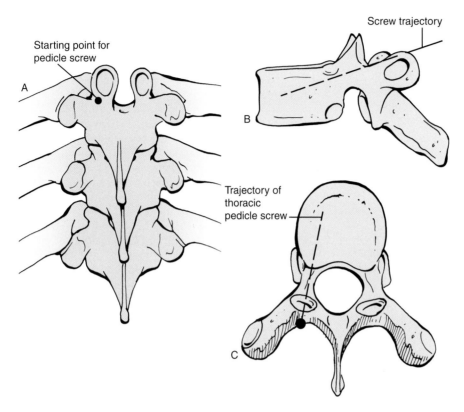

**Figure 15-2**  (**A**) The entry portal for a thoracic pedicle screw is at the inferolateral aspect of the facet joint, near the junction of the superomedial edge of the transverse process. This location can be appreciated further by viewing the lateral (**B**) and axial (**C**) views of the thoracic vertebra. The portal sits in the "valley" between the transverse process and the lamina (**C**).

niated disc, and 25% had imaging evidence of a deformed spinal cord. Patients with Scheuermann's kyphosis had a 38% incidence of disc or vertebral irregularities, which may have represented disc herniations; only 29% of patients were found to have an annular tear. All patients available for long-term follow-up (26 months) remained asymptomatic. Discs causing less than 10% canal compromise tended to get bigger, whereas discs causing 20% or more compromise appeared to resorb. The radiographic finding of thoracic spondylosis is common, but it would be difficult to measure specifically. In most cases, thoracic spondylosis is asymptomatic and never comes to clinical attention.

## CLASSIFICATION

The categorization of thoracic disease may be helpful in determining treatment. There is no gold standard classification system. In general, three groups can be recognized:

- Thoracic disc herniations
- Thoracic stenosis
- Thoracic spondylosis

There can be overlap between these groups because their etiologies are interrelated.

### Herniations

Thoracic disc herniations can be organized by many features. The location, which may be central, paracentral, or foraminal, is important to note. Central herniations are most likely to produce spinal cord compression and myelopathy. They are the least likely to cause radicular pain, although this may occur. Paracentral discs lie off the midline and can cause spinal cord and root compression. Foraminal discs can cause isolated root compression (Fig. 15-3). The surgical approach for this type is distinct and is discussed subsequently.

Discs also may be distinguished by the presence of calcifications. Calcified discs are more likely to be symptomatic than noncalcified discs. They may be associated with adhesions between the disc and the dura, making surgical excision more difficult.

The level of herniation is important. Upper disc herniations are the least common, whereas herniations at the thoracolumbar junction (T11-12 and T12-L1) are the most common. It is believed that the transition between the stiffer thoracic and more mobile lumbar vertebrae is a contributing factor to accelerated degeneration in this region. Most (about 60%) thoracic disc herniations occur between T8 and L1.

### Stenosis

Stenosis denotes central or foraminal narrowing that is not related to a soft disc herniation. Stenosis may be developmental or acquired. Developmental stenosis is usually idiopathic and represents a congenitally narrowed spinal canal.

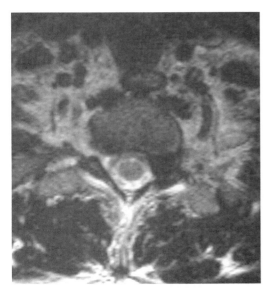

**Figure 15-3**  Axial MRI shows a foraminal thoracic disc herniation at T1-2.

## TABLE 15-1  INITIAL VERSUS PRESENTING SYMPTOMS

| Initial Symptoms (before Initial Evaluation) | % of Cases | Presenting Signs or Symptoms | % of Cases |
|---|---|---|---|
| Pain | 57 | Radicular pain only | 9 |
| Sensory | 24 | Sensory only | 15 |
| Motor | 17 | Motor only | 6 |
|  |  | Motor and sensory | 61 |
|  |  | Brown-Séquard (SCI) | 9 |
| Bladder | 2 | Bladder or sphincter | 30 |

SCI, spinal cord injury.
Adapted from Arce CA, Dohrmann GJ. Herniated thoracic disks. Neurol Clin 1985;3:383–392.

It is a predisposition to neurologic dysfunction but usually is not sufficient alone to cause symptoms. Congenital stenosis is common in patients with achondroplasia. Acquired stenosis usually is related to the later stages of degenerative disc disease. This may be superimposed on a congenitally narrowed canal.

Another type of acquired stenosis is that from ossification of the posterior longitudinal ligament. This rare disorder is more frequent in Asians. Adhesion between the ossified ligament and the dura make surgical excision demanding.

### Spondylosis

Degeneration of the thoracic spine without neural involvement is common and usually asymptomatic. There are no formal classification systems to organize thoracic spondylosis. With the stability of the ribs, degenerative instability or spondylolisthesis is uncommon in the thoracic spine.

## DIAGNOSIS

### History

The most common initial symptoms with thoracic disc disease are the following:

- Pain (57% of patients)
- Sensory complaints (24% of patients)
- Motor complaints (17% of patients)
- Bladder complaints (2% of patients)

Initial symptoms should be distinguished from the complaints at presentation, which are more severe and include

bladder symptoms in 30% of patients and motor or sensory symptoms in 61% of patients (Table 15-1).

Pain can be axial or radicular. Radicular complaints down the arm and leg are uncommon. Radiculopathy usually presents as a bandlike pain along the chest or abdomen. The level of complaint may correlate to the anatomic region of disease, although most patients exhibit T10 findings regardless of the level of disease.

Questions about possible mechanisms of injury might indicate a traumatic etiology. Twisting or heavy lifting can be the inciting event and suggests an acute soft disc herniation. Preinjury back pain suggests underlying disc disease.

History suggesting myelopathy (upper motor neuron findings or long tract signs) must be noted. Weakness in the legs, instability, gait disturbances, and imbalance can be clues. In some situations, patients can present with complete or incomplete spinal cord injury related to a minor injury. These cases have a poor prognosis. Neurologic compression in the upper (T2-5) levels can lead to Horner's syndrome, characterized by a drooping eyelid, pupillary constriction, and dry eye or infrequently pain radiating down the arm.

### Physical Examination

A full physical examination, including an in-depth neurologic evaluation, is required. Specific attention is directed toward the reflex examination. Hyperreflexia in the lower extremities with normal findings in the upper extremities suggests thoracic level spinal cord compression. Other findings indicating thoracic myelopathy are gait imbalance (i.e., wide-based), clonus, and an up-going plantar response (positive Babinski's sign). Abdominal and cremasteric reflexes also should be noted. The examiner specifically must examine for pathologic cervical level reflexes, such as Hoffmann's sign, to rule out cervical myelopathy, which can be missed with a focal exam. Objective weakness or sensory loss in the trunk or lower extremities also can be present. Spinal cord injury may be complete or incomplete.

Radicular findings are difficult to determine at the thoracic level. Regardless of the level of thoracic disc herniation, T10 dermatomal findings are the most common. More often, dysesthesia rather than anesthesia occurs.

## Differential Diagnosis

A wide variety of disorders may manifest similar to thoracic disc disease. Back or flank pain can be associated with renal or gastrointestinal conditions. Zoster pain can present in a dermatomal distribution, feigning the bandlike syndrome of thoracic radiculopathy. Systemic neurologic disorders, such as multiple sclerosis, amyotrophic lateral sclerosis, and Stickler's syndrome, also can confuse the diagnosis. Surgeries performed for radiologic evidence of thoracic disc herniations with these underlying disorders often lead to a poor neurologic outcome. Tumors, with and without neural involvement, also can present similar to thoracic disc disease. Cardiac pain may radiate to or from the thoracic spine and may be the first sign of ischemia.

## Natural History

Information regarding the natural history of thoracic disc disease is sparse. Clinically, approximately 77% of patients with radiculopathy have some symptomatic resolution of symptoms with conservative treatment. Symptoms are correlated poorly with imaging evidence. The radiologic resolution of thoracic disc herniations seems to correlate with initial size: Discs that cause less than 10% of canal compromise tend to stay the same, whereas discs compromising more than 20% of the canal tend to get smaller with time. CT-myelography seems to be no better than MRI in predicting symptoms. A possible advantage of CT is superior detection of calcifications within the disc, which have a higher rate of being symptomatic than noncalcified discs.

## Radiographs

Spinal alignment is noted on plain radiographs, including high-quality anteroposterior and lateral views. Kyphotic deformities, especially with Scheuermann's disease, are associated with a higher rate of thoracic disc herniations. The kyphosis may potentiate spinal cord compression with small disc bulges or osteophytes (Fig. 15-4). Radiographic hallmarks of spondylosis are vertebral body osteophytes, disc space narrowing, and facet hypertrophy. Infrequently, listhesis of the thoracic vertebrae can be noted. This finding is rare because of the extra stability provided by the ribs. "Stippling" within the disc space can suggest calcifications. As stated previously, 45% to 71% of calcified discs are symptomatic, a much higher frequency than noncalcified discs.

## Advanced Imaging

CT-myelography is a useful substitute for MRI if the latter is not possible. With better bone detail, a clearer picture of "hard" discs (i.e., bony osteophytes) is afforded. Facet involvement also is well visualized. CT is the modality of choice to detect ossification of the posterior longitudinal ligament or ossification of the ligamentum flavum, a rare

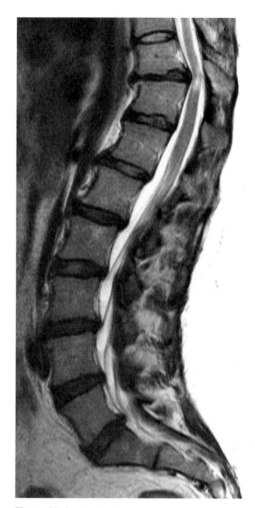

**Figure 15-4**  Kyphosis can exaggerate the compressive effects of small herniated discs. In this patient, posterior vertebral body osteophytes also contributed to canal compromise.

cause of myelopathy in the thoracic spine (Fig. 15-5). CT is useful for detecting intradiscal calcifications.

MRI offers superior soft tissue visualization. It may "overdiagnose" thoracic disc herniations because the rate of abnormal findings in asymptomatic individuals is high. Because of the smaller spinal canal in the thoracic region, however, smaller herniations (compared with lumbar disc herniations) can cause significant symptoms. The integrity of the disc, including the presence of annular tears, bulges, or frank herniations, and the ligaments, including the anterior longitudinal ligament, posterior longitudinal ligament, flavum, and facet capsule, can be noted on MRI. Edema within the spinal cord may be appreciated, suggesting profound neurologic damage.

MRI is an excellent preoperative planning tool. It clearly shows the location of the disc. Most (70% to 90%) are central or paracentral discs; foraminal discs are infrequent. A disc fragment rarely is found within the dural sac. In contrast to cervical and lumbar levels, sequestered fragments are extremely infrequent. The level of disc herniation also is determined. The most common symptomatic levels of herniation are T11-L1, representing the biomechanical

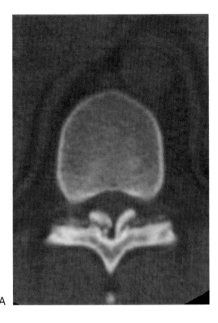 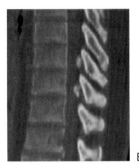

**Figure 15-5** (**A, B**) Ossification of the yellow ligament is an extremely rare cause of thoracic stenosis. On axial CT, the ossified ligament's insertion onto the anterior aspect of the lamina can be seen.

transition zone of the thoracolumbar junction. The most common overall (symptomatic and asymptomatic) region is the T8-L1 area. Calcifications within the disc can appear as hypointensities on T1-weighted and T2-weighted images within the nucleus (Fig. 15-6).

# TREATMENT

## Nonoperative Treatment

Nonoperative treatment is indicated in patients without signs or symptoms of spinal cord compression. This includes patients with signs of root compression or pure axial back pain. Patients with evidence of spinal cord compression by physical examination and imaging are treated better with surgical decompression. The best results for surgi-

cal decompression for myelopathy are early in its presentation while the patient is still highly functional and ambulatory.

Pain is addressed initially with nonsteroidal medications, unless these are contraindicated because of gastrointestinal or renal issues. Mild narcotics should be reserved for severe pain and should not be continued for extended periods. A brief course of rest may help acute pain episodes. Some physicians advocate a short course of oral steroids. Bracing may be of most symptomatic benefit in patients with spinal deformity. The efficacy of this maneuver depends on the flexibility of the curve. Hyperextension bracing may relieve compressive forces across the disc. Extended periods of bracing should be avoided to minimize muscle deconditioning. Rehabilitative efforts through formal physical therapy can be helpful. Emphasis on strengthening, flexibility, and range of motion are beneficial.

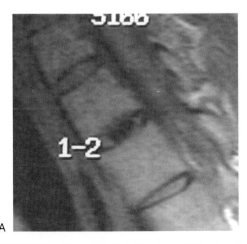 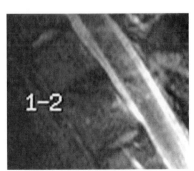

**Figure 15-6** (**A and B**) Calcifications within the disc appear as hypointensities within the nucleus on T1-weighted and T2-weighted images.

Epidural injections have been advocated in the cervical and lumbar spine for the temporary symptomatic treatment of radiculopathy. Some practitioners have found injections to be useful in the thoracic spine for similar indications. Epidural steroids in patients with thoracic level myelopathy and stenosis can be dangerous and are not indicated routinely. Intercostal nerve blocks, analogous to selective nerve root blocks in the neck and low back, may offer some relief for thoracic radiculopathy.

## Surgical Treatment

Surgery for axial back pain associated with thoracic disc disease, whether herniation or spondylosis, is highly controversial. Most of these patients should be treated with observation and nonsurgical modalities. The goal for treating nerve root or spinal cord compromise is decompression. This can be performed through various approaches. Bone or disc or both that are believed to be the offending elements are removed.

### Thoracic Disc Excision

A basic tenet of thoracic disc excision is to choose an approach according to the location of the pathology. The disc should be accessed with no manipulation of the spinal cord. For this reason, standard posterior laminectomy is not advisable. Options include anterior and posterior approaches.

**Anterior Excision.** The anterior disc space may be accessed from a direct anterior exposure. In the high thoracic spine (T1-2), this can be performed with a modified low anterior cervical approach, including a medial claviculectomy. Safe access to the T2-3 disc space is usually possible; however, this should be determined by carefully examining a preoperative sagittal MRI study. The inferior limit to access is the manubriosternal body junction. If it lies proximal to the disc level in question, an alternative approach should be sought. The disadvantages of this approach are the risk for damage to the recurrent laryngeal nerve and thoracic duct (left side). Patients should be advised preoperatively of the cosmetic effects of removing the medial half of the clavicle and manubrium.

The transsternal technique is the "open heart" approach. It is best for exposure of T1-4 when other approaches are not advisable; this should be determined preoperatively. A radiographic marker can be placed within the axilla to determine the most proximal extent of exposure through a thoracotomy. Only if the proposed level cannot be reached in this manner should transsternal exposure be planned. The approach should be performed by an experienced thoracic surgeon.

The transthoracic approach (thoracotomy) uses intercostal dissection to gain lateral access to the thoracic disc spaces from T4-12. A right-sided or left-sided technique can be used, depending on the location of the disc herniation. A double-lumen endotracheal tube should be used. Associated morbidity may be related to lung deflation, lung injury, and intercostal neuralgia from retractor compression.

The advantages of anterior approaches are as follows:

- Direct access to the disc space
- Access to central and paracentral disc herniations
- Direct visualization of spinal cord compression and subsequent decompression
- Ability to perform interbody fusion
- Safer approach for removal of most calcified discs

The disadvantages include the associated morbidity from exposure, including the risk for pulmonary, vascular, and lymphatic injury. Thoracotomies require a postoperative chest tube. Foraminal disc pathology is not well addressed using anterior approaches.

Another important potential disadvantage of the anterior approach is the possibility of spinal cord ischemia from ligation of segmental arteries. The "watershed" region of the thoracic spine is about T4-9, although this can vary. The artery of Adamkiewicz, or great medullary artery, is usually a branch of an intercostal or lumbar artery in the T10-12 region. It then anastomoses with the anterior spinal artery in the spinal canal through a neural foramen. It is present on the left 80% of the time. The artery travels cranially within the spinal canal to supply the so-called watershed area. Sacrifice of this artery can cause acute ischemia of the thoracic spinal cord at this level. In performing an anterior discectomy, the segmental vessels should be spared, which usually is possible unless more extensive bone resection is required. If the segmental artery must be sacrificed, it should be ligated within the midvertebral body. This leaves the anastomosis of the radicular artery with the intercostal artery patent, allowing the possibility of retrograde flow. Intraoperatively the proposed segmental artery can be compressed temporarily, while monitoring evoked potentials for signs of neurologic compromise. A preoperative arteriogram of the spinal vasculature has been used by some authors to determine the level of the great medullary artery preoperatively.

Thoracoscopic approaches also have been advocated. This technique has a learning curve and should be attempted only by properly trained and experienced clinicians. Through multiple thoracic portals, the disc space is accessed and dissected. In most cases reported, the indications have been more for axial pain than for neurologic decompression. The advantages seem to be related to avoidance of an open thoracotomy. Intercostal neuralgia has been associated with large rigid cannulae; neuralgia can be minimized with flexible devices.

**Posterior Approaches.** Although laminectomy/laminotomy is useful for lumbar disc excision, it usually is not for thoracic disc excision. The spinal cord cannot be mobilized or retracted as the cauda equina. This limitation has prompted numerous posterior alternatives for access to thoracic disc herniations without the need for neural retraction.

*Costotransversectomy* can be used to remove centrolateral (paracentral) and lateral disc herniations. The side of the disc herniation is approached. The medial rib, associated transverse process, and pedicle are removed (Fig. 15-7). By maintaining an extrapleural dissection, placement of a postoperative chest tube is avoided. This technique allows direct access to the posterior and posterolateral disc space.

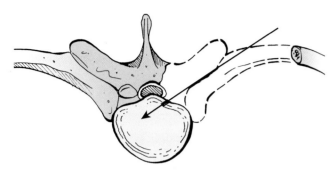

**Figure 15-7**  Costotransversectomy necessitates resection of the pedicle, hemilamina, facet joint, and medial rib on the affected side. This allows decompression without manipulation of the cord.

It is difficult, and possibly dangerous, to remove central disc herniations from this approach. Calcified discs may be approached better by anterior excision. The aorta may be injured with right-sided costotransversectomy. This technique is difficult in obese patients.

The *transpedicular approach* typically involves removal of the pedicle and facet to gain access to the disc space. It is best reserved for lateral or paracentral discs. Some surgeons have used this approach successfully for central disc herniation, but this is technically demanding and requires specially designed curets. By the nature of the procedure, the operation is potentially destabilizing. Visualization is limited without a significant amount of bone removal. Le Roux et al described a modification of the approach that entails work through the pedicle (transpedicular decompression). The authors reported excellent results in lateral and central discs.

Another modification of this approach has been developed and is called the *transfacet approach*. This approach creates a window in the facet joint at the level and side of the disc herniation (Fig. 15-8). It is ideal for foraminal disc fragment excision, regardless of calcifications. By keeping the periphery of the facet intact, the procedure theoretically is less destabilizing. Other advantages include decreased blood loss and shorter operative times. Disadvantages include difficulty assessing the decompression through the small bone window, difficult exposure in obese patients, and inability to decompress centrally.

**Fusion.**  The decision to fuse the spine after disc excision is influenced by the number of discs removed and the amount of bone resected. One-level or two-level anterior discectomies usually can be left unfused, whereas multiple-level discectomies may benefit from fusion. The presence of listhesis, instability, or kyphosis is an indication for fusion (see Fig. 15-4). The thoracolumbar junction (T12-L1) is an area of transition that might benefit from fusion even after a one-level discectomy. This determination is made by intraoperative assessment of stability and imaging evidence of angulation or translation.

The use of instrumentation is controversial. It usually is not necessary for three consecutive levels of discectomy (which is rarely performed). After corpectomy, the role of anterior instrumentation must be weighed against the decision to use supplemental posterior fixation. Extensive posterior facetectomy and rib excision may result in instability that might benefit from fusion.

## Reported Results

Currier et al reported results of 19 cases of central or centrolateral thoracic disc herniations treated by anterior discectomy through an open thoracotomy. All patients had neurologic evidence of myelopathy. Primary disc excisions (16 of 19) yielded statistically significant improvements in motor recovery. In these cases, outcomes were rated as six excellent, six good, and three fair. Three patients who had undergone a previous laminectomy responded poorly to surgery. All patients were fused despite being one-level operations. The authors' justification included the more extensive bony resection performed. Their technique avoided dissection within the neural foramina with the intention of avoiding injury to the medullary artery anastomosis. They also stated that motion at the degenerated segment would produce pain and instability postoperatively. Bohlman and Zdeblick reported their results in 19 cases; in half, they used a transthoracic approach, and in the other half they used a costotransversectomy. Five patients were treated for back pain alone and had no signs of neurologic involvement. Two of these patients had continued pain, with one remaining disabled with workers' compensation. Only one patient who had preoperative myelopathy (treated by costotransversectomy) did not have neurologic improvement. Two patients in the costotransversectomy group had a transient paraparesis. Fusion was not performed routinely. The authors' technique maintained the anterior portion of the disc space and anterior longitudinal ligament (Fig. 15-9).

Stillerman et al used the transfacet, pedicle-sparing technique in six patients, three of whom had calcified discs. Myelopathy and pain resolved in all patients. No patient underwent fusion. Reviewing their results with the transpedicular approach in 20 patients, Roux et al found the only factor that influenced outcome was the duration of symptoms preoperatively.

Regan et al reported their extensive experience with thoracoscopic excision of herniated thoracic discs. An initial report in 1995 noted a long learning curve and various possible complications, including intercostal neuralgia, atelectasis, excessive epidural bleeding, and temporary paraparesis. A follow-up series of 29 cases with 12- to 24-month follow-up showed that 76% of patients were satisfied with the operation, 20% reported no change, and 4% were worse. The most common indication was axial or radicular pain, with only two patients reported to have mild or moderate myelopathy preoperatively. The authors did not report the neurologic recovery in these patients. Building on their series, the same group later published results of 100 patients who underwent the procedure. Only eight patients had thoracic myelopathy, and although improvements in Oswestry scores were reported, the authors did not document specifically neurologic recovery. Discography was used to aid diagnosis of painful disc herniations. Overall the surgeons showed modest improvements in pain in most patients. Future analysis must show that thoracoscopic techniques are cost-ef-

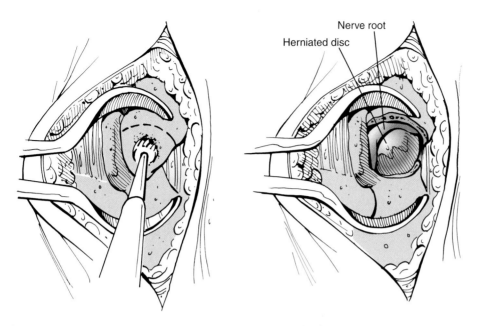

**Figure 15-8** The pedicle-sparing transfacet approach is ideal for foraminal disc herniation causing radiculopathy. The nerve is displaced superiorly by the extruded disc material. A microscope can be helpful during excision.

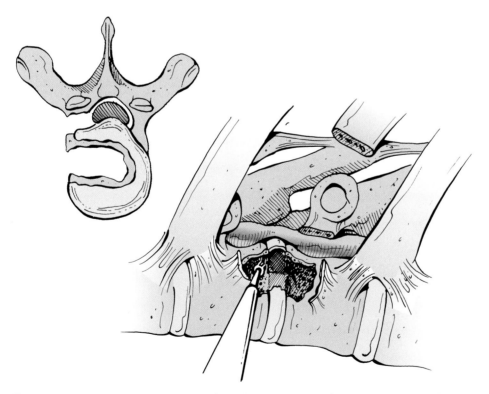

**Figure 15-9** Leaving the anterior aspect of the disc intact, parts of the posterior vertebral body can be removed to allow greater exposure. This technique can preserve anterior column stability.

fective. Their role in decompression of the spinal canal for neurologic decompression has not been well established.

# Thoracic Stenosis

Degenerative narrowing of the thoracic spinal canal can occur from spondylosis. Osteophytes along the posterior border of the vertebral body at the disc space can encroach on the free space for the spinal cord. Facet hypertrophy, also thought to arise from the degenerative process, can decrease the posterior space for the cord. Degenerative changes can be superimposed on a congenitally narrowed canal. Other documented, but unusual, causes of thoracic stenosis are ossification of the posterior longitudinal ligament and ossification of the ligamentum flavum (see Figure 15-5 A, B).

Anterior or posterior techniques can be used to decompress the spinal canal. There is little agreement about the gold standard treatment. Conceptually, anterior compressive structures should be removed by anterior techniques, such as discectomy and corpectomy. An anterior technique allows direct access and visualization of anterior spinal cord. Posterior pathology, such as ossification of the ligamentum flavum or facet overgrowth, is addressed better with posterior surgery, such as laminectomy and foraminotomy. An important consideration in planning a laminectomy is the alignment of the spine. In the cervical spine, lordotic alignment optimizes the effectiveness of posterior decompression. Although laminectomy may be an effective decompressive procedure in normokyphotic thoracic spines, it may not be as effective in hyperkyphotic spines. The decision to fuse should be based on the amount of destabilization created iatrogenically during the operation, the degree of preoperative kyphosis, and the presence of listhesis or instability.

In the few series reported on the surgical treatment of thoracic stenosis, the results generally are worse than after surgery for the cervical or lumbar stenosis. Palumbo et al treated 12 patients with either an anterior or a posterior decompression. The approach was based on the location of the compressive pathology. Five of 12 patients endured

neurologic deterioration, one of whom was motor intact preoperatively. No attempt at discectomy was made through the posterior approach. With greater than 2-year follow-up in all patients, the authors noted that results tended to deteriorate with time. In only six patients treated with laminectomy, Barnett et al reported more encouraging results. All showed some neurologic improvement. These findings are limited by low patient numbers. Similarly, Smith and Godersky found that seven of seven patients responded well—neurologically and in pain level—after a laminectomy and facetectomy for degenerative thoracic stenosis secondary to spondylosis. Follow-up was less than 1 year in this series.

# SUGGESTED READING

Albrand OW, Corkill G. Thoracic disc herniation: treatment and prognosis. Spine 1979;4:41–46.

Currier BL, Eismont FJ, Green BA. Transthoracic disc excision and fusion for herniated thoracic discs. Spine 1994;19:323–328.

El-Kalliny M, Tew JM, Loveren HV, et al. Surgical approaches to thoracic disc herniations. Acta Neurochir (Wien) 1991;111:22–32.

Larson SJ, Holst RA, Hemmy DC, et al. Lateral extracavitary approach to traumatic lesions of the thoracic and lumbar spine. J Neurosurg 1976;45:628–637.

LeRoux PD, Haglund MM, Harris AB. Thoracic disc disease: experience with the transpedicular approach in twenty consecutive patients. Neurosurg 1993;33:58–66.

Mack MJ, Regan JJ, McAfee PC, et al. Video-assisted thoracic surgery for the anterior approach to the thoracic spine. Ann Thorac Surg 1995;59:1100–1106.

Morgan H, Abood C. Disc herniation at T1-2: report of four cases and literature review. J Neurosurg 1998;88:148–150.

Palumbo MA, Hilibrand AS, Hart RA, et al. Surgical treatment of thoracic spinal stenosis. Spine 2001;26:558–566.

Regan JJ, Ben-Yishay A, Mack MJ. Video-assisted thoracoscopic excision of herniated thoracic disc: description of technique and preliminary experience in the first 29 cases. J Spinal Disord 1998;11:183–191.

Singounas EG, Kypriades EM, Kellerman AJ, et al. Thoracic disc herniation: analysis of 14 cases and review of the literature. Acta Neurochir (Wien) 1992;116:49–52.

Videman T, Battie MC, Gill K, et al. Magnetic resonance imaging findings and their relationship in the throracic and lumbar spine. Spine 1995;20:928–935.

Yablon JS, Kasdon DL, Levine H. Thoracic cord compression in Scheuermann's disease. Spine 1988;13:896–898.

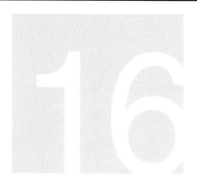

# LUMBAR STENOSIS

## DILIP K. SENGUPTA
## JEFFREY S. FISCHGRUND

With the availability of modern imaging facilities, lumbar spinal stenosis increasingly is being recognized as a cause of low back pain and radiculopathy in elderly patients. Surgical treatment for spinal stenosis increased in the United States by eightfold from 1979 to 1992, from 7.8 to 61 procedures per 100,000 persons 65 years old and older. There has been no long-term prospective, randomized, controlled study, however, to establish the superiority of surgical treatment over the natural history of this disease.

## DEFINITION AND CLASSIFICATION

*Spinal stenosis* is defined as any condition involving narrowing of the spinal canal or neural foramen. There are many forms of lumbar spinal stenosis. The most common is *degenerative stenosis,* which occurs in virtually the entire adult population as a result of the natural process of aging.

Lumbar spinal stenosis can be classified as follows:

- Congenital/developmental stenosis

  Idiopathic (hereditary)
  Achondroplastic

- Acquired stenosis

  Degenerative
  Combined congenital and degenerative stenosis
  Sponylolytic/spondylolisthetic
  Iatrogenic—postlaminectomy, postfusion
  Posttraumatic
  Metabolic—Paget's disease, fluorosis

Degenerative lumbar spinal stenosis is a narrowing of the spinal canal or intervertebral foramina or both caused by bone or ligament hypertrophy (or both) in local, segmental, or generalized regions. The narrowing results in compression of spinal nerves and nerve roots, causing a constellation of symptoms, including lower back pain, neurogenic claudication, and lower extremity pain.

Congenital lumbar stenosis is relatively rare and usually presents at an early age, often between 30 and 40 years old. Acquired lumbar spinal stenosis is more common and generally develops when patients are 60 years old or older. The incidence of degenerative lumbar stenosis is not influenced by sex, race, or ethnicity, and it is not associated with any particular occupation or body habitus.

## CLINICAL PRESENTATION

Patients often are elderly, of either sex, and present with progressively increasing leg pain. They usually have associated low back pain. As always, low back pain from sources other than the spine needs to be considered, such as abdominal aortic aneurysm, pelvic tumors, and hip osteoarthrosis. Posture and gait should be noted. Frequently, stenotic patients stand with hip hyperextension and knee flexion to compensate for increased lumbar flexion. Gait may be antalgic, broad-based with instability, or show a Trendelenburg lurch. There is usually no demonstrable neurologic deficit at rest; however, subtle findings may appear after exercise.

Symptoms include dull-to-severe aching pain in the lower back or buttocks, which radiates into one or both thighs and legs (60% bilateral pain). The pain, numbness, weakness, or paresthesia involving the lower extremities typically develops with walking or other activities. This condition is known as *neurogenic claudication.*

Neurogenic claudication must be differentiated from vascular claudication. In vascular claudication, peripheral pulses are diminished or absent, calf/leg pain is not relieved by leaning forward, and pain relief is slower after resting. Vascular claudicant calf pain often occurs at night, awakening the patient from sleep and prompting "dangling" the legs from the side of the bed to gain relief. In contrast, neurogenic claudication pain typically is relieved by stooping forward, and relief usually is quicker after stopping than with vascular disease. Vascular claudication often produces burning calf pain, whereas neurogenic claudication may produce pain associated with tingling, numbness, and weakness. Although walking uphill produces vascular claudicant pain quickly, patients with lumbar stenosis often report that walking uphill is less painful than walking downhill. Activities that encourage a flexed lumbar posture are tolerated better by stenotic patients. Patients often feel relief by holding onto a shopping cart while ambulating (the "shopping cart" sign). Similarly, exercise endurance while pedaling a stationary bicycle can be nearly normal in patients with lumbar stenosis, whereas patients with vascular claudication quickly experience typical lower extremity symptoms.

# PATHOGENESIS

The cause of neurogenic claudication is not fully understood. One component may be ischemia of the nerve roots induced by exercise demands. Mechanical neural impingement is another important factor. This impingement can occur centrally, in the lateral recesses, or in the neural foramina. Facet joint hypertrophy and ligamentum flavum infolding caused by loss of disc space height frequently are present. Asymmetric collapse, rotatory and lateral listhesis, anterolisthesis, or retrolisthesis can compromise further the dimensions of the spinal canal and foramina.

# NATURAL HISTORY

Lack of longitudinal prospective studies documenting the clinical course of the disorder in untreated lumbar spinal stenosis patients makes it difficult to gain a clear picture of the natural history of lumbar stenosis. Although some patients experience a rapid decline in physical function and a rapid increase in symptom severity, for most progression is slow.

Johnsson et al studied the "natural course" of lumbar spinal stenosis in 32 patients observed over 49 months. Based on a visual analogue pain scale, 15% improved, 70% remained unchanged, and 15% deteriorated at 4 years. Based on clinical examination, however, 41% improved, 41% remain unchanged, and 18% were worse. The authors concluded that observation seems to be an important alternative to surgical treatment because severe progression is unlikely.

# NONOPERATIVE TREATMENT

Considering the low likelihood of rapid deterioration and the possibility of spontaneous improvement, nonoperative treatment is an important option. Activity modification is the mainstay of nonsurgical treatment. Flexion exercises and aerobic conditioning should follow a short period of rest for symptom flare-ups. Stationary bicycle riding, aquatic exercises, and partially unloaded treadmill exercise are helpful. A lumbar corset may decrease motion and reduce pain; however, prolonged bracing may lead to paraspinal muscle weakness and should be avoided.

Pain medications, such as acetaminophen and nonsteroidal antiinflammatory drugs, are often helpful, but are not without associated risks of gastrointestinal ulceration and renal impairment, especially in elderly patients. The selective cyclooxygenase-2 inhibitors may be safer in regards to gastrointestinal complications. Use of narcotics should be limited to control of acute flare-ups to minimize constipation, drug dependence, and mental function impairment. Antidepressants in low doses occasionally are helpful as an adjuvant to pain medication, particularly in controlling neuropathic pain. Calcitonin treatment in lumbar spinal stenosis has been established to be beneficial in a randomized, placebo-controlled, double-blind, crossover study with 1-year follow-up.

Trigger point and facet joint injections may be helpful in a few cases. Epidural steroid injections are used more frequently, but they are controversial. Rosen et al reported temporary relief of radicular pain in 50% of patients. In contrast, in a prospective, randomized, double-blind study, Cuckler et al failed to establish any efficacy of injecting methylprednisolone acetate over physiologic saline. The caudal route of epidural injection in elderly patients with spinal stenosis is technically easier than injecting through arthritic posterior elements of the spine, but it has the disadvantage of failure of the drug to reach beyond a level of tight stenosis.

Other modalities of nonsurgical treatment include manipulation, acupuncture, stress reduction, ultrasound, transcutaneous electrical nerve stimulation, thermal modalities, and traction. These modalities, although anecdotally beneficial in a few patients, cannot be recommended based on the available data.

## Results of Nonoperative Treatment

Amundsen et al reported a prospective 10-year follow-up study of 68 patients treated nonoperatively. Twenty patients eventually underwent surgery because of early deterioration between 3 and 27 months (median 3.5 months). Of the remaining 48 cases, good outcome was observed in more than 70%. The authors could not identify any predictor of successful outcome after conservative treatment. They found that delayed surgical intervention in patients who failed a trial of conservative care still could be expected to have a good result.

Simotas et al studied 49 patients with lumbar spinal stenosis treated conservatively for 16 to 55 months. Treatment included exercise, analgesics, and epidural steroid injections. Of patients, 18% underwent surgery, 14% worsened, 24% remain unchanged, and nearly 50% had mild or sustained improvement. The authors concluded that aggressive nonoperative treatment remains a reasonable option.

Onel et al described a more aggressive nonoperative treatment regimen that included an intensive 1-month inpatient rehabilitation program, calcitonin injections, oral calcium supplementation, heat, ultrasound therapy, and active exercises in 145 patients. The authors reported 91% of patients became pain-free, whereas 5% failed to have satisfactory improvement. Only two patients went on to surgical treatment. Duration of follow-up and long-term results were not reported.

## Surgery Versus Nonoperative Treatment

The Maine Lumbar Spine Study was a multicenter, prospective observational study of a cohort of 67 surgically treated and 52 conservatively treated patients with 4-year follow-up. Surgically treated patients had more severe symptoms. Despite this difference, patient satisfaction at 4 years was higher with surgical treatment (63%) compared with nonsurgical treatment (42%), even after adjustment for other independent predictors of outcome. The relative benefit of surgery declined over time, however, whereas the outcomes for nonsurgically treated patients who improved were relatively stable over 4 years.

In the long-term prospective study reported by Amundsen et al, a cohort of 100 patients was followed for more than 10 years. Within this cohort, 31 patients were randomized to either conservative (n = 18) or surgical (n = 13) treatment. Surgically treated patients had a better outcome.

# SURGICAL TREATMENT

## Indications for Surgery

Surgical treatment is indicated in patients who have intractable pain, who have failed an appropriate nonoperative course, and who have spinal stenosis as the cause of their symptoms. Progressive neurologic deficit in radicular distribution and presence of bladder and bowel dysfunction are relatively uncommon in spinal stenosis. Except in these two situations, surgery for spinal stenosis is an elective procedure. Delayed surgery does not seem to worsen the outcome. Predominant low back pain is not alleviated reliably with surgical decompression because isolated back pain is not a good indication for surgery. Most patients with lumbar spinal stenosis present because of pain and activity limitations. Treatment decision making should be driven by the patient's assessment of how these factors are affecting his or her daily life.

## Preoperative Evaluation

The exact anatomic diagnosis of the pain generator is the key to a successful outcome after surgery. The decision for the extent of surgery, unilateral or bilateral decompression, number of levels, and need for fusion depends on proper identification of the location of stenosis and instability.

Plain radiographs may not establish the diagnosis of spinal stenosis, but signs of disc degeneration, disc height loss, osteophytes, hypertrophic facet arthropathy, and degenerative spondylolisthesis should be noted. The radiographic study should include standing anteroposterior and lateral views, which may show associated scoliosis, and flexion/extension lateral views, which may show segment instability. Congenital stenosis is noted by short pedicles in lateral views and a narrow interpedicular distance on anteroposterior views.

Computed tomography (CT) is helpful in diagnosing the degree and location of the stenosis. CT has several limitations, however. Viewing of soft tissues generally is inadequate. The morphology of the canal may be different in recumbent compared with standing or sitting posture. In the presence of deformity, the CT scan may be difficult to interpret.

The value of CT is enhanced greatly when combined with intrathecal contrast myelography. Central canal stenosis may be diagnosed correctly by direct measurement of the canal diameter in only 20% cases without contrast enhancement versus 83% after contrast images. Often in elderly patients with a pacemaker or other metal implants contraindicating magnetic resonance imaging (MRI), CT-myelography is a reliable preoperative imaging study. High-grade stenosis may limit visualization of the distal regions; however, this often may be overcome by flexion of the spine for a few minutes before imaging.

MRI is the imaging study of choice in most cases. MRI is noninvasive, permits visualization of the soft tissues, and allows surveillance of the entire spine. The bone canal is imaged better with CT, however. MRI and contrast-enhanced CT are comparable in their ability to show spinal stenosis, but MRI is more sensitive in showing disc degeneration.

Lumbar spinal stenosis can be classified radiologically as mild, moderate, or severe. There is no consensus on criteria for these definitions. Speciale et al reported only a fair level of interobserver reliability (average κ score 0.26) in grading the severity of spinal stenosis on the basis of MRI. It cannot be overemphasized that radiologic severity of stenosis does not correlate with clinical severity. Surgical treatment is indicated only when the patient has symptoms not responding to conservative treatment and has concordant radiologically demonstrable stenosis.

In the presence of multiple-level stenosis with predominantly radicular symptoms, it may be difficult to identify the level generating symptoms. Selective nerve root block may help in identifying the pain source and may provide at least temporary pain relief when combined with steroid.

Somatosensory evoked potential studies often are useful and more sensitive than electromyography to identify the level of nerve root compression to implicate one level over another. Somatosensory evoked potentials have a significant rate of false-positive readings and should be considered in conjunction with imaging studies.

## Operative Setup and Preparation

Appropriate preoperative medical and psychological evaluations are essential, particularly in elderly patients with multiple comorbidities. For extensive surgical procedures, it may be preferable to donate 2 to 3 U of autologous blood before surgery. Use of cell saver to avoid homologous transfusion may not be cost-effective.

Spinal anesthesia has the advantage of less frequent postoperative pulmonary complications, and it is adequate for routine decompression of one or two levels that requires less than 2 hours of operating time. If the patient coughs during surgery, it may cause major nerve root prolapse even through a small dural tear, making repair more difficult.

Other intraoperative measures include antibiotic prophylaxis, sequential compression pump devices (calf "squeezers"), and antiembolic stockings to help prevent deep vein thrombosis. Patients should be positioned on the table with adequate padding of the pressure points. The abdomen should be hanging freely to reduce intraabdominal pressure. The head of the table should be elevated during prolonged surgery to prevent facial edema. Pressure to the eyes must be avoided. Use of loupes, a headlight, or a microscope depends on the surgeon's preference. Adequate illumination and magnification are essential.

# TYPICAL VERSUS COMPLEX SPINAL STENOSIS

Hansraj et al suggested a therapeutic classification of degenerative spinal stenosis. *Typical* spinal stenosis is degenerative stenosis without radiographic evidence of instability (i.e., less than grade I degenerative spondylolisthesis, less than 20 degrees of degenerative scoliosis) and no history of previous lumbar surgery. These patients may be treated by decompression alone. *Complex* spinal stenosis is defined as cases associated with degenerative spondylolisthesis exceeding grade I, degenerative scoliosis with curves exceeding 20 degrees, postoperative radiographic evidence of instability, or postlaminectomy junctional stenosis. These cases often benefit from decompression and fusion with or without instrumentation. Algorithm 16-1 is a systematic treatment alogrithm to aid in effective and appropriate surgical decision making.

## Typical Spinal Stenosis

Lee et al classified degenerative spinal stenosis according to the anatomic location of neurologic compression:

- *Central* canal stenosis often is associated with congenital short pedicle.
- *Lateral recess* of the spinal canal is divided into three zones:

The *entrance zone* is the most cephalad part, located medial to or underneath the superior articular process. This zone has only anterior and posterior walls. The medial and lateral aspects are open. The anterior wall is the posterior surface of the disc, and the posterior wall is the facet joint (Fig. 16-1).

The *mid zone* is located under the pars interarticularis part of the lamina and below the pedicle. The anterior border of this zone is the posterior aspect of the vertebral body. The posterior border is the pars interarticularis, the lateral border is the pedicle, and the medial border is open to the central spinal canal. The mid zone contains the dorsal root ganglion (see Fig. 16-1).

The *exit zone* is the area surrounding the intervertebral foramen. The posterior border is the lateral aspect of the facet joint of the lower level, and the anterior border is the disc of the lower level (see Fig. 16-1). Stenosis may involve one or more of the three zones.

## Central Canal Stenosis

Central canal stenosis is treated by decompressive lumbar laminectomy at the stenotic segment. The decompression should begin away from the area of maximal stenosis and progress from caudad to cephalad. The lamina is removed

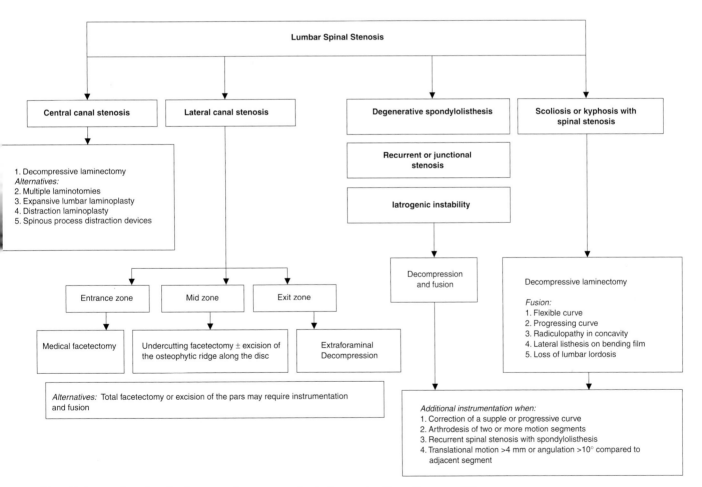

**Algorithm 16-1**   An algorithm for the surgical treatment of spinal stenosis. (From Sengupta DK, Herkowitz HN. Lumbar Spinal Stenosis: Treatment Strategies And Indications For Surgery. Orthop Clin North America 2003;34:281–295.)

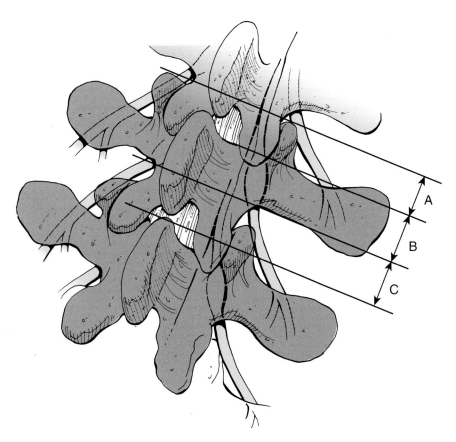

**Figure 16-1** The lateral spinal canal in the lumbar spine showing the different zones. (**A**) Entrance zone. (**B**) Mid zone. (**C**) Exit zone. (Redrawn with modification from Lee CK, Rauschning W, Glenn W. Lateral lumbar spinal canal stenosis: classification, pathologic anatomy and surgical decompression. Spine 1988;13:313–320.)

out to the most medial portion of the articular facets. Care should be taken to preserve the pars. At the end of the procedure, it is important to check if adequate decompression was obtained by palpating the nerve root canals with a "hockey-stick" or a ball-point probe. If the nerve root path is tight, further decompression is indicated as described subsequently.

### Lateral Recess Stenosis

When the stenosis is confined to the lateral recess, the nerve root may be decompressed by laminotomy. The spine is approached by midline incision, but only the symptomatic side is exposed. The nature of the decompressive procedure depends on the location of the stenosis.

### Entrance Zone Stenosis

Decompression of entrance zone stenosis requires medial facetectomy. Partial excision of the medial margin of the superior facet may be done with a Kerrison rongeur or with an osteotome. If the ridge is too thick, it may be thinned with a bur. Without significantly compromising stability, 50% of the facet joint can be removed bilaterally. After satisfactory completion of the procedure, the nerve root should be able to be displaced by 1 cm medially, the root canal should allow free passage of a probe, and evoked potentials may show an improvement (Fig. 16-2).

### Mid Zone Stenosis

The dorsal root ganglion, which is the thickest and most pressure-sensitive section of the nerve root, lies within the mid zone. Total facetectomy and excision of the pars ensure complete decompression but destabilize the segment. Partial decompression may be achieved by removing the anterior half of the superior facet and the lamina with an osteotome. In the presence of spondylolysis, abundant soft tissue from the pseudocapsule of the pars defect usually causes the compression and may be removed by a curet or rongeur (Fig. 16-3).

### Exit Zone Stenosis

Exit zone stenosis may be caused by hypertrophic osteophytes from the facets or osteophytic ridge along the disc and causes entrapment of the exiting nerve root. The L4 nerve root may be entrapped by a hypertrophic superior articular facet of L5 or an osteophytic ridge along the L4-5 disc. In the presence of degenerative listhesis with an intact pars, the exiting nerve root may be entrapped between the pedicle of the vertebra above and the superior margin of the vertebra and disc below. A conservative approach to decompress the nerve root in this zone may involve medial facetectomy, discectomy, or impaction of the osteophytic ridge along the disc with a bone tamp. Total facetectomy and removel of the pars ensure adequate decompression but induce instability requiring stabilization and fusion.

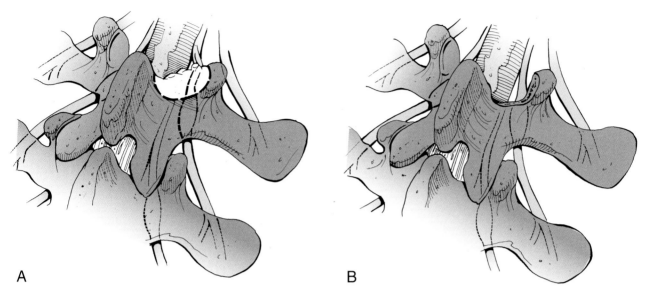

**Figure 16-2**  The extent of decompression for entrance zone stenosis. A partial excision of the medial margin of the superior facet and removal of osteophytes along the superior margin of the lamina usually are necessary. (**A**) Before decompression. (**B**) After decompression. (Redrawn with modification from Lee CK, Rauschning W, Glenn W. Lateral lumbar spinal canal stenosis: classification, pathologic anatomy and surgical decompression. Spine 1988;13:313–320.)

Stenosis *beyond the exit zone* may be approached best by the paraspinal muscle-splitting approach described by Wiltse. The perforating posterior branch of the lumbar artery is located immediately lateral to the facet joint and may be ligated or controlled with bipolar cautery. The nerve root should be decompressed by removing the transverse process, part of the pedicle, and osteophytes from the facet joints (Fig. 16-4).

### Less Invasive Decompression Techniques

Because spinal stenosis affects elderly patients who have multiple comorbidities, many less invasive procedures have been developed.

**Multiple Laminotomies.**  Some authors prefer to do laminotomies, as an alternative to laminectomy, to preserve the midline structures. Multiple laminotomies may be associated with a lower incidence of postoperative instability but are associated with a higher incidence of neurologic sequelae and require longer operating time. Multiple laminotomies may be indicated for mild-to-moderate degenerative stenosis or low-grade degenerative spondylolisthesis. Total laminectomy is preferred for patients with severe degenerative stenosis or higher grade degenerative spondylolisthesis.

**Expansive Lumbar Laminoplasty.**  Tsuji et al were the first to report expansive lumbar laminoplasty, a variant of a procedure initially developed for the cervical spine. The purpose was to preserve stability, particularly in younger active subjects, while achieving decompression. Matsui et al reported results of 27 patients treated with open door-type expansive lumbar laminoplasty. They observed 80% good or excellent results in an average follow-up of 5.6

years. Only one case required additional surgery, which involved discectomy at a caudal adjacent level.

**Distraction Laminoplasty.**  O'Leary and McCance reported a technique of modification of routine laminectomy that allows decompression of the lumbar canal with maximal bone preservation. The technique involves the application of a distraction force, in conjunction with an undercutting laminoplasty. This maneuver allows removal of the medial 20% of the facet joints and the inner one third of the lamina. Clinical outcomes were not reported.

**"Porthole" Approach.**  Kleeman et al described a technique of open laminectomy through a micro-discectomy-like approach. In a prospective series of 54 consecutive cases, they reported good or excellent outcomes in 96% of patients at 4 years. No progression of slip was reported, even in cases with preoperative degenerative spondylolisthesis.

**Spinous Process Distraction Devices.**  Different spinous process distraction implants have been devised, including X-Stop (St. Francis Medical Technologies, Inc, Concord, CA) and Wallis system, a polyetheretherketone-based system described by Senegas and others. These devices distract the spinous processes at the stenotic segment, essentially to hold the spine in flexion, which is the most comfortable posture in patients with spinal stenosis. The decompression is indirect. The hypertrophied ligamenta flava are unfolded by intersegmental distraction. Implantation can be performed under a short local anesthetic period. The procedures currently are recommended for elderly patients with comorbid conditions that may preclude conventional decompression surgery.

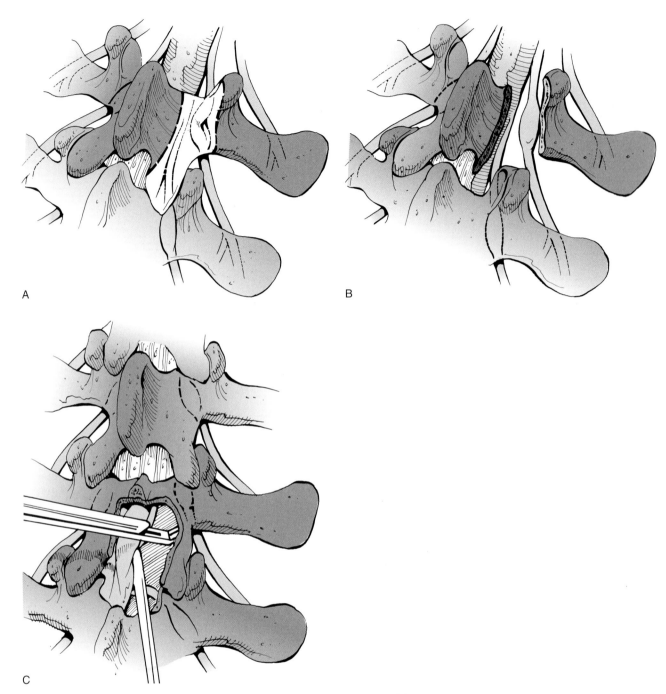

**Figure 16-3**   The extent of decompression for mid zone stenosis. (**A** and **B**) Total laminectomy and total removal of the inferior articular facet ensure adequate decompression but may lead to a significant amount of instability of a motion segment. The osteophytes and hypertrophic ligamentum flavum under the pars interarticularis can be excised and curettaged without sacrificing the facet joint or an entire lamina. Careful undercutting of the facet and removal of the bone from the undersurface of the lamina overlying the root canal can be performed with a Kerrison rongeur (**C**). This can achieve neural decompression, while minimizing destabilization of the spine. (Redrawn with modification from Lee CK, Rauschning W, Glenn W. Lateral lumbar spinal canal stenosis: classification, pathologic anatomy and surgical decompression. Spine 1988;13:313–320.)

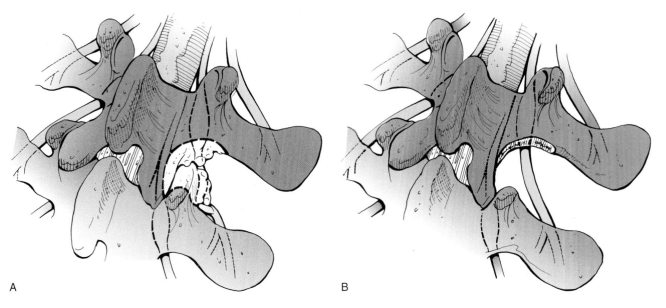

**Figure 16-4** The extent of decompression for exit zone stenosis. This procedure is performed best using a lateral-to-medial approach, as shown here. (**A**) Before decompression. (**B**) After decompression. (Redrawn with modification from Lee CK, Rauschning W, Glenn W. Lateral lumbar spinal canal stenosis: classification, pathologic anatomy and surgical decompression. Spine 1988;13:313–320.)

## Results of Surgical Decompression

Most authors report greater than 85% good-to-excellent results after decompressive lumbar laminectomy, but the benefits seem to decline over time. In a prospective study, Atlas et al reported 63% of patients were satisfied at 4 years; the benefit of surgery declined over time. Katz et al also reported progressive deterioration of initially good results, with 23% undergoing revision surgery at 7- to 10-year follow-up. In a subsequent study, these authors found that patients' own assessments of their health and comorbidity were the most powerful preoperative predictors of good outcome after surgery. Hansraj et al reported patient satisfaction in 95% of the 103 cases treated with decompression alone for typical lumbar stenosis. Only four patients went on to revision surgery during the first year; however, no additional revision surgery was performed at 2 to 5 years. In a metaanalysis, Niggemeyer et al found that the least extensive surgical procedure could obtain the best results if the correct diagnosis and determination of the symptomatic levels were made and operation was done relatively early. Female gender, compensation or litigation, negative preoperative diagnostic nerve root block, previous surgery, obesity, and smoking have been suggested to be predictors of poor outcome after surgery.

## Complex Spinal Stenosis

Spinal stenosis associated with instability or deformity or recurrent stenosis after previous decompression has been described as *complex* stenosis. Fusion and instrumentation often are employed in these cases. Although there seems to be a consensus on the role of decompression for lumbar

spinal stenosis, recommendations for fusion or stabilization are less clear. The goals of fusion are relief of mechanical back pain from a degenerated disc or elimination of instability. The goals of stabilization are to promote fusion and to correct deformity.

Generally, fusion with or without stabilization is recommended after laminectomy for lumbar stenosis in the following situations:

- Degenerative spondylolisthesis
- Iatrogenic instability after decompression
- Recurrent stenosis (at same or adjacent level of previous decompression)
- Degenerative scoliosis or kyphosis

### Degenerative Spondylolisthesis

**Decompression Alone.**    Previously, decompression alone was the "standard" surgical treatment for degenerative spondylolisthesis with spinal stenosis. More recently, improved clinical results have been documented with the addition of posterolateral fusion.

**Decompression and Fusion.**    In a classic prospective randomized study, Herkowitz and Kurz reported 50 cases of spinal stenosis with degenerative spondylolisthesis treated with either decompression alone or decompression and posterolateral fusion. The study showed significantly better outcomes in the fusion group. Although the pseudarthrosis rate was 36%, the clinical results were good or excellent in all the patients in this group. It has been postulated that even with a nonunion, the clinical benefit of substantially decreasing motion (albeit not complete) are significant.

Since this landmark study, subsequent studies have supported these findings.

Solid fusion may prevent recurrent stenosis. Postacchini and Cinotti retrospectively compared 16 cases of degenerative spondylolisthesis treated with decompression alone versus 10 cases with an added arthrodesis. The decompression group had more bone regrowth and a significantly poorer outcome than the arthrodesis group. It has been suggested that solid fusion may promote resorption of compressive osteophytes that were not removed at the time of the initial decompression.

**Selective Fusion.** When is it necessary to fuse decompressed segments? In a prospective randomized study of 45 patients with spinal stenosis without instability, Grob et al found no difference in outcomes between decompression alone, decompression with selective fusion, or decompression with fusion of all the segments. These authors concluded that arthrodesis was not justified in the absence of radiographically documented instability. Other authors have reported similar findings (Fig. 16-5).

**Role of Instrumentation to Enhance Fusion.** Many studies have addressed the role of instrumentation, but there remains no consensus. The key issues are:

- Whether instrumentation improves fusion rate
- If it does, whether clinical outcome also is improved

Zdeblick reported a higher fusion rate with use of instrumentation in a prospective randomized study in 124 patients (including 56 with degenerative or isthmic spondylolisthesis). Bridwell et al compared instrumented versus uninstrumented fusion in 44 patients with degenerative stenosis and spondylolisthesis. The instrumented group showed a much higher fusion rate, better functional outcome, and improved restoration of sagittal alignment compared with the uninstrumented group (87% versus 30%). In an historical cohort study of 2684 patients with degenerative spondylolisthesis, Yuan et al observed a significantly quicker and more reliable fusion in the instrumented group and a better clinical outcome.

Fischgrund et al performed a prospective, randomized, controlled study comparing decompressive laminectomy and arthrodesis with or without instrumentation for degenerative lumbar spondylolisthesis. All patients underwent decompressive laminectomy, with 35 having fusion with pedicle screw supplementation and 33 undergoing uninstrumented posterolateral fusion. After a minimum 24-month follow-up, Fischgrund et al found an 83% fusion rate in the instrumented group versus a 45% fusion rate in the uninstrumented group. There was no detectable significant

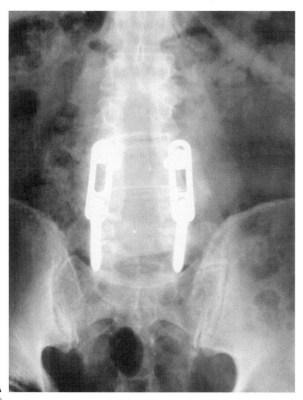
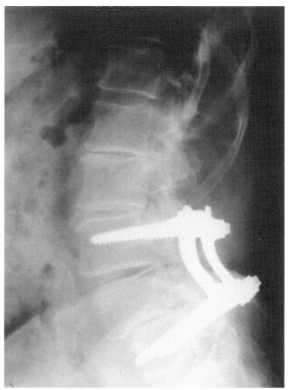

A                                                                                                                    B

**Figure 16-5** (A, B) A 68-year-old man with multiple-level central and lateral canal stenosis and degenerative spondylolisthesis at L4-5 was treated surgically by decompressive laminectomy from L2-S1 levels. At operation, adequate decompression at L3-4 required substantial bilateral facet joint resection. A selective fusion of L3-5 with instrumentation was performed in addition to the decompression. (From Sengupta DK, Herkowitz HN. Lumbar Spinal Stenosis: Treatment Strategies And Indications For Surgery. Orthop Clin North America 2003;34:281–295.)

difference in the clinical outcome. These authors concluded that instrumentation improves fusion rate but does not improve the clinical outcome.

**Reduction of Spondylolisthesis.**    Reduction of listhesis may improve sagittal alignment and improve fusion rate by decreasing tension on the posterior fusion mass. The procedure is technically difficult, is associated with a higher rate of neurologic complications, and often needs an additional segment of fusion to achieve biomechanical stability. Montgomery and Fischgrund prospectively evaluated a technique of passive reduction in a series of patients undergoing decompressive laminectomy and fusion for degenerative spondylolisthesis. They found an average decrease in listhesis by 24% by comparing an intraoperative prone radiograph with a preoperative flexion radiograph. This postural reduction may obviate the need for fusion of an extra level (usually one extra cranial level) and reduces the risk of complication associated with active reduction maneuvers.

### Iatrogenic Instability

How much of the facet joint may be excised during decompression before causing instability is uncertain, but it generally is believed that less than half of both sides or all of one facet at a given level may be tolerated without significant instability. In a biomechanical study in cadaver spines, Abumi et al showed that removal of greater than 50% of each facet joint led to instability. When facet excision is greater than 50% in each side (or >50% of the total facets—25% of one and 75% of the other), an instrumented fusion may be indicated.

Clinical instability after decompression is uncommon. Hazlett and Kinnard reported that only 4 of 33 patients who underwent unilateral or bilateral complete facet excisions in addition to disc excision were unstable. White and Wiltse found only a 2% incidence of postdecompression spondylolisthesis in 182 patients. Some authors believe that the development of postoperative spondylolisthesis is related to facet joint orientation and dimensions, rather than the absolute amount of joint removed.

### Recurrent and Junctional Stenosis

Repeat decompression for recurrence of stenosis at a previously decompressed level often necessitates additional resection of the pars interarticularis and facet joints. If stability is compromised, an instrumented fusion is recommended.

With lack of long-term prospective data, the true incidence of adjacent segment stenosis is unknown. In a retrospective study with long-term follow-up, Lehman et al observed adjacent segment disease in 42% of cases. Recurrent stenosis may be produced by laminar regrowth. Postacchini and Cinotti reported some degree of bone regrowth in 88% of cases after laminectomy or laminotomy with or without fusion; 40% were symptomatic from either moderate or severe stenosis.

Whitecloud et al reported a study of 14 patients with adjacent level stenosis treated with decompression and fusion. They found an 80% pseudarthrosis rate with uninstrumented fusion compared with only 17% with instrumentation.

Patel et al reviewed 42 cases operated on for adjacent level stenosis. They found that symptoms developed more frequently and earlier if the initial surgery involved instrumentation compared with uninstrumented fusion. Adjacent segment stenosis was found to be more frequent in the proximal segment. Although all patients underwent a revision laminectomy, 33 of the 42 had extension of the fusion to the adjacent level.

## SUGGESTED READING

Abumi K, Panjabi MM, Kramer KM, et al. Biomechanical evaluation of lumbar spinal stability after graded facetectomies. Spine 1990; 15:1142–1147.

Bridwell KH, Sedgewick TA, O'Brien MF, et al. The role of fusion and instrumentation in the treatment of degenerative spondylolisthesis with spinal stenosis. J Spinal Disord 1993;6:461–472.

Caputy AJ, Luessenhop AJ. Long-term evaluation of decompressive surgery for degenerative lumbar stenosis. J Neurosurg 1992;77: 669–676.

Feffer HL, Wiesel SW, Cuckler JM, Rothman RH. Degenerative spondylolisthesis: to fuse or not to fuse. Spine 1985;10:287–289.

Herron LD, Mangelsdorf C. Lumbar spinal stenosis: results of surgical treatment. J Spinal Disord 1991;4:26–33.

Johnsson KE, Rosen I, Uden A. The natural course of lumbar spinal stenosis. Clin Orthop 1992;82–86.

Katz JN, Lipson SJ, Chang LC, et al. Seven- to 10-year outcome of decompressive surgery for degenerative lumbar spinal stenosis. Spine 1996;21:92–98.

Lee CK, Rauschning W, Glenn W. Lateral lumbar spinal canal stenosis: classification, pathologic anatomy and surgical decompression. Spine 1988;13:313–320.

Mardjetko SM, Connolly PJ, Shott S. Degenerative lumbar spondylolisthesis: a meta-analysis of literature 1970-1993. Spine 1994;19: 2256S–2265S.

# LUMBAR DISC HERNIATIONS, DISCOGENIC BACK PAIN, AND CAUDA EQUINA SYNDROME

## CHRISTOPHER M. BONO

## LUMBAR DISC HERNIATIONS

### Pathoanatomy

The disc is the anterior border of the spinal canal at the facet joint level. It is covered by the thin posterior longitudinal ligament, which is concentrated centrally and leaves the posterolateral disc bare. This anatomy is thought to contribute to posterolateral (or paracentral) herniations being the most common herniations. Nerve roots branch from the cauda equina one level above their exiting foramen. The L5 nerve root leaves the cauda equina approximately at the level of the L4 vertebral body, then descends to pass beneath the L5 pedicle, where it turns lateral to exit the spinal canal.

The location of the disc herniation determines which root is primarily affected. The *central zone* is delineated by the lateral borders of the cauda equina. The *lateral recess* is between the lateral border of the cauda equina and the medial border of the pedicle. Within the lateral recess, fragments that migrate medial to the nerve root are termed *axillary herniations*. The *foraminal zone* is between the medial and lateral borders of the pedicle. Herniations beyond the lateral border of the pedicle are within the far-lateral or *extraforaminal zone*. Herniations in the foraminal or extraforaminal zones usually affect the exiting nerve, whereas in the other zones the descending (or traversing) nerve root is affected. Fragments can displace cranially or caudally.

### Pathophysiology

The exact inciting event leading to disc herniation is unknown. Some investigators believe that an acute traumatic episode leads to displacement of the disc, although this most likely is related to force imparted onto a previously degenerated disc, which has developed a focal annular weakness. In support of this idea, acute sciatica from disc herniation often is predated by a history of previous back pain. Postural variations can influence intradiscal pressures. The highest pressures have been recorded in patients with the torso forward flexed with weight in hand.

The relationship between disc herniation and sciatica is not completely understood. In animals and humans, pure compression of a noninflamed nerve produces sensory and motor changes without pain, whereas pain is elicited with manipulation of inflamed nerves. These findings suggest that herniated discs large enough to cause mechanical compression of a nerve root may produce focal deficits, but that associated sciatic-type pain is produced only if the nerve root is irritated or inflamed concurrently. Neurochemical factors, such as IgG, IgM, and tumor necrosis factor-$\alpha$, also may have a role in the production of sciatic pain. There is evidence of systemic inflammatory responses to disc herniations as well.

### Classification of Disc Herniations

Disc herniations can be described by their morphology, as follows:

- *Protruded*—eccentric bulging through an intact anulus fibrosus
- *Extruded*—crosses the anulus but is in continuity with the remaining nucleus

- *Sequestered*—not continuous with the disc space (free fragment)
- *Contained*—subligamentous (by posterior longitudinal ligament or the outer anulus)
- *Uncontained*—cross the posterior longitudinal ligament or outer anulus

## History and Symptoms

Pain is the most common complaint. Some patients describe a specific incident (e.g., fall, twist, heavy lifting). Radicular pain is more typical and often the more "treatable" of the complaints. Lower lumbar or lumbosacral disc herniations can lead to the classic symptoms of pain radiating below the knee, following a dermatomal distribution. S1 radicular pain may radiate to the back of the calf or the lateral aspect or sole of the foot. L5 radicular pain can lead to symptoms on the dorsum of the foot. L2 and L3 radiculopathy can produce anterior or medial thigh and groin pain. Groin pain also may indicate L1 pathology. It is important to ask questions pertaining to bowel and bladder function.

## Physical Examination

Gait should be observed. A sciatic list may be present, usually manifest as the patient leaning away from the side of leg pain. Axillary herniations may cause a list toward the side of herniation. A footdrop or foot slippage gait may occur with an L4 or L5 paresis. A Trendelenburg gait suggests hip abductor weakness (L5).

Tenderness to palpation of one or two levels is more consistent with bone or disc pathology than tenderness at multiple levels. Paraspinal muscle spasm can be noted in addition to tenderness. A neurologic exam is requisite in all patients with suspected herniated discs. Motor, sensory, and reflex examination should be thorough.

### Specific Tests

The *straight-leg raise test* is performed with the patient in the supine position. The test is considered positive if sciatic pain is reproduced between 35 and 70 degrees of elevation. More than 70 degrees of elevation causes no further stretch of the nerve roots. The straight-leg raise test is best for eliciting L4, L5, or S1 radiculopathy. It is not useful for upper lumbar roots, for which a femoral stretch test (performed in the prone position) should be used. If raising the *contralateral leg* reproduces symptoms in the ipsilateral side, this suggests a herniated disc. *Lasègue's sign* is a modification of the straight-leg raise test and involves dorsiflexion of the foot, which aggravates pain.

## Diagnostic Imaging

Plain radiographs cannot show a herniated disc. They can show changes, however, that suggest a herniated disc, such as a scoliotic list or osseous signs of disc degeneration. These changes include osteophytes, disc space narrowing, subtle changes in translation, facet hypertrophy, or changes in sagittal alignment.

### Magnetic Resonance Imaging

The disc is readily visualized using magnetic resonance imaging (MRI). Free fragments can be differentiated from extruded disc herniations and a symmetric bulge from a contained protrusion. The size and type of disc herniation can be determined reliably using MRI. In a postoperative patient with continued or recurrent symptoms, MRI best is delayed until 6 months after surgery, if symptoms allow. The main challenge is differentiating scar from new-onset disc. Although gadolinium-enhanced T1-weighted MRI (which highlights scar but not disc) is considered the gold standard, more recent evidence suggests that sophisticated T2-weighted images (obtained with high-powered magnets) might supplant the need for gadolinium-enhanced MRI.

### Computed Tomography

Before the advent of MRI, CT was the imaging modality of choice for evaluation of herniated discs. CT performed with intrathecal contrast injection (i.e., CT-myelography) is nearly as sensitive as MRI in detecting herniated discs.

## Treatment

### Nonoperative Treatment

Bed rest should be limited to no more than 2 to 3 days. Longer periods of inactivity can potentiate prolonged disability and continued or augmented pain. Exercise therapy and physical rehabilitation should be included in the nonoperative care of herniated discs. Treatment goals are to restore strength, flexibility, and function that were lost secondary to pain, splinting, and spasm. Nonsteroidal anti-inflammatory drugs are first-line agents. In the acute setting, short-term narcotic use, such as a single dose of a morphine-derivative analgesic, can be useful for severe pain, but should not be prescribed in an extended manner. So-called muscle relaxants frequently are prescribed, but these agents have more significant sedative effects than production of muscle relaxation. Selective transforaminal steroid injections can produce symptomatic short-term relief in many patients. In a restrospective study, 77% of patients who were considered surgical candidates but were interested in an injection had clinical resolution and had "avoided" surgery at an average follow-up of 1.5 years.

### Operative Treatment

**Indications.** An absolute indication for lumbar discectomy is a progressive neurologic deficit. In this circumstance, operative intervention may be considered conservative care, provided that no medical contraindications exist. A neurologic deficit most commonly is associated with a cauda equina syndrome.

The relative requirements for an elective discectomy vary but include the following:

- Radiologic identification of compressive pathology that is concordant with the patient's physical signs and symptoms
- Patient's strong desire to return to work or activity
- Failure of at least 6 weeks of nonoperative management,

including observation and therapy with or without selective injections

**Techniques.** There are many techniques of surgical discectomy. Standard open discectomy is the most common surgical approach. It involves careful incision planning, laminotomy or partial laminectomy to provide adequate visualization of the pathologic condition, gentle retraction of the neural elements, and direct excision of the herniation. As an adjunct to open discectomy, some investigators advocate the use of a microscope for better visualization and minimizing incision size. Alternatives to interlaminar techniques have been developed for excision of foraminal and extraforaminal lateral disc herniations (more common in elderly patients), which involve exposures between the transverse processes and lateral to the pars interarticularis.

Various percutaneous methods of treatment have been developed. Some methods entail placement of the cutting device intradiscally to decompress the disc space to retract the herniated fragment. Other methods involve directly visualizing the neural elements and disc using an endoscope. Chemical digestion of the disc (i.e., chemonucleolysis) previously was popular, but enzyme-related complications and results inferior to open discectomy have limited its continued popularity in the United States.

**Postoperative Care.** After an uncomplicated, simple open discectomy, the patient usually is discharged on postoperative day 1 or 2. The activity level recommended varies among surgeons. Concerns are that aggressive movements and load can predispose to reherniation or excessive scarring. This concern has led many surgeons to limit lifting and bending after discectomy for about 3 to 4 weeks. Although this is probably the predominant practice, there is little literature to support such extended periods of protected activity. Unrestricted activity protocols have shown comparable success and reherniation rates.

**Surgical Outcomes.** The outcomes of surgical discectomy are reliable when one adheres to strict preoperative selection criteria. In a careful review of the literature, many factors were shown to affect surgical outcome. In one study, patients with larger herniations had a better outcome after discectomy than patients with small (<6 mm) fragments. Patients with highly positive straight-leg raise test results and younger patients with large disc herniations also tend to have better results. Good or excellent clinical results of open discectomy for paracentral and intraforaminal disc herniations are reportedly about 80%. Patients should be advised that the operation is intended primarily to relieve leg pain, not back pain. Central discs are associated with poorer outcomes (50% good or excellent). In experienced hands, endoscopic discectomy can yield results as satisfying as open discectomy. There is insufficient evidence to conclude that using a microscope leads to superior clinical results.

Psychological and social factors have been shown by many authors to influence surgical results of lumbar discectomy profoundly. Patients who are self-confident, only mildly depressed, and generally optimistic are more likely to do well. Other predictors of good results are a high preoperative pain index, a higher education level, an overall satisfaction with life, and the perception that the patient's job was of light or suitable duty. In one study, the best predictor of outcome was the psychological score as measured by the Minnesota Multiphasic Personality Inventory.

**Complications.** Complications of discectomy are summarized as follows:

- *Recurrent herniation* can occur in 0% to 12% of cases. Some investigators have recommended aggressive disc curettage to decrease reherniation rates; however, this can lead to a higher rate of postoperative back pain. The results of surgical discectomy for a recurrent disc are comparable to primary surgery.
- *Wound infections* have been reported in 0% to 3% of cases.
- *Epidural abscess* is rare, with reported rates of 0.3%, and should be managed with surgical evacuation.
- *Pyogenic discitis* may occur after discectomy 2.3% of the time.
- *Vascular injuries* are exceedingly rare.
- Incidental *dural tears* occur in 0% to 4% cases.
- *Instability* is rare after discectomy. Preservation of the facet joints is helpful in avoiding this complication.

# DISCOGENIC BACK PAIN

Diagnosis and treatment of discogenic low back pain are difficult and controversial. The difficulty stems primarily from the facts that (1) there is no objective test to determine origin of low back pain, and (2) radiologic abnormalities, such as disc degeneration and lumbar spondylosis, are common in asymptomatic patients. An explosion of interest has occurred in the basic scientific understanding of the biochemical and biomechanical changes associated with disc degeneration.

The term *internal disc derangement* has been introduced more recently. This term refers to a pathologic mechanical or chemical condition of the disc that leads to low back pain. The exact mechanism is elusive; however, innervation of the posterior anulus by branches of the sinuvertebral nerve has been well documented. This is the suggested pathway of nociceptive pain transmission from the disc.

## Diagnosis

### Clinical Presentation

The diagnosis of internal disc derangement is difficult. Clinical presentation is that of low back pain with or without leg pain that often is present for years but highlighted by increasingly more frequent acute episodes of pain. Back symptoms are predominant. Leg pain infrequently extends below the knee. Flexion usually aggravates pain more than extension.

### Imaging Findings

Plain radiographs often are negative but may show disc space collapse, end plate sclerosis, or osteophytes. MRI is more useful. On T2-weighted images, the disc appears dark, an indication that it has lost its normal water content. The predictive value of the so-called high-intensity zone within the posterior anulus (which represents a peripheral annular tear) for low back pain is questionable. Bone edema can be noted around the end plate (Modic changes). The role of discography is controversial (see Chapter 3).

## Treatment

### Nonoperative Modalities

Nonoperative treatment modalities include the following:

- Activity modification
- Medications, including nonsteroidal antiinflammatory drugs
- Epidural steroid injections
- Physical therapy, with a focus on lumbar extension exercises, paraspinal muscle strengthening, stretching, and generalized conditioning

### Invasive Modalities

Intradiscal electrothermal therapy has been introduced more recently. This modality involves percutaneous insertion of a heating coil into the disc to coagulate collagenous tissue and nociceptive nerve endings within the posterior anulus. Clinical results have varied, with one report showing about 50% pain reduction in about 50% of patients treated. Two more recently presented randomized prospective studies comparing intradiscal electrothermal therapy with nonoperative care showed modest (1 to 2 points on visual analogue scale) benefits.

Fusion is the most common method of surgical treatment of chronic discogenic low back pain. Results have varied widely in the reported literature. Even in carefully selected patients, posterolateral fusion is successful in only about 50% of cases. Interbody fusion techniques, such as posterior lumbar interbody fusion and anterior lumbar interbody fusion, have produced better clinical results, with reported success rates of 75% to 90%.

On the forefront of technology are motion-sparing procedures, such as total disc arthroplasty and nuclear replacement. From preliminary data, it seems that total disc arthroplasty can be as successful as interbody fusion. The long-term benefits of preserving motion on decreasing the incidence of adjacent segment degeneration remain to be seen.

## CAUDA EQUINA SYNDROME

Cauda equina syndrome most commonly occurs from a herniated lumbar disc, but it also can develop secondary to tumor, abscess, or hematoma. It is more common with central herniation (27% of central herniations), although it can occur with paracentral or lateral herniations as well. It is more frequent in men in their 30s. An L4-5 disc is the usual culprit. Cauda equina syndrome should be considered a true surgical urgency because the neurologic results are affected by the time to decompression. The clinical diagnosis of cauda equina syndrome relies on many components, including perineal sensory deficit (so-called saddle anesthesia), bowel or bladder incontinence, new-onset lower extremity sensory deficit, and a new or progressive motor deficit. In addition to a meticulous physical examination, evaluation of cauda equina syndrome should include measurement of a bladder postvoid residual. Normally, postvoid residual should be less than 50 to 100 mL. The postvoid residual is often abnormal preoperatively and can be an important parameter to follow postoperatively.

Decompression and discectomy can be via a laminotomy or through a formal laminectomy. Proponents of laminectomy believe this provides superior visualization of the dura and avoids excessive traction. Adequate exposure is particularly relevant for removal of central disc herniations. Discectomy is performed best within 48 to 72 hours of the onset of symptoms; this leads to better sensory, motor, urinary, and rectal function recovery. Motor strength may continue to improve for 1 year after surgery. Although the postvoid residual usually decreases to less than 110 mL by 6 weeks, bladder function may continue to improve for 16 months. Early surgery does not seem to affect substantially the resolution of postoperative pain compared with delayed intervention. Preoperative neurologic status seems to be the greatest predictor of recovery.

## SUGGESTED READING

Ahn UM, Ahn NU, Buchowski JM, et al. Cauda equina syndrome secondary to lumbar disc herniation. Spine 2000;25:1515–1522.

Atlas SJ, Deyo RA, Keller RB, et al. The Maine Lumbar Spine Study, Part II: 1-year outcomes of surgical and nonsurgical management of sciatica. Spine 1996;21:1777–1786.

Croissant PD. Extreme-lateral lumbar disc herniation. J Neurosurg 1996;84:1077.

Jonsson B, Stromqvist B. Clinical characteristics of recurrent sciatica after lumbar discectomy. Spine 1996;21:500–505.

Lee CK, Vessa P, Lee JK. Chronic disabling low back pain syndrome caused by internal disc derangements: the results of disc excision and posterior lumbar interbody fusion. Spine 1995;20:356–361.

Parker LM, Murrell SE, Boden SD, et al. The outcome of posterolateral fusion in highly selected patients with discogenic low back pain. Spine 1997;21:1909–1916.

Saal JA, Saal JS, Herzog RJ. The natural history of lumbar intervertebral disc extrusions treated nonoperatively. Spine 1990;15:683–686.

Schecter NA, France MP, Lee CK. Painful internal disc derangements of the lumbosacral spine: discographic diagnosis and treatment by posterior lumbar interbody fusion. Orthopedics 1991;14:447–451.

Weber H. Lumbar disc herniation: a controlled, prospective study with ten years of observations. Spine 1983;8:131–140.

# 18

# LUMBAR SPONDYLO-LISTHESIS

**JOHN M. BEINER**
**JONATHAN N. GRAUER**
**BRIAN K. KWON**
**TODD J. ALBERT**

The term *spondylolisthesis* comes from the Greek *spondylo,* meaning "vertebra," and *olisthesis,* meaning "movement or slipping." Spondylolisthesis describes the pathologic state of one vertebra slipping on another; this can be forward (anterolisthesis) or backward (retrolisthesis). In the lumbar spine, the etiology of spondylolisthesis is varied. *Spondylolysis,* a term that comes from the Greek *spondylo* plus *lysis,* or "break," indicates a defect in the pars interarticularis region. Spondylolisthesis can occur after the development of a lytic defect, after degeneration of the intervertebral disc and facet joints, or from a variety of other causes.

The investigation into spondylolisthesis dates back to the 18th century. A large body of literature exists that attempts to describe the pathogenesis, natural history, and treatment of this extremely common disorder. This chapter describes the classification of spondylolisthesis and summarizes the important aspects of the clinical presentation and treatment options of the various types of lumbar spondylolisthesis. The focus is on the two most common types of spondylolisthesis—isthmic and degenerative. The most well-known system of classifying lumbar spondylolisthesis evolved from the cooperative endeavors of three prominent surgeons, Wiltse, Newman, and Macnab. The *Wiltse classification,* as it is commonly known, divides the disorder into five types (Fig. 18-1):

- *Type I—dysplastic or congenital.* This type is due to the presence of congenital abnormalities of the upper sacrum or the posterior arch of L5.
- *Type II—isthmic.* The lesion is in the pars interarticularis. Three types can be recognized: IIA, lytic-fatigue fracture of the pars; IIB, elongated but intact pars; and IIC, acute fracture of the pars.
- *Type III—degenerative.* This type is due to long-standing instability, arthritic changes, and degeneration of the disc and facet joints.
- *Type IV—traumatic.* Acute fractures in areas of the bone hook other than the pars (often the pedicles) allow translational instability of the motion segment.
- *Type V—pathologic.* There is generalized or localized bone disease (metabolic or neoplastic).

- *Type VI* (this type has since been added by convention)*—iatrogenic.* This is due to aggressive resection of the facet joints or intervertebral disc, or both, leading to the creation of instability in the lumbar spine.

## ANATOMY

Some anatomic factors bear consideration when determining the etiology of spondylolisthesis. In the normal lordotic posture of the lumbar spine, axial load is shared between the intervertebral discs (approximately two thirds) and the facet joints (one third). This distribution can vary depending on posture and loading conditions. The oblique orientation of the facet joints results in limitation of axial and sagittal rotations within the lumbar spine. This facet angle changes from a relative sagittal orientation in the upper lumbar spine to a more coronal orientation in the lower lumbar vertebrae. Most importantly, in the lower lumbar spine, the facet joints provide significant resistance to anterior shear in flexion, especially with increased lumbar lordosis. At the level of L5-S1, the strong iliolumbar ligaments provide additional restraint to forward flexion and lateral motion. This restraint may cause stress concentration at the superjacent (L4-5) motion segment.

In the 1960s, Newman conducted an observational study, performing a comprehensive analysis of the etiologic factors involved in spondylolisthesis. His theories formulated many of the concepts that since have withstood critical analysis. The normal lordosis of lumbar spine in animals that walk erect leads to a constant downward and forward thrust to the lower lumbar vertebrae. This tendency to forward slipping is counteracted by the facets, pedicles, neural arches, and normal bone structure. These anatomic observations form the basis for the Wiltse classification system: the slip may occur secondary to a defect in the facets, a defect in the neural arch or pedicle, or from a structural inadequacy of bone.

Much has been made of the nature of the lytic defect in the pars, the morphologic changes in the facets that accom-

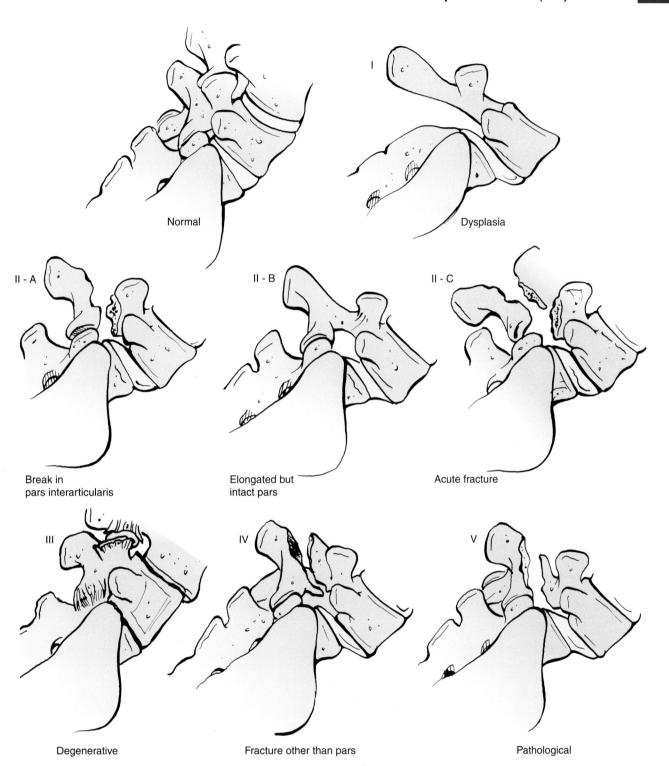

Normal

I

Dysplasia

II - A

Break in
pars interarticularis

II - B

Elongated but
intact pars

II - C

Acute fracture

III

Degenerative

IV

Fracture other than pars

V

Pathological

**Figure 18-1**    Schematic drawing of the modified Wiltse classification of lumbar spondylolisthesis.

pany arthritis, and the predisposing factors in each case. These studies are reviewed in subsequent sections.

# CONGENITAL/DYSPLASTIC SPONDYLOLISTHESIS

Dysplastic spondylolisthesis is considered the only true congenital form of spondylolisthesis. There is a 2:1 female-to-male ratio. These slips account for approximately 14% to 21% of all spondylolisthesis cases. These congenital abnormalities of the lumbosacral junction, including dysplasia of the fifth lumbar and sacral neural arches and facets, compromise the normal buttress function of the posterior elements. Gradual forward displacement of the fifth lumbar vertebra on the sacrum occurs. Displacement is early but usually does not progress beyond 50%.

The pars interarticularis may remain unchanged, or it may elongate or separate. An elongated pars is difficult to distinguish from isthmic subtype B on plain radiographs (see later); a broken pars may be difficult to distinguish from subtype A. These may be discerned, however, during surgery.

When the posterior neural arch is intact, as is the case in most of these patients, two phenomena are observed. The slip is limited in its extent because of impingement of the neural arch on the anterior structures. At the same time, significant neurologic findings are evident with relatively low-grade slips (25% to 35%), resulting from the compression of the cauda equina by the posterior arch of L5 as it is carried forward with the body of L5.

Dysplastic spondylolisthesis is divided into three subtypes, based on the orientation of the facets:

- In *subtype A,* the dysplastic facets have a transverse, or horizontal, orientation. Spina bifida of L5 is common, and early symptoms of the slip, such as hamstring tightness, are relatively common. Fusion for this subtype often is required because of the unstable nature of the motion segment.
- In *subtype B,* the facets have an asymmetric sagittal orientation, and the neural arch is likely to be intact. Associated symptoms of hamstring tightness, leg pain, and even cauda equina syndrome are common. Management requires decompression and fusion for the best clinical outcome.
- *Subtype C* groups other causes of congenital malformations of the lumbosacral junction. Treatment is based on the nature of the abnormality and the severity of clinical symptoms.

# ISTHMIC SPONDYLOLISTHESIS

## Incidence and Etiology

Isthmic, or spondylolytic, spondylolisthesis involves a defect in the pars interarticularis (with normal facets) that permits the forward slippage. It is the most common type of spondy-

lolisthesis. Isthmic spondylolisthesis is divided into three subtypes (Fig. 18-2):

- Spondylolytic fatigue fracture of pars
- Elongated but intact pars
- Traumatic (acute pars fracture)

The sex ratio is the opposite of the congenital type: males predominate in a 2:1 ratio. Much attention has been devoted to the incidence and etiology of this type of spondylolisthesis. It is most common at the L5 level, leading to L5-S1 slip.

Genetic and environmental causes seem to contribute to isthmic spondylolisthesis. Relatives of patients have a reported incidence of 28% to 69%, which is much higher than in the general population. It is rare in individuals of African descent (2.8%), higher in individuals of northern European descent (6.4%), and highest in Alaskan Inuits (26% to 50%). This high incidence is thought to be due to a combination of genetic and environmental causes; Alaskan natives have been observed to stoop over while harvesting seal blubber, possibly changing the stresses on the lumbar spine. The incidence continues to increase in this population until age 34, in contrast to other populations, lending evidence for an environmental contribution.

Spondylolysis rarely is found in newborns; in most studies, it is reported only after walking begins. It has not been reported in quadrupeds or chronically bedridden adults. The incidence increases dramatically between age 5 years and adolescence. Wiltse found a 5% incidence of spondylolysis in children 5 to 7 years old, increasing to 6% to 7% by age 18. Patients with Scheuermann's kyphosis and certain athletes seem to have a higher incidence. Football linemen, gymnasts, butterfly swimmers, weight lifters, rowers, divers, wrestlers, and tennis players all have been noted to use excessive lumbar extension, contributing to the theory of a fatigue fracture. Wiltse defined the basic lesion in isthmic spondylolysis as a fatigue fracture of the pars, and most authors are in accord.

The literature supports the following conclusions regarding the etiology and pathogenesis of spondylolytic spondylolisthesis:

- There seems to be a genetic predisposition or *diathesis.*
- Mechanical stresses from environmental or occupational factors influence the development of a type of fatigue fracture in susceptible or high-risk individuals.
- These fatigue fractures develop at an earlier age, after relatively minor trauma, and persist relative to other known fatigue fractures.
- The presence of a lytic defect adds to instability and contributes to the development of a spondylolisthesis to a varying degree.
- Females are more prone to severe displacement and more frequently need stabilization to treat their instability and lessen their symptoms.
- Less than 20% of patients with a spondylolysis develop symptoms of any kind related to the spondylolysis.

## Natural History

The natural history depends on the subtype. True traumatic pars fractures are rare and usually heal with conservative

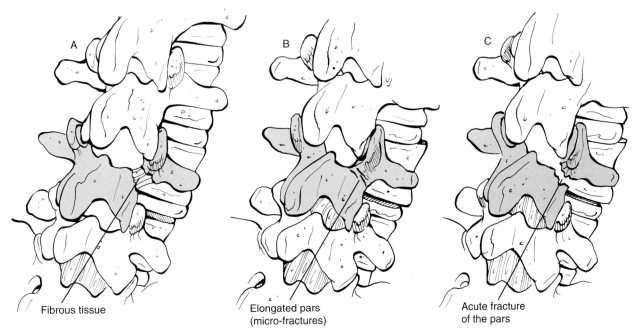

Fibrous tissue

Elongated pars
(micro-fractures)

Acute fracture
of the pars

**Figure 18-2**   Isthmic spondylolisthesis subtypes: (**A**) Spondylolytic fatigue fracture of pars. (**B**) elongated but intact pars. (**C**) traumatic (acute pars fracture).

treatment, without undergoing olisthesis. The percentage of patients with spondylolysis who develop spondylolisthesis was evaluated in a longitudinal study by Fredrickson et al. They found that in patients with lytic defects of the pars, most slips occurred before adulthood: 68% of 5-year-old children had an associated slip, increasing only slightly to 74% in adulthood. Saraste followed 255 patients with isthmic spondylolisthesis for 20 years and found that 40% of adults did not have progression, 40% progressed less than 5 mm, and only 15% progressed more than 1 cm. Slip progression has been found to correlate with a poor outcome in terms of pain and deformity. The literature supports the conclusion that low percentages of slips progress, but there is little agreement as to which factors predict progression. In general, isthmic slips that progress do so farther than degenerative slips, which are limited by the bone anatomy.

Some radiographic indices, such as slip angle (see later), have been reported to predict progression by some authors but not by others. Floman, echoing Taillard, postulated that slip progression after skeletal maturity almost always is related to disc degeneration at the slip level. Slip progression in his study always was accompanied by disc degeneration at the level below the pars defect. The presence of this pathology in the disc may explain the late onset of symptoms associated with the slip. Wiltse pointed out, however, that when the disc collapses, there is little further progression.

## Clinical Findings

Although spondylolysis and olisthesis develop in late childhood or early adolescence, symptoms are relatively uncommon in children. Teenagers and young adults may experience a dull aching back pain, which is aggravated by athletic activity, particularly repetitive flexion/extension motion. This pain may radiate down into the buttocks or posterior thighs. Radicular pain is uncommon in adolescents and more common in adults, and this is usually in the L5 distribution owing to nerve compression by the hypertrophic callus at the pars defect or owing to the foraminal stenosis accompanying the spondylolisthesis, commonly at the L5-S1 level. Objective signs on examination include postural changes, such as a flattening of the buttocks and increased lumbar lordosis. A waddling gait may reflect vertical rotation of the pelvis and short steps due to an inability to extend the hips. The characteristic crouched gait is seen more commonly in high-grade slip with associated hamstring tightness. A step-off at the lumbosacral area may be evident. Uncommonly, there is weakness of the extensor hallucis longus muscle secondary to compression of the fifth nerve root. Compression of this root is an important concept; the root is compressed by the fibrocartilaginous material at the site of the pars defect, made worse by the stretching from the slip (Fig. 18-3).

## Radiographic Evaluation

Traditional views of the lumbar spine include anteroposterior, lateral, and oblique projections. The defect is seen as the "collar" on the "Scotty dog" (Fig. 18-4). In patients with a defect, collimated lateral views show it 84% of the time. Oblique views are controversial; one study reported that they show a lytic defect in less than 4% of cases not seen on the lateral view, with more than twice the gonadal radiation. Further imaging to identify a lytic defect should be with a bone scan using single-photon emission computed tomography (SPECT) (Fig. 18-5). SPECT also can help determine

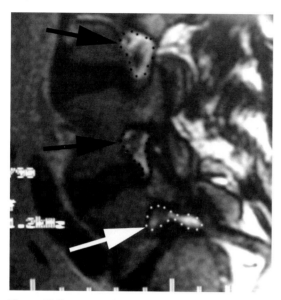

**Figure 18-3**  T1-weighted sagittal MRI of a patient with isthmic spondylolisthesis at L5-S1. Note the open intervertebral foramen (*black arrows* and *outlines*), in contrast to the narrowed foramen at L5-S1 (*white arrow* and *outline*). Compression of the exiting L5 nerve root is shown.

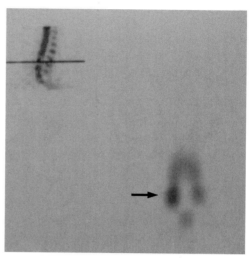

**Figure 18-5**  SPECT with uptake at the site of a lytic pars defect.

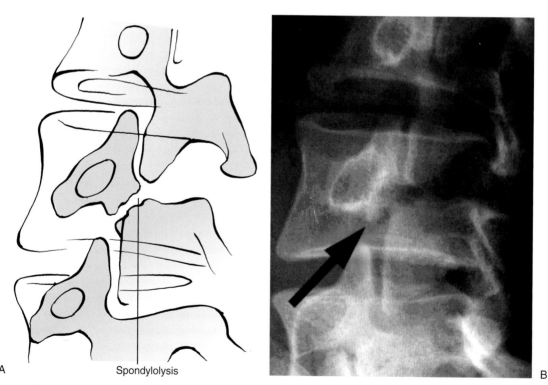

A    Spondylolysis    B

**Figure 18-4**  Illustration (**A**) and oblique radiograph (**B**) of a lytic pars defect classically described as a collar on the "Scotty dog."

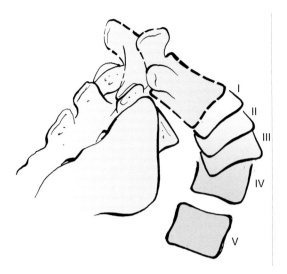

**Figure 18-6** Schematic drawing of the Meyerding classification of spondylolisthesis, based on the percentage of slippage of the vertebral bodies (I = 0% to 24%, II = 25% to 49%, III = 50% to 74%, IV = 75% to 99%). Stage V is 100% olisthesis, or spondyloptosis.

whether a defect is acute or chronic. To maximize the chances of observing an olisthesis, standing lateral radiographs should be obtained.

Special measurements of the deformity have evolved from Wiltse and other authors, using a standard lateral radiograph in the standing position. The two most common measurements are the grade of the slip and the slip angle. The Meyerding grading classification is used most commonly to express the slip as a percentage of the anteroposterior measurement of the body of S1 (Figs. 18-6 and 18-7). This classification divides the sacrum into quadrants I

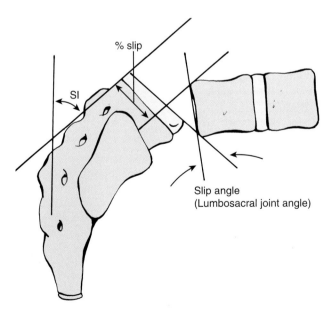

**Figure 18-7** Calculation of the slip angle as a measure of kyphosis and of the percent slip of one vertebral body on the other.

through IV and expresses the grade of the slip according to how far the body of L5 has slipped forward on the sacrum. Grade V is used for spondyloptosis, or 100% slip. The slip angle, the angle formed by lines drawn along the posterior border of the sacrum and along the anterior body of L5, measures the kyphosis associated with the deformity (see Fig. 18-7). The slip angle has been found by some to predict progression of the slip. In particular, Saraste found that risk factors for slip progression included dysplastic etiology, slip angles greater than 40 degrees, Meyerding grades III or higher, female patients, and the presence of a rounded-off or domed S1.

## Treatment

The treatment options for a patient with spondylolysis or spondylolisthesis range from observation, restriction of athletic activities, bracing or casting, and open repair of a pars defect to decompression, fusion, and possible reduction of the slip. The natural history of these disorders is paramount in selecting the best treatment option; many of these patients, particularly adults with the disorder, do not require active treatment, much less operative intervention, for a successful outcome. Adults with continued back pain and L5 radicular symptoms can be treated effectively with a decompression and fusion procedure.

The following guidelines for treatment have been proposed for spondylolysis/spondylolisthesis in pediatric patients:

- *Incidental pars defect*—observe with radiographs annually in a growing child; no restrictions
- *Up to 25% slip*—no limitation in activity; observe with radiographs semiannually
- *Up to 50% slip in an asymptomatic patient*—observe with radiographs semiannually; consider restriction of high-risk athletic activity and avoiding an occupation with heavy labor
- *Up to 50% slip in a symptomatic patient*—conservative treatment with activity modification, physical therapy, or bracing/casting (particularly if SPECT documents an acute pars fracture); observe with radiographs semiannually until maturity, then annually
- *Greater than 50% slip*—consider surgical intervention

Other, less specific indications for surgical intervention include persistence of major symptoms for an extended period despite conservative care, postural symptoms/deformities not relieved by physical therapy, progressive neurologic deficit, progressive slipping beyond 25% to 50%, and a high slip angle in a young patient (because this indicates a high likelihood of slip progression). Repair of the pars defect in cases of spondylolysis without slip has been advocated. Bradford and Iza reported good results with bone grafting and fixation using wiring between the transverse and spinous processes. Other techniques involve direct screw fixation and bone grafting of the defect. The advantage of these techniques lies in preserving the affected and adjacent motion segment as long as no olisthesis is present. In an older patient with a spondylolisthesis, the competency of the intervertebral disc must be questioned, however, and a fusion is a better operation. Pars repair is contraindicated when a slippage has occurred.

A one-level L5-S1 posterolateral fusion is performed for patients with low-grade slips unresponsive to conservative care. As described by Wiltse, this fusion can be performed through a midline incision, bilateral lateral fascial incisions, and a paramidline muscle-splitting approach to the spine. Abnormal motion is eliminated, but decompression is not performed with this technique. Postoperatively, patients should be braced with a lumbosacral orthosis or body cast with a leg extension to improve fusion rates. The role of more aggressive surgical techniques also has been explored. If more than 50% slippage is present, many authors advocate extension of the fusion to L4 owing to the technical difficulty of accessing the L5 transverse process without exposure of the L4 process. Extension to L4 also improves the success of fusion by increasing the surface area for the fusion mass.

Decompression of the L5 or S1 nerve root is controversial. If significant radicular symptoms exist, most authors advocate resection of the hypertrophic fibrocartilaginous mass at the pars defect, decompressing the L5 root. The basis of the decompression is the Gill procedure. Gill described removal of the loose lamina, with further resection of the pars area as above. Wiltse, using a midline exposure, believed initially that this did not cause further instability. After observing slip progression in this patient population postoperatively, Wiltse later changed to his paramidline approach and included a fusion in the operation. Rates of slip progression after decompression without fusion have been reported to be 27%, particularly in patients younger than 30 years old. Wiltse went on to report that most radicular symptoms from compression of the L5 root and the associated back pain and hamstring tightness completely resolve with a successful fusion.

Results from anterior interbody fusions in the treatment of symptomatic adult isthmic spondylolisthesis have been shown to be equivalent to posterolateral fusion with instrumentation. These and other observations indicate that the motion segment instability causes irritation of the nerve root, rather than compression. We routinely add a transforaminal lumbar interbody fusion to the normal posterolateral fusion in these patients to maximize success of a solid arthrodesis. In the absence of severe neurologic injury (cauda equina syndrome, significant motor weakness), decompression is not necessary and may worsen results. In a prospective, randomized trial comparing single-level fusion with or without decompression for isthmic spondylolisthesis in adults, Caragee found that the addition of decompression to arthrodesis significantly increased the pseudarthrosis rate and led to more unsatisfactory results. Although it is tempting to compensate for the instability caused by decompression using instrumentation as an adjunct to fusion, Caragee did not find any decrease in the pseudarthrosis rate with the addition of pedicle screw fixation.

The role of instrumentation in these patients also is controversial, and to some extent this is tied up in the question of whether a reduction should be performed. The use of pedicle screw instrumentation is extremely common in these patients. It may be used to stabilize the fusion, obviating postoperative bracing, or to maintain or achieve a reduc-

tion on the operating table. Moller and Hedlund conducted a prospective randomized trial of instrumentation in the treatment of adult isthmic spondylolisthesis and found that supplemental pedicle screw fixation prolonged the operative time and increased total blood loss but did not affect the clinical outcome or fusion rate.

The purported advantages of reduction of these slips are reduced pseudarthrosis rate (owing to increased surface area for fusion), a decrease in the rate of slip progression postoperatively, preserved motion segments, and reduced clinical deformity. Most modern systems require extension to L4 to pull the L5 vertebral body (via its pedicle screw) backward in the sling created by the screws in S1 and L4. The clinical outcome has not been shown to improve after these reductions, however, and the complication rates are higher than reported for in situ fusions, albeit with the use of older reduction techniques. In a retrospective review of patients who underwent reduction of high-grade slips, Hu et al found overall good clinical results but a 25% significant complication rate. Another retrospective study of patients treated with posterior reduction, interbody fusion, and segmental fixation reported a high fusion rate, no loss of reduction, and minimal complications. It remains to be shown whether the newer techniques of reduction decrease the complication rate for this part of the procedure.

In an adult patient with an isthmic spondylolisthesis, a formal reduction rarely is indicated. Bradford listed the following criteria for patients who may be candidates for an attempted reduction:

- Vertebral slippage greater than 60%
- Slip angle greater than 50 degrees
- Symptoms uncontrollable by nonoperative means
- Age between 12 and 30 years

These criteria leave room for surgical decision making. There has been no study in adults, however, documenting an improved clinical outcome with reduction of the slip. In our practice, we routinely combine a transforaminal lumbar interbody fusion with decompression and posterolateral fusion. A partial reduction often is obtained during preparation of the interbody space and fusion procedure; further reduction is not attempted routinely, unless significant external deformity exists or there is greater than a grade II olisthesis.

## Complications

The pseudarthrosis rate varies in the literature from 0% to 25%, with most studies reporting fewer than 15% but a higher rate with more severe slips. The rates of slip progression seem to be higher after a Gill procedure and disruption of the posterior ligamentous complex. Neurologic complications have been chiefly in the form of radicular symptoms after reduction of high-grade slips, most commonly from the root of L5. Complete reduction is not necessary, and because most strain in L5 occurs in the last stages of reduction, this should be avoided. Attention instead should focus on correcting the lumbosacral kyphosis, which may decompress the nerve root. Cauda equina syndrome also has been reported, with or without reduction of the slip.

# DEGENERATIVE SPONDYLOLISTHESIS

## Etiology and Pathogenesis

Degenerative spondylolisthesis, previously called *pseudospondylolisthesis*, also has been called *spondylolisthesis with an intact neural arch*. This condition affects predominantly older individuals, after age 40, and is thought to derive from a combination of facet arthritis and degenerative disc disease. It occurs most often at the L4-5 level. In a landmark study, Rosenberg reported on the incidence and predisposing factors in 20 cadavers and 200 patients with degenerative spondylolisthesis. This condition occurs five to six times more commonly in women and three times more often in individuals of African descent. The predominance in women is thought to be due to the influence of a generalized ligamentous laxity. The increased incidence in blacks is thought to be related to anatomic factors, which include less lumbosacral lordosis than in other populations and a high incidence of sacralization of L5.

The pathogenesis of degenerative spondylolisthesis involves an increase in stress borne by the posterior elements as a result of degeneration of the intervertebral disc combined with abnormal stress concentration on the L4-5 motion segment. Facet morphology may influence development of slips. In contrast to the coronal orientation at L5-S1, the facets at L4-5 have a tendency toward a more sagittal alignment. This alignment decreases the facets' ability to resist forward flexion forces, increasing the tendency to slip and accelerating facet arthritis. When disc degeneration occurs, the motion segment settles into an anterolisthesis; this rarely progresses past grade II and in general is less than that seen in isthmic slips.

## Clinical Presentation

The clinical presentation of degenerative spondylolisthesis is intertwined closely with that of spinal stenosis, which commonly accompanies a degenerative spondylolisthesis. Patients typically complain of lumbago-type low back pain that commonly radiates into the buttocks or lateral thighs, proximal weakness or "drop spells" because they are prone to collapse while walking, and intermittent claudication symptoms. These claudication symptoms notably are not relieved simply by standing still; patients often describe the need to sit down or lean on something (classically the shopping cart) to relieve the pain. This lumbar flexion effectively increases the diameter of the spinal canal and intervertebral foramen, which relieves the pressure on the nerves or cauda equina. This is a useful distinction in assessing any contribution by vascular causes; vascular claudication usually occurs after a repeatable distance and is relieved by stopping and standing still.

True radicular symptoms occur in about half of patients, usually corresponding to L5. Compression of the L5 nerve root is common with degenerative spondylolisthesis. This compression results from overgrowth of the facet at the L4-5 level, compressing the traversing nerve root posterolaterally between the superior facet and the posterosuperior border of the L5 vertebral body (the lateral recess).

In contrast to patients with isthmic spondylolisthesis, the clinical examination in patients with degenerative slips often reveals normal or even hypermobility of the lumbar spine in flexion, with a notable lack of stiffness. This phenomenon is thought to be related to a generalized ligamentous laxity in these patients, which predisposes them to a slip. Extension maneuvers may exacerbate the pain owing to narrowing of the canal and foramina. Cauda equina syndrome is rare with this disorder but a history of such should be solicited aggressively because the onset can be insidious, and urinary continence issues, such as hesitancy, dribbling, and poor control, can overlap with common genitourinary conditions in this age group.

## Radiographic Findings

Plain radiographs should include a standing lateral projection (Fig. 18-8), which can show a spondylolisthesis not detected on supine films in 15% of patients. Flexion/extension lateral radiographs may show a dynamic slip, but this is relatively rare and may not influence treatment. Axial imaging by computed tomography (CT), with or without myelography, traditionally has been the imaging modality of choice for degenerative slips associated with spinal stenosis. CT gives excellent detail of the source of compression, facet joint morphology, and pedicle orientation and an idea of bone stock present. Magnetic resonance imaging (MRI) is used increasingly for this disorder, often in combination with CT-myelography, to evaluate the soft tissue structures further. MRI reveals nerve root compression, disc pathology, facet joint synovial cysts, yellow ligament hypertrophy,

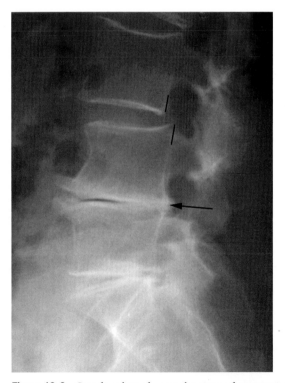

**Figure 18-8** Standing lateral x-ray showing a degenerative spondylolisthesis at L3-4, above a relatively stiff degenerative segment at L4-5 (*arrow*).

and other soft tissue sources of compression that may not be apparent on CT or CT-myelography. MRI is a noninvasive imaging modality, avoiding painful lumbar or cervical injections and the side effects of myelography (e.g., headache and nausea), which can occur in 20% of patients.

## Natural History

Several excellent studies on the natural history of degenerative spondylolisthesis call attention to the fact that this disorder may not be as aggressive as previously thought. About 25% to 30% of patients may experience progression of the slip, but rarely to more than 30% of the subjacent vertebra. Progression of the slip does not correlate with clinical symptoms.

## Nonoperative Treatment

The initial conservative treatment for low back or radicular symptoms associated with degenerative spondylolisthesis is rest not to exceed 1 to 2 days, nonsteroidal antiinflammatory drugs, and activity modification. This supportive therapy is supplemented by physiotherapy emphasizing flexion exercises and back strengthening, progressing to aerobic conditioning. Use of a stationary bicycle is encouraged; the seat and handlebars can be set up to allow lumbar flexion during aerobic conditioning, expanding the canal and neural foramen and allowing greater exercise tolerance with less irritation of nerve roots. We also routinely use epidural steroid injections for this disorder, similar to the treatment of spinal stenosis without a slip. These injections are more effective for relief of radicular-type pain and less effective for back pain.

## Operative Treatment

Herkowitz and Kurz reported the following indications for surgical intervention:

- Persistent or recurrent leg pain despite a minimum of 3 months of conservative treatment
- Progressive neurologic deficit
- Significant reduction in the quality of life
- Confirmatory imaging studies consistent with the clinical findings

Surgical treatment can take the form of simple decompression, decompression and posterolateral fusion with or without instrumentation, or anterior or posterior interbody fusion.

The role of adjunctive fusion in these patients, by whatever means, has been the subject of many studies. Lombardi et al reported results of 47 patients with degenerative spondylolisthesis who underwent decompression with or without fusion. They found that patients who had a radical decompression fared poorly; patients who underwent spinal fusion fared the best. Poor results from these and other authors after decompression alone are related to the progression of slip in these patients postoperatively and to the persistence of instability at the level. Approximately 25% to 50% of patients who undergo decompression without fusion

experience a progression of their slip; this postoperative progression seems to correlate variably with outcome. Bone regrowth after decompressive laminectomy in patients with degenerative slips also is higher in patients who are not fused, contributing to recurrence of symptoms.

The controversy surrounding the addition of adjunctive fusion, with or without instrumentation, persists despite several prospective, randomized trials examining these variables in the treatment of degenerative spondylolisthesis. In 1991, Herkowitz and Kurz published their results in patients with associated spinal stenosis. They showed statistically better clinical outcomes in patients who underwent fusion. Zdeblick compared noninstrumented fusions with semirigid and rigid instrumented fusions in 124 patients, 56 of whom had spondylolisthesis, and found better fusion rates in the rigidly instrumented group. Better clinical results also were found in the instrumented groups. Bridwell reported on 44 patients divided into three groups: (1) no fusion, (2) noninstrumented posterolateral fusion, and (3) instrumented posterolateral fusion using pedicle screws. Instrumentation significantly improved fusion rates, functional outcome, and sagittal alignment.

A meta-analysis of the literature on degenerative spondylolisthesis was performed in 1994 (Mardjetko et al). This study examined the issues of fusion and the use of instrumentation as an adjunct. In patients undergoing decompression without arthrodesis, 69% had a satisfactory outcome. Progressive slipping after decompression was noted in most reports. The addition of arthrodesis increased the satisfactory outcome to 90%, with 86% achieving solid fusion. In this meta-analysis, five studies were identified as suitable for examining the value of instrumentation; the authors reported a strong trend ($p = 0.08$) toward increased fusion with pedicle instrumentation, but minimal difference in clinical outcome.

Since this meta-analysis, several more prospective, randomized trials examining these issues have been published. The Volvo award winner for 1997 (Fishgrund et al.) examined instrumentation in this population; the authors found a significantly higher fusion rate in the instrumented group (82% versus 45%), but no significant difference in clinical outcomes with the use of instrumentation. They concluded that at least in the short-term, successful arthrodesis does not influence patient outcome. Later, with longer follow-up, the patients with pseudarthrosis did not do as well, however, as the patients with a solid fusion. This finding prompted the authors to advocate the routine use of instrumentation to increase the fusion rates. Another Volvo award winner (Thomsen et al., 1997) studied posterolateral spinal fusions for spondylolisthesis or "segmental instability." The authors found that if neural decompression was performed, instrumentation significantly improved functional outcomes. Other comparisons between the instrumented and noninstrumented groups, including fusion rates, did not show significant differences. They observed "significant symptoms related to misplacement of a screw" in 4.8% of patients and concluded that routine use of pedicle screw fixation alone is not justified as an adjunct to posterolateral lumbar fusion.

The symptoms due to degenerative spondylolisthesis are multifactorial and depend heavily on the presence of associated spinal stenosis. A long trial of conservative therapy and injections should be granted the patient before operative intervention is undertaken. Surgery should consist of decompression and fusion. The use of pedicle instrumentation should be tailored to the instability and the extent of decompression. We believe that the use of instrumentation in patients at risk of instability or pseudarthrosis is warranted to increase fusion rates and improve stability, in turn improving outcome.

## TRAUMATIC SPONDYLOLISTHESIS

Documented acute fractures of the pars interarticularis are rare. Wiltse noted that forced marches in recruits laden with gear have been known to produce pars fractures and to generate a typical "fluffy callus" at the site that almost always heals. He also noted several cases of traumatic spondylolisthesis, all with an easily recognizable history—of falling backward on a curb, with a blow to the lumbar area—and a break in the pars evident on radiography. Wiltse emphasized that some patients may have a "chronic diathesis," which predisposes them to injury to the pars with relatively minor trauma, but this is better termed an *isthmic slip* than a true traumatic pars fracture, which requires a great deal of force. Traumatic olistheses also are seen with bilateral pedicle fractures and separation of the posterior elements in major trauma.

## PATHOLOGIC SPONDYLOLISTHESIS

Generalized bone disease, such as osteoporosis, Paget's disease, and osteomalacia, can weaken the posterior elements to the extent that allows spondylolisthesis. Little has been published on this condition; most authors group these cases with degenerative spondylolisthesis.

## IATROGENIC SPONDYLOLISTHESIS

Resection of more than 50% of each facet joint, the pars, or one entire facet joint predisposes the spine to instability. Although this predisposition varies clinically depending on the amount of preexisting disc degeneration and associated instability, if the decompression requires sacrifice of these important stabilizing structures, the addition of an arthrodesis to enhance stability is required. Instrumentation can be used to augment a posterolateral fusion.

## SUGGESTED READING

Amato M, Totty WG, Gilula LA. Spondylolysis of the lumbar spine: demonstration of defects and laminar fragmentation. Radiology 1984;153:627–629.

Baker D, McHollick W. Spondyloschisis spondylolisthesis in children. J Bone Joint Surg 1956;38A:933–934.
Bradford DS. Closed reduction of spondylolisthesis: an experience in 22 patients. Spine 1988;13:580–587.
Bradford DS, Iza J. Repair of the defect in spondylosis or minimal degrees of spondylolisthesis by segmental wire fixation and bone grafting. Spine 1985;10:673–679.
Bridwell K. Sedgewick T, O'Brien M, et al. The role of fusion and instrumentation in the treatment of degenerative spondylolisthesis with spinal stenosis. J Spinal Disord 1993;6:467–472.
Caragee EJ. Single-level posterolateral arthrodesis, with or without posterior decompression, for the treatment of isthmic spondylolisthesis in adults: a prospective, randomized study. J Bone Joint Surg 1997;79A:1175–1180.
Fishgrund JS, Mackay M, Herkowitz HN, et al. Degenerative lumbar spondylolisthesis with spinal stenosis: a prospective, randomized study comparing decompressive laminectomy and arthrodesis with and without spinal instrumentation. Spine 1997;22:2807–2812.
Floman Y. Progression of lumbosacral isthmic spondylolisthesis in adults. Spine 2000;25:342–347.
Fredrickson BE, Baker D, McHolick WJ, et al. The natural history of spondylolysis and spondylolisthesis. J Bone Joint Surg 1984;66A:699–707.
Grobler L, Robertson P, Novotny J, Pope M. Etiology of spondylolisthesis: assessment of the role played by lumbar facet joint morphology. Spine 1993;18:80–92.
Herkowitz HN, Kurz LT. Degenerative lumbar spondylolisthesis with spinal stenosis: a prospective study comparing decompression with decompression and intertransverse progressive arthrodesis. J Bone Joint Surg 1991;73A:802–808.
Hu SS, Bradford DS, Tansfeldt EE, Cohen M. Reduction of high-grade spondylolisthesis using Edwards instrumentation. Spine 1996;21:367–371.
Johnsson K, Wilner S, Johnsson K. Postoperative instability after decompression for lumbar spinal stenosis. Spine 1986;11:107–110.
Kim NH, Lee JW. Anterior interbody fusion versus posterolateral fusion with transpedicular fixation for isthmic spondylolisthesis in adults: a comparison of clinical results. Spine 1999;24:812–817.
Lombardi J, Wiltse L, Reynolds J, et al. Treatment of degenerative spondylolisthesis. Spine 1985;10:821–827.
Mardjetko SM, Connolly PG, Schott S. Degenerative lumbar spondylolisthesis: a meta-analysis of the literature 1970–1993. Spine 1994;10:2256S–2265S.
Moller H, Hedlund R. Instrumented and non-instrumented posterolateral fusion in adult spondylolisthesis—a prospective randomized study: II. Spine 2000;25:1716–1721.
Newman PH. The etiology of spondylolisthesis. With a special investigation by K.H. Stone. J Bone Joint Surg 1963;47B:39–59.
Roberts FF, Kishore PR, Cunningham ME. Routine oblique radiography of the pediatric lumbar spine: is it really necessary? AJR Am J Roentgenol 1978;131:297–298.
Rosenberg NJ. Degenerative spondylolisthesis. Predisposing factors. J. Bone Joint Surg 1975;57A:467–474.
Saraste H. Long-term clinical and radiological follow-up of spondylolysis and spondylolisthesis. J Pediatr Orthop 1987;7:631–638.
Thomsen K, Christensen FB, Eiskjaer SP, et al. The effect of pedicle screw instrumentation on functional outcome and fusion rates in posterolateral lumbar spinal fusion: a prospective, randomized clinical study. Spine 1997;22:2813–2822.
Zdeblick T. A prospective randomized study of lumbar fusion. Spine 1993;18:983–991.

# CONGENITAL DEFORMITY

**PETER O. NEWTON**
**GARY S. SHAPIRO**

Congenital spinal deformities are caused by anomalous embryologic vertebral development that can lead to severe malalignment of the trunk, depending on the type and location of defect in the spine. These deformities can be more difficult to treat than idiopathic curves owing to the frequency of associated medical problems, their presence in extremely young patients, and increased curve rigidity. The most likely times of increasing deformity match the phases of normally rapid spinal growth (first 2 to 3 years and during adolescence).

Congenital anomalies of the spine can be grouped into two basic types of malformations based on the development of the vertebral elements:

■ Defects of formation
■ Defects of segmentation

Both types of malformation can be present, creating a mixture of deformities at different levels in the spine. This chapter focuses on congenital scoliosis and kyphosis.

# CONGENITAL SCOLIOSIS

## Pathogenesis

### Etiology

Congenital scoliosis is a lateral curvature of the spine caused by developmental vertebral anomalies that produce deviations in spinal alignment. These deficiencies occur in the first trimester of intrauterine development and commonly are associated with cardiac and urologic abnormalities that develop during the same period. The vertebral anomalies are present at birth, but the clinical deformity may not become evident until later as the child grows, classifying it as congenital scoliosis. This condition should not be confused with infantile idiopathic scoliosis, in which the scoliosis also develops early in life, yet all the vertebral elements are normal in shape. The etiology is unknown in humans; however, in animal studies, congenital scoliosis has occurred after exposure to toxic elements during the fetal period.

### Epidemiology

Congenital scoliosis is relatively uncommon, but the true incidence in the population is unknown because only some patients progress to warrant an investigation and a subsequent radiograph. Wynne-Davies analyzed the families of 337 patients with congenital spinal anomalies. She showed that isolated hemivertebrae or similar localized defects were sporadic events that carried no risk to subsequent siblings. In patients with multiple anomalies, however, there is a 5% to 10% risk that siblings also will be affected. The Minneapolis group found 1% of patients with congenital spinal deformity had a relative with the problem.

## Classification

Congenital deformities are classified based on the developmental anomaly of the spine, each with its own natural history (Fig. 19-1). These anomalies include the following:

■ Failures of vertebral formation (*type I*)
■ Failures of segmentation between the vertebrae (*type II*)
■ Types I and II combined (*type III* or *mixed*)

Vertebral anomalies may occur on either the left or the right side of the body or involve the anterior or posterior elements, resulting in scoliosis or kyphosis/lordosis. Combined defects are common, so coronal and sagittal planes need to be evaluated.

## Pathophysiology

A hemivertebra is the classic example of failure of formation (type I). These triangular-shaped vertebrae form only on one side of the spine and can be subclassified as follows:

■ Vertebrae that have disc and growth potential on the superior and inferior ends of the vertebra—*fully segmented*
■ Vertebrae that have disc and growth potential on either the superior or the inferior end only—*semisegmented*
■ Vertebrae that are fused to the vertebrae above and below—*nonsegmented*

Active growth from the end plate/disc produces progressive scoliosis with the risk and rate of progression greatest for the fully segmented hemivertebrae and least for the nonsegmented hemivertebrae. Hemivertebrae are said to be *incarcerated* when they lie within the confines of the curve and vertebral column or *unincarcerated* when they extend laterally beyond the contour of the adjacent vertebrae (Fig.

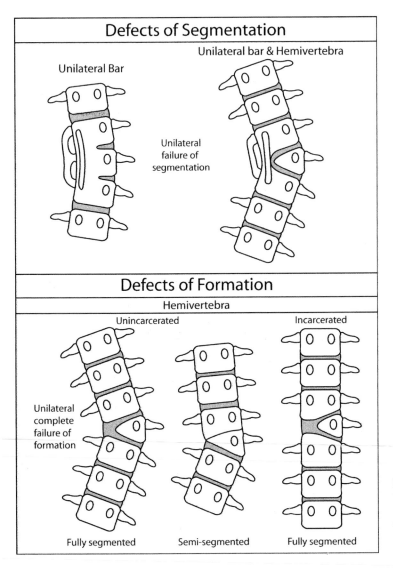

**Figure 19-1**   Diagrammatic representation of classification system of congenital scoliosis. (Modified from McMaster MJ. Congenital scoliosis. In: Weinstein SL, ed. The pediatric spine: principles and practice, 2nd ed. Lippincott Williams and Wilkins, Philadelphia, 2001, Chapter 7, p. 163.)

19-2). Of the various types of hemivertebrae, the fully segmented unincarcerated hemivertebra has the greatest potential for progression with growth. Rib deficiencies tend to match the vertebral deficiencies, and a mismatch of the number of ribs (right versus left) should lead to suspicion for congenital anomalies. The term *hemimetameric shift* defines two hemivertebrae that are present on opposite sides of the spine and separated by at least one normal vertebra. In this case, global balance of the spine in the coronal plane often is maintained.

Failure of segmentation (type II) may occur on one or both sides of the spine, causing a bar of bone bridging the disc spaces, the pedicles, or the facet joints. These anomalies inhibit longitudinal growth and result in little deformity if they occur circumferentially around the spine (block vertebra). A unilateral unsegmented bar causes a growth tether that generally results in marked scoliosis (Fig. 19-3). Unilateral unsegmented bars are seen most commonly in the thoracic spine. Radiographically a failure of segmentation often is seen best as conjoined pedicles or ribs, or both.

Mixed congenital deformities (type III) are important to understand because the *highest likelihood for progression is when there is a unilateral bar with a hemivertebra on the opposite side.* The radiographs of a mixed congenital malformation may be difficult to interpret fully. A newborn or infant radiograph (if available) is often the most useful for identifying the malformations.

The likelihood of any single case of congenital scoliosis developing a progressive deformity is difficult to know. There are features, however, of the malformation that allow educated predictions. McMaster and Ohtsuka studied the natural history of 251 patients followed past age 10 without treatment. Three fourths of the patients' curves progressed substantially, and this progression seems related to curve location and type of anomaly. The annual rates of curve progression for each of the congenital anomalies are presented in Table 19-1.

*Block vertebrae progress the least (<1 degree per year), whereas hemivertebrae with a contralateral unsegmented bar progress the most (>10 degrees per year).* Deformities of the

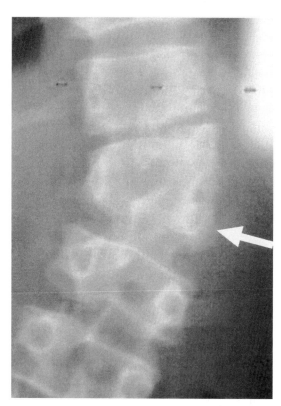

**Figure 19-2** Radiograph showing a semisegmented hemivertebra (*arrow*).

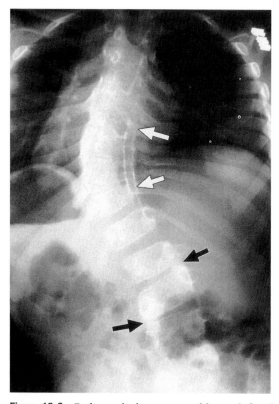

**Figure 19-3** Radiograph shows a typical bar with fused pedicles (*white arrows*). *Black arrows* show narrowing of the disc spaces, also suggesting bar formation.

thoracic spine are in general at greater risk for progression than deformities in the lumbar spine.

## Diagnosis

### History and Physical Examination

**Clinical Features.** The evaluation should begin with the child's birth history, developmental milestones, family history, and complete review of systems. Of patients with congenital spinal malformations, 33% have genitourinary abnormalities, 25% have Klippel-Feil syndrome (cervical vertebral fusion), 15% have intraspinal anomalies (diastematomyelia, tethered cord), and 10% have congenital heart disease. Given the frequency of these associated lesions, the history and exam should include these areas.

The physical exam includes a careful assessment of trunk shape and neurologic function. The effect of the spinal malformation on the trunk may be visible as a shift of the head or trunk off midline, a rotational prominence of the ribs, or a sagittal plane deformity such as kyphosis. Specific findings that suggest an intraspinal lesion include skin lesions on the back (e.g., hairy patches, dimples, masses, nevi, lipomas) and lower extremity abnormalities (e.g., clubfoot, vertical talus, cavovarus foot, thigh or calf atrophy, reflex asymmetry, leg-length discrepancy).

**Radiologic Features.** The radiographic assessment is based largely on sequential frontal and lateral radiographs, upright if the child is mature enough to sit or stand. Congenital scoliosis must be followed closely during the times of rapid spinal growth using serial radiographs. The interval of observation (6 months to 2 years) varies by the age of patient and type of deformity, with more frequent radiographs for children age 0 to 3 years and 9 to 14 years and children with lesions most likely to progress. Interobserver variability in Cobb measurement of congenital scoliosis may be 10 degrees. Measuring the compensatory curve, if present, provides another means to assess curve progression.

At the time of initial evaluation, the genitourinary system should be screened with a renal ultrasound. Magnetic resonance imaging of the entire spine and brain should be obtained to rule out malformations, such as a tethered cord or diastematomyelia, if anything in the history or physical exam suggests an abnormality or the patient is to undergo surgical treatment of the deformity. A preoperative three-dimensional computed tomography (CT) scan can be helpful to visualize the bone elements of the spine, and multiplanar reformatted images have proved useful in identifying anomalies not seen on standard CT (Fig. 19-4).

## Treatment

### Surgical Indications and Contraindications

In general, brace treatment has not been shown to be effective in preventing progression of congenital scoliosis. Occasionally, it may be helpful in rebalancing the trunk or in reducing a compensatory curve. Exercises, spinal manipula-

## TABLE 19-1 ANNUAL RATES OF CURVE PROGRESSION FOR EACH OF THE CONGENITAL ANOMALIES*

| Site of Curvature | Block Vertebra | Wedge Vertebra | Hemivertebra | | Unilateral Unsegmented Bar | Unilateral Unsegmented Bar and Contralateral Hemivertebrae |
| --- | --- | --- | --- | --- | --- | --- |
| | | | Single | Double | | |
| Upper thoracic | <1°–1° | †–2° | †–2° | 2°–2.5° | 2°–4° | 5°–6° |
| Lower thoracic | <1°–1° | 2°–2° | 2°–2° | 2°–3° | 5°–6.5° | 6°–7° |
| Thoracolumbar | <1°–1° | 1.5°–2° | 1.5°–2° | 5°–† | 6°–9° | >10°–† |
| Lumbar | <1°–† | <1°–† | <1°–† | † | >5°–† | † |
| Lumbosacral | † | † | <1°–1.5° | † | † | † |

\* The shaded areas represent the likelihood of spinal fusion based on the predicted increase in deformity. ☐ No treatment required. ▨ May require spinal surgery, ☐ Require spinal fusion
† Too few or no curves. Ranges represent the degree of derotation before and after 10 years of age.
*From McMaster MJ, Ohtsuka K. The natural history of congenital scoliosis: a study of two hundred and fifty-one patients. J Bone Joint Surg 1982;64A:1144.*

tion, electrical stimulation, special diets, and shoe lifts are not effective in preventing progression.

Operative treatment often is necessary to limit progressive congenital scoliosis. Because operative reduction of the curve magnitude in congenital scoliosis is more complex (with greater risk) and less effective than in idiopathic scoliosis, early intervention is suggested when progression is appreciated. Surgical intervention in some cases may come at a relatively young age (1 to 3 years).

Treatment options include the following:

▪ Posterior fusion (with or without instrumentation)
▪ Combined anterior and posterior fusion
▪ Convex hemiepiphysiodesis (anterior or posterior hemiarthrodesis)
▪ Hemivertebra excision

The options must be considered carefully for each individual patient, with knowledge of the risks and benefits of each approach.

The most important aim of surgery is to halt progression. The surgeon, patient, and parents must understand that, by design, surgical treatment halts the growth of the spine. This knowledge generates concern about shortening; however, continued growth without surgery would not lead to increased height, but instead would result in worsening spinal alignment. It also has been shown that these children are small for their age and remain short, even if they do not require surgery. Ultimate standing height is maximized by allowing the unaffected segments of the spine to grow normally. Because the ultimate goal is to halt progression, in situ fusion commonly is performed. If instrumentation is used to add stability, the corrective force must be applied with extreme caution, if at all, because neurologic risk seems to be higher in these patients. Even with limited correction, however, the internal support decreases the need for postoperative external immobilization in many cases.

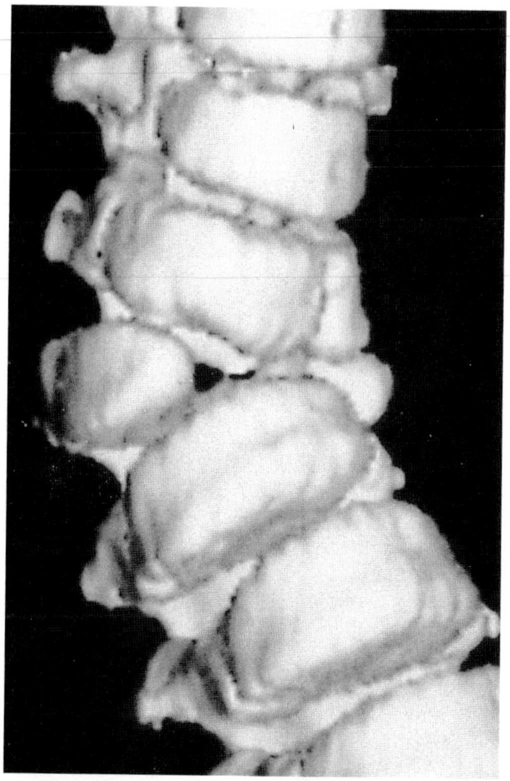

### Choice of Approach

One may approach the spine anteriorly or posteriorly or both ways. The choice depends on the type of curve, magnitude, location, age of the patient, and experience of the surgeon.

Posterior in situ fusion is the simplest approach and is designed to arrest the deformity at its current degree. It

**Figure 19-4** Three-dimensional CT scan shows an unincarcerated fully segmented hemivertebra. (From Newton PO, Wenger DR, Lovell. Idiopathic and congenital scoliosis. In: Winter's pediatric orthopaedics, 5th ed. Lippincott Williams and Wilkins, Philadelphia, 2001, p. 732.)

involves placement of bone graft (autograft or allograft or both) along the lamina, facets, and transverse processes of the vertebrae to be fused. A brace or cast is worn for 4 to 6 months postoperatively. Instrumentation provides children older than about 3 years the potential for added stability, although postoperative immobilization due to limited fixation in an immature spine is recommended.

Anterior fusion procedures usually are employed in cases in which substantial anterior vertebral growth is expected (Risser 0 and open triradiate cartilage) and often are combined with a posterior fusion. The advantages of the anterior approach include halting anterior spinal growth (which may lead to the additional "crankshaft deformity") and increasing the flexibility of the spine in cases in which correction is planned. There seems to be an increased risk of spinal cord injury owing to disruption of the blood supply to the cord from dividing segmental vessels during anterior surgery in patients with congenital deformity (particularly kyphosis). Monitoring of the spinal cord with sensory and motor potentials is recommended. An anterior and posterior combined fusion is used most commonly for young patients with highly progressive deformities (e.g., fully segmented hemivertebrae or hemivertebrae with a contralateral bar). Block vertebrae, semisegmented hemivertebrae, and wedge vertebrae are less likely to require anterior procedures because of their limited growth potential.

### Partial Fusion, Growth Modulation, and Hemiepiphysiodesis

Convex hemiarthrodesis (hemiepiphysiodesis) involves performing a fusion only on the convex side of the curve, usually anteriorly and posteriorly. The goal of this procedure is to create a bone tether (convex fusion mass) that would allow subsequent growth on the concave side, ultimately reducing the deformity. One level above and one level below a hemivertebra often are included in the hemiarthrodesis to encourage correction. This technique is best reserved for failures of formation with less than 50 degrees of deformity in patients younger than 5 years old.

### Hemivertebra Excision

Hemivertebra excision allows for acute deformity correction and is coupled with stabilization by arthrodesis. This procedure is technically demanding with greater neurologic risk but has been shown to be safe and effective in experienced hands. It is safest below the level of the conus (tip of the cord) and has the most pronounced effect on truncal imbalance when performed in the lower lumbar region. The procedure may be performed as simultaneous or staged anterior and posterior procedures and via an isolated posterior exposure. Spinal cord monitoring and a Stagnara wake-up test are required to ensure neurologic function after the realignment. Care must be taken not to compress neural elements when the gap created by the bone excision is closed. Instrumentation appropriate to the size of the patient is used, often with a body cast as well.

### Results and Outcome

The results for in situ fusion for congenital vertebral deformity show that localized fusion is effective in preventing progression of the deformity. The complication rates are low because the spine is not manipulated, and instrumentation is not used. The cosmetic improvement in trunk shape is limited, but this remains the gold standard for most congenital spinal deformities.

Hemivertebra excision carries a low neurologic risk in experienced hands and depends on the location of the defect. Correction rates on average of 60% to 70% can be achieved. A successful outcome depends on careful exposure and protection of the neural elements combined with secure internal fixation.

The effectiveness of convex hemiarthrodesis has been mixed. In many cases, the hemiarthrodesis functions as an in situ fusion limiting progression but not achieving correction. The greatest chance for true correction by modifying growth exists for the youngest patients with smaller deformities (patients <5 years old with a hemivertebra and <50 degrees of curvature).

### Postoperative Management

Close medical management by a multidisciplinary approach is necessary. If associated medical conditions are identified preoperatively, most postoperative complications can be avoided. Neurovascular checks are vital to identify any neurologic deficit. Because of the immature nature of the patients, it often is necessary to use casts and braces while the fusion is maturing. In patients younger than 3 years old, the cast may need to include an arm or leg, or both. The length of time necessary for immobilization usually is 3 to 4 months.

## CONGENITAL KYPHOSIS

Kyphotic deformities are less common than scoliotic deformities but have a higher likelihood of developing neurologic impairment. Congenital kyphosis is a deformity in which there is an abnormal posterior convex angulation of a segment of the spine caused by anomalous vertebrae.

### Classification

The classification is similar to congenital scoliosis, with failures of formation (type I), failures of segmentation (type II), and mixed deformities (type III) (Fig. 19-5).

### Pathophysiology

Failures of formation produce the most severe angular kyphosis and the highest likelihood of paraplegia, especially when located between T4 and T9 (vascular watershed area). It is the second most common cause of paraplegia after the infectious spinal deformities. Type I deformities can result in kyphosis and scoliosis if the greatest absence of vertebral body is anterolateral. Defects of segmentation (type II) occur most often in the lower thoracic spine and thoracolumbar junction. They are less progressive and rarely cause paraplegia. Surgery is required (in situ fusion or correction by osteotomy) if there is a significant deformity or if progres-

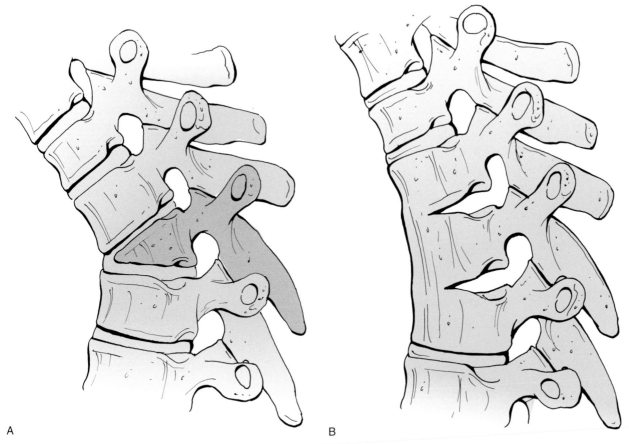

**Figure 19-5**   Diagrammatic representation of classification system of congenital kyphosis. (**A**) Defect of formation. (**B**) Defect of segmentation.

sion occurs. Mixed (type III) deformities often progress rapidly and require surgery.

Progression occurs in most patients (95%) with type I and III defects. The severity of kyphosis and likelihood of progression are related directly to the amount of vertebral body missing. Conservative treatment is ineffective, and early surgical treatment is suggested. The surgical approach is based on the age of the patient, type of vertebral anomaly, size of the deformity, and presence or absence of spinal cord compression.

## Treatment

### Surgical Indications and Contraindications

Kyphosis less than 40 degrees to 50 degrees can be treated by posterior in situ fusion; however, in deformities larger than this, a combined anterior-posterior fusion is recommended. Anterior "strutting" within the concavity is biomechanically superior to a posterior fusion mass under tension.

If there is a neurologic deficit (e.g., weakness, bowel or bladder dysfunction, hyperreflexia), the patient should undergo anterior decompression, not laminectomy alone. An anterior approach is the method of choice for decompressing the spinal cord by removing the posterior remnant of the vertebral body. Preoperative halo traction is contraindicated because this stretches the spinal cord even tighter over the apical bone.

### Results and Outcome

The results of posterior fusion for curves less than 50 degrees are excellent. The kyphosis in patients with continued anterior growth may improve over time, especially in younger patients. The results of posterior fusion alone, with or without instrumentation, are poor in stabilizing a deformity greater than 50 degrees. The most successful results in patients with curves greater than 50 degrees occur in those treated with anterior disc excision, strut grafting, and arthrodesis combined with a posterior arthrodesis. Correction obtained in published series is roughly 30%.

Neurologic risks are higher than in congenital scoliosis because of a frequent reduction in the cross-sectional area of the canal and stretching of the spinal cord induced by reduction. The results for improvement of preoperative neurologic deficits vary from complete recovery to no recovery at all, depending on the chronicity of the deficit and severity of the compression.

## SUMMARY

Congenital spinal deformities arise from an embryologic failure of formation or segmentation of the vertebral elements. There are frequently associated malformations of the cardiac, urologic, and neurologic structures. Progression of a deformity is an indication for surgical stabilization, most often by in situ arthrodesis.

# SUGGESTED READING

Apel DM, Marrero G, King J, et al. Avoiding paraplegia during anterior spinal surgery: the role of somatosensory evoked potential monitoring with temporary occlusion of segmental spinal arteries. Spine 1991;16:S365–S370.

Beals RK, Robbins JR, Rolfe B. Anomalies associated with vertebral malformations. Spine 1993;18:1329–1332.

Callahan BC, Georgopoulos G, Eilert RE. Hemivertebral excision for congenital scoliosis. J Pediatr Orthop 1997;17:96–99.

Drvaric DM, Ruderman RJ, Conrad RW, et al. Congenital scoliosis and urinary tract abnormalities: are intravenous pyelograms necessary? J Pediatr Orthop 1987;7:441–443.

Goldberg CJ, Moore DP, Fogarty EE, et al. Long-term results from in situ fusion for congenital vertebral deformity. Spine 2002;27:619–628.

King AG, MacEwen GD, Bose WJ. Transpedicular convex anterior hemiepiphysiodesis and posterior arthrodesis for progressive congenital scoliosis. Spine 1992;17:S291–S294.

Wynne-Davies R. Congenital vertebral anomalies: aetiology and relationship to spina bifida cystica. J Med Genet 1975;12:280–288.

# ADOLESCENT DEFORMITY

**MAYA E. PRING**
**DENNIS R. WENGER**

## ADOLESCENT IDIOPATHIC SCOLIOSIS

Adolescent idiopathic scoliosis (AIS) is a structural lateral curvature and rotation of the spine that occurs in patients just before or during puberty. If congenital, neuromuscular, infectious, and pathologic conditions (discussed in other chapters) have been ruled out, the curvature is considered to be *idiopathic,* or of unknown origin. Curves can progress to cause significant trunk deformity and eventually cardio-respiratory compromise. Nationwide school screening programs have been started to identify scoliosis in an early phase so that progression can be prevented with bracing or corrected with surgery before the development of these late complications.

## Pathogenesis

### Etiology

There seems to be a genetic basis to AIS because there frequently is a positive family history; however, the expression is variable, and a specific gene has not been identified yet. Harrington showed that there was a 27% incidence of scoliosis in girls whose mother had a curve greater than 15 degrees. A genetic survey of patients with AIS indicated that 11% of first-degree relatives have scoliosis; this decreases to 2.4% of second-degree relatives and 1.4% of third-degree relatives. Studies of monozygotic twins have shown concordance of 73%.

More recent studies have suggested that hormonal factors, such as melatonin, growth hormone, and calmodulin, may play a role. Studies also have looked at disorders of connective tissue; neurologic abnormalities; and proprioception, muscle, and growth differences as the cause. No study has shown conclusive evidence as to the underlying etiology of AIS, however, and the term *idiopathic* remains appropriate.

### Epidemiology

Prevalence studies indicate that 2% to 3% of adolescents have AIS. Small curves (<10 degrees) occur equally in adolescent boys and girls. The female-to-male ratio is 4:1 for large curves, however, and females have a 10 times greater risk of curve progression compared with males. Approximately 10% of cases that are detected with school screening require eventual treatment with a brace or surgery. Most adolescent idiopathic curves have their apex to the right. A thoracic curve with the apex to the left should undergo further work-up (i.e., magnetic resonance imaging) to rule out other causes of scoliosis.

### Curve Progression

The risk of curve progression is affected directly by the skeletal maturity of the patient and the magnitude of the curve (Table 20-1):

- Skeletally immature patients with large curves are at the greatest risk of curve progression.
- Double-curve patterns have a higher risk of progression than single-curve patterns.
- Curves with loss of thoracic kyphosis also are at increased risk of progression and are more likely to develop pulmonary compromise.

Although most progression occurs during growth spurts, curves can continue to progress at a slower rate when the patient is skeletally mature. In adults, small curves (<30 degrees) are unlikely to progress. Curves of 30 degrees to 50 degrees may progress an additional 10 degrees to 15 degrees, and large curves (>50 degrees) continue to progress at a rate of approximately 1 degree/yr.

### TABLE 20-1 PROBABILITY OF CURVE PROGRESSION BASED ON RISSER SIGN AND MAGNITUDE OF CURVE

| Risser Sign | 5–19° Curves | 20–29° Curves |
| --- | --- | --- |
| 0, 1 | 22% | 68% |
| 2, 3, 4 | 1.6% | 23% |

From Lonstein JE, Carlson JM. The prediction of curve progression in untreated idiopathic scoliosis during growth. J Bone Joint Surg, 1984; 66A:1067.

## Classification

The pattern of AIS is determined by the location of the apical vertebra, which is the most horizontal and laterally placed vertebral body or disc. The King and Moe (Table 20-2) classification was the standard for curve evaluation and management decisions before the advent of modern imaging and surgical treatment options. This classification is limited because it evaluates the curve in only one dimension and because it has been shown to have poor interobserver and intraobserver reliability. There are four main patterns:

- Thoracic
- Lumbar
- Thoracolumbar
- Double major

Lenke et al presented a more comprehensive classification system for AIS that has improved interobserver and intraobserver reliability. This system is treatment based and evaluates the spine in two dimensions—coronal and sagittal (Table 20-3). Six curve patterns (1 through 6) are modified further based on characteristics of the lumbar curve (A, B, or C) and the presence or absence of thoracic kyphosis (−, N, or +).

- The lumbar curve modifier is determined by where the central sacral vertical line intersects the lumbar apical vertebral body.
- The stable vertebra is the most proximal lower thoracic or lumbar vertebra that is bisected most closely by the central sacral vertical line (Fig. 20-1).
- Curves are considered structural if the Cobb angle is greater than 25 degrees on side bending films.
- Each patient is described by a designation such as *1B+* (curve type/lumbar modifier/thoracic sagittal modifier) that thoroughly describes the curve.

## TABLE 20-2 CURVE PATTERNS AS DESCRIBED BY KING AND MOE

| Location | Type | Description |
| --- | --- | --- |
| Thoracic | I | Principal lumbar, secondary thoracic curve |
| | II | Principal thoracic, secondary lumbar curve |
| | III | Thoracic curve only (apex $\geq$ T10) |
| | IV | Long thoracic curve (extends to L4) |
| | V | Double thoracic curve |
| Double major | | Equally structural thoracic & lumbar curves |
| Lumbar | | Apex in lumbar spine |
| Thoracolumbar | | Apex at thoracolumbar junction |

Adapted from King HA, Moe JH, Bradford DS, et al. The selection of fusion levels in thoracic idiopathic scoliosis. J Bone Joint Surg, 1983; 65A:1302.

## TABLE 20-3 CURVE PATTERNS AS DESCRIBED BY LENKE et al

| Type | Proximal Thoracic | Main Thoracic | Thoracolumbar/Lumbar | Curve Type |
| --- | --- | --- | --- | --- |
| 1 | Nonstructural | Structural (major*) | Nonstructural | Main thoracic |
| 2 | Structural | Structural (major*) | Nonstructural | Double thoracic |
| 3 | Nonstructural | Structural (major*) | Structural | Double major |
| 4 | Structural | Structural (major*) | Structural | Triple major |
| 5 | Nonstructural | Nonstructural | Structural (major*) | Thoracolumbar/lumbar |
| 6 | Nonstructural | Structural | Structural (major*) | Thoracolumbar/lumbar; main thoracic |

| Modifiers | | | |
| --- | --- | --- | --- |
| **Lumbar Spine Modifier** | **Location of Central Sacral Vertical Line at Lumbar Apex** | **Thoracic Sagittal Modifier** | **Sagittal Profile T5–12** |
| A | Between pedicles | − | Hypokyphotic <10° |
| B | Touches apical body | N | Normal 20–40° |
| C | Lateral to body | + | Hyperkyphotic >40° |

From Lenke LG, Betz RR, Harms J, et al. Adolescent idiopathic scoliosis: a new classification to determine extent of spinal arthrodesis. J Bone Joint Surg, 2001; 83A(8): 1169.

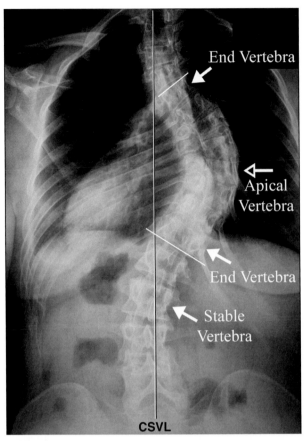

**Figure 20-1** Radiograph showing the central sacral vertical line (CSVL), apical vertebra, stable vertebra, and end vertebrae. The stable vertebra is the most proximal lower thoracic or lumbar vertebra that is bisected most closely by the CSVL.

Based on a multicenter review, the most common curve type is main thoracic, comprising 51% of curves, followed by double thoracic (20%), thoracolumbar/lumbar (12%), and double major curves (11%). Common usage of this more comprehensive classification system may be limited to scoliosis centers because of its relative complexity.

# DIAGNOSIS

## Screening

School nurses and pediatricians who routinely screen adolescents for scoliosis refer many patients to orthopaedic surgeons. Screening is performed using the Adams forward bending test. With the patient bending forward from the waist, the examiner views the patient from behind for thoracic asymmetry, from in front for lumbar asymmetry, and from the side for assessment of kyphosis. A rib prominence seen with the forward bending test is from rotation of the spine and can be measured with a scoliometer. An angle of trunk rotation measurement of 7 degrees with the scoliometer is the current recommendation for further work-up. With this level of screening, approximately 10% of children referred require treatment. There is concern that this cutoff leads to overreferral and unnecessary x-rays; however, the

7-degree cutoff prevents missing children with curves that are likely to progress.

## History

When evaluating patients who have been referred for possible scoliosis, in addition to routine history questions (age, gender, past medical history, family and social history), it is important to determine the following: age at onset of menarche in girls, family history of scoliosis, and current height of other first-degree family members (to determine potential for growth remaining). Any history of neuromuscular conditions, presence of skin lesions (neurofibromatosis), back pain, or neurologic symptoms such as bowel and bladder dysfunction should prompt further diagnostic work-up.

## Physical Examination

A general evaluation of maturity includes height, presence of axillary or pubic hair, and breast development. The skin should be examined for café au lait spots, which may indicate neurofibromatosis, and for signs of dysraphism (patch of hair or dimple over spine). Leg lengths need to be measured because leg-length discrepancy is a frequent cause of spinal asymmetry. Hamstring tightness can indicate a spinal cord problem, such as tethering, and should be checked during the forward bending test. A screening neurologic exam includes strength testing, deep tendon reflexes, Babinski's sign, abdominal reflexes, and examination for clonus.

The patient should be examined for pelvic and shoulder height asymmetry, scapular prominence, breast and flank fold asymmetry, and the presence of a kyphotic deformity. The forward bending test allows the examiner to evaluate the degree and severity of rotational deformity. The combination of these measurements allows the examiner to begin to understand the curve in three dimensions.

## Radiologic Features

For routine scoliosis screening, a standing posteroanterior x-ray (which protects the breasts from the excess radiation exposure of an anteroposterior x-ray) on a 36-inch cassette should include the cervical spine and the pelvis. Including the iliac apophyses allows for evaluation of the Risser sign, which is an indicator of growth remaining (Fig. 20-2). A lateral x-ray of the spine is obtained if there is concern for a round-back deformity or spondylolisthesis, but it is not necessary for routine scoliosis screening. Magnetic resonance imaging should be obtained if the curve is atypical (apex to the left), if there is associated back pain (concern for infection or malignancy), or if there is any neurologic abnormality (concern for intraspinal process, such as syrinx, tethering, or tumor).

On the posteroanterior film, the apical vertebra is used to describe the location of the curve. The Cobb method is used to measure the curve: The end plates of the most tilted vertebrae at the top and bottom of the curve are marked, and lines perpendicular to these end plates are drawn. The angle of intersection of these two lines is the Cobb angle (Fig. 20-3). Curves less than 10 degrees are considered spinal asymmetry, which is a normal variation. Curves greater than 10 degrees are considered scoliosis and should be followed to monitor for progression. Frequency of follow-

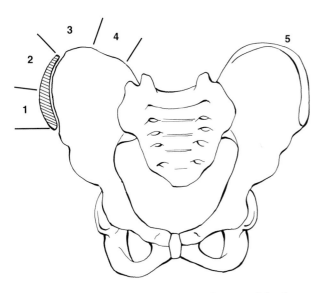

**Figure 20-2** Risser sign—progressive ossification of the iliac apophyses is a soft indicator of skeletal maturity. Risser 1(beginning of ossification) usually is visualized around the time of menarche. Risser 4 (entire apophysis visualized but not fused to crest) signifies the patient is past peak height velocity and is nearing the end of spinal growth. Risser 5—the entire apophysis has fused to the crest.

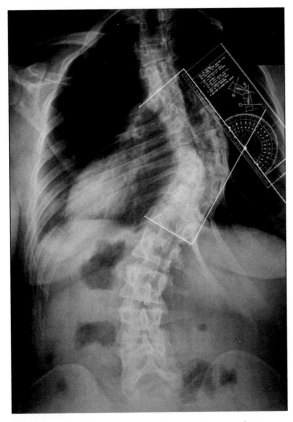

**Figure 20-3** Cobb technique of measuring a scoliotic curve.

up is determined by level of maturity and the degree of curve; immature patients with larger curves need to be followed more closely (every 4 to 6 months), whereas older patients with small curves can be followed yearly until they are past their period of peak growth velocity. If surgery is considered, a lateral x-ray of the spine is obtained to assess the lateral contour, and bending films are obtained to assess the stiffness of the curves. On bending films, a curve that remains greater than 25 degrees is considered structural.

## Treatment

Treatment is based on the maturity of the patient, the magnitude of the curve, and the progression of the curve over time. Options for treatment include the following:

- Observation
- Bracing
- Surgery

Physical therapy, exercise, manipulation, and electrical stimulation have been shown to have little or no measurable effect on curve progression. A general treatment algorithm is presented in Table 20-4.

### Observation

Patients with minimal asymmetry (curve <10°) should be monitored clinically by the primary care physician and referred for x-ray only if there is curve progression based on the forward bending test. Patients with curves measuring 10 degrees to 20 degrees can be monitored with an exam and a posteroanterior x-ray every 6 to 12 months until skeletal maturation occurs. Skeletally immature patients with curves of 20 degrees to 30 degrees should be followed every 4 to 6 months to monitor closely for curve progression. Of patients referred for scoliosis, 90% require only observation.

### Bracing

If the curve measures 30 degrees to 45 degrees or greater than 25 degrees with documented progression of greater than 5 degrees, bracing should be considered in a skeletally immature patient. Patients who have reached skeletal maturity are not candidates for brace wear because braces help to prevent progression but in general do not correct scoliosis.

Several brace types can be prescribed. All braces are custom molded with pads that provide an external force on the ribs and trunk to correct rotation and curve of the spine. The current standard is a thoracolumbosacral orthosis (TLSO) (Boston brace, Wilmington brace, or Miami brace) for curves with the apex below T7 and a cervicothoracolumbosacral orthosis (CTLSO) (Milwaukee brace) for more proximal curves. It is much more difficult to convince a teenager to wear a CTLSO because the chin extension makes the brace difficult to hide under clothes. The psychological impact of bracing is difficult to measure, but it can have an adverse effect on self-esteem at a time when social acceptance is important.

Ideally a brace is worn 23 hours a day to slow the progression of the curve. Some authors have suggested a 16-hour per day schedule. The Charleston bending brace, which is designed to be worn only at night to improve compliance, has been shown to be effective in some studies. Most experts

## TABLE 20-4 GENERAL TREATMENT ALGORITHM FOR ADOLESCENT IDIOPATHIC SCOLIOSIS

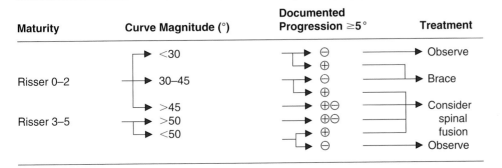

| Maturity | Curve Magnitude (°) | Documented Progression ≥5° | Treatment |
|---|---|---|---|
| Risser 0–2 | <30 | ⊖ | Observe |
| | | ⊕ | Brace |
| | 30–45 | ⊖ | |
| | | ⊕ | |
| | >45 | ⊕⊖ | Consider spinal fusion |
| Risser 3–5 | >50 | ⊕⊖ | |
| | <50 | ⊕ | |
| | | ⊖ | Observe |

believe, however, that brace efficacy is dose related: The more hours per day the brace is worn, the greater the chance for curve control.

The brace should be worn until the patient is skeletally mature, which is approximately 2 years postmenarchal for girls and when boys are Risser 4 to 5 by x-ray. X-rays should be checked every 4 to 6 months during brace wear. We recommend alternating x-rays in and out of the brace to assess for curve progression and adequacy of brace fit with a minimum of radiation exposure. The brace may need to be adjusted or remade as the adolescent grows. If the curve progresses beyond 40 degrees despite brace wear, surgical stabilization should be considered.

### Surgical Intervention

Indications for surgical intervention include the following:

- Progression of the curve despite use of brace
- Curve greater than 40 degrees in a skeletally immature patient
- Curve greater than 50 degrees in a skeletally mature patient

It is important to recognize the variation in patient appearance and emotional acceptance, which are not based on x-ray curve magnitude. Some patients with smaller curves are unwilling to accept the cosmetic deformity of scoliosis or the social stigma of wearing a brace. These patients may be candidates for surgery before the curve reaches 45 degrees. This is particularly true for lumbar curves, in which a 35-degree curve may produce a marked trunk shift. Likewise, some patients with large curves refuse surgery. Each patient must be treated individually to obtain the best outcome emotionally and physically. When the surgeon and patient have agreed that surgical intervention is warranted, many options are available. The surgical approach and fusion can be posterior, anterior, or anterior and posterior.

**Posterior Spinal Fusion.** Posterior spinal fusion with instrumentation is the gold standard for most scoliosis curves. It has the longest track record, going back to 1960 when Harrington introduced metal implants for curve correction. Cotrel and Dubousset developed a modern universal instrumentation system (CD) that uses rods, hooks, and screws to correct scoliosis mechanically through translation, rotation, and distraction in three dimensions (Fig. 20-4). The CD system has been modified, and many variations now are available. This mechanical correction must be maintained ultimately by spinal fusion produced by decortication, facet excision, autograft, or allograft.

Posterior spinal fusion can be extended to the pelvis or sacrum if necessary; however, it is rare that patients with IAS require fusion below L4. Every effort should be made to stop the fusion at L3 if possible to leave lumbar motion segments. Fusion to L4 or L5 has led to an increased incidence of late low back pain. The levels fused during posterior spinal surgery depend on the curve and the flexibility of curves above or below. The structural curves always should be fused; compensatory curves often can be left out of the fusion mass. Moe recommended that the neutral vertebra (vertebra with symmetric pedicles on posteroanterior x-ray) should be included in the fusion.

**Anterior Spinal Fusion.** Anterior spinal fusion can be used to correct single thoracic, lumbar, and thoracolumbar curves (Fig. 20-5) but cannot be used for double structural curves. Anterior spinal fusion can be done through an open incision or endoscopically. The video-assisted endoscopic approach is becoming more common as techniques and instrumentation improve, but this technique has the steepest learning curve for the surgeon.

Because anterior spinal fusion can increase kyphosis, it should not be used for patients with excessive preoperative thoracic kyphosis, and it must be used cautiously when trying to preserve or enhance lordosis. All levels within the curve should be fused; instrumentation and fusion should extend from the transitional neutral vertebra above to the transitional neutral vertebra below the curve. This extension may allow a shorter segment of fusion than posterior spinal fusion. Anterior spinal fusion can be accomplished through an open thoracotomy, retroperitoneal approach, anterior thoracolumbar approach, or endoscopically (either laparoscopically or thoracoscopically). After disc removal and structural bone grafting at each level (with autograft ribs, allograft, or cages), a bicortical screw is placed in each vertebral body, and a single rod is used for correction. Newer systems use double screws at each level and double rods to improve stability and possibly to decrease the pseudarthrosis rate, which has been shown to be higher with ante-

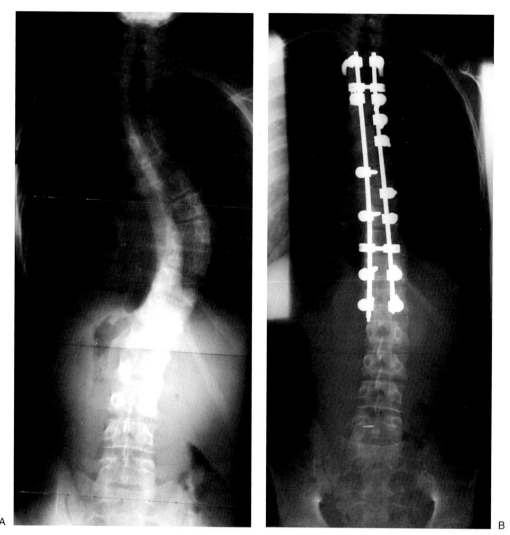

A

B

**Figure 20-4** Preoperative (**A**) and postoperative (**B**) x-rays of a patient treated with segmental posterior spinal instrumentation and fusion for scoliosis.

rior fusions. A double-rod system also may obviate the need for postoperative bracing.

**Combined Anterior and Posterior Spinal Fusion.** Large, stiff curves may require anterior release before posterior fusion. This procedure can be done through an open or thoracoscopic approach and involves removing the disc at each segment within the curve to be fused. The stiffness of the curve is determined on the preoperative bending films. Curves that do not change or change very little with bending are unlikely to correct adequately with posterior fusion alone; anterior release and sometimes anterior instrumentation improve the correction.

In skeletally immature patients who undergo posterior spinal fusion, the anterior spine can continue to grow and create a crankshaft phenomenon as the anterior spine rotates around the posterior fusion mass. Young patients (Risser 0 or 1) who are at risk of developing problems from the crankshaft phenomenon frequently undergo a combined anterior and posterior spinal fusion. This procedure can be done in a single setting or staged days to months apart,

depending on the condition of the patient and surgeon preference.

Lenke et al developed treatment recommendations for curves requiring surgery based on their classification system (Table 20-5). After any type of spinal fusion, thoracoplasty or partial rib resections can be done on the convex side of the curve to reduce a prominent rib hump and to improve the associated deformity.

**Surgical Risks.** The most devastating complication associated with scoliosis surgery is neurologic damage, ranging from a mild neuropathy to paraplegia. Intraoperative monitoring during surgery can help protect a child from permanent injury. Many centers use neuromotor evoked potential (NMEP) or somatosensory evoked potential (SSEP) monitoring intraoperatively. NMEPs monitor the motor pathways and are more sensitive and reliable than SSEPs, which monitor only the sensory pathways in the dorsal columns of the spinal cord. The Stagnara wake-up test is the gold standard for monitoring motor function if there is any intra-

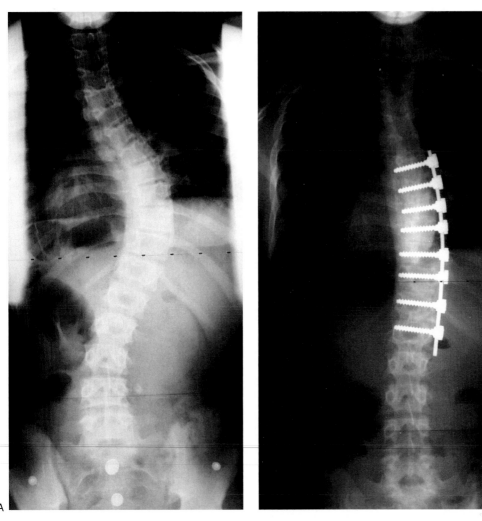

**Figure 20-5**   Preoperative (**A**) and postoperative (**B**) x-rays of a patient treated with anterior instrumentation and fusion for scoliosis. This thoracic curve showed hypolordosis, which was corrected by the kyphogenic anterior instrumentation.

## TABLE 20-5  SURGICAL TREATMENT BASED ON CURVE TYPE

| Curve Type | Structural Regions | Regions to Be Fused | Approach |
|---|---|---|---|
| 1—MT | MT | MT | PSF or ASF |
| 2—DT | PT, MT | PT, MT | PSF |
| 3—DM | MT, TL/L | MT-TL/L | PSF |
| 4—TM | PT, MT, TL/L | PT, MT, TL/L | PSF |
| 5—TL/L | TL/L | TL/L | ASF or PSF |
| 6—TL/L, MT | TL/L, MT | TL/L, MT | PSF |

ASF, anterior spinal fusion; DM, double major; DT, double thoracic; MT, main thoracic, PSF, posterior spinal fusion; PT, proximal thoracic; TL/L, thoracolumbar lumbar; TM, triple major.
From Lenke LG, Betz, RR, Clement D, et al. Curve prevalence of a new classification of operative adolescent idiopathic scoliosis. Spine 2002; 27: 604–611.

operative concern; this allows alteration of hardware or curve correction with the patient still under anesthesia.

Surgery can be complicated by early or late infection. There also is a risk of pseudarthrosis, hardware failure, and postoperative back pain. Later in life, there is a concern for degenerative changes above and below the levels fused.

**Postoperative Management.** Postoperative plans can vary depending on the patient and surgeon. After posterior fusion, with good fixation and bone quality, most patients do not require bracing. Anterior spinal fusion alone frequently requires external support with a custom-molded TLSO for 6 to 12 weeks postoperatively. In our institution, patients are mobilized the day after surgery. If bracing is necessary, the patient is molded and fitted with the brace before discharge from the hospital. Patients with spine fusion for AIS typically are discharged by postoperative day 4 to 7. They are encouraged to walk as much as tolerated for the first 3 months, with no lifting, twisting, or bending permitted. After 3 months, activity usually is progressed to jogging and bicycling. After 12 months, if x-rays show adequate fusion, patients are allowed to return to noncontact sports. It is recommended that patients avoid contact sports for at least another year.

# SCHEUERMANN'S KYPHOSIS

Increased thoracic kyphosis, commonly seen in adolescents, ranges from flexible or postural round-back deformity to a true rigid deformity with bony and soft tissue changes. In 1920, Scheuermann described the deformity as having characteristic changes on x-ray, including vertebral wedging and end plate irregularity. In addition to trunk deformity, Scheuermann's kyphosis in the thoracic spine frequently causes back pain that is modest early in the disease process but tends to increase as patients approach skeletal maturity. The less common lumbar form of Scheuermann's disease often causes severe back pain but little deformity. Adults also may experience back pain; Bradford reported that adults with Scheuermann's kyphosis have a higher incidence of disabling back pain than the normal population. Scheuermann's kyphosis is known to progress during growth periods, but it also can progress during adult life, and it is worsened by senile progression into kyphosis with advanced age. Physicians should recognize and manage Scheuermann's kyphosis appropriately to prevent progression, limit deformity, and minimize pain or discomfort.

## Pathogenesis

### Etiology

Many hypotheses about the underlying causes of Scheuermann's kyphosis have been suggested, yet the true etiology remains unknown. Scheuermann originally hypothesized that aseptic necrosis of the ring apophyses led to an arrest of growth and anterior wedging of the vertebrae, but this hypothesis has not been confirmed. Scheuermann later noted an increased incidence of Scheuermann's kyphosis in patients carrying heavy loads, suggesting a mechanical disruption—a theory supported by several other authors. Schmorl and Junghans noted the radiographic finding of Schmorl's nodes and hypothesized that a weakening of the cartilaginous end plate allowed the intervertebral disc to penetrate the bone and disrupt normal growth. It since has been shown, however, that Schmorl's nodes are present in many different types of spinal deformity and are not limited to Scheuermann's kyphosis.

Because extreme hamstring tightness is common in Scheuermann's kyphosis, Lambrinudi proposed that the hamstring tightness is the primary factor in the etiology owing to the creation of posterior pelvic tilt and resultant increased spine flexion above to maintain sagittal balance.

Scheuermann's kyphosis is associated with several disease processes, including endocrine abnormalities, hypovitaminosis, inflammatory disease, neuromuscular disorders, dural cysts, and spondylolysis, but no direct cause-and-effect relationship between these conditions and Scheuermann's kyphosis has been established.

Histologic exam of vertebrae from patients with Scheuermann's kyphosis has shown grossly disorganized endochondral ossification. Bradford et al suggested that a change in calcium metabolism and resultant osteoporosis is the primary cause of the vertebral wedging.

There seems to be a strong genetic predisposition for the development of Scheuermann's kyphosis. Halal et al studied five families with a high incidence of this deformity and suggested that it is inherited in an autosomal dominant fashion with a high degree of penetrance and variable expressivity. Ascani and Montanaro reported that affected patients have elevated levels of growth hormone and advanced bone age compared with chronologic age. A report of identical twins with thoracolumbar Scheuermann's kyphosis suggested that genetics and mechanical factors play a role; the twin who was more active in strenuous activities had a worse deformity.

It is likely that there is a complex interaction of hereditary and environmental factors that result in kyphotic deformity. Further studies need to be done to determine more definitively the etiology and biology of Scheuermann's kyphosis.

### Epidemiology

Scheuermann's kyphosis usually becomes apparent between 10 and 14 years of age with a prevalence of 0.4% to 8% of the general population. Generally, boys and girls seem to be affected equally, although some studies show a slight gender bias toward either boys or girls. An associated mild scoliosis is noted in 20% to 30% of patients, but this lateral curve rarely progresses to require treatment. Progression of kyphosis has been documented during the growth spurt and later in adult life. In contrast to idiopathic scoliosis, the risk for kyphosis progression currently is unknown and warrants further study. There have been rare reports of acute paraparesis in patients with severe Scheuermann's kyphosis, which is thought to be secondary to thoracic disc herniation, dural cysts, or the canal compromise from the deformity.

### Classification

There are two forms of Scheuermann's kyphosis—type I and type II. The classic thoracic type (type I) has an apex between T7 and T9 and is associated with increased lumbar lordosis. The thoracolumbar or lumbar type (type II) has a lower apex, which frequently is associated with reduced upper thoracic kyphosis or thoracic lordosis. Type II Scheuermann's kyphosis occurs more frequently in males in a slightly older age group (15 to 18 years). This form tends to be more painful but rarely leads to progressive deformity.

## Diagnosis

### History

In addition to the standard history (age, gender, past medical history, and family history), one should determine maturity: age at menarche for girls, presence of pubertal hair, history of a growth spurt, current patient height, and the height of first-degree family members. Further assessment includes evaluation of pain or any neurologic symptoms.

### Physical Examination

General body habitus and maturity or Tanner stage should be evaluated. The skin should be examined for café au lait spots, axillary and inguinal freckling (which may indicate neurofibromatosis), and signs of dysraphism (skin markings, dimpling, hair on the back). The adolescent should be examined for asymmetry of shoulders, pelvis, and muscular development. Tightness of the hamstrings is common and can be evaluated with the straight-leg raise test or forward bending test. The patient should be examined for hip flexion contracture or fixed pelvic tilt with the Thomas test. A neurologic exam needs to be done on every patient with a spinal deformity.

The spinal deformity should be understood in three dimensions. In a forward bending test, the kyphotic deformity is accentuated, and the apex appears as a sharp angulation, in contrast to the smooth curve of a patient with postural kyphosis. A forward bending test also exposes any associated scoliosis. The hyperextension test helps the examiner understand the rigidity of the curve. A curve that is flexible or reduces significantly with hyperextension is typically postural and not Scheuermann's kyphosis, although in younger children a flexible round-back deformity may be the first sign of evolution to true Scheuermann's kyphosis.

### Radiologic Features

The Scoliosis Research Society has described normal thoracic kyphosis as 20 degrees to 40 degrees. Standing radiographs of the entire spine of a patient with Scheuermann's kyphosis typically have the following characteristic features (Fig. 20-6):

- Anterior wedging (>5 degrees) of three or more consecutive vertebral bodies
- Increased kyphosis (>45 degrees), which can be measured by the modified Cobb method on the lateral x-ray
- Irregularity of vertebral end plates
- Schmorl's nodes—depressions in the vertebral bodies that represent disc herniation into the end plate

In 20% to 30% of patients, the posteroanterior x-ray shows an associated mild scoliosis in the area of the kyphosis. The scoliotic apex usually corresponds with the kyphotic apex. A lateral x-ray should be examined for spondylolisthesis in addition to kyphosis. In the later stages of Scheuermann's kyphosis, x-rays often reveal changes consistent with degenerative arthritis, including decreased intervertebral disc spaces, marginal osteophytes, and ankylosis.

## Treatment

Scheuermann's kyphosis can be treated with observation, physical therapy, bracing, and, rarely, surgery, depending on the degree of deformity and patient acceptance. It is important to understand how each patient is affected mentally and physically by a kyphotic deformity. This assessment should be made over time because the symptoms of Scheuermann's kyphosis are inconsistent, and there are no certain rules regarding who should have bracing or surgery.

### Conservative Management

Because Scheuermann's kyphosis is not a life-threatening problem until severe deformity is present, all patients with mild-to-moderate kyphosis (<75 degrees) should have a trial of conservative treatment to control symptoms and

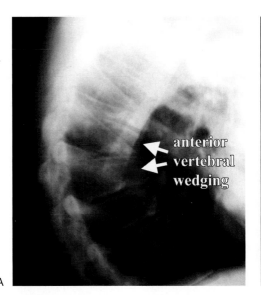

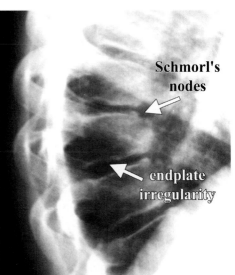

**Figure 20-6**  (**A** and **B**) Radiographs showing typical bone changes associated with Scheuermann's kyphosis.

minimize deformtiy. Physical therapy should emphasize hamstring stretching, trunk strengthening exercises, and postural improvement. Ideally the surgeon and family should find a physical therapist who has a special interest in posture and the relationship between trunk appearance and self-esteem.

### Bracing

A kyphosis brace applies three point bending forces that decrease thoracic kyphosis. In skeletally immature patients with thoracic kyphosis greater than 45 degrees and less than 75 degrees, bracing can be considered. Attempts to brace curves greater than 75 degrees have led to a high failure rate, and this is not recommended. To influence a type I deformity, a CTLSO or modified Milwaukee brace provides the best extension force, but wear compliance with this brace tends to be poor. More cosmetically acceptable underarm braces commonly are used now, but these require expert orthotic design and alteration to be effective.

There are mixed reports regarding brace efficacy in the literature. Acute application of a brace can influence the deformity and improve kyphosis by 40% to 50%; however, several articles have shown at least partial loss of this correction when brace wear is stopped. It is recommended that a brace be worn full-time (23 hours per day) for 12 to 18 months, then part-time to full-time (depending on the severity of the kyphosis) until the patient reaches skeletal maturity. If a teenager strongly refuses to wear a brace out of the house (a frequent reaction in a peer-conscious age group), a vigorous exercise program combined with nighttime brace wear can be considered. All kyphosis braces require careful orthotist attention to ensure fit and to recontour the posterior bars and pads every 2 months to gain further correction progressively. There is no indication to brace skeletally mature patients.

### Surgical Intervention

Tribus suggested five reasons to consider surgical treatment of type I (thoracic) Scheuermann's kyphosis, as follows:

- Pain
- Progressive curve
- Neurologic compromise
- Cardiopulmonary compromise
- Trunk deformity

Rarely, thoracic disc herniation, epidural cysts, or a severe kyphosis (>100 degrees) can cause neurologic deficit in patients (usually adults) with Scheuermann's kyphosis. Neurologic deficits are the only absolute indication for surgery. Relative indications include kyphosis greater than 75 degrees and kyphosis greater than 60 degrees associated with pain that is not alleviated by nonoperative measures. The goals of surgery include correction of the deformity and relief of pain. Surgical correction of the deformity always includes spinal fusion.

**Posterior Spinal Fusion.**    Historically, fusion was achieved with a posterior approach and Harrington compression instrumentation. With larger rigid curves, however, this approach led to a high pseudarthrosis rate, frequent loss of correction, and unacceptable hardware fail-

ures, including broken rods and hooks pulling through the lamina.

Modern segmental posterior instrumentation, such as the CD system, provides much better fixation. Modern instrumentation includes cross-linked rods attached to hooks and screws that can correct the deformity in three dimensions; this allows correction of any associated scoliosis in addition to the kyphosis. There still are occasional problems with junctional kyphosis developing at the ends of the instrumented segment. Otsuka recommends posterior fusion alone only if the curve bends out to less than 50 degrees on a hyperextension lateral radiograph.

**Combined Anterior and Posterior Spinal Fusion.**    Anterior release and fusion at the apex of the deformity in addition to posterior fusion has provided significantly better results with regard to immediate and long-term correction of large kyphotic deformities and now is the standard of care for large, rigid deformities (Fig. 20-7). The anterior procedure can be done open or endoscopically before the posterior instrumentation.

Debate remains regarding selection of fusion levels in Scheuermann's kyphosis. It is clear from the literature that too short a fusion leads to junctional kyphosis developing at the proximal and distal ends of the rods. The criteria to determine the fusion levels in Scheuermann's kyphosis are not as well established as they are for scoliosis. Current recommendations are to include the proximal end vertebra (determined by the modified Cobb method) and to extend the fusion past the transitional zone to the first lordotic disc distally. Lowe also recommended limiting correction of the kyphosis to 50% of the original deformity or less to prevent junctional kyphosis. Overcorrection should be avoided. Patients with type II Scheuermann's kyphosis almost never require surgery.

**Risks of Surgery.**    Reported complications of surgical correction of Scheuermann's kyphosis include death, gastrointestinal obstruction, hardware failure, pseudarthrosis, progression of the deformity, hemothorax, pneumothorax, pulmonary emboli, and persistent postoperative back pain. The most feared complication is neurologic injury, including paralysis. Vascular insult to the cord and mechanical damage have led to paraplegia. Correction of kyphosis carries a higher than usual risk of neurologic injury, which is related directly to the amount of correction. Intraoperative neurologic monitoring is crucial during any surgery to correct kyphosis because the thoracic cord is at risk during correction and instrumentation. NMEPs and SSEPs are used in most spine centers. The Stagnara wake-up test is the gold standard for motor monitoring if there are any concerns during surgery. If monitoring or the wake-up test indicates a neurologic deficit, any corrective maneuvers should be reversed.

There are significant risks to surgical correction of thoracic kyphosis that must be weighed carefully when considering surgery because the natural history of Scheuermann's kyphosis still is not yet well defined. Corrective kyphosis surgery has benefited immensely from new developments in spine instrumentation (e.g., pedicle screws, in situ bending). Perhaps even more than idiopathic scoliosis, surgical management of Scheuermann's kyphosis requires treatment by experienced spinal deformity surgeons.

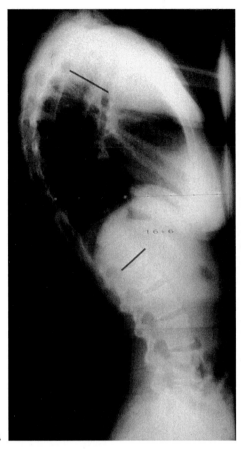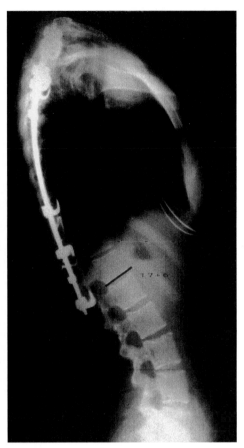

A                                                                                    B

**Figure 20-7**  Preoperative (**A**) and postoperative (**B**) x-rays of a patient treated with posterior instrumentation and fusion.

**Postoperative Management.**  Most patients undergoing surgical correction of Scheuermann's kyphosis require postoperative bracing for approximately 3 to 6 months. Patients typically are mobilized the day after surgery to help prevent atelectasis and gastrointestinal obstruction. They usually are hospitalized for 4 to 7 days and are encouraged to ambulate several times a day for the first 3 months. No bending, stooping, or lifting is allowed for at least 3 months. No sports are allowed for the first year after surgery. After 1 year, patients may return slowly to normal activities if x-rays show consolidation of the fusion and minimal progression of the kyphosis.

# SUGGESTED READING

Ascani E, Montanaro A. Scheuermann's disease. In The Pediatric Spine, DS Bradford, RM Hensinger, eds. New York: Thieme, 1985: 307–324.

Bagnall KM, Raso VJ, Hill DL, et al. Melatonin levels in idiopathic scoliosis. Diurnal and nocturnal melatonin levels in girls with adolescent idiopathic scoliosis. Spine 1996;21:1974–1978.

Barrack RL, Whitecloud, TS, 3rd, Burke, SW, et al. Proprioception in idiopathic scoliosis. Spine 1984;9:681–685.

Barrack RL, Wyatt MP, Whitecloud TS, 3rd, et al. Vibratory hypersensitivity in idiopathic scoliosis. J Pediatr Orthop 1988;8:389–395.

Beals RK. Nosologic and genetic aspects of scoliosis. Clin Orthop 1973;93:23–32.

Bell M, Teebi AS. Autosomal dominant idiopathic scoliosis? Am J Med Genet 1995;55:112.

Bradford DS, Ahmed KB, Moe JH, et al. The surgical management of patients with Scheuermann's disease: a review of twenty-four cases managed by combined anterior and posterior spine fusion. J Bone Joint Surg Am 1980;62:705–712.

Bradford DS, Brown DM, Moe JH, et al. Scheuermann's kyphosis: a form of osteoporosis? Clin Orthop 1976;118:10–15.

Bradford DS, Moe JH. Scheuermann's juvenile kyphosis. A histologic study. Clin Orthop 1975;110:45–53.

Bradford DS, Moe JH, Montalvo FJ, et al. Scheuermann's kyphosis and roundback deformity. Results of Milwaukee brace treatment. J Bone Joint Surg Am 1974;56:740–758.

Bradford DS, Moe JH, Montalvo FJ, et al. Scheuermann's kyphosis. Results of surgical treatment by posterior spine arthrodesis in twenty-two patients. J Bone Joint Surg Am 1975;57:439–448.

Branthwaite MA. Cardiorespiratory consequences of unfused idiopathic scoliosis. Br J Dis Chest 1986;80:360–369.

Brooks HL, Azen SP, Gerberg E, et al. Scoliosis: a prospective epidemiological study. J Bone Joint Surg Am 1975;57:968–972.

Bunnell WP. The natural history of idiopathic scoliosis before skeletal maturity.

Bushell GR, Ghosh P, Taylor TK. Collagen defect in idiopathic scoliosis. Lancet 1978;2:8080.

Bylund P, Jansson E, Dahlberg E, et al. Muscle fiber types in erector spinae muscles. Fiber types in idiopathic and other forms of scoliosis. Clin Orthop 1987;214:222–228.

Carr AJ, Ogilvie DJ, Wordsworth BP, et al. Segregation of structural collagen genes in adolescent idiopathic scoliosis. Clin Orthop 1992; 274:305–310.

Cobb JR. Outline for the study of scoliosis. Instructional Course Lectures, The American Academy of Orthopedic Surgeons 1948;5: 261–275.

Cochran T, Irstam L, Nachemson A. Long-term anatomic and functional changes in patients with adolescent idiopathic scoliosis treated by Harrington rod fusion. Spine 1983;8:576–584.

Cotrel Y, Dubousset J, Guillaumat M. New universal instrumentation in spinal surgery. Clin Orthop 1988;227:10–23.

Czeizel A, Bellyei A. Barta O. et al. Genetics of adolescent idiopathic scoliosis. J Med Genet 1978;15:424–427.

De George FV, Fisher RL. Idiopathic scoliosis: genetic and environmental aspects. J Med Genet 1967;4:251–257.

Deacon P, Flood BM, Dickson RA. Idiopathic scoliosis in three dimensions. A radiographic and morphometric analysis. J Bone Joint Surg Br 1984;66:509–512.

Dickson RA, Lawton JO, Archer IA, et al. The pathogenesis of idiopathic scoliosis. Biplanar spinal asymmetry. J Bone Joint Surg Br 1984;66:8–15.

Dubousset J, Herring JA, Shufflebarger H. The crankshaft phenomenon. J Pediatr Orthop 1989;9:541–550.

Durham JW, Moskowitz A, Whitney J. Surface electrical stimulation versus brace in treatment of idiopathic scoliosis. Spine 1990;15: 888–892.

Green NE. Part-time bracing of adolescent idiopathic scoliosis. J Bone Joint Surg Am 1986;68:738–742.

Hadley-Miller N, Mims B, Milewicz DM. the potential role of the elastic fiber system in adolescent idiopathic scoliosis. J Bone Joint Surg Am 1994;76:1193–1206.

Halal F, Gledhill RB, Fraser C. Dominant inheritance of Scheuermann's juvenile kyphosis. Am J Dis Child 1978;132:1105–1107.

Harrington PR. The etiology of idiopathic scoliosis. Clin Orthop 1977; 126:17–25.

Herndon WA, Emans JB, Micheli LJ, et al. Combined anterior and posterior fusion for Scheuermann's kyphosis. Spine 2000;25: 1028–1035.

Hilibrand AS, Blakemore LC, Loder RT, et al. The role of melatonin in the pathogenesis of adolescent idiopathic scoliosis. Spine 1996; 21:1147–1152.

Kane WJ, Moe JH. A scoliosis-prevalence survey in Minnesota. Clin Orthop 1970;69:216–218.

King HA, Moe JH, Bradford DS, et al. The selection of fusion levels in thoracic idiopathic scoliosis. J Bone Joint Surg Am 1983;65: 1302–1313.

Klein DM, Weiss RL, Allen JE. Scheuermann's dorsal kyphosis and spinal cord compression: case report. Neurosurgery 1986;18: 628–631.

Lambrinudi C. Adolescent and senile kyphosis. Brit Med J 1934;2: 800–804.

Lenke LG, Betz RR, Clements D, et al. Curve prevalence of a new classification of operative adolescent idiopathic scoliosis: does classification correlate with treatment? Spine 2002;27:604–611.

Lenke LG, Betz RR Harms J, et al. Adolescent idiopathic scoliosis: a new classification to determine extent of spinal arthrodesis. J Bone Joint Surg Am 2001;83-A:1169–1181.

Lesoin F, Leys D, Rousseaux M, et al. Thoracic disk herniation and Scheuermann's disease. Eur Neurol 1987;26:145–152.

Lonstein JE, Carlson JM. The prediction of curve progression in untreated idiopathic scoliosis during growth. J Bone Joint Surg Am 1984;66:1061–1071.

Lowe TG. Double L-rod instrumentation in the treatment of severe kyphosis secondary to Scheuermann's disease. Spine 1987;12: 336–341.

Lowe TG. Scheuermann disease. J Bone Joint Surg Am 1990;72: 940–945.

Lowe TG, Kasten MD. An analysis of sagittal curves and balance after Cotrel-Dubousset instrumentation for kyphosis secondary to Scheuermann's disease. A review of 32 patients. Spine 1994;19: 1680–1685.

Lowe TG, Peters JD. Anterior spinal fusion with Zielke instrumentation for idiopathic scoliosis. A frontal and sagittal curve analysis in 36 patients. Spine 1993;18:423–426.

Machida M, Dubousset J, Imamura Y, et al. Melatonin. A possible role in pathogenesis of adolescent idiopathic scoliosis. Spine 1996;21: 1147–1152.

Misol S, Ponseti IV, Samaan N, el al. Growth hormone blood levels in patients with idiopathic scoliosis. Clin Orthop 1971;81:122–125.

Moe JH. Modern concepts of treatment of spinal deformities in children and adults. Clin Orthop 1980;150:137–153.

Montgomery F, Willner S. The natural history of idiopathic scoliosis: incidence of treatment in 15 cohorts of children born between 1963 and 1977. Spine 1997;22:772–774.

Montgomery SP, Erwin WE. Scheuermann's kyphosis—long-term results of Milwaukee brace treatment. Spine 1981;6:5–8.

Murray PM, Weinstein SL, Spratt KF. The natural history and long-term follow-up of Scheuermann kyphosis. J Bone Joint Surg Am 1993;75:246–248.

Newton PO, Shea KG, Granlund KF. Defining the pediatric spinal thoracoscopy learning curve: sixty-five consecutive cases. Spine 2000;25:1028–1035.

Otsuka NY, Hall JE, Mah JY. Posterior fusion for Scheuermann's kyphosis. Clin Orthop 1990;251:134–139.

Papagelopoulos PJ, Klassen RA, Peterson HA, et al. Surgical treatment of Scheuermann's disease with segmental compression instrumentation. Clin Orthop 2001;386:139–149.

Price CT, Scott DS, Reed FR Jr, et al. Nighttime bracing for adolescent idiopathic scoliosis with the Charleston Bending Brace. Preliminary report. Spine 1990;15:1294–1299.

Price CT, Scott DS, Reed FR Jr, et al. Nighttime bracing for adolescent idiopathic scoliosis with the Charleston Bending Brace: long-term follow-up. J Pediatr Orthop 1997;17:703–707.

Risenborough EJ, Wynn-Davies R. A genetic survey of idiopathic scoliosis in Boston, Massachusetts. J Bone Joint Surg Am 1973;55: 974–982.

Rogala EJ, Drummond DS, Gurr J. Scoliosis: incidence and natural history: a prospective epidemiological study. J Bone Joint Surg 1978;60A:173–176.

Sachs B, Bradford D, Winter R, et al. Scheuermann kyphosis. Follow-up of Milwaukee brace treatment. J Bone Joint Surg Am 1987;69: 50–57.

Scoles PV, Latimer BM, Digiovanni BF, et al. Vertebral alterations in Scheuermann's kyphosis. Spine 1991;16:509–515.

Speck GR, Chopin DC. The surgical treatment of Scheuermann's kyphosis. J Bone Joint Surg Br 1986;68:189–193.

Stone B, Beekman C, Hall V, et al. The effect of an exercise program on change in curve in adolescents with minimal idiopathic scoliosis. A preliminary study. Phys Ther 1979;59:759–763.

Taylor TC, Wenger DR, Stephen J, et al. Surgical management of thoracic kyphosis in adolescents. J Bone Joint Surg Am 1979;61: 496–503.

Tribus CB. Scheuermann's kyphosis in adolescents and adults: diagnosis and management. J Am Acad Orthop Surg 1998;6:36–43.

van Linthoudt D, Revel M. Similar radiologic lesions of localized Scheuermann's disease of the lumbar spine in twin sisters. Spine 1994;19:987–989.

Weinstein SL. Idiopathic scoliosis. Natural history. Spine 1986;11: 780–783.

Weinstein SL. Adolescent idiopathic scoliosis: prevalence and natural history. Instr Course Lect 1989;38:115–128.

Weinstein SL, Ponseti IV. Curve progression in idiopathic scoliosis. J Bone Joint Surg 1983;65A:447–455.

Weinstein SL, Zavala DC, Ponseti IV. Idiopathic scoliosis: long-term follow-up and prognosis in untreated patients. J Bone Joint Surg Am 1981;63:702–712.

Wenger DR, Frick SL. Scheuermann kyphosis. Spine 1999;24: 2630–2639.

Winter RB, Lovell WW, Moe JH. Excessive thoracic lordosis and loss of pulmonary function in patients with idiopathic scoliosis. J Bone Joint Surg Am. 1975;57:972–977.

Wynne-Davies R. Familial (idiopathic) scoliosis. A family survey. J Bone Joint Surg Br. 1968;50:24–30.

# ADULT DEFORMITY

CHARLES C. EDWARDS II
KEITH H. BRIDWELL

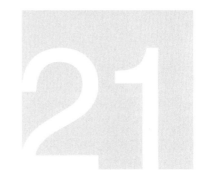

Patients with adult spinal deformities usually seek treatment because of a combination of symptoms, including back pain, radiculopathy, progression of deformity, and global imbalance. The spinal deformity is categorized according to whether the predominant malalignment occurs in the coronal (scoliosis) or sagittal (kyphosis/lordosis) plane. An important distinction for coronal and sagittal deformities is whether the deformity developed de novo in adulthood or had its onset before skeletal maturity with progression over time. This chapter discusses the evaluation and treatment for adult scoliosis and iatrogenic sagittal deformities in ambulatory patients who do not have a paralytic or congenital etiology.

## NORMAL ALIGNMENT

An important prerequisite to the treatment of spinal deformity is a thorough understanding of the spine's normal architecture and alignment. In the coronal plane, the spine is normally straight. A vertical line (*plumb*) from the tip of the dens (C2) on a standing anteroposterior radiograph should nearly bisect each distal vertebra below, including the sacrum. Significant deviation of the vertebra from this vertical line indicates a scoliotic deformity. By tradition, coronal curvature of the spine is termed *scoliosis* if the Cobb measurement is greater than 10 degrees. Normal alignment in the sagittal plane is defined less easily owing to marked variation in global and regional parameters. In evaluating global sagittal balance, the center of the C7 body is a useful reference. It is usually visible on long cassette radiographs, and a plumb line drawn through the center of the C7 body usually intersects with the posterior-superior body of S1 (Fig. 21-1). Normal thoracic kyphosis in adults has a broad range (20 degrees to 60 degrees) with a mean value that tends to increase with age. The apex of thoracic kyphosis usually falls between T6 and T8. Normal lumbar lordosis (L1-S1) ranges from approximately 30 degrees to 80 degrees. Two thirds of the lumbar lordosis usually exists between L4 and the sacrum with 40% at L5-S1. Eighty percent of the lumbar lordosis occurs through wedging of the intervertebral discs, whereas only 20% is derived from the trapezoidal shape of the vertebral bodies.

## ADULT SCOLIOSIS

There are two major categories of patients who have adult scoliosis:

- Adults with a deformity dating back to adolescence with or without superimposed degenerative changes (*adult idiopathic scoliosis*)
- Older adults with degenerative de novo scoliosis who did not have any deformity before age 40 (*adult de novo scoliosis*)

These two types of adult scoliosis are clinically distinct from the adolescent idiopathic variety (Table 21-1). With advancing age, the normal spinal degenerative process may contribute to the progression of an adult idiopathic scoliosis curve or the development and progression of a de novo scoliosis deformity.

### Natural History

The natural history of scoliosis curves that were not treated before skeletal maturity is variable. Smaller curves and curves in patients with good overall spinal alignment may progress little over time. Conversely, larger curves and curves associated with global imbalance may progress at a rate of 1 degree or more per year during adulthood. In general, thoracolumbar and lumbar curves are more likely to progress than more stable thoracic curves. With advancing age, the rate of progression may increase as patients undergo degenerative changes in discs, facets, and ligaments. Older patients with de novo degenerative scoliosis curves may progress at a rate of 3.3 degrees per year.

### Clinical Manifestations

Curve progression typically is appreciated by the patient as a loss of trunk height, a change in trunk contour, or a shift in the position of the head relative to the pelvis (global balance). Although both types of adult scoliosis may increase in magnitude, the change for degenerative idiopathic curves tends to be clinically noticeable, whereas for degenerative de novo curves, the change tends to be more radiographic.

De novo degenerative scoliosis is distinct from adult idio-

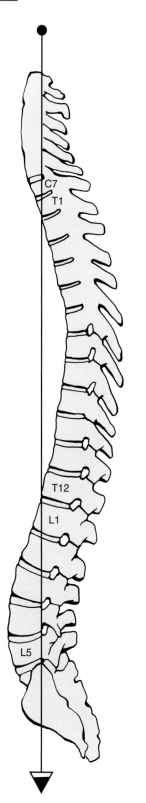

**Figure 21-1** Sagittal alignment showing the C7 plumb and its typical relationship relative to the sacrum.

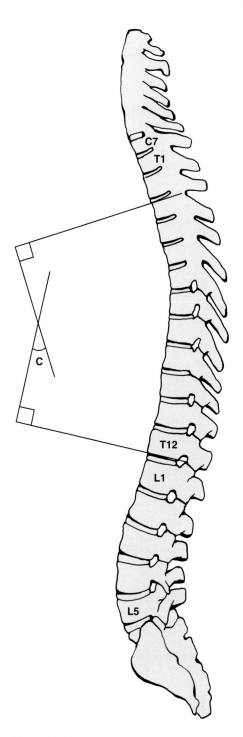

**Figure 21-2** Sagittal alignment of the spine showing the Cobb method of quantifying spinal deformities.

**TABLE 21-1  COMPARISON OF CLINICAL CHARACTERISTICS ASSOCIATED WITH ADOLESCENT AND ADULT SCOLIOSIS**

|  | Adolescent Scoliosis | Adult Scoliosis |
|---|---|---|
| Presenting complaints | Cosmesis, (+) screening | Back pain, leg pain, global imbalance |
| Physical findings | Partially flexible curve, neurologically intact | Typically rigid curve, painful motion, lumbar radiculopathy |
| Radiographic findings | Preserved disc height, minimal listhesis or degeneration | Loss of disc height, listhesis, sclerosis and osteophyte formation |
| Progression | Rapid during years of peak growth | Gradual over decades |

pathic scoliosis in that patients have no history of previous spinal deformity. It occurs in the lumbar spine in the absence of any significant thoracic deformity. Mild-to-moderate de novo adult scoliosis deformities may be well tolerated, especially when global balance is maintained. Larger curves and curves with advanced degeneration tend to be symptomatic.

Adult scoliosis patients typically present with reports of back pain, leg pain, or progressive deformity. Axial discomfort arises from advanced degeneration of spine motion segments and paraspinal muscle fatigue resulting from the body's attempt to maintain regional and global balance. Degeneration of the disc, facet complex, and segmental listhesis also can result in stenosis of the canal, lateral recess, or foramen causing claudicatory symptoms or radiculopathy or both. Stenosis and neural compression occur most frequently in the areas of greatest force concentration within the spine. These areas are principally the concavity of the scoliotic curve or within the remaining segments between the distal aspect of the thoracolumbar or lumbar curve and the sacrum (fractional curve) (Fig. 21-3).

## Nonsurgical Treatment

Nonoperative management for adult scoliosis is similar to that recommended for symptomatic lumbar disc degeneration. Initially, nonsteroidal antiinflammatory drugs, exercise, weight management, and, in some cases, orthotic devices are recommended. None of these measures has been shown to arrest the progression of deformity or relieve symptoms resulting from neurologic compression. A trial of nonoperative measures is indicated, however, in patients who have mild deformities or who have sizable deformities but for a variety of organic and psychosocial reasons are not candidates for surgical intervention.

## Surgical Intervention

### Indications

The four principal indications for the surgical treatment of adult scoliosis are as follows:

▪ Large deformity based on Cobb measurement, vertebral rotation, coronal balance, and the sagittal plane

▪ Documented deformity progression
▪ Function limiting axial or radicular pain that is poorly responsive to nonoperative measures
▪ Pulmonary dysfunction related to the spinal deformity

In addition, a good overall state of health, a stable emotional state, and an intact social support structure ideally should be present. Modifiable risk factors for the development of perioperative complications should be optimized before surgery is undertaken (e.g., smoking, malnutrition, skin compromise, steroid use).

### Surgical Decision Making

The optimal surgical strategy is individualized for each patient based on their specific complaints, physical and radiographic findings, and overall state of health. Radiographic evaluation includes long cassette anteroposterior and lateral views to assess regional and global balance. Flexibility radiographs in the coronal and sagittal plane provide valuable insight into the rigidity of the curve. When it is difficult to assess degenerative changes at the lumbosacral junction, a true anteroposterior radiograph (the Ferguson anteroposterior view) of the lumbosacral joint with the beam angled up to the degree of lumbosacral lordosis is helpful.

Evaluation of the spinal stenosis is achieved best with myelography followed by computed tomography (CT). Myelography may be obtained in supine and standing positions to define the dynamic nature of the stenosis. Thin (1-mm) CT axial slices provide for a precise assessment of the central canal, lateral recess, and foramen. Magnetic resonance imaging (MRI) is helpful for assessing the disc degeneration and foraminal stenosis, especially at the distal lumbar segments. For the central canal and lateral recess, MRI is not as helpful for defining the extent of stenosis as CT-myelography. Many surgeons find provocative discograms helpful in deciding where to stop a fusion distally. To date, there is no universal agreement, however, on the reproducibility and reliability of discograms.

The optimal surgical strategy is one in which the patient's complaints are addressed adequately with the smallest magnitude of surgery, while minimizing the potential for perioperative and subsequent complications (Table 21-2). For adult idiopathic scoliosis without significant spinal degeneration, an anterior-only or posterior-only fusion is indi-

## TABLE 21-2 DEGENERATIVE SCOLIOSIS: SURGICAL STRATEGIES

| Symptoms | Decompression | Fusion |
|---|---|---|
| Neurologic symptoms, no severe back pain, mild deformity | Focal decompression with preservation of stabilizing structures | Often not necessary |
| Severe back pain and/or significant deformity | Not indicated | Segmental instrumentation and fusion |
| Severe back pain, deformity, neurologic symptoms | Decompression | Posterior only or circumferential instrumentation and fusion |
| Severe imbalance | At levels of osteotomy | Posterior only versus circumferential instrumentation and fusion |

cated. For degenerative scoliosis, a variety of surgical strategies are possible depending on the patient's constellation of symptoms (see Table 21-2). If the patient's complaints can be localized to a specific level, a focused treatment strategy of limited decompression or fusion, or both, may be employed. A focused intervention often is best suited for patients with mild scoliotic deformities, hyperstable spines, or significant comorbidities who would not tolerate more extensive reconstruction procedures. This strategy must be considered carefully in terms of its effect on segmental stability, regional alignment, and the potential for subsequent deformity progression.

Young adults with scoliosis usually do not have a significant amount of lumbar degeneration. The principles of selecting fusion levels for these patients are similar to those for patients with adolescent scoliosis. The highest and lowest instrumented vertebrae should be stable (intersected by the center sacral line) and nonrotated (neutral), and the sagittal profile, especially lumbar lordosis, should be corrected to as near normal as possible.

In older adult patients, the fractional curve in the distal lumbar spine typically has degenerative changes and becomes increasingly stiff. Segments to be included in the fusion include segments with subluxation, spinal stenosis, and posterior column deficiencies due to previous laminectomies or spondylolysis. Whether to include distal segments with mild-to-moderate disc degeneration is controversial. Provocative discography may provide the answer in select cases, but the procedure is not universally accepted. In general, segments in the distal lumbar spine with only mild degenerative changes do not need to be included in the fusion if there is no underlying degenerative deformity, central, lateral recess, or foraminal stenosis. After surgical treatment, the cephalad and caudad ends of the fusion should be neutral and stable. In most cases, it is preferable for the top and bottom of the fusion to end up parallel to the shoulders and the sacrum.

The question frequently arises as to whether a long fusion should stop at L5 or the sacrum (Table 21-3). Indications for extension to the sacrum include advanced degeneration of the L5-S1 disc, oblique take of L5 on the sacrum, previous L5-S1 decompression, or presence of spondylolysis. In the absence of these conditions, stopping the fusion at L5 should be considered.

Preservation of a "healthy" L5-S1 motion segment offers multiple theoretical advantages. With a long fusion to L5, challenges involved with obtaining and maintaining lumbosacral fixation and fusion are negated. Adjunctive anterior discectomy and fusion procedures selectively may be avoided, and postoperative bracing requirements are decreased. The smaller magnitude of surgery involved with arthrodesis to L5 also theoretically may lead to a decreased incidence of perioperative complications.

L5 and the sacrum have unique limitations as a distal fusion level. For long fusions stopping at L5, the remaining lumbosacral motion segment is subjected to supraphysiologic forces and may undergo accelerated degeneration. A "transition syndrome" at L5-S1 may result in pain, radiculopathy, and forward shift in sagittal balance. Conversely, long fusions to the sacrum are limited by the larger initial scope of surgery required, an increased risk of perioperative morbidity, and the increased possibility for the subsequent development of pseudarthrosis. The decision of whether to stop a long fusion at L5 or the sacrum should be evaluated on a case-by-case basis with consideration of the preoperative sagittal balance, degenerative status of the L5-S1 disc, and medical status of the patient.

In terms of the sagittal plane, the upper and lower instrumented vertebrae should extend into areas of lordosis. It almost always is a mistake to stop a fusion at the apex of a sagittal kyphosis, because a progressive junctional kyphosis commonly follows.

## TABLE 21-3 ADVANTAGES OF TERMINATING A LONG FUSION AT L5 VERSUS THE SACRUM

| L5 | Sacrum |
|---|---|
| Preserved lumbosacral motion | No potential for subsequent L5–1 disc degeneration |
| Lower incidence of nonunion | Better operative deformity correction |
| Less surgery | Superior maintenance of correction over time |
| Less bracing | |

## Surgical Approaches

Factors that determine whether a posterior fusion or circumferential fusion are needed include the following:

- Length of the fusion
- Curve flexibility
- Quality of the posterior bone for fixation and fusion
- Patient's sagittal balance

Spinal segments with rigid kyphosis or rotatory subluxation usually are treated best with circumferential surgery. In these cases, anterior structural grafting of a distracted disc space tends to create a ligamentotaxis effect to help reduce subluxations. Retensioning the anulus and the posterior longitudinal ligament also often normalizes alignment. The presence of a previous laminectomy or the need for a concurrent extensive decompression results in a decreased surface area for posterior fusion and is another relative indication for a circumferential fusion. Anterior surgery increases the amount of correction achieved and the likelihood of obtaining a solid fusion (see Fig. 21-3). The poten-

tial benefits of a supplemental anterior procedure must be balanced on a case-by-case basis, however, against the added operative time, operative risks, and recovery.

Osteotomies for deformity correction should be considered for patients with severe, out-of-balance, or highly inflexible curves. Three basic types of osteotomies exist:

- Osteotomies that involve posterior element wedge resection (Smith-Peterson osteotomy)
- Posterior wedge resection in association with anterior discectomy and structural grafting (circumferential osteotomy)
- Posterior three-column wedge resection (pedicle subtraction or decancellation osteotomy)

Although osteotomies are best suited for the correction of sagittal imbalance, coronal deformity correction also may be achieved by resecting additional bone in the coronal plane from the side of the convexity. If circumferential procedures are contemplated, it is usually advisable to start with the anterior approach. The exceptions to this principle

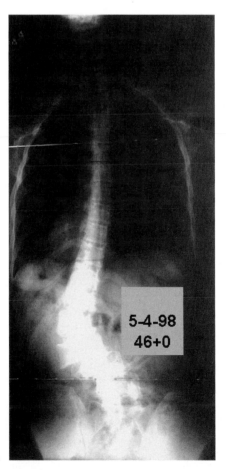
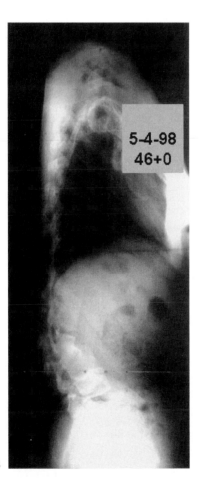
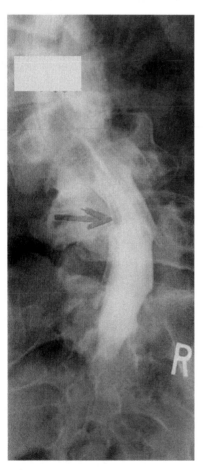

A                                    B                                    C

**Figure 21-3** Anteroposterior (A) and lateral standing (B) radiographs of a 46-year-old woman with a known history of untreated adolescent idiopathic scoliosis who experienced the progressive onset of back discomfort, left leg radicular symptoms, and worsened cosmesis over the past few years. Standing anteroposterior myelogram (C) shows decreased dye filling in the area of the lateral recess on the left side at L5. A combination of factors, including facet hypertrophy (inferior facet of L4 and superior facet of L5), scoliosis, listhesis, and capsular hypertrophy, contributes to the stenosis at the L4-5 level. *Figure continues.*

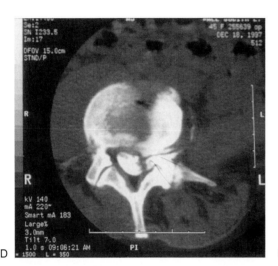

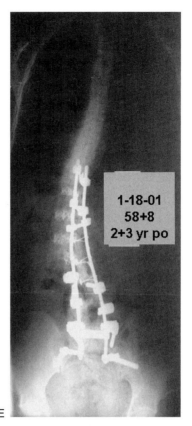

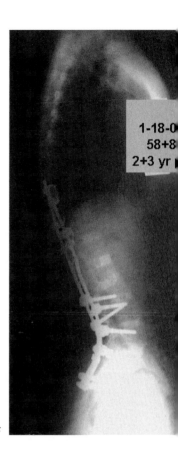

D                                                          E                                          F

**Figure 21-3** (*Continued*) Displacement of the cauda equina and compression of the left L5 nerve root shown on the postmyelogram CT scan (**D**) account for the left leg radicular symptoms experienced by the patient. Standing anteroposterior (**E**) and lateral (**F**) radiographs 2.3 years status post spine decompression and reconstruction. The patient underwent a two-stage procedure beginning with anterior discectomies and fusion from T11 to the sacrum using a combination of structural interbody cages, fresh frozen femoral rings, and autogenous autograft. One week later, the patient underwent a posterior decompression at L4-5 and instrumented fusion from T10 to the sacrum with significant deformity correction. The decision was made to fuse to the sacrum owing to the presence of advanced L5-S1 disc degeneration. Posterior Smith-Peterson osteotomies were performed to improve the sagittal alignment beyond that achieved with anterior discectomies and structural grafting alone. At more than 2 years after surgery, the patient's regional coronal and sagittal alignment are much improved, and global balance is well maintained. The leg pain has resolved. *Figure continues.*

are cases with severe stenosis in which the canal could be compromised further by an anterior grafting and extension at the level of an already stenotic canal.

### Grafting Choices

Forms of bone grafting anteriorly include morcellized or structural autogenous bone (rib or iliac crest), morcellized or structural allograft (fresh frozen femoral rings), and mesh cages filled with morcellized autograft or allograft. Advantages of fresh frozen femoral rings and mesh cages are that anterior structural support is provided, and the disc space is held open to increase lordosis and theoretically to expand the foramen. Morcellized autogenous bone is recommended for posterior fusion. The role of bone-stimulating factors, such as bone morphogenetic protein, in stimulating bone formation in the presence of a long adult deformity fusion is investigational at this time.

### Spinal Fixation

Segmental fixation always should be used when performing an arthrodesis for adult deformity. Fixation at each level provides for not only better correction, but also superior maintenance of correction and theoretically a higher rate of fusion. The benefits of segmental fixation are most pronounced in older patients with osteoporosis who are at especially increased risk for subsequent implant pull-out/failure and loss of alignment. The use of cement augmentation in association with pedicle screw placement and prophylactic vertebroplasty of adjacent unfused levels has been advocated in these cases, but these methods have not been widely adopted.

It may be possible to use only anterior segmental spinal instrumentation for certain lumbar and thoracolumbar curves in young and flexible patients. For most patients, some form of posterior segmental spinal instrumentation

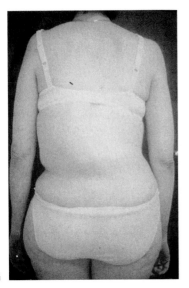
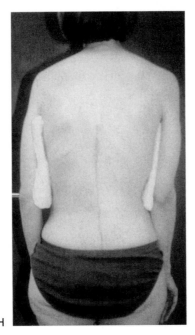
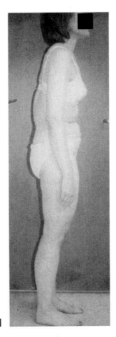
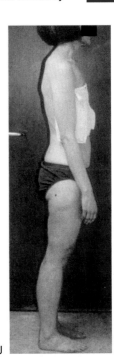

G     H     I     J

**Figure 21-3** *(Continued)* Preoperative lateral photograph (**G**) shows forward shift in global sagittal balance and marked thoracolumbar kyphosis. H: Postoperative lateral photograph (**H**) shows restoration of a normal spine sagittal alignment. Preoperative posterior photograph (**I**) shows a left thoracolumbar prominence and asymmetric abdominal creases. Postoperative posterior photograph (**J**) shows significant improvement in the chest wall and abdominal crease symmetry. Global coronal balance is maintained. The patient's preoperative back and radicular complaints have resolved, and her function has improved greatly.

should be used, however. Constructs using pedicle screws in the lumbar spine and either pedicle screws or hooks in the thoracic spine with cross-link placement is the current state-of-the-art. With long fusions to the sacrum, it is mandatory to have four points of fixation in the sacrum. Alternatives include bilateral S1 and S2 screws, sacral screws with supplemental iliac screws, sacral screws with two intrasacral rods, or bilateral S1 screws with a Galveston-type technique in the ilium.

With long fusions to the sacrum, the likelihood of obtaining a successful fusion is greater if the sagittal C7 plumb line falls through or behind the sacrum. Many patients with progressive degenerative scoliosis have had previous decompressions and have decreased posterior bone stock. This situation often is a relative indication for a circumferential fusion procedure. Anterior structural grafting at L4-5 and L5-S1 also improves maintenance of alignment and successful fusion by reducing the mechanical stress on the bone-implant interface.

# FIXED SAGITTAL IMBALANCE

Sagittal deformity in adults results from a loss of normal lumbar lordosis, an increase in thoracic kyphosis, or both. Mild changes in regional sagittal alignment typically are well compensated for by an alteration in the alignment of another region of the spine and with mild hip flexion. To maintain a relatively erect posture (head over sacrum), these

patients usually have to hyperextend their necks and stand with knees and hips slightly flexed. When these compensatory mechanisms are exceeded, patients become symptomatic, and a change in global alignment (forward shift in the sagittal C7 plumb) ensues. The combination of clinical and radiographic findings associated with a forward shift in global balance that exceeds the body's compensatory mechanisms is termed *fixed sagittal imbalance.*

Fixed sagittal imbalance can be severely disabling. Efforts to maintain an erect posture result in early fatigue, pain, poor cosmesis, and functional limitations. In cases of previous spine fusion, accelerated degeneration of adjacent motion segments also can result in the development of mechanical back pain and neurologic compression. Adjacent segment degeneration is especially prevalent when a fusion ends at an area of focal hypolordosis or hyperkyphosis.

## Etiology

Multiple causes of sagittal imbalance exist. With normal aging, the intervertebral disc gradually loses hydration and decreases in height. Because 80% of lumbar lordosis is derived from the discs, loss of disc height at multiple levels results in shortening of the anterior column and diminished lordosis. In cases of trauma, fusion of the thoracolumbar or lumbar spine in kyphosis often leads to regional and global imbalance. Deformity correction procedures that involve shortening of the anterior column or, alternatively, procedures that lengthen the posterior column (Harrington scoliosis correction) also often result in loss of normal lordosis. The loss of lordosis associated with the treatment of idiopathic scoliosis with posterior distraction instrumentation may result in a subset of fixed sagittal imbalance termed *flat back syndrome.*

Fusion for degenerative conditions also may lead to sagittal imbalance when lumbar segments are fused in kyphosis. Great care should be taken when performing lumbar arthrodesis procedures to maintain a lordotic sagittal alignment over the fused segments. This alignment is achieved best by positioning the patient on the operating table with the hips fully extended. Additional lordosis may be added by administering compression across the posterior implants or by performing an osteotomy if necessary.

With long adult fusions, global sagittal balance may deteriorate over time for a few reasons, including nonunion, loss of distal fixation at L5 or the sacrum, or accelerated degeneration at a motion segment above or below the existing fusion. Vertebral fracture at the level above a long adult fusion also can lead to increased thoracic kyphosis and the development of positive sagittal imbalance.

## Patient Assessment

A careful history and physical examination is essential to identify the specific factors resulting in symptoms. An assessment of global balance is made by having the patient stand erect with the hips and knees fully extended. Flexibility at different regions of the spine is assessed with either active or passive bending maneuvers and radiographs. Sagittal deformities that seem stiff on initial evaluation may show remarkable flexibility if subjected to gentle supine bending over a bolster over 5 to 10 minutes. Physical examination should include an assessment of hip range of motion because a hip flexion contracture may occur in patients with fixed sagittal imbalance.

Long cassette (36-inch) radiographs of the patient standing erect with hips and knees extended provide for quantitative assessment of global sagittal balance (C7 plumb relative to the posterior cortex of the body of S1). Short cassette radiographs and "cone-down" views of an area of particular interest provide additional information regarding local anatomy and the extent of disc and facet degeneration. Radiographs in standing, flexion/extension, and passive extension over a bolster show the amount of motion present at the kyphotic or previously fused levels and the amount of compensatory motion available at adjacent levels. These "dynamic" views also may show the presence of any pathologic motion, such as listhesis, hypermobility, or motion within a previously fused segment.

MRI provides additional information regarding the degree of disc degeneration that may be important in determining the distal extent of the fusion. Myelography followed by CT with thin (approximately 1 mm) axial slice images is a superior means of characterizing the location and magnitude of cauda equina and nerve root compression. Standing myelograms, in particular, are helpful in defining the extent to which dynamic stenosis is present.

The patient's age, state of health, nutritional status, respiratory function, and expectations need to be assessed carefully for each patient in whom surgical intervention is being considered. The surgeon has the responsibility to weigh honestly the likelihood for significant improvement against the potential for perioperative complications and late morbidity. In some patients with fixed sagittal imbalance, the risks of surgery and the modest likelihood of significant functional improvement make surgical intervention ill advised.

## Surgical Planning

Surgical goals in the management of adult kyphotic deformities are as follows:

- Restoring normal regional sagittal alignment
- Establishing global sagittal balance
- Minimizing the potential for complications and late failure

After corrective surgery, a plumb line dropped from C7 on a sagittal standing radiograph should fall through or behind the lumbosacral disc (Fig. 21-4).

For flexible sagittal deformities that completely reduce on bending radiographs, a posterior instrumented fusion without osteotomies may be sufficient. The most effective means of achieving significant sagittal deformity correction is through the performance of spinal osteotomies, however, at one or more levels. Three classes of osteotomies commonly are employed:

- Posterior column wedge resection (Smith-Peterson)
- Combination of posterior column wedge resection osteotomy with anterior discectomy and structural grafting
- Three-column wedge resection procedure (pedicle subtraction, eggshell)

The osteotomy always should shorten the posterior column and ideally is performed at the apex of the deformity.

Smith-Peterson osteotomies are performed by resecting a chevron V portion of the posterior elements at the level of the facet joint (Fig. 21-5). The ligamentum flavum and a portion of the lamina and spinous processes also are removed to provide for a complete posterior column defect. The amount of facet and lamina removed depends on the amount of angular correction desired. A good rule of thumb is that for every 1 mm of posterior element removed, 1 degree of sagittal correction is achieved. Undercutting the ventral surface of the lamina and facets is advised to minimize the potential for the development of iatrogenic central, lateral recess, or foraminal stenosis after osteotomy closure. The osteotomy is closed by compressing the posterior elements proximal and distal to the osteotomy and maintaining the reduction with spinal implants. With the middle column as its fulcrum, the disc space hinges open with widening of the anterior disc space. Smith-Peterson osteotomies may be performed at multiple adjacent levels. Advantages of this type of osteotomy are that it may be performed rapidly; it involves minimal blood loss; it does not necessitate neural element manipulation; it is performed safely at cord, conus, or cauda levels; and it provides for a harmonic lordotic correction. Smith-Peterson osteotomies are limited, however, by the following:

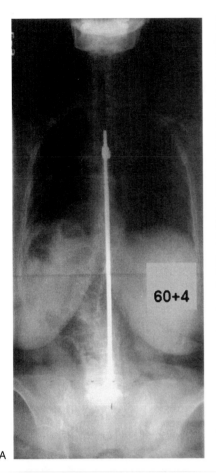

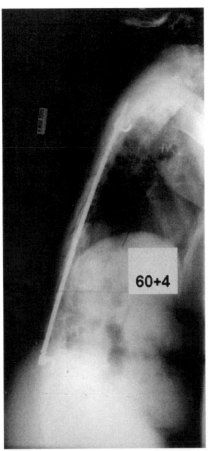

A

B

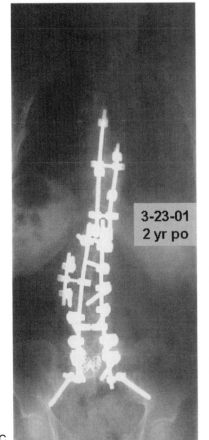

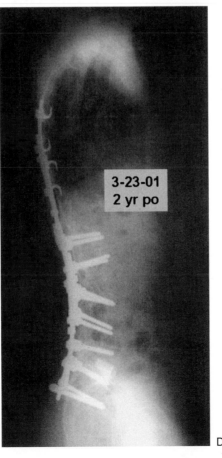

C

D

**Figure 21-4** Anteroposterior (**A**) and lateral standing (**B**) radiographs of a 60-year-old woman who was treated for idiopathic scoliosis as a teenager with a posterior Harrington instrumented fusion from T4-L5. Her chief complaints on presentation were back discomfort and loss of ambulatory endurance. She experienced regular back fatigue, radicular leg pain, and an increasingly forward-pitched posture. Anteroposterior and lateral preoperative standing radiographs show a Harrington distraction rod from T4-L5, loss of lumbar lordosis, and a significant forward shift in the global sagittal balance. Anteroposterior (**C**) and lateral (**D**) radiographs show status post spinal reconstruction. Arthrodesis was extended to the sacrum with an anterior L5-S1 discectomy and fusion using a structural mesh cage and cancellous iliac crest autograft followed by posterior instrumented fusion using sacral and iliac screws. Additional sagittal correction was achieved with a pedicle subtraction osteotomy at L2. *Figure continues.*

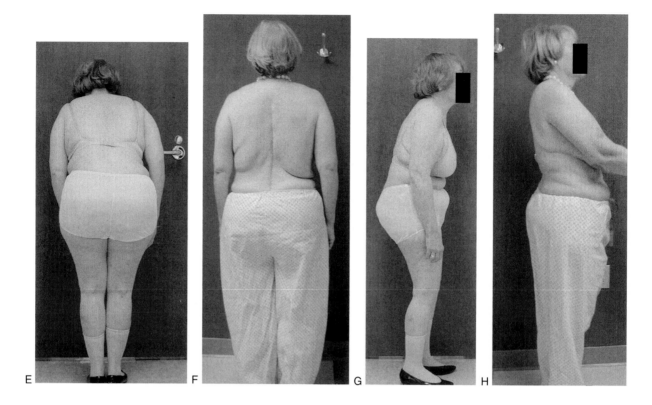

E  F  G  H

**Figure 21-4** *(Continued)* (**E-H**) Clinical photographs show preoperative (**E** and **G**) sagittal imbalance, decreased lumbosacral lordosis, and a tendency to stand with hips slightly flexed. At 3 years postoperatively (**F** and **H**), the patient stands with hips extended, head centered over the pelvis, and has normal lumbosacral lordosis.

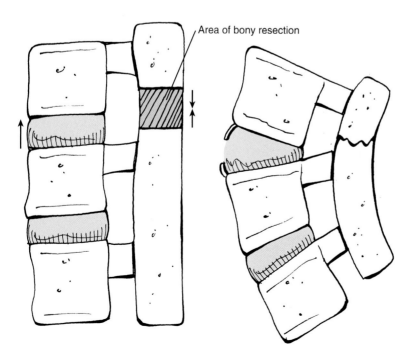

Area of bony resection

**Figure 21-5** Schematic depicting a Smith-Peterson spinal osteotomy. The hatched portion of the posterior elements is resected, and the posterior elements are compressed, increasing the amount of lordosis.

- The modest amount of correction that can be achieved at each level (10 degrees to 15 degrees)
- A single (posterior) column is relied on for fusion
- Lengthening of the anterior spinal column and adjacent vascular structures

In general, Smith-Peterson osteotomies without anterior surgery are best suited for younger patients with modest deformities in whom sagittal correction at several levels is desirable. The presence of a mobile disc also is beneficial because it accommodates anterior column distraction and posterior column shortening.

Smith-Peterson osteotomies combined with anterior releases and grafting offer certain advantages. When the discs are relatively immobile, anterior releases and morcellized grafting can increase the amount of correction subsequently achieved at a given level. Anterior morcellized grafting also is beneficial for fusion, especially in cases of previous nonunion, or for poor fusion candidates.

Anterior structural grafting after Smith-Peterson osteotomies is beneficial if one of three situations arises:

- Broad anterior disc space gapping is present after closure of the osteotomy.
- Sagittal restoration is incomplete after completion of the osteotomies.
- In the presence of a long fusion to the sacrum, anterior structural grafting at L4-5 and L5-S1 helps to maintain the correction and protect the posterior fixation.

If a patient with fixed sagittal imbalance has undergone previous anterior and posterior spinal fusion, circumferential osteotomies or a transpedicular osteotomy is needed.

Transpedicular three-column (pedicle subtraction) osteotomies involve the resection of a bone wedge extending from the posterior elements through the pedicles and into the anterior cortex of the vertebral body (Fig. 21-6). As the posterior and middle column bone defects are closed, the anterior vertebral cortex length remains unchanged, and the disc shape remains unchanged. With closure of the osteotomy, anterior, middle, and posterior bone surfaces are in contact, providing a significant surface area for fusion. The level of the osteotomy generally should be at the area of greatest focal kyphosis. Although pedicle subtraction osteotomy may be performed at thoracic levels, selection of a level below L1 limits the potential for spinal cord or conus compression. Either L2 or L3 is usually the best level for a pedicle subtraction osteotomy for three reasons:

- L2 and L3 are the normal apex of lumbar lordosis.
- The levels are typically distal to the cord and conus.
- Remaining vertebrae caudal to the osteotomy provide sufficient distal fixation sites without mandating arthrodesis extension to the sacrum.

A distal osteotomy level also has the benefit of producing a greater correction global balance than a more proximal osteotomy for the same amount of sagittal angular correction. In general, 30 degrees to 35 degrees of correction may be generated from a single pedicle subtraction osteotomy. With a 30-degree to 35-degree correction, the sagittal C7 plumb usually shifts posteriorly 12 to 15 cm (see Fig. 21-4).

Advantages of the pedicle subtraction osteotomy include the following:

- Ability to produce significant correction at a single level
- High likelihood of maintenance of reduction and successful osteotomy fusion due to three columns of bone contact
- Avoidance of the need for a supplemental anterior approach

Pedicle subtraction osteotomies are technically demanding. Significant mobilization of the dura is required, with the potential for dural tears and spinal fluid leaks. Bleeding from epidural veins and osteotomy surfaces can be brisk. The surgeon may have to go back and forth between multiple osteotomy sites using thrombin packing and bone wax where necessary to control bleeding.

Correction of sagittal deformities requires involved surgical procedures, which carry an attendant increased risk for complications. Although nonunion at the level of the osteotomy is uncommon for pedicle subtraction osteotomy if done through a previous fusion mass, nonunion may occur at any level after Smith-Peterson procedures. Degenerated levels above and below a pedicle subtraction osteotomy are at risk for nonunion and should be addressed with circumferential fusion. Procedures that require more than 10 to 12 hours of operating time should be staged. Administration of total parenteral nutrition between stages has been shown to reduce morbidity associated with infectious complications of the wound, urinary system, and respiratory system. Medical complications, including pneumonia, venous thrombosis, and postoperative ileus, are common and are managed best with an aggressive preventive strategy and postoperative team approach.

## RESULTS AND COMPLICATIONS

Reconstructive surgery for adult spinal deformity should not be regarded as a "cure." Although a high degree of satisfaction is reported after these procedures, patients often continue to experience some degree of discomfort, although markedly less than preoperatively. When solid arthrodesis is achieved, the patient's function may return to near-normal levels, with restrictions only on heavy lifting, repetitive activities, and contact sports. Correction of adult spinal deformity has been shown to have positive effects on self-image, pain, and function as measured by the Scoliosis Research Society outcomes instrument.

The physiologic age of the patient and the distal extent of the fusion have significant bearing on the scope of surgery required and how well it is tolerated by the patient. Elderly patients tend to have more preoperative medical comorbidities and less physiologic reserve than younger adults. As a result, older patients are at greater risk for medical complications, such as pneumonia, postoperative ileus, deep venous thrombosis, and infection. Osteoporotic bone, common in older adult deformity patients, makes obtaining and maintaining secure implant fixation more challenging. Multiple points of fixation, anterior interbody structural grafting, and use of a postoperative brace help "protect" the corrected position of the spine while fusion takes place.

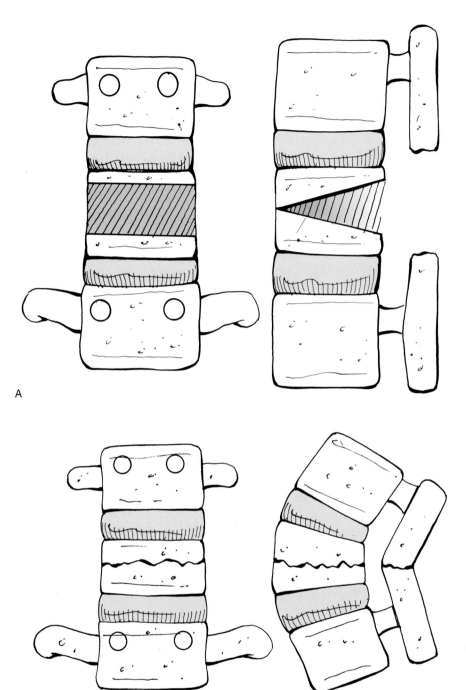

**Figure 21-6** (**A**) Schematic depicting a pedicle subtraction osteotomy. After the posterior element resection has been performed, the pedicles are cannulated, and a wedge of the vertebral body is decancellated. When the vertebral body is decancellated sufficiently, the triangular portion of cortical bone is resected from the lateral aspect of the vertebral body bilaterally. Finally, a rectangular portion of the posterior cortex of the vertebral body is resected. Closure of the osteotomy may occur spontaneously with gravity or may require lordotic force application through patient repositioning or posterior instrumented compression. (**B**) Schematic depiction of pedicle subtraction osteotomy closure with restoration of regional lordosis. Ideally, bone-to-bone posterior element contact is achieved after closure of the osteotomy. The central canal, lateral recess, and foramen should be evaluated during and after osteotomy closure to confirm that stenosis has not occurred inadvertently.

## Nonunion

Pseudarthrosis occurring after long adult deformity fusions (5% to 30%) often is recognized by a shift in spinal alignment, new onset of pain, or radiographically by loosening at the bone-implant interface or implant failure. Pseudarthrosis may present early or late depending on the rigidity of the implant construct used, the level involved, and the demands of the patient. With the use of segmental fixation points and more rigid implant systems, it is becoming increasingly common for a pseudarthrosis to go unrecognized for 5 years or more after surgery. Multiple risk factors for pseudarthrosis have been identified (Table 21-4). Areas particularly prone to the development of pseudarthrosis are the lumbosacral junction, the thoracolumbar junction, and segments that have undergone decompression. For long fusions to the sacrum, four points of fixation in the sacrum and ilium provide the greatest resistance to implant loss of fixation. Anterior discectomies and interbody fusion with either structural cages or femoral ring allografts provide additional biomechanical stability and surface area for fusion. Consideration should be made for performing anterior discectomies and structural grafting at levels that are at increased risk.

## Neurologic Complications

Neurologic deficits after reconstruction for adult spinal deformity are uncommon, occurring in less than 5% to 15% of cases. Risks are greater for cases with severe rigid curves that are managed through anterior and posterior approaches and with correction of a severe kyphotic deformity. Direct injury to neural elements can result from instrumentation (hooks, wires, and screws) or from indirect injury caused by ischemic insult or neurapraxia due to distractive forces. In these cases, consideration should be given to a staged correction to provide for stress relaxation of the tensioned structures and accommodation of neural elements to any borderline ischemia. In the case of osteotomies, nerve root or dural constriction may result if the edges of the osteotomy site are not undercut carefully to allow for adequate space for the neural elements after correction of the deformity. Neurologic sequelae may be detected intraoperatively with the use of neurophysiologic monitoring, including somatosensory evoked potentials, motor evoked potentials, and selective nerve electromyography. Although these modalities are relatively efficacious for detecting spinal cord and conus dysfunction, select cauda equina nerve root compression (especially unilateral) may go unnoticed. Early detection provides the opportunity to intervene and possibly to reverse the offending process. Despite many monitoring advances, a wake-up test remains the gold standard.

## Infection

Postoperative wound infection is reported to occur in 2% to 6% of patients undergoing posterior spinal fusion. Infection after anterior spinal fusion is far less common. Nutritional depletion has been shown to predispose to the development of infection. Total parenteral nutrition is recommended in patients who are malnourished (decreased albumin, prealbumin, and transferrin) preoperatively. In addition, elderly patients and patients at risk for nutritional depletion who are undergoing staged procedures should be administered parenteral nutrition between stages.

## CONCLUSIONS

Surgical reconstruction and recovery for adult scoliosis is more challenging than what is observed with pediatric patients. Most adults with flexible thoracic and thoracolumbar deformities fare well with posterior surgery alone. Adults with decompensated deformities, rigid curves, and involvement of the lumbosacral junction often benefit from combined anterior discectomies and fusion and posterior segmental instrumented fusion. Sagittal malalignments are corrected reliably using a combination of spinal osteotomies and segmental fixation. Although complications commonly occur, studies show a significant improvement in patient-reported pain and function and a high degree of satisfaction in most adult deformity patients after spinal reconstruction.

## SUGGESTED READING

Bernhardt M, Bridwell KH. Segmental analysis of the sagittal plane alignment of the normal thoracic and lumbar spines and thoracolumbar junction. Spine 1989;14:717.

Dickson JH, Mirkovic S, Noble PC, et al. Results of operative treatment of idiopathic scoliosis in adults. J Bone Joint Surg 1995;77A: 513–523.

Edwards CC, Bridwell KH, Patel A, et al. Thoracolumbar deformity arthrodesis to L5 in adults: the fate of the L5-S1 disk. Spine 2003; 28:2122–2131.

Farcy JPC, Schwab FJ. Management of flatback and related kyphotic decompensation syndromes. Spine 1997;22:2452–2457.

Gelb DE, Lenke LG, Bridwell KH, et al. An analysis of sagittal plane alignment in 100 asymptomatic middle and older aged volunteers. Spine 1995;12:1351–1358.

Jackson RP, McManus AC. Radiographic analysis of sagittal plane alignments and balance in standing volunteers and patients with low back pain matched for age sex and size: a prospective controlled clinical study. Spine 1994;9:1611.

Kuklo TR, Bridwell HH, Lewis SJ, et al. Minimum two-year analysis of sacropelvic fixation and L5/S1 fusion utilizing S1 and iliac screws. Spine 2001;26:1976–1983.

LaGrone MO, Bradford DS, Moe JH, et al. Treatment of symptomatic flatback after spinal fusion. J Bone Joint Surg 1988;70A:569–580.

Weinstein SL, Ponseti IV. Curve progression in idiopathic scoliosis. J Bone Joint Surg 1983;65A:447–455.

## TABLE 21-4  RISK FACTORS FOR PSEUDARTHROSIS AFTER LONG FUSIONS FOR ADULT SPINAL DEFORMITY

| Factor | Effect on Pseudarthrosis Potential |
|---|---|
| Age | ↑ |
| Comorbidities | ↑ |
| Smoking | ↑ |
| Revision surgery | ↑ |
| Fusion to the sacrum | ↑ |
| Posterior bone defect from decompression | ↑ |
| Number of levels fused | ↑ |
| Posterior-only surgery | ↑ |
| Nonsegmental fixation | ↑ |

# INFLAMMATORY SPONDYLO-ARTHROPATHY

## ANDREW V. SLUCKY

## RHEUMATOID ARTHRITIS

### Pathogenesis

According to the *immune-complex theory,* expression of a new synovial antigen triggers the body to produce rheumatoid factor (RF), an IgM molecule directed against the autologous IgG antibody of the expressed aberrant synovial antigen. Approximately 80% of patients with active rheumatoid disease are positive for IgM anti-IgG; however, the presence of RF alone in the synovial fluid does not produce rheumatoid arthritis. Several other autoantibodies have been identified in rheumatoid arthritis with specificity greater than 90%, including antikeratin, anticitrullinated peptides, anti-RA33, anti-Sa, and anti-p68. T cell-mediated mechanisms also have been implicated. Granulation tissue formed within the reactive synovium by proliferating fibroblasts and inflammatory cells is called the *pannus,* which invades and destroys local articular structures.

### Epidemiology

Rheumatoid spondylitis primarily affects the cervical spine, but uncommonly may involve the thoracic, lumbar, and sacroiliac regions. Depending on the applied diagnostic criteria, cervical involvement in rheumatoid arthritis ranges from 25% to 95%. Approximately 10% of rheumatoid patients present with spondylitis as the initial disease manifestation. Cervical spine subluxations are observed in 43% to 86% of patients, more commonly in men despite greater general disease incidence in women.

Cervical involvement occurs early in the disease process, and the subsequent severity is correlated closely with the extent and severity of the peripheral disease activity. Neurologic impairment caused by cervical instability reportedly ranges from 11% to 58%. A postmortem study of rheumatoid patients identified unrecognized medullary compression as the cause of death in 10% of patients.

### Pathophysiology

The destructive process of rheumatoid arthritis is characterized by a proliferative synovial inflammation, the *pannus,* and progressive erosion of adjacent cartilage and bone. Erosion of bone results in cyst formation and osteoporosis. Extension of the pannus into the adjacent disc space results in spondylodiscitis.

The synovial cell populations that contribute most to the articular destruction are the fibroblast-like *synoviocytes* and *synovial tissue macrophages.* Considerable evidence has accumulated suggesting that rheumatoid synovial fibroblasts are transformed cells that have acquired proliferative and invasive properties and are susceptible to significant up-regulation by interleukin-1 or tumor necrosis factor-α. These synoviocytes have been identified as producing the important degradative enzymes collagenase, stromelysin, and cathepsins involved in articular destruction.

Macrophages in rheumatoid synovial tissue are characterized by significant increased expression of the proinflammatory cytokines interleukin-1 and tumor necrosis factor-α. Although they may participate directly in articular matrix degradation, their suggested predominant role may be in amplifying the pathogenic cascade via cytokine-mediated up-regulation of synoviocyte proteolytic enzyme production and resultant articular destruction.

Destruction of the spinal motion segment and adjacent disc and ligament structures by the rheumatoid inflammatory process may result in segmental instability and neurologic compromise. Additionally, proliferation of the pannus into the epidural space may result in direct neural element compression compounded by the presence of proinflammatory factors.

### Classification

The upper cervical spine (occiput through C2) is most affected in rheumatoid arthritis, owing to the predominance of synovial articulations. The axial plane orientation of the C1-2 facets, without bone interlocking, further predisposes the rheumatoid-compromised motion segment to instability.

Three deformity patterns commonly have been identified in the rheumatoid-affected cervical spine:

- Atlantoaxial subluxation (AAS)
- Vertical subluxation of the odontoid (VS)
- Subaxial subluxation (SAS)

AAS is most common and has been reported to occur in

49% of patients. The subluxation is usually anterior, although lateral subluxation (>2 mm) occurs in 20% of patients, and posterior subluxation occurs in 7%.

VS occurs in 38% of patients and is the result of destructive erosion of the occipitoatlantal and atlantoaxial joint complexes leading to vertical translation of the odontoid and settling of the occiput. Direct odontoid compression on the brainstem or excessive kyphosis (flexion) of the cervicomedullary junction can lead to significant neurologic compromise or death.

SAS is the least common, occurring in 10% to 20% of patients. SAS occurs at multiple levels, most commonly at C2-4, resulting in kyphosis and a "stepladder" appearance. Neurologic compromise occurs directly from facet pannus extension or indirectly from segmental subluxation. Progressive SAS after upper cervical fusion has been reported in 36% of rheumatoid patients undergoing occipitocervical fusion and 5.5% of patients undergoing atlantoaxial fusion.

## Diagnosis

### Clinical Features

Neck pain, classically at the occipitocervical junction, is reported in 40% to 88% of patients and frequently is associated with occipital headaches due to greater occipital nerve (C2) irritation or referred pain from the posterior ramus of C1 nerve root. Ear pain or facial pain may be present, owing to C2 sensory contributions to the greater auricular nerve or nucleus of the spinal trigeminal tract.

Myelopathic symptoms, such as hand paresthesias, weakness, loss of endurance, loss of dexterity, and gait imbalance, may be subtle and should be reviewed in context relative to historical patient function. Neck motion may result in electric shock-like sensations of the torso or extremities (Lhermitte's sign). Urinary retention or incontinence may be the first indication of myelopathy in the advanced rheumatoid patient. Vertebrobasilar insufficiency or cervicomedullary compression may present with visual disturbances, vertigo, tinnitus, or dysphagia.

As previously mentioned, physical exam findings of myelopathy may be difficult to assess secondary to rheumatoid peripheral extremity involvement. Hyperreflexia, Hoffmann's sign, Babinski's sign, and clonus sign may be difficult to elicit secondary to peripheral joint mutilation. Presence of a scapulohumeral reflex (Shimuzu's sign) may indicate compression proximal to C4.

History and physical exam findings can be categorized according to the Ranawat classification of rheumatoid myelopathy, which has proved useful in planning treatment and prognosticating outcome:

- *Grade I*—no neural deficit
- *Grade II*—subjective weakness, hyperreflexia
- *Grade IIIA*—objective weakness, long-tract signs, ambulatory
- *Grade IIIB*—objective weakness, long-tract signs, non-ambulatory

Alternatively the degree of cervical myelopathy can be classified according to the Japanese Orthopaedic Association scale with modification to Western parameters.

Laboratory tests include complete blood count, erythrocyte sedimentation rate (ESR), RF, and antinuclear antibody. RF is positive in 80% of patients with active disease; antinuclear antibody is positive in 20% to 60% of patients. ESR typically is greater than 30 mm, depending on disease activity and degree of anemia.

### Radiographic Features

Anteroposterior, open-mouth (odontoid), lateral, and flexion/extension lateral radiographs must be obtained at some point in the historical evaluation of the rheumatoid patient. Radiographs are required on any patient requiring endotracheal intubation or cervical manipulation. Fifty percent of patients with radiographic abnormalities are asymptomatic at initial presentation. Of patients undergoing peripheral extremity procedures (arthroplasty), 61% show radiographic abnormalities on preoperative cervical screening radiographs.

Radiographic determinants of instability include the following (Fig. 22-1):

- Anterior atlantodental interval (AADI) and posterior atlantodental interval (PADI) for AAS
- McGregor's line, Ranawat index, and Redlund-Johnell measurement for VS
- Subaxial canal diameter for SAS

The AADI is measured on a lateral view from the anterior odontoid to the posterior surface of the anterior C1 ring; the PADI is measured from the posterior odontoid to the anterior surface of the posterior C1 ring. Normal AADI in adults is less than 3 mm; greater than 10 mm indicates instability and risk of neurologic compromise. Normal PADI is greater than 14 mm; less than 14 mm is associated with increased risk of neurologic deficit. The PADI seems to be a better predictor of paralysis than the AADI (Fig. 22-2).

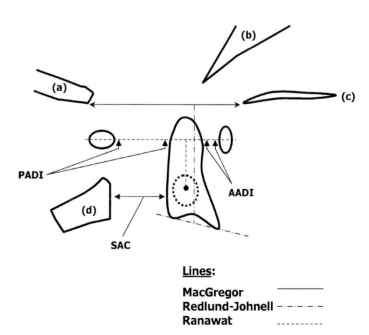

**Lines:**

MacGregor ——————
Redlund-Johnell –·–·–·–
Ranawat ----------

**Figure 22-1** Radiographic parameters of cervical rheumatoid arthritis: (a) occiput, (b) clivus, (c) hard palate, (d) C2 arch.

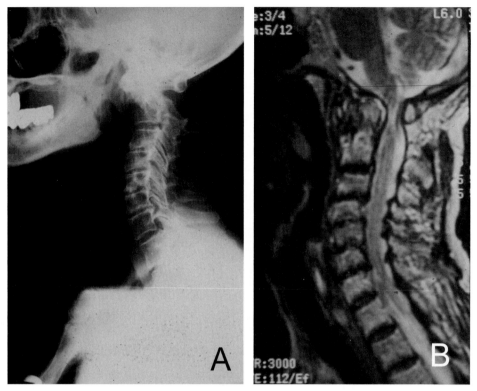

**Figure 22-2** Rheumatoid arthritis of the cervical spine. (**A**) Lateral radiograph demonstrating atlantoaxial subluxation (AAS) instability pattern. (**B**) Sagittal MRI, T2-weighted image. Note C1-C2 leval canal compromise and pannus formation.

VS can be difficult to assess, owing to the altered vertebral morphology in rheumatoid patients. MacGregor's line is a line drawn on lateral view from the hard palate to the base of the occiput. VS is defined as migration of the superior odontoid greater than 4.5 mm above MacGregor's line. The Redlund-Johnell measurement is useful in cases of odontoid mutilation and is determined by measuring the distance between the midpoint of the inferior margin of the body of the axis (C2) to MacGregor's line. A value of less than 34 mm in men and 29 mm in women is considered abnormal. The Ranawat index is derived on the lateral view as the distance between the center of the C2 pedicle and a line intersecting the anterior and posterior arches of C1. A distance of less than 15 mm for men and 13 mm for women is regarded as significant for VS.

SAS can be accessed on lateral and dynamic lateral views. Subluxation of greater than 20% of the lateral vertebral width or 4 mm of listhesis is considered significant. Additionally, patients with subaxial canal diameters, as measured from the posterior vertebral cortex to ventral laminar surface, of less than 13 mm are at increased risk for neurologic deficit.

Computed tomography, combined with thin-section sagittal reconstruction, is useful in delineating rheumatoid-altered bone anatomy and in assessing rotatory or lateral subluxation. Additionally, clear visualization of the vertebral artery foramen assists in preoperative planning about the C1-2 complex.

Magnetic resonance imaging (MRI) allows for excellent visualization of soft tissue and neurologic structures, including spinal cord parenchyma, rheumatoid pannus, and epidural space compromise (space available for the cord [SAC]). Minimal SAC is 13 mm at C1-2 and 12 mm at the subaxial regions. Upper cervical pannus thickness greater than 3 mm has been correlated with neural compression. MRI, particularly a supervised flexion view, is useful in assessing VS and the spinal cord configuration. Patients with a cervicomedullary angle of less than 135 degrees, as measured by intersecting lines of the anterior cervical spinal cord and medulla surfaces, show significant VS and probable neurologic compromise.

A diagnostic algorithm is provided to help guide workup and treatment (Algorithm 22-1).

## Treatment

A diagnostic algorithm can be helpful to guide treatment. The goals of treatment in rheumatoid involvement of the cervical spine are:

- To avoid development of irreversible neurologic deficit
- To prevent sudden death caused by unrecognized neural compression
- To avoid unnecessary surgery, given that 50% of patients with radiographic evidence of instability remain asymptomatic

### Nonoperative Treatment

Aggressive medical management of the systemic disease presentation is the cornerstone of rheumatoid arthritis

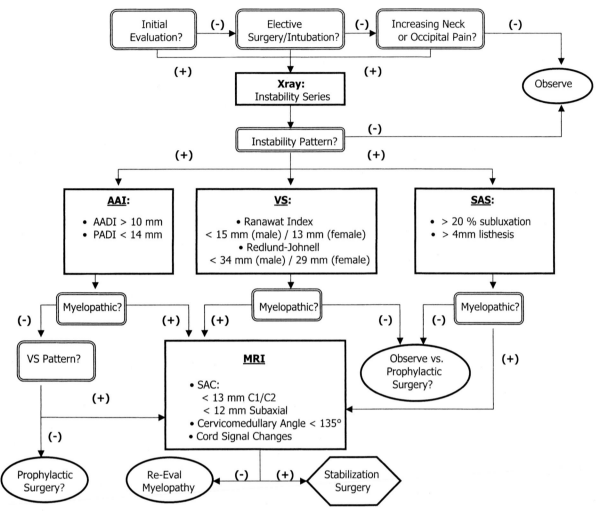

**Algorithm 22-1**  Ranawat classification of rheumatoid myelopathy. AADI, anterior atlantodental interval; AAS, atlantoaxial subluxation; PADI, posterior atlantodental interval; SAC, space available for the cord; SAS, subaxial subluxation; VS, vertical subluxation of the odontoid.

treatment. The clinical course of spinal involvement is correlated directly to the severity of the systemic disease presentation. Nonoperative treatment is supportive with use of soft collars, physical therapies, patient education, and close monitoring of neurologic status.

## Operative Treatment

Operative indications for surgery are based on the presenting neurologic condition, with a poorer prognosis associated with more significant neurologic deficits. Ambulation seems to be an important prognostic hallmark, with some studies reporting at least one grade of improvement in 58% of surgically treated Ranawat grade IIIA patients versus 20% in Ranawat grade IIIB patients. Operative goals include the following:

- Stabilization of the C1-2 complex
- Prevention of further deformity
- Reduction of pain
- Stabilization or reversal of myelopathy

Absolute indications for surgery include development of neurologic deficit (Ranawat grade II) and radiographic evidence of spinal instability (PADI <14 mm, AADI >10 mm, SAC <13 mm, evidence of VS, or spinal cord diameter in flexion <6 mm). Relative indications include intractable neck pain (typically cervicooccipital) and radiographic instability.

Prophylactic surgical treatment of the asymptomatic patient (Ranawat grade I) with radiographic instability is controversial. The natural history of radiographic instability is that progression occurs in a predictable pattern of reducible AAS to reducible combined AAS and VS to irreducible VS. Numerous authors advocate early stabilization of AAS to prevent progression to irreducible VS and the increased morbidity associated with such advanced disease. The prognostic value of radiographic studies for myelopathy development is variable. Several studies report no conclusive correlation between AADI and neurologic status. PADI seems more useful with a reported sensitivity of 97% for paralysis with PADI less than 14 mm and a negative predictive value for paralysis of 94% with PADI greater than 14 mm. MRI findings of subarachnoid encroachment are sensitive in that affected patients with neurologic findings show a 12 times risk of progressive neurologic deterioration.

Surgical treatment of AAS includes attempted subluxation reduction and posterior fusion using either Gallie or Brooks wiring techniques, transarticular screw fixation, or a combination of screws and wiring. Posterior wiring techniques require an intact posterior C1 and C2 lamina. Safe sublaminar wire passage may be compromised by inadequate subluxation reduction. Typically, supplemental postoperative halo fixation is required. Reported fusion rates are 67% to 90% and are increased with halo fixation. Higher fusion rates are reported with the Brooks wiring technique. Several studies have shown spontaneous pannus resorption subsequent to solid posterior fusion. Anterior transoral decompression is reserved for patients with persistent neurologic deficit and no evidence of pannus resorption on postoperative MRI.

Surgical treatment of VS requires posterior occipitocervical fusion. As with AAS, improved reduction, neurologic recovery, and higher rates of fusion are reported with plate and screw techniques. Irreducible deformity may require C1 laminectomy or odontoid resection to achieve adequate decompression. Surgical treatment of SAS is achieved best with posterior lateral mass reduction and screw and plate fixation. If the subluxation is not reduced adequately, complementary anterior decompression and fusion is indicated.

## Results and Outcome

Reportedly 76% to 100% of rheumatoid patients with cervical involvement and myelopathy show progressive neurologic deficit and paralysis if left untreated. One third experience sudden death due to neurologic compromise, typically with VS.

Neurologic improvement with surgical treatment has been reported in 27% to 100% of patients. Variably, 95% of patients improved one Ranawat grade after treatment of AAS; 76%, after combined AAS and VS; and 94%, after isolated SAS. Universally, ultimate neurologic outcome is determined by the preoperative neurologic condition, with only 20% of Ranawat grade IIIB patients showing one grade of postoperative improvement versus 58% of Ranawat grade IIIA patients. Pain relief has been reported in 80% to 100% of patients with solid fusion.

Surgical complications include death, infection, nonunion, and adjacent segment subluxation. Morbidity and mortality are higher in more neurologically compromised patients. Postoperative mortality has been reported to be 13% in Ranawat grade IIIB patients. Improved perioperative techniques of fiberoptic intubation, meticulous soft tissue surgical technique, and biomechanically sound constructs have reduced postoperative morbidity significantly. Mean fusion rates of 83% have been reported, with the highest rates shown by plate and screw techniques. Nonunion rates are increased in patients with advanced mutilating disease and osteoporosis. Neurologic compromise resulting from cervical spine surgery is uncommon and associated with inadvertent subluxation during operative positioning or canal compromise during sublaminar wire passage.

# PSORIATIC ARTHRITIS

## Pathogenesis

The inflammatory nature of psoriatic arthritis, with deposition of cellular infiltrates and immunoglobulins in skin and joint lesions, supports an immunologic mechanism of disease origin. Autoantibodies, leukotrienes, increased levels of complement activation fragments, and T-cell activity imbalance all have been described as possible causative factors, although the exact mechanism is unknown.

## Epidemiology

Cutaneous psoriasis occurs in 1% to 3% of the population with typical presentation in the 20s or 30s. Variably, 6% to 40% of patients with cutaneous lesions develop psoriatic arthritis; 15% of patients develop arthritis manifestations before developing cutaneous lesions. The male-to-female ratio is approximately 1:1. Ten percent of patients with psoriatic arthritis show spinal involvement.

## Pathophysiology

Joint and spinal motion segment destruction occurs through a combination of proliferative synovial destruction and inflammatory ankylosis. In contradistinction to ankylosis spondylitis, discovertebral erosion and axial ankylosis occur in a patchy, asymmetric involvement with mixed marginal and nonmarginal syndesmophyte presentation. Proliferative synovial destruction of the diarthrodial joints of the upper cervical spine can result in instability patterns similar to rheumatoid arthritis. The major predictor of disease involvement is the duration of disease at presentation.

## Classification

Moll and Wright described five clinical patterns of psoriatic arthritis presentation, as follows:

- Asymmetric oligoarthritis
- Distal arthritis
- Arthritis mutilans
- Symmetric polyarthritis
- Spondyloarthropathy

Approximately 10% of patients with psoriatic arthritis show spondyloarthropathy. Variably, 35% to 75% of this subset show principally cervical spine involvement.

Blau and Kaufman described two types of spinal presentation:

- *Type I*—inflammatory response with diarthrodial erosion or joint subluxation, or both, without evidence of ankylosis
- *Type II*—vertebral ankylosis with apophyseal joint fusion and mixed marginal/nonmarginal syndesmophyte formation

As with rheumatoid arthritis, patients with type I presentation are at risk for segmental instability or neurologic deficit.

## Diagnosis

### Clinical Features

Clinical presentations of psoriatic spondyloarthropathy include presence of cutaneous lesions and axial spine symptoms. Typical age of onset is in the 20s or 30s. Physical manifestations of psoriatic spondyloarthropathy include axial pain, stiffness, and diminished range of motion. Laboratory findings include mildly elevated ESR and C-reactive protein, particularly in cases of erosive disease. RF is characteristically negative. Approximately 20% of patients with psoriasis are HLA-B27 positive, whereas 60% to 80% of patients with radiographic evidence of psoriatic spondyloarthropathy are HLA-B27 positive. Of patients, 10% to 20% have elevated serum uric acid levels.

### Radiographic Features

Radiographic presentation follows two forms:

- *Type I* presentation—erosive destruction of the spinal diarthrodial joints without overt segmental ankylosis (Fig. 22-3).
- *Type II* presentation—similar to ankylosing spondylitis with spontaneous apophyseal joint fusion and syndesmophyte formation

## Treatment

The initial management of psoriatic spondyloarthropathy is similar to that of rheumatoid arthritis. Refractory cases may require adjunct drug therapies, including gold, penicillamine, methotrexate, and cyclosporine. Steroids should be used judiciously, given reports of an erythrodermic picture and significant cutaneous lesion flares with dose reductions. Surgery is reserved for patients with segmental instability or neurologic deficit or both.

# REITER'S SYNDROME

## Pathogenesis

The prevailing view of Reiter's syndrome is that of a postinfective reactive arthritis in susceptible individuals. Commonly, Reiter's syndrome presents within 1 month of a defined infectious event, commonly a urethritis or enteritis.

## Epidemiology

Reiter's syndrome typically affects individuals in their 20s or 30s. Postvenereal disease seems to affect men more than women; enteric forms affect men and women equally. Approximately 1% to 2% of enteric-affected individuals develop Reiter's syndrome. Approximately 50% of Reiter's syndrome patients manifest symptom recurrence at intervals 3 weeks to 20 years after initial presentation. Twenty percent of patients exhibit progressive degenerative disease in the peripheral joints and axial spine. HLA-B27 histocompatibility antigen is present in 60% to 85% of patients and seems to correlate with the severity and chronicity of Reiter's syndrome.

## Pathophysiology

The pathogenesis of Reiter's syndrome is unclear but seems to involve an inflammatory initiation by an "infection trigger," gastrointestinal in nature, in susceptible individuals.

## Diagnosis

### Clinical Features

The classic clinical presentation of Reiter's syndrome is one of the following within 2 to 4 weeks of infectious exposure:

- Urethritis (80%)
- Conjunctivitis
- Unilateral polyarthritis
- Mucocutaneous lesions

Spinal involvement includes complaints of low back pain and stiffness in 50% of affected patients. The lumbar spine is involved in 29% of cases; the cervical spine rarely is involved. Spinal pain is characterized by morning stiffness, rest pain, and improvement with exercise. Variably, 30% to 80% of patients develop asymmetric sacroiliitis, especially early in the disease. HLA-B27-positive patients are more likely to show radiographic changes.

### Radiographic Findings

Spinal changes are characterized by nonmarginal syndesmophytes with asymmetric distribution. Spinal involvement

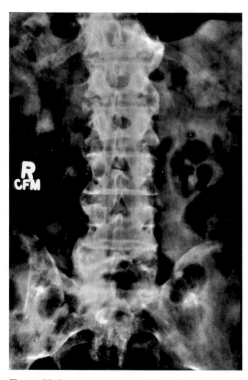

**Figure 22-3**  Psoriatic spondylitis of the lumbar spine. Note the patchy pattern of asymmetric non-marginal syndesmophytes. (Courtesy of B. Gehlman, MD)

is progressive in an ascending fashion with skip lesions. Sacroiliitis is asymmetric and less severe than with ankylosing spondylitis.

### Treatment

Reiter's syndrome is a systemic disease without cure. General treatments include antiinflammatory agents and physical therapies. Surgical treatment typically involves joint arthroplasty at end-stage disease presentation. Spinal surgery is uncommon.

# ENTEROPATHIC SPONDYLOARTHROPATHY

Enteropathic arthritis describes the occurrence of arthritis in patients with inflammatory bowel disease (i.e., ulcerative colitis or Crohn's disease). The reported incidence of HLA-B27 in patients with inflammatory bowel disease and spondyloarthropathy is 50% to 75%. The occurrence of ankylosing spondylitis is highest in patients with HLA-B27 phenotype and is more prone to develop with greater severity, at a younger age, in women with inflammatory bowel disease. Two forms of axial arthropathy present with inflammatory bowel disease:

- Ankylosing spondylitis indistinguishable from idiopathic variants
- Asymptomatic sacroiliitis

Inflammatory bowel disease patients with ankylosing spondylitis generally are HLA-B27 positive, and asymptom-

atic patients generally are HLA-B27 negative. In symptomatic patients, clinical and radiographic findings are identical to those of ankylosing spondylitis, including low back pain, stiffness, spondylitis, and marginal syndesmophyte formation. The peripheral arthritis is nondeforming radiographically.

Clinical treatment is contingent on disease manifestation. Peripheral arthritis responds to suppression of bowel disease, including sulfasalazine and colectomy. The axial condition is independent of the bowel disease course. Surgical treatment indications are the same as described for ankylosing spondylitis.

# DIFFUSE IDIOPATHIC SKELETAL HYPEROSTOSIS

Diffuse idiopathic skeletal hyperostosis (DISH) is a systemic arthropathy of unknown etiology first described by Forestier in 1950 as *senile ankylosing hyperostosis of the spine.*

### Pathogenesis

DISH is characterized by a spinal and peripheral enthesopathy affecting the insertion of soft tissue structures and ligaments into bone (the enthesis) with resultant osteophyte formation. The most commonly affected anatomic areas are the spine, shoulder, elbow, knee, and calcaneus. In contrast to ankylosing spondylitis, DISH affects middle-aged and older age groups, shows no HLA-B27 association, and has no findings of apophyseal or sacroiliac joint ankylosis. In

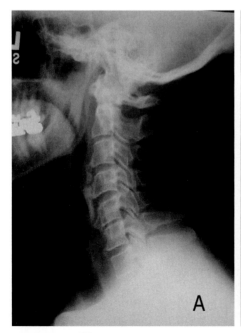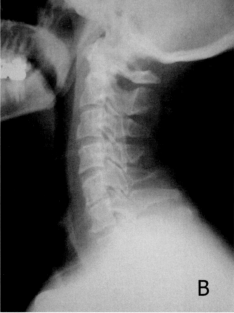

**Figure 22-4**   Diffuse idiopathic skeletal hyperostosis (DISH) of the cervical spine in a 55-year-old man with severe dysphagia. (a) Preoperative lateral radiograph. Note significant, non-contiguous osteophyte formation in the cervical region. (b) Postoperative lateral radiograph 6 months after osteophyte resection.

differentiating DISH from ankylosing spondylitis or degenerative disc disease, classification criteria include the following:

- Preservation of intervertebral disc space height
- Ossification of at least four consecutive vertebral bodies
- Absence of sacroiliac or apophyseal joint ankylosis
- Absence of vacuum phenomenon or vertebral body marginal sclerosis

## Diagnosis

Clinical features of DISH are relative to the anatomic localization. Thoracic and lumbar involvement is characterized by thoracolumbar stiffness or pain, although of no greater frequency than in age-matched spondylosis patients. Laboratory values are generally unremarkable. Prolific anterior osteophyte formation may evoke clinical symptoms of dysphagia, aspiration, stridor, Horner's syndrome, or thoracic outlet syndrome. Dysphagia is reported in 17% to 28% of cervical DISH patients. Symptoms do not always correlate with osteophyte mass. Endotracheal intubation or endoscopic procedures may be difficult. Concurrence with ossification of posterior longitudinal ligament may show significant myelopathy (Fig. 22-4).

## Treatment

Less than 10% of patients require surgical resection of the anterior cervical osteophyte for dysphagia. DISH concurrence with ossification of posterior longitudinal ligament and myelopathy may require canal decompression. Fusion stabilization with posterior approaches may be deferred secondary to anterior osteophyte stability. As with ankylosing spondylitis, DISH patients with extensive cervical involvement can incur catastrophic neurologic compromise from forceful trauma subsequent to fracture instability of the compromised motion segment. Surgical treatment requires fracture reduction and multisegmental stabilization as with ankylosing spondylitis.

## SUGGESTED READING

Amor B. Reiter's syndrome: diagnosis and clinical features. Rheum Dis Clin North Am 1998;24:677–688.

Blau RH, Kaufman RL. Erosive and subluxing cervical spine disease in patients with psoriatic arthritis. J Rheumatol 1987;14:111–117.

Boden SD, Dodge LD, Bohlmann HH, Rechtine GR. Rheumatoid arthritis of the cervical spine: A long-term analysis with predictors of paralysis and recovery. J Bone Joint Surg 1993A;75:1282–1297.

De Keyser F, Elewaut D, De Vos M, et al. Bowel inflammation and the spondyloarthropathies. Rheum Dis Clin North Am 1998;24:785–813.

Keat A. Reiter's syndrome and reactive arthritis in perspective. N Engl J Med 1983;309:1606–1615.

Mata S, Fortin PR, Fitzcharles MA, et al. A controlled study of diffuse idiopathic skeletal hyperostosis: clinical features and functional status. Medicine 1997;76:104–117.

Moll JM, Wright V. Psoriatic arthritis. Sem Arthrits Rheum 1973;3:45–78.

Oda T, Fujiwara K, Yonenobu K, et al. Natural course of cervical spine lesions in rheumatoid arthritis. Spine 1995;20:1128–1135.

Ranawat CS, O'Leary P, Pellicci P, et al. Cervical spine fusion in rheumatoid arthritis. J Bone Joint Surg 1979;61A:1003–1010.

# ANKYLOSING SPONDYLITIS

**EDWARD D. SIMMONS**
**YINGGANG ZHENG**

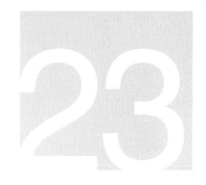

Ankylosing spondylitis is a seronegative inflammatory arthritis of the spine with an unknown etiology. It affects about 0.2% to 0.3% of the U.S. population and is more common in men than women. It presents in its early stages with inflammatory arthritic pain typically involving the sacroiliac joints that spreads to involve other portions of the spine. Early on, there is normal or mildly limited range of motion. As the disease progresses, however, with ossification of the spinal ligaments, the spine eventually may fuse in a kyphotic position. This can involve the lumbar, thoracic, and cervical areas of the spine. It also may affect the hip joints.

The inflammatory process also causes sacroiliitis, noted by erosion and sclerosis of the bone adjacent to the sacroiliac joints. Occasionally, this erosive sclerotic process extends into the intervertebral disc and adjacent bone, and is termed *spondylodiscitis*. It has a reported incidence of 5% to 6% and is most common in the lower thoracic spine. Spondylodiscitis frequently is asymptomatic, noted on routine radiographic studies, but it may become symptomatic with minor injury or stress.

Ankylosing spondylitis is a different disease than rheumatoid arthritis, with a different serology. Rheumatoid arthritis is more common in women and tends to affect the joints of the appendicular skeleton, whereas ankylosing spondylitis is more common in men and usually affects the spine and major joints. The following features commonly are used for the diagnosis of ankylosing spondylitis:

- Pain and stiffness begin in the sacroiliac joints and subsequently spread to the lumbar, thoracic, and cervical regions. The symptoms are of at least 3 months' duration and are improved by exercise but not relieved by rest.
- Spinal motion in the coronal and sagittal planes becomes limited.
- There is decreased chest expansion relative to normative values for age and sex.
- Radiographic evidence of arthritic changes in the sacroiliac joints is considered the hallmark of ankylosing spondylitis. In addition, there is ossification of the ligaments of the spine and squaring of the lumbar vertebrae.
- As the disease progresses, spinal deformity may result from loss of the normal cervical and lumbar lordosis and increasing thoracic kyphosis, resulting in flexion deformity of the spine. It also may affect the hip joints.
- The HLA-B27 antigen test is positive in 90% of patients.

## SPINAL OSTEOTOMY FOR CORRECTION OF FLEXION DEFORMITY

It is well recognized that severe flexion deformities of the spine may occur in patients with ankylosing spondylitis. Despite emphasis on early recognition and current advances in medical treatment, patients still are seen with advanced kyphotic deformities of the trunk, who are severely disabled and who present a major challenge for definitive surgical correction.

For lumbar flexion deformity, two types of osteotomies may be used:

- Smith-Peterson type (removal of a V-shaped wedge of bone from the posterior spinal column)
- Thomasen type (removal of bone from all three spinal columns through a posterior approach by a combination of laminectomy, pedicle resection, and posterior decancellation of the vertebral body, also called *pedicle subtraction osteotomy*)

We prefer the Smith-Peterson osteotomy for ankylosing spondylitis.

Smith-Peterson et al reported their experience of lumbar osteotomy for ankylosing spondylitis in 1945. This is the first description of surgical correction for kyphotic deformity in ankylosing spondylitis. The initial procedure as reported by Smith-Peterson et al was done under general anesthesia with the patient lying prone. This procedure was revised further by LaChappelle, Herbert, Nunziata, Wilson and Turkell, Law, and others. To avoid difficulties with the use of the prone position for a patient with kyphotic deformity, Adams recommended that surgery be done with patients on their sides, and he used a three-point rack to manipulate the spine for correction.

The initial recommendation of Smith-Peterson et al was to perform a single-stage posterior wedge resection of the midlumbar spine in a "V" fashion with controlled fracturing of the ossified anterior longitudinal ligament. A midline resection was carried upward and outward through the superior facet of the vertebrae above and the inferior facet of the vertebrae below in an oblique fashion. The obliquity of the osteotomy was to allow locking of the vertebrae after correction in an effort to prevent displacement. This technique is the basis for our current procedure.

In a few patients with ankylosing spondylitis, flexion deformity of the spine occurs primarily in the cervical region. This deformity can be severely disabling with restriction of the field of vision. Multiple, undiagnosed, healed fractures of the cervical spine are often the cause of flexion. Surgical correction is fraught with great potential hazards. It was reported that isolated attempts to correct this deformity under general anesthesia resulted in a high rate of disastrous neurologic complications. The current technique of correction under local anesthesia has allowed for satisfactory correction with relative safety.

The techniques described subsequently allow for the osteotomy to be done from a single-stage posterior approach in the lumbar or cervical spine and allow for a high degree of correction to be obtained in a safe manner with the least morbidity to the patient. The results can be gratifying in terms of overall improvement in functional status and quality of life.

## Relevant Surgical Anatomy

The preferred level for lumbar osteotomy is L3-4, which is the normal center of lumbar lordosis, below the termination of the conus medullaris. The spinal canal volume is relatively capacious at this level. These factors decrease the neurologic risk of an osteotomy at L3-4 compared with more proximal levels, where the presence of the distal spinal cord and conus within the spinal canal increases the risk of neurologic injury. A computed tomography (CT) scan should be obtained to evaluate the spinal canal preoperatively and to assess for spinal stenosis.

The reasons for greater vascular safety of osteotomies done at L3-4 or L4-5 are the increased mobility of the aortic bifurcation and iliac arteries related to lower limb motion. The reasons for greater vascular risk of osteotomies at higher levels are that the aorta becomes less mobile proximally; the renal arteries arise at L2-3, tethering the aorta; and the segmental vessels increase in size proximally.

There are seven vertebra and eight pairs of nerve roots in the cervical spine. The cervical osteotomy is carried out at C7-T1, which is just below the entry point of the vertebral arteries at C6 and above the fixed thoracic spine. Because it is at the base of the neck, it also provides for the maximal amount of head position correction per osteotomy angle (this being a geometric part of the longer lever arm of action). This site protects the vertebral arteries from the likelihood of injury during osteotomy (Fig. 23-1). The spinal canal of C7-T1 is relatively spacious, and the cervical spinal cord and the eighth cervical nerve roots have reasonable flexibility. Injury to the C8 nerve root also would cause less disability than injury to more proximal cervical nerve roots.

## Indications for Spinal Osteotomy

Indications for cervical spine osteotomy are flexion deformities leading to impairment of the visual field to see ahead (horizon), difficulty with personal hygiene, and compromised function. Difficulty with swallowing is common. The most severe case of this is the "chin on chest" deformity. Because cervical osteotomy has high potential risks, it is most important that the patient must have the earnest desire

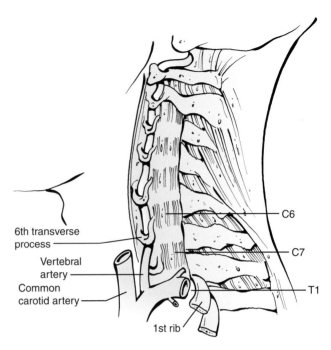

**Figure 23-1** Diagram showing position of vertebral artery and veins in front of the transverse process of the seventh vertebra entering into spine through transverse foramen of the sixth vertebra. (From Simmons EH. The cervical spine in ankylosing spondylitis. In: Bridwell KH, DeWald RL, eds. The textbook of spinal surgery, 2nd ed. Vol 1. Philadelphia: Lippincott-Raven, 1997:1144, with permission.)

to accept these risks and the rehabilitative measures required for correction.

Lumbar osteotomy commonly is done for surgical correction of lumbar hypolordosis or kyphosis giving rise to a fixed flexion deformity. The indications are variable and depend on the extent of the deformity, the degree of functional impairment, the age and general condition of the patient, the feasibility of correction, and the commitment of the patient to the risks and necessary rehabilitation measures.

Kyphotic deformity of the thoracic spine in ankylosing spondylitis usually does not reach proportions that require surgical correction. Combined anterior and posterior approaches are necessary. The diaphragm must not be violated because these patients breathe solely with their diaphragms owing to absence of motion through the costovertebral joints.

## Contraindications for Spinal Osteotomy

Contraindications for spinal osteotomy include patients who are not suitable candidates for medical reasons and patients in whom the severity of the deformity does not warrant the procedure. Severe osteopenia also is a relative contraindication.

## Assessment of Spinal Flexion Deformity

In assessing patients for possible surgical correction, it is important to recognize the primary site of flexion deformity.

Although all areas of the spine may be involved, there is usually one particular region that is primarily responsible for the overall malalignment and functional handicap. If any major correction is to be attempted, the correction must be done at the site of the main deformity.

Accurate assessment and measurement of flexion deformity are required in planning surgical treatment and in evaluating its results. The most effective and consistent measure of trunk flexion deformity is the chin-brow to vertical angle. This is a measure of the angle from a line extending from the chin to the brow measured to the vertical, when the patient stands with the hips and knees extended and the neck in neutral or fixed position (Fig. 23-2). Based on this measurement, the size of the wedge in the spine to be removed posteriorly is determined. For lumbar flexion deformity, this angle is transposed to a lateral radiograph of the lumbar spine with the apex of the angle at the posterior longitudinal ligament of the L3-4 disc space.

Cervical radiographs should be obtained, including anteroposterior, neutral, flexion/extension lateral (if any motion persists), and swimmer's views. These radiographs outline the shape and size of the spinous processes of C6, C7, and T1, allowing these processes to be recognized more readily at surgery (Fig. 23-3A). Flexion/extension lateral radiographs rule out the presence of instability at the craniocervical junction. A CT scan centered at the C7-T1 level should be obtained preoperatively. The CT scan provides evidence of previous compression fracture and allows assessment of the size of the spinal canal at the proposed site of osteotomy so that any area of stenosis can be decompressed adequately (Fig. 23-3B). In addition, preoperative magnetic resonance imaging may be considered for complex cases (Fig. 23-4).

## Preoperative Preparation

Careful medical assessment is carried out, including pulmonary function tests and electrocardiography. Many patients have concomitant medical illnesses and cardiac problems and must be evaluated carefully preoperatively from a medical standpoint. A physiotherapy program of deep breathing and extremity exercises is given, as will be used postoperatively. Psychological preparation includes preoperative visits by the anesthesiologist and the surgeon, to explain the whole procedure to the patient and gain his or her confidence.

## General Anesthesia for Lumbar Osteotomy

The patient is intubated fiberoptically while awake. The patient is positioned on the operating table prone in the knee-chest position. The position is adjusted until the patient is comfortable, avoiding any strain on the neck or elsewhere. Spinal cord monitoring is done throughout the procedure.

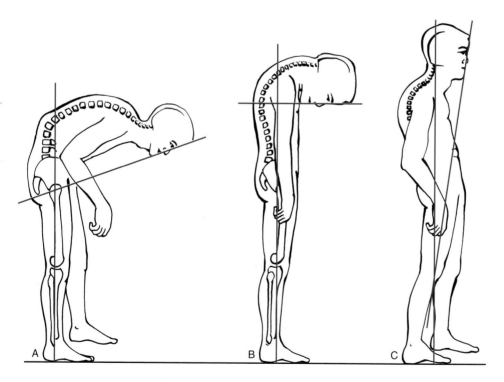

**Figure 23-2** The chin-brow to vertical angle is used to measure the degree of flexion deformity of the spine in ankylosing spondylitis, which is from the brow to the chin to the vertical line with the hips and knees extended and the neck in its fixed or neutral position. (**A**) For thoracolumbar deformity. (**B**) For cervical deformity. (**C**) For postoperative assessment. (From Hammerberg KW. Ankylosing spondylitis, *and* Simmons EH. The cervical spine in ankylosing spondylitis. In: Bridwell KH, DeWald RL, eds. The textbook of spinal surgery, 2nd ed. Vol 1. Philadelphia: Lippincott-Raven, 1997:1114, 1136, with permission.)

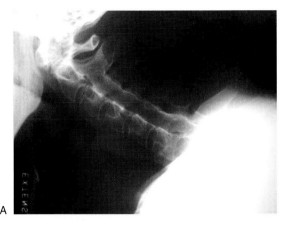
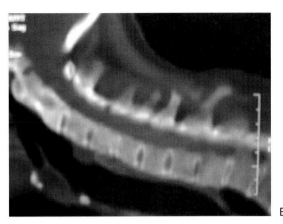

A    B

**Figure 23-3** (**A**) Lateral radiograph of a patient with cervical flexion deformity. (**B**) Lateral CT scan of the cervical spine of the same patient showing the spinal canal.

It is important to have valid preoperative tracings for comparison with findings during surgery. When the hips are extended to produce anterior osteoclasis with extension of the lumbar spine, the knees should be kept flexed to avoid any sciatic nerve tension that would alter the evoked spinal responses if posterior tibial nerve stimulation is used at the ankles.

Routine monitoring of vital signs and spinal cord monitoring are done throughout the procedure. A wake-up test also can be used if necessary. Pulse oximetry, carbon dioxide analyzer, and systemic blood gases are used to monitor the

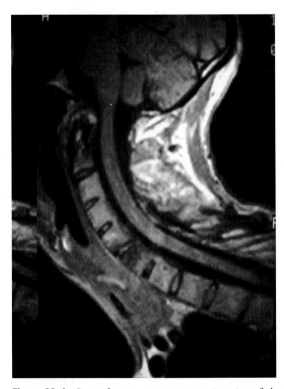

**Figure 23-4** Lateral magnetic resonance imaging of the cervical spine of a patient with cervical flexion deformity showing the spinal canal and cord.

patient. A Doppler apparatus is fixed to the patient's chest to detect any possible air embolisms.

## Techniques

After fiberoptic intubation with the patient awake (as described earlier), the patient is placed in the prone position on an adjusted Tower or Andrews table. The patient must be positioned carefully on the operating table in a flexed knee-chest position. Careful positioning also is necessary because these patients have fixed ankylosed spines, and undue pressure in any one particular area must be avoided. The thoracic chest support often must be elevated considerably to accommodate the patient on the operating table.

The osteotomy is done at the L3-4 level. A midline exposure is made, and the proposed osteotomy site is confirmed radiographically because operative localization is difficult owing to the fused confluent nature of the posterior elements of the spine.

The resection is carried out. The interspinous ligaments usually are ossified, and the osteotomy can be started with large bone cutters to trim away the intervening bone and spinous processes in a V-shaped fashion. The laminae can be thinned out with Leksell rongeurs and the bone fragments maintained for autogenous bone graft. A high-powered bur can be used alternatively; however, if this is used exclusively, less bone is available for the bone grafting.

When the spinal canal is opened, the dura is stripped carefully from the bone with a seeker and protected with cottonoid patties. In many long-standing cases, the dura is atrophic, similar to that of long-standing spinal stenosis. Rarely the dura may be adherent to the laminae, making its separation difficult. The entire L4 lamina is removed along with a portion of the L3 and L5 laminae with undercutting of the laminae to bevel them so that there is no impingement on closure of the osteotomy site. The cauda equina must be decompressed well laterally out to the level of the pedicles. The entire superior L4 facet is removed, and the L3-4 neuroforamina are exposed widely laterally and undercut with a medium-angle Kerrison rongeur to prevent any impingement on closure of the osteotomy site.

The precise amount of bone removed posteriorly is calculated to arrive at the amount of correction desired. On closure of the osteotomy with osteoclasis of the spine anteriorly, the lateral masses should meet with good bone surface contact. The pedicles also must be undercut, removing the superior edge of the L4 pedicle and inferior edge of the L3 pedicle to allow adequate room for the nerve root during extension of the spine.

Before the osteoclasis, the pedicle screws are inserted in L1, L2, L3, L5, and S1. The pedicle screws are inserted in a standard fashion, using anatomic and image-guided techniques as required. It is not usually possible to have screws in L4 because they impinge on the L3 screws after extension correction of the spine.

The osteoclasis is carried out by extending the foot-end of the table, bringing the hips and thighs up into an extended position. On doing so, pressure also can be applied manually by pushing downward at the L3-4 site, causing a fulcrum for the osteoclasis to occur. An audible and palpable osteoclasis of the spinal column often is present, and the lateral masses then come together in apposition. The lower extremities and hips now are kept in an extended position, preferably with the knees flexed, so as to avoid any tension on the sciatic nerve roots. Rods are cut and contoured to the appropriate length and shape for each side of the spine, then fitted into the pedicle screws and secured (Fig. 23-5). Posterolateral and posterior bone grafting is

done using the autologous local bone graft fragments from the decompression.

A well-molded plaster shell is applied extending from head to knee. The patient is strapped into the shell and transferred in the shell to a Roto-rest bed. This is an essential part of the procedure.

After extension osteotomy, the rigid thoracic kyphosis is more prominent than the pelvis, and if the patient is lying on a flat surface, forces tend to push the thorax forward and allow the pelvis and lower lumbar spine to move posteriorly. If the trapdoor of the bed is removed for a bowel movement, the spine would be unsupported. A well-contoured, padded rigid posterior plastic shell provides a contoured, well-fitted surface on which the rigid trunk can lie protecting the osteotomy site. A nasogastric suction tube is placed before the patient leaves the operating room. It is maintained until the patient is passing gas, with normal gastric function.

For the successful maintenance of correction, the most important factor is to correct the deformity completely, shifting the weight-bearing line posterior to the osteotomy site so that gravity helps maintain the correction with stimulation of bone formation across the osteotomy site. Postoperatively the patient is fitted with a thoracolumbosacral orthosis brace and mobilized with physical therapy.

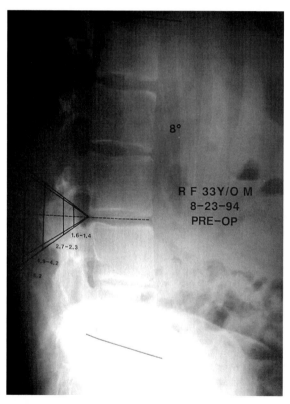
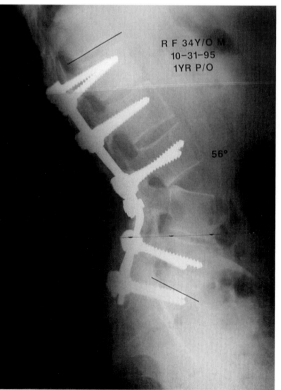

**Figure 23-5**   The chin-brow angle of a patient with lumbar flexion deformity was 70 degrees, and the lumbar lordosis was decreased to 8 degrees. (**A**) Lateral radiograph of lumbar spine showing the measured angle superimposed with the apex at the L3-4 disc space. (**B**) Postoperative lateral radiograph shows the angle of correction obtained after closure of the resected defect posteriorly with an opening anterior osteoclasis at the L3-4 disc level. Pedicle screws are placed bilaterally at L1, L2, L3, L5, and S1 with rods. *Figure continues.*

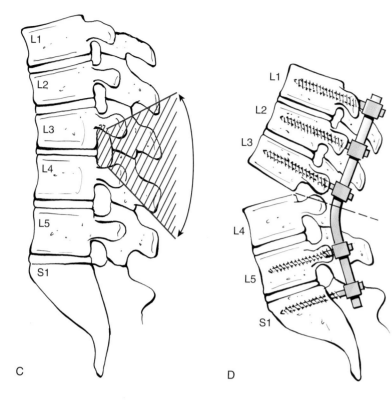

C    D

**Figure 23-5** (*Continued*) The 56 degrees of normal lumbar lordosis has been created with solid fusion mass. (**C** and **D**) Diagrams showing areas of posterior resection for L3-4 osteotomy and pedicle screw fixation with osteoclasis.

## Results and Potential Complications

One concern about extension osteotomy of the lumbar spine is the possibility of injury to the major vessels, particularly the abdominal aorta. We reviewed all the reported cases of major vascular injury associated with resection/extension osteotomy of the lumbar spine for ankylosing spondylitis, and the level at which the osteotomy was performed in each case was documented. In all cases, with injury to the abdominal aorta, the osteotomy was done at T12-L1, L1-2, or L2-3. There is no reported case of aortic injury with osteotomy performed at L3-4 or L4-5.

A major and consistent complication of lumbar osteotomy is gastric dilation and abdominal ileus. When the spine is extended with the costal margin moving away from the pelvis, the superior mesenteric artery is stretched over the third part of the duodenum, producing a functional block to the outlet of the stomach, predisposing to gastric dilation. If this hazard is not anticipated, patients may vomit a large amount. With a stiff rigid neck in the supine position, there is a risk of aspiration, which could prove fatal. It is necessary to have a nasogastric tube in position postoperatively with suction drainage until intestinal motility is established and the patient is passing gas.

The potential complications of any spinal procedure can occur. Major neurologic problems are relatively infrequent but can be a major problem when they occur. Potential complications specific to this procedure include intraspinal hematoma, intestinal obstruction, problems related to instrumentation due to osteopenia, and difficulty with surface landmarks in terms of inserting the instrumentation. Removal of too little or too much bone posteriorly can result in too little or too great a correction. Careful preoperative planning is necessary to determine the amount of correction desired and the appropriate amount of bone removal.

## Pitfalls of Lumbar Osteotomy

The clinician needs to be aware of the following pitfalls of lumbar osteotomy:

- The nasogastric tube always should be left in place postoperatively for at least several days, until proven intestinal motility has occurred. Failure to do so may result in emesis and aspiration due to the inability of the patient to rotate the neck and clear the airway.
- Extra assistance usually is required at the time of the osteoclasis to assist in extending the hips and repositioning the patient adequately on the operating table.
- The positioning of the patient must be evaluated carefully before, during, and after the procedure to be certain there is no undue pressure on the facial area or eyes and there is appropriate padding and positioning of the upper extremities.

## ANKYLOSING SPONDYLITIS OF CERVICAL SPINE

Ankylosing spondylitis presenting with a solid fused cervical spine may place increased stress at the craniocervical junction. Inflammation may cause erosion of the transverse ligament and associated hyperemia at its bony attachments. As these conditions progress, atlantoaxial subluxation and dislocation may occur.

## Posterior Surgical Techniques for Fixation of Atlantoaxial Instability

Four techniques commonly are used for fixation of atlantoaxial instability:

- Gallie technique with a modified H graft (most commonly used) (Fig. 23-6)
- Brooks technique with a bone block graft and sublaminar wires
- Transarticular fixation with screws (Fig. 23-7)
- Halifax clamp-type device

## Cervical Spine Fracture in Ankylosing Spondylitis

Undiagnosed fracture of the cervical spine is often the cause of progressive flexion deformity. Sudden pain with minor trauma (e.g., car accident), with or without forward flexion of the cervical spine, often indicates a fracture even though the trauma was relatively trivial. An undiagnosed fracture can go on to settle and heal in a forward flexed position. When such a fracture is recognized, a halo should be applied with traction to restore the alignment of the head and the neck to its *prefracture position*. If the head was in a previously flexed position, pulling it with traction into a neutral alignment may cause neurologic injury. When the appropriate alignment has been obtained, the patient should be immobilized in a halo vest for 4 months. A high union rate is associated with this protocol. If pseudarthrosis develops, posterior fusion or anterior cervical fusion can be undertaken.

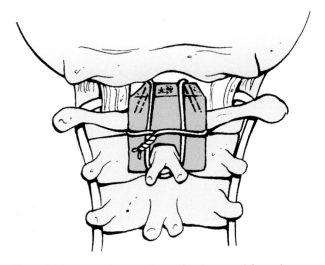

**Figure 23-6** Gallie fusion. The graft is harvested from the posterior iliac crest and fashioned to allow maximal bony contact with C1 and C2. Posterior view shows the graft in position. The loop of wire shown has been passed under the posterior arch of C1, then is pulled inferiorly over the C1 lamina and graft and around the C2 spinous process, which must be preserved. The free ends of the wire are crossed over the graft and twisted. (Modified from Drummond DS. Congenital anomalies of the pediatric cervical spine. In: Bridwell KH, DeWald RL, eds. The textbook of spinal surgery, 2nd ed. Vol 1. Philadelphia: Lippincott-Raven, 1997:965, with permission.)

## Technique of Cervical Osteotomy

The operation is carried out under local anesthesia with intravenous sedation, with the patient awake and in the sitting position using a dental chair. This approach allows the best form of active spinal cord monitoring and immediate assessment of the patient's vital functions and neurologic status. A halo-vest is applied to the patient preoperatively, and a 9-lb weight of traction is applied in direct line with the neck to stabilize the head throughout the procedure.

Besides routine monitoring measures for vital signs, pulse oximetry, carbon dioxide analyzer, and systemic blood gases are used for patient monitoring. A Doppler apparatus is fixed to the patient's chest to detect any possible air embolisms. The anesthesiologist may administer oxygen to the patient during the procedure by a facemask or nasal catheter. The patient is allowed to listen to the radio or other music throughout the procedure and usually converses with the anesthesiologist.

The cervical osteotomy is done at C7-T1, and the posterior portion of the angle is centered over the posterior arch of C7. This site is below the entry point of the vertebral arteries, which typically enter at the foramen transversarium at C6. This approach protects these vessels from the likelihood of injury during osteotomy at C7-T1. The spinal canal of C7-T1 is relatively spacious, and the cervical spinal cord and the eighth cervical nerve roots have reasonable flexibility. Also, any injury to the C8 nerve root would cause less disability than injury to other cervical nerve roots.

The entire posterior arch of C7 with the inferior portion of C6 and the superior portion of T1 are removed. The eighth cervical nerve roots are identified at the C7-T1 neuroforamen and are decompressed widely, removing the overlying bone at the foramen, decompressing widely laterally through the lateral recesses (Fig. 23-8).

The cervical pedicles need to be undercut with a Kerrison rongeur to allow ample room for the eighth cervical nerve root when the osteotomy site is closed. The amount of bone to be resected is assessed carefully preoperatively and intraoperatively to avoid any compression of the nerve roots on closure of the osteotomy. The residual portions of the laminae of C6 and T1 must be beveled carefully and undercut to avoid any impingement or kinking of the spinal cord on closure of the osteotomy site.

After adequate removal of bone, the osteoclasis procedure is done. The patient is given an intravenous dose of short-acting barbiturate, usually methohexital sodium (Brevital Sodium) or thiopental sodium (Pentothal). The surgeon grasps the halo and brings the neck into an extended position, with closure of the osteotomy site posteriorly as the osteoclasis occurs anteriorly. An audible snap and sensation of osteoclasis usually are noted. The lateral masses and osteotomy site laterally should be well approximated. With the surgeon holding the head in the corrected position, the assistants attach the vest to the halo with the upright supports anteriorly.

The posterior elements of the spine can be decorticated at the C7-T1 area, then autogenous bone graft is packed on each side over the decorticated areas. The local bone

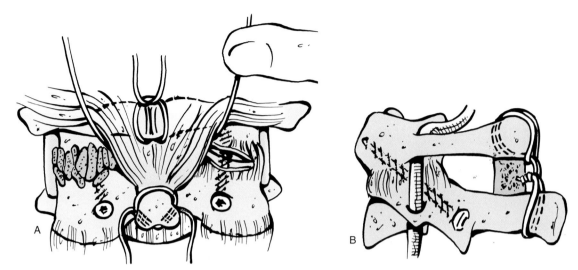

**Figure 23-7**   C1-2 transarticular fixation and posterior interspinous bone block graft and wiring. (**A**) After reduction, transarticular C1-2 screws are placed, and joints are packed with cancellous bone. (**B**) Lateral view of the transarticular technique. Fixation and grafting are enhanced by an intraspinous graft as shown here. (From Aebi M. Surgical treatment of cervical spine fractures by AO spine technique. In: Bridwell K, DeWald RL, eds. The textbook of spinal surgery. Philadelphia: JB Lippincott, 1991:1086, with permission.)

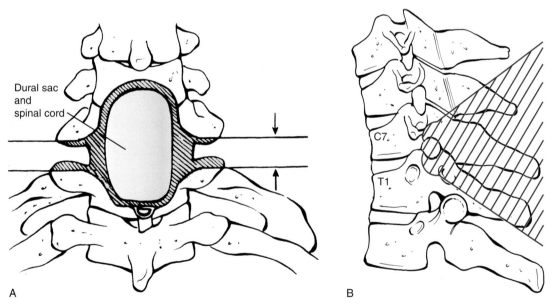

**Figure 23-8**   (**A**) Diagrammatic outline of the posterior view of the area of cervical resection. The lines of resection of the lateral fused joints are beveled slightly away from each other, extending posteriorly so that the two surfaces are parallel and in apposition after correction. The pedicles must be undercut to avoid impingement on the C8 nerve roots. The midline resection is beveled on its deep surface above and below to avoid impingement against the dura after extension correction. (**B**) Lateral diagram of the area of resection. (Modified from Simmons EH. The cervical spine in ankylosing spondylitis. Bridwell KH, DeWald RL, eds. The textbook of spinal surgery, 2nd ed. Vol 1. Philadelphia: Lippincott-Raven, 1997:1143, 1144, with permission.)

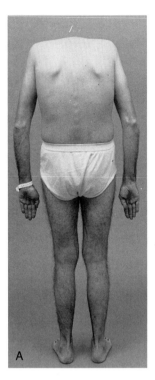
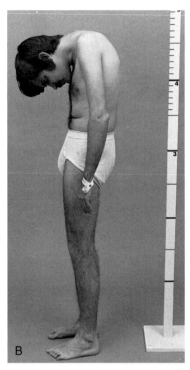
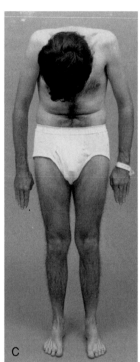

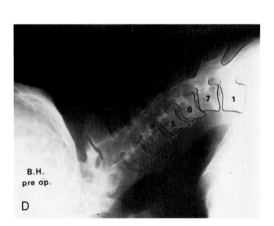

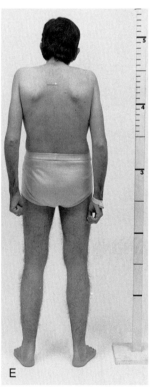
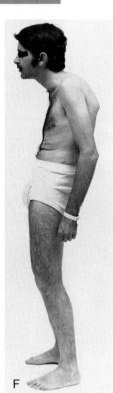
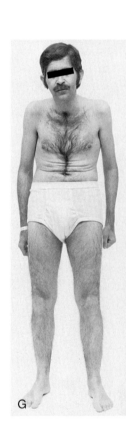

**Figure 23-9** (**A**) Posterior view of a man with rigid flexion deformity of the cervical spine of such magnitude that the head is not visible from behind. (**B**) Lateral view shows his chin rigidly fixed against his chest, with marked restriction of the field of vision and interference with the ability to open his mouth. (**C**) Anterior view shows complete restriction of the field of vision. (**D**) Lateral view x-ray of cervical spine shows complete ossification of posterior joints and previous subluxation of C6-7. (**E-G**) Postoperative posterior, lateral, and anterior views of patient shows correction of deformity with nearly normal chin-brow to vertical angle. (From Simmons EH. The cervical spine in ankylosing spondylitis. In: Bridwell KH, DeWald RL, eds. The textbook of spinal surgery, 2nd ed. Vol 1. Philadelphia: Lippincott-Raven, 1997:1148, with permission.)

**TABLE 23-1  THE KEY POINTS OF SINGLE-LEVEL CERVICAL AND LUMBAR OSTEOTOMY**

| | Cervical | Lumbar |
|---|---|---|
| Osteotomy level | C7-T1 | L3–4 |
| Vascular anatomy | Below the entry point of the vertebral arteries at the foramen transversarium of C6 | Normal center of lumbar lordosis. Increased mobility of the aortic bifurcation and iliac arteries |
| Neuroanatomy | C8 nerve root at C7-T1 neuroforamen and the spinal canal is relatively spacious | Below the conus medullaris and spinal canal volume is relatively spacious |
| Patient's position | Sitting position | Prone position |
| Anesthesia | Awake and local | General anesthesia |
| Approach | Posterior | Posterior |
| Spinal cord monitoring | No | Yes |
| Skull traction | Yes | No |
| Decompression extent | Entire posterior arch of C7 with the inferior portion of C6 and the superior portion of T1 are removed | Entire L4 lamina is removed along with the inferior portion of L3 and the superior portion of L5 laminae |
| Fixation | Halo-vest | Pedicle screw and rods |

removed from the posterior decompression is used for the bone graft.

The wound is closed in layers and dressed. The posterior upright supports also are connected to the halo, and these all are secured fully.

## Postoperative Care of Cervical Osteotomy

The patient is awake and can be helped to stand and walk to a revolving circular (CirOlectric) bed, which is in a vertical position. The bed can be tilted to the horizontal position, and the patient is taken to the surgical intensive care unit. When the patient is sufficiently mobile to get in and out of a regular bed, he or she is transferred to a regular bed with or without a trapeze attachment. The patient is instructed to leave the vest and halo intact and is left in this for 4 months. When the vest and halo are removed, lateral tomography or CT evaluation centered at C7-T1 is necessary to evaluate the radiographic union. Further bracing with a sternal occipital mandibular immobilization brace can be done for an additional 2 months (Fig. 23-9).

## Potential Pitfalls and Complications of Cervical Osteotomy

Potential pitfalls include osteotomy at the wrong level. If osteotomy is performed proximal to C7, injury to the vertebral arteries may occur. If osteotomy is performed below C7-T1, little or no correction is obtained. Radiographic confirmation always is necessary. Other pitfalls include inadequate or excessive removal of bone, resulting in too little or too great correction.

Neurologic injuries may occur. The dura may unfold in the region of the osteotomy and result in kinking of the spinal cord. If this problem is noted, the dura can be opened carefully to relieve compression. Most C8 nerve root problems resolve as long as they are partial. Some postoperative distraction through the halo vest can be carried out if C8 nerve root compression is noted postoperatively.

Other potential complications include air embolism because this surgery is performed in the sitting position. A Doppler monitor with sound amplification is fixed to the patient's chest preoperatively and can be monitored during the procedure. To prevent air embolisms, the wound should be filled with irrigation fluid and wet sponges during procedure.

Table 23-1 summarizes the key points of single-level cervical and lumbar osteotomy.

## SUGGESTED READING

Adams JC. Technique, dangers, and safeguards in osteotomy of the spine. J Bone Joint Surg 1952;34B:226–232.
Brooks AL, Jenkins ED. Atlantoaxial arthrodesis by the wedge compression methods. J Bone Joint Surg 1978;60A:279–284.
Calin A. Ankylosing spondylitis. In: Kelly WN, Harris ED, Ruddy S, Sledge CB, eds. Textbook of rheumatology. Philadelphia: WB Saunders, 1981:1017.
Herbert JJ. Vertebral osteotomy for kyphosis, especially in Marie-Strumpell arthritis: a report on 50 cases. J Bone Joint Surg 1959;41A:291.
LaChapelle EH. Osteotomy of the lumbar spine for correction of kyphosis in a case of ankylosing spondylarthritis. J Bone Joint Surg 1959;28A:270.
McMaster PE. Osteotomy of the spine for fixed flexion deformity. Pacific Med Surg 1965;73:314.
Simmons ED, Capicotto PN. Clinical cervical deformity and postlaminectomy kyphosis. In: White AH, Schofferman JA, eds. Spine care. St. Louis: Mosby, 1995:1633–1650.
Thomasen E. Vertebral osteotomy for correction of kyphosis in ankylosing spondylitis. Clin Orthop 1985;194:142–152.
Urist MR. Osteotomy of the cervical spine: report of a case of ankylosing rheumatoid spondylitis. J Bone Joint Surg 1958;40A:833–843.
Wills DG. Anesthetic management of posterior lumbar osteotomy. Can Anesth Soc J 1985;83:248–257.

# OSTEOPOROSIS OF THE SPINE

**EERIC TRUUMEES**

Osteoporosis is the most common metabolic bone disorder. With the aging of populations worldwide, it is becoming more pervasive. Similar to the intimal damage to arteries caused by hypertension, the destruction of bone caused by osteoporosis is clinically silent until an acute event occurs. With hypertension, the acute event is stroke or myocardial infarction, whereas with osteoporosis the acute event is fracture. Although a great deal of attention has been paid to osteoporotic fractures of the hip, osteoporotic fractures of the spine were thought to be benign, self-limited entities. With further study, an increasing list of acute and chronic sequelae are being ascribed to spinal insufficiency fractures, even in patients who never present to their physician for evaluation.

The spine care physician frequently is asked to treat patients with spinal osteoporosis. Osteoporosis may cause symptoms directly through one of three common fracture types:

- Vertebral compression fractures (VCF)
- Osteoporotic burst fractures
- Sacral insufficiency fractures

Alternatively, osteoporosis may complicate the treatment plan of other spinal interventions, such as instrumented stabilization of a degenerative spondylolisthesis. Although fractures are the main manifestation of spinal osteoporosis, the clinician must have a solid understanding of the biology and biomechanics of osteoporosis in treating any spinal condition in an osteoporotic patient population.

## PATHOGENESIS

### Etiology

Bone is a composite material composed of mineral, proteins, water, and cells. The exact composition of bone varies with anatomic site, age, diet, and presence of disease. Osteoporosis results from loss of the crystalline (inorganic) and collagenous (organic) phases of bone. In general, the mineral phase represents 60% to 70% of bone's dry weight and is composed mainly of an analogue of the naturally occurring mineral *hydroxyapatite* ($Ca_{10}(PO_4)_6(OH)_2$). Loss of the mineral phase weakens the bone to compressive load-

ing. The organic matrix of bone represents approximately 30% of its dry weight, and 90% of this matrix is collagen. Collagen is a protein of extremely low solubility comprising three polypeptide chains of 1000 amino acids. Loss of the organic matrix of bone makes it more brittle.

Bone is dynamic and well organized. Apatite crystal arrangement is modulated at the molecular level, and strain patterns of the trabecular network are modulated at the organ level. The close modulation of the molecular, cellular, and tissue properties of bone result in a relatively lightweight tissue with a tensile strength close to that of cast iron. At the microscopic level, bone consists of two forms: *woven* (or primitive) and *lamellar* bone. Lamellar bone begins to form 1 month after birth, and by age 4 years, most normal bone is lamellar. Lamellar bone is characterized by highly organized, stress-oriented collagen, which gives it anisotropic properties; that is, the mechanics of loading lamellar bone depend on the direction of force application. Typically, bone is strongest parallel to the long axis of the collagen molecules.

In the mature skeleton, lamellar bone is found in two forms: *trabecular* (spongy or cancellous) and *cortical* (dense or compact). Trabecular bone exhibits much greater metabolic activity, with eight times greater turnover. This trabecular bone represents 20% of the total bone mass and is found in the metaphyses and epiphyses of long bones and in the cuboid bones (including the vertebrae). In trabecular bone, spicules form a three-dimensional branching lattice aligned to applied mechanical stresses. Conversely, cortical bone has a fairly uniform density. Cortical bone forms the "envelope" of cuboid bones and the diaphysis of long bones and constitutes 80% of total bone mass.

Bone contains three main cell types: *osteoblasts, osteocytes,* and *osteoclasts.* Osteoblasts and osteocytes arise from the same lineage but differ in location and function. Osteoblasts produce osteoid, or bone matrix; line the surface of bone; and follow osteoclasts in cutting cones. Osteocytes are osteoblasts encased in a mineralized matrix but are in chemical contact with the osteoblasts on the bone surface by cellular processes through canaliculi. Osteoblasts receive the endocrine signals, then transmit them to the osteocytes. Strain-generated signals within the bone are regulated by osteocytes and are passed on to the osteoblasts. Osteoclasts are the major resorptive cells of bone and are characterized by large size (20 to 100 μm) and multiple nuclei. These cells are derived from pluripotent cells of bone marrow and bind to the bone surface through cell attachment proteins (integrins).

Throughout life, the body constantly remodels bone by removing old bone and creating new bone. In osteoporosis, there is a decrease in the rate of bone formation relative to the rate of destruction. In contradistinction, osteomalacia represents a dysregulation of bone mineralization in the context of normal osteoid production. Given the lower rates of formation in osteoporosis, the overall mineral density of the bone decreases. With unbalanced osteoclast activity, the normal connectivity of bone trabeculae is lost. The bone is weakened in a material and in an architectural sense. Although there are many environmental, genetic, and pharmacologic factors affecting the development of osteoporosis, the root etiology of this dysregulation is not yet understood and is probably multifactorial.

## Epidemiology

There are 35 million people at risk for osteoporosis in North America alone. This number is expected to triple over the next 3 decades with the aging of the population. VCFs are the most common manifestation of spinal osteoporosis and are estimated to affect one third of all North Americans at some point during their lifetime. Outnumbering hip and wrist fractures combined, there are 700,000 VCFs per year in the United States. In a population-based European study, a12% prevalence of spinal fractures was recorded in men and women age 50 to 79 years. The direct medical costs associated with these fractures have been estimated at $13.8 billion annually in the United States alone. By 2030, annual direct costs are projected to exceed $60 billion, or $164 million per day. Indirect costs in lost productivity are higher.

## Pathophysiology

Osteoporosis is a disease state characterized by a decrease in the organic and the inorganic phases of bone. With age, everyone loses bone mass at approximately 0.5% per year, but not everyone develops osteoporosis. The two most important determinants for the development of osteoporosis are peak bone mass and the rate of bone loss.

Peak bone mass is achieved in the early 30s. The most effective way to prevent the devastating complications of VCF is to increase peak bone mass in pubertal patients. Disorders such as anorexia and exercise-induced amenorrhea lead to profound osteoporosis. Several studies have documented increasing rates of osteoporosis among young women. Lack of weight-bearing exercise and changes in dietary habits have been implicated.

After peak bone mass, bone is lost gradually with age. The rate of loss is accelerated through decreased exposure to gonadal hormones (i.e., menopause); genetic, environmental, and nutritional conditions; and chronic disease states. Estrogen deficiency is implicated directly in accelerated bone loss at 2% to 3% per year for 10 years. The mechanism of bone loss resulting from normal aging is poorly understood, but its rate is equivalent in women and men.

## TABLE 24-1  RISK FACTORS FOR OSTEOPOROSIS

- Advanced age
- Endocrine risk factors
  - Hypercortisolism
  - Hyperthyroidism
  - Hyperparathyroidism
  - Hypogonadism
- Other disease states
  - Tumors
  - Chronic disease
  - Expression of abnormal collagen or bone matrix genes
- Activity level
  - Immobilization or inactivity
- Dietary issues
  - Calcium-deficient diet
- Alcohol (>80 g/d)
- Body mass index <22 kg/m$^2$
- Smoking

Other endocrinopathies and risk factors associated with osteoporosis are listed in Table 24-1.

## Classification

Osteoporosis and related fractures have been classified. Stages of bone loss are classified by the t-score (see later). Bone mineral density more than 1 SD below the mean young adult value is defined as *osteopenia*. When the density is more than 2.5 SD below the mean, the patient has osteoporosis. Bone mineral density more than 2.5 SD below the mean with fragility fractures is termed *severe osteoporosis*.

Osteoporosis also is divided into three etiologic categories:

- *Type I (postmenopausal)*—affects women more often than men (hypogonadic men get this form of osteoporosis as well). Patients are affected in their 50s and 60s, and fractures of trabecular bone (wrist and spine) predominate.
- *Type II (senile)*—affects men and women equally, occurs in the 70s and 80s, and increasingly affects cortical bone.
- *Type III (secondary)*—medications and disease states contribute.

Most commonly, endogenous or exogenous cortisol is deleterious to bone mass due to:

- Decreased calcium absorption across the intestinal lumen
- Increased calcium loss from kidney
- Direct inhibition of bone matrix formation (secondary hyperparathyroidism)

Alternate-day dosing of corticosteroids decreases bone damage. Calcium, vitamin D, and antiosteoporotic medications counter some of the deleterious effects.

When fractures occur, these are classified morphologically. Just as osteoporotic fractures of the proximal femur are divided anatomically into femoral neck and intertro-

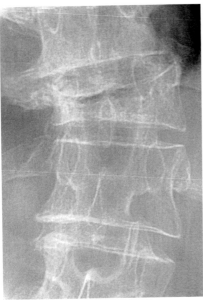
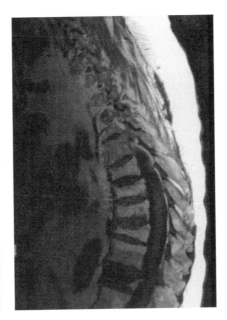
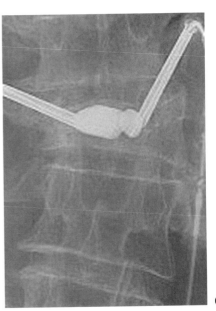

A,B                                                                                                   C

**Figure 24-1**  A 74-year-old man with secondary osteoporosis and degenerative scoliosis complained of severe midback pain and balance difficulties after a fall from a stepladder. Anteroposterior radiograph (**A**) shows osteopenia and a lateral vertebral compression fracture. Pain failed to respond to 4 weeks of management with narcotics and a Cash brace, and MRI was obtained. T1-weighted image (**B**) shows decreased signal intensity in T12. Increased signal was noted on T2 image (not shown). The patient was point tender over this level. Based on his continued pain and functional limitation, he was offered kyphoplasty. Anteroposterior fluoroscopic image during early balloon inflation (**C**) shows differential inflation on the more compressed side. The patient reported continued improvement for the next 2 weeks and ultimately returned to his baseline 3/10 visual analogue pain scale pain level. He was started on alendronate (Fosamax), calcium, and vitamin D.

chanteric fractures and are subdivided based on fracture pattern, axial skeleton injuries first are described based on spinal level and then on fracture pattern. The most common injury is VCF. There are a wide range of fracture patterns, including failure of the superior, inferior, and both end plates. Lateral compression deformities may worsen preexisting coronal plane deformities (Fig. 24-1A). In the lumbar spine, these fractures may include collapse of the central portion of the superior and inferior end plates and has been termed a *biconcave* or *codfish vertebra*. In the thoracic spine, the anterior portion of the superior end plate most typically is involved and leads to a wedge-compression fracture. A senile burst fracture represents increased axial loading and failure of the middle column (posterior vertebral body) with retropulsion of bone into the spinal canal. Sacral insufficiency fractures may occur in the context of insufficiency fractures of the pelvis with concomitant pubic ramus fractures or as isolated injuries.

# DIAGNOSIS

## Clinical Features

Symptoms of osteoporosis usually are not evident until low-energy (fragility) fractures occur. The most common sites for these fractures are the spine, ribs, hips, and wrists. The patient reports localized pain in these areas. Diffuse bone pain is a feature of osteomalacia and is not seen with osteoporosis (Table 24-2). Before fracture, osteoporosis is identified based on screening studies in at-risk populations. All physicians, including orthopaedic and spine surgeons, must ensure that their at-risk patients have been screened and, if necessary, treated for osteoporosis (Table 24-3). Patient outcomes after primary prevention greatly exceed that of fracture stabilization.

When a patient has sustained a fracture related to osteoporosis, the work-up begins with a careful history. Fracture occurs in the context of minimal to no trauma and leads to focal, intense, deep midline spine pain. Fracture pain must be differentiated from muscular pain, which more typically is diffuse pain or paravertebral. Symptoms should be primarily mechanical and vary with activity and loading. It is necessary to understand the time course of the patient's symptoms and the course of any previous fractures. The physician should ask about associated thoracic or lumbar radicular complaints. Past medical history, including a history of cancer, tuberculosis, or systemic infection, is investigated to ascertain appropriate treatment of underlying osteoporosis. Patients with night pain, fevers, chills, unusual weight loss, or bowel or bladder changes require more intense investigation.

On physical examination, the patient's general condition

## TABLE 24-2  COMPARISON OF OSTEOPOROSIS AND OSTEOMALACIA

|  | Osteoporosis | Osteomalacia |
|---|---|---|
| Definition | Bone mass decreased | Bone mass variable |
| Mineralization | Normal | Decreased |
| Age of onset | Generally elderly | Any age |
| Etiology | Endocrine abnormality | Vitamin D deficiency |
|  | Age | Abnormality of vitamin D pathway |
|  |  | Idiopathic hypophosphatemia |
|  |  | Renal tubular acidosis |
|  |  | Hypophosphatasia |
| Symptoms | Pain referable to fracture | Generalized bone pain |
| Signs | Tenderness at fracture | Generalized tenderness |
| Laboratory findings |  |  |
| Serum Ca$^{++}$ | Normal | Low or normal (high hypophosphatasia) |
| Serum P | Normal | Low or normal (high renal osteodystrophy) |
| Alkaline phosphatase | Normal | Elevated ($\times$ hypophosphatasia) |
| Urinary Ca$^{++}$ | High or normal | Normal or low (high in hypophosphatasia) |
| Bone biopsy | Normal | Abnormal |

and sagittal spinal balance are assessed. Body shape, difficulty breathing, and obesity each affect the likelihood of effective bracing. Associated rib tenderness should be sought because coexisting and iatrogenic rib fractures are common. Acute VCFs and burst fractures typically are point tender over the spinous process. A complete neurologic exam should be conducted. Although major neurologic deficits are rare (0.05%), many patients have significant stenosis or neuropathic changes. Sacral insufficiency fractures cause pain over the sacral body, in the sacroiliac joint regions, or in a bandlike distribution across the low back. Maneuvers that stress the sacroiliac joint, such as Gaenslen's sign or Patrick's test, increase this pain.

Laboratory evaluation in osteoporosis is used mainly to exclude other causes of osteopenia, such as osteomalacia. Laboratory studies may be abnormal in osteomalacia, which should be suspected when the product of the serum calcium level multiplied by the serum phosphate level remains chronically less than 25 mg/dL. Serum alkaline phosphatase levels are elevated, and 24-hour urinary calcium excretion may be less than 50 mg. Occasionally, serum blood tests alone are insufficient to exclude the diagnosis of osteomalacia, at which time a transiliac bone biopsy may be indicated.

Bone biopsy also is indicated in patients younger than 50 years old with idiopathic osteopenia, in patients when osteomalacia is highly suspected, or in chronic renal failure patients with skeletal symptoms. Two weeks before the biopsy, tetracycline is administered twice each day for 3 days. This dose is repeated in the 3 days immediately before biopsy. The tetracycline binds to newly mineralized osteoid and permits the determination of mineralization rates. In osteoporosis, a normal mineralization pattern of two distinct bands of fluorescence, representing the tetracycline labels, is noted. With impaired mineralization, a single band of fluorescence is encountered.

Bone biomarker assays increasingly are being requested to provide complementary information to densitometry. Markers of bone formation, such as bone-specific alkaline phosphatase (an osteoblast enzyme) and osteocalcin (a bone matrix protein), and bone resorption, such as urinary collagen degradation products (cross-linked telopeptides and pyridinolines), offer improved prediction of future fracture risk and a sensitive means to monitor therapy effectiveness. In patients with unusual fracture patterns or histories suggesting malignancy or infection, laboratory evaluation may include sedimentation rates, differential blood counts, C-reactive protein assays, tumor antigens, and protein electrophoresis.

## TABLE 24-3  INDICATIONS FOR DUAL-ENERGY X-RAY ABSORPTIOMETRY SCREENING FOR OSTEOPOROSIS

Postmenopausal women >65 years old
Women <65 years old with ≥1 risk factors
Patients with fragility fractures
Women considering therapy in which bone mineral density would affect decision
Women on hormone replacement therapy for prolonged periods
Patients with osteopenia on x-rays
Patients with diseases known to place them at risk for osteoporosis

## Radiologic Features

Although plain radiographs are useful in symptomatic patients, they are the least accurate and precise method of assessing bone density. A decrease in bone mass of at least 30% is necessary to detect osteopenia. More accurate measurements of bone mass are crucial in the diagnosis and treatment of osteoporosis. Noninvasive bone densitometry provides information about the specific site measured, and density measurements in the lumbar spine correlate well with the incidence of vertebral fracture. The first widely available densitometry test was dual-photon absorptiometry, which measured axial skeletal bone mineral density via soft tissue signal attenuation using radioisotopes. Since the 1990s, dual-energy x-ray absorptiometry (DEXA) has become the standard. This x-ray-based modality has significant advantages over dual-photon absorptiometry, including:

- Superior precision (1% to 2% at spine, 3% to 4% at femur)
- Lower radiation dose
- Shorter examination time
- Higher image resolution
- Greater technical ease

DEXA scores are used to assess baseline bone density in at-risk patients and to track response to therapy. The t-score compares the patient's bone mineral density with mean values for healthy same-gender young adults. For each 1 SD below the norm, fracture risk increases 1.5-fold to 3-fold. A t-score of $-1$ implies a 30% chance of fracture. The z-score compares bone mineral density with age-matched controls. A z-score less than $-1.5$ warrants a more extensive work-up for underlying causes of the bone loss. DEXA values are falsely increased with scoliosis, compression fractures, bone spurs, extraosseous calcification, and vascular disease.

Quantitative computed tomography (CT) generates a cross-sectional image of a vertebral body and allows preferential measurement of trabecular bone density. Because the rate of turnover in trabecular bone is eight times that in cortical bone, quantitative CT is a sensitive indicator of bone density in highly vulnerable skeletal areas. Quantitative CT involves the simultaneous scanning of tubes containing standard solutions of a bone mineral equivalent. A standard calibration curve is calculated, and vertebral trabecular bone density is extrapolated. Measurements are taken from centers of vertebral bodies, and values from T12 to L4 are averaged to yield a mean bone density. This method allows exclusion of osteophytes and aortic calcifications and is accurate to within 5% to 10%. Cost and radiation dose are higher, however, than with DEXA. Ultrasound is an attractive means of measuring bone density because it does not expose a patient to ionizing radiation. Although these methods are rapid and inexpensive, they are not as precise as DEXA and are useful mainly for initial screening.

In patients with known fractures, the goals of imaging are to determine the following:

- Extent of vertebral collapse
- Location and extent of any lytic process
- Visibility and degree of pedicular involvement
- Presence of cortical destruction
- Presence of epidural or foraminal stenosis
- Age or acuity of the fracture

Several of these goals are achieved through plain radiog-

raphy. With standing radiographs, overall sagittal and coronal spinal balance is apparent. Thoracolumbar fractures are discovered readily, but sacral fractures are difficult to see. Determination of the age or acuity of the fracture is more difficult. Comparison films, including old chest radiographs, may be helpful, but apparent sclerosis may represent healing or merely compressed bone. Spot films, particularly at the thoracolumbar junction, aid visualization. During early patient management for acute fracture, plain radiographs should be followed serially over the short term to assess for further collapse.

Plain radiographs should be scrutinized for signs of posterior cortical compromise, such as widened pedicles and greater than 50% height loss. End plate erosion suggests infection or pedicular destruction ("winking owl" sign) as seen in malignancy. Fractures above T6 are more likely to represent neoplasm.

The canal involvement and fracture acuity are determined more readily with magnetic resonance imaging (MRI) (Fig. 24-2). The edema seen in acute fractures is reflected by increased signal on T2 or short tau inversion recovery sequences. Acutely, fractures show decreased T1 signal, and T1 and T2 marrow signal changes normalize over time (see Fig. 24-1B). MRI may reveal several key features that differentiate malignant from osteoporotic compression fractures, including pedicular and soft tissue extension.

Avascular necrosis of the vertebral bone (Kümmell's disease) is an increasingly recognized cause of chronic, unheal-

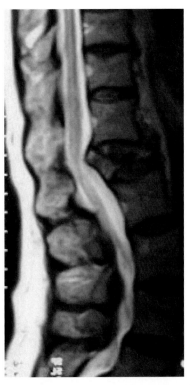

**Figure 24-2** A 63-year-old woman with postmenopausal osteoporosis was admitted to the hospital with bladder incontinence and severe back pain after a slip and fall injury. MRI showed an L1 osteoporotic burst fracture with conus compression.

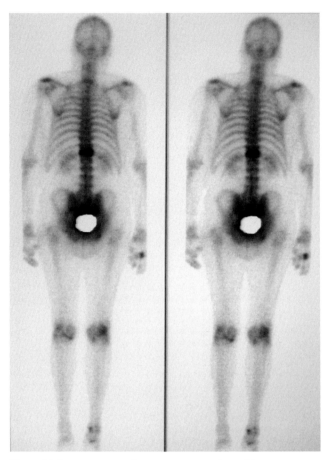

**Figure 24-3**    Bone scan shows intense uptake at T11 in a patient with 4 months of pain after sustaining a vertebral compression fracture.

ing compression fractures. This continuing collapse of the vertebra after minor trauma is particularly common in patients with known risk factors for avascular necrosis, such as previous radiation therapy or long-term corticosteroid use. On MRI, these fractures show the "double line sign" of discrete fluid collections within a vacuum cleft with areas of diminished T2 signal surrounding the cleft.

In patients unable to undergo MRI, CT offers high bone and soft tissue contrast and clearly delineates posterior cortical compromise. Fracture acuity may be determined by bone scan (Fig. 24-3). MRI and CT show sacral insufficiency fractures. On bone scan, these lesions may have the classic H configuration or may appear as a linear band of increased uptake in the region of the sacral ala (Fig. 24-4C).

## Diagnostic Work-up Algorithm

The goals of evaluation in osteoporosis are:

- To identify decreased bone mineral density
- To exclude the osteopenia of malignancy, osteomalacia, or secondary osteoporosis
- To assess bone turnover state

Evaluation algorithms begin with a screening DEXA scan. In patients with t-scores less than $-1.5$, further evaluation is undertaken. For younger patients and women with a questionable menstrual history, a hormonal profile, including sex hormones, thyroid-stimulating hormone, thyroxine, and parathyroid hormone (PTH), should be ordered. Standard chemistries include serum calcium, phosphate, alkaline phosphatase, creatinine, and a 24-hour urine calcium excretion. If no clearly identifiable cause of osteopenia is found, an iliac crest bone biopsy and marrow aspiration are indicated.

In osteopenic patients presenting with back pain, the physician should obtain a good history, perform a thorough physical exam, and evaluate plain radiographs. In patients with red flags, neurologic involvement, or long-standing pain, MRI is recommended. In patients unable to undergo MRI, CT and bone scan are ordered.

## TREATMENT

### Treatment of Osteoporosis

Treatments for osteoporosis have had variable success because of delayed and inaccurate diagnosis, insufficient understanding of the disease process, and inadequate follow-up. The primary goal of treatment is to decrease fracture risk (Table 24-4). Optimal treatment begins before the first fracture and focuses on the material and structural properties of bone by calcium and physiologic vitamin D administration and mild weight-bearing exercise. These measures are intended to decrease bone resorption and to mineralize osteoid, but they do not increase total bone mass. Studies have shown that individuals taking calcium supplements have a quarter of the hip fractures of individuals with low calcium intake, but excess calcium may be harmful. Other early management addresses fracture risk by fall prevention. Household obstacles should be removed. Tai chi (an Asian form of exercise) has been favored because it improves patient balance.

In menopausal women, estrogen supplementation may be appropriate. Estrogen receptors have been identified in bone-forming cells. Estrogen acts to block the action of PTH on osteoblasts and marrow stromal cells, and estrogen supplementation decreases bone loss by acting to counter the effect of unopposed PTH activity. Without estrogen, osteoblasts and marrow stromal cells secrete increased levels of interleukin-6, which stimulates the osteoclasts to resorb bone. Estrogen does not alter bone formation rates appreciably, but it does increase bone mass slightly by slowing resorption. More recent studies seem to show increased rates of coronary artery disease, stroke, pulmonary embolus, and cancer in women on hormone replacement therapy. The potential of untoward side effects of estrogen has increased interest in selective estrogen receptor modulators, such as raloxifene (Evista). These agents seem to have similar bone-preserving effects as estrogen without oncogenic or adverse cardiac effects.

More aggressive pharmacologic management in patients with fractures or with femoral t-scores less than $-2.5$ should be undertaken. Calcitonin, via subcutaneous

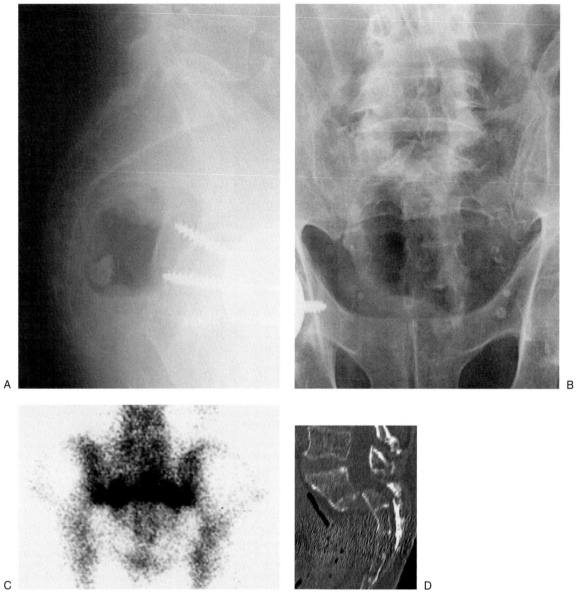

**Figure 24-4**   An 84-year-old man complained of severe sacral pain after "sitting down too hard." He was point tender over the sacral body, and his pain increased with Patrick's test. Initial antero-posterior (**A**) and lateral (**B**) radiographs show only osteopenia. Scintigraphy in patients with sacral insufficiency fractures generally shows intense uptake, often in an "H" pattern, over the sacrum (**C**). This patient was mobilized gradually, but sustained a second episode of falling into his hard kitchen chair. New lateral radiographs showed complete displacement of the S1-2 segment. CT scan with sagittal reconstructions shows a transverse fracture through S1-2 (**D**). *Figure continues.*

injection or nasal spray, decreases osteoclastic bone resorption. Over the short term, calcitonin enhances bone formation, leading to a slight net bone accretion. With long-term treatment, osteoblastic activity slows, and bone mass stabilizes.

Bisphosphonates dramatically suppress bone resorption and decrease the risk for hip and spinal fractures. These agents directly stabilize the bone crystal, making it more resistant to osteoclastic bone resorption. They also inhibit osteoclast activity. Bisphosphonates preserve bone architecture and overall density. Weekly forms of these agents afford better compliance with no increase in toxicity.

Intermittent administration of PTH is anabolic and leads to early, dramatic increases in bone mass, especially in trabecular bone. The long-term safety and efficacy of these protocols have not yet been established, and clinical trials are under way. Ultimately, for patients with severe osteoporosis, combination therapies linking an anabolic agent with an antiresorptive agent along with calcium and vitamin D supplementation may be ideal.

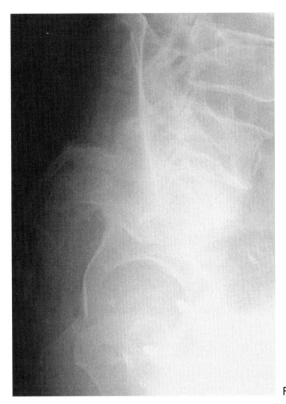

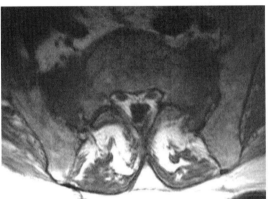

E                                                                                          F

**Figure 24-4**  (*Continued*) MRI typically shows an abnormal signal pattern through the sacral ala (**E**). After his second fall, the patient reported urinary retention and ultimately was admitted to the hospital for pyelonephritis. He had toe flexor weakness. He underwent a laminectomy and noted improvement in neurologic symptoms (**F**).

## Management of Osteoporotic Fractures

The goals of osteoporotic spinal fracture management include the following:

- Decreased pain
- Early mobilization
- Preservation of sagittal and coronal spinal stability
- Prevention of late neurologic compromise

During the initial painful interval, patients presenting to their physicians typically are offered pain medications and braces. Limited activity and often bed rest are advised or self-imposed. In patients with osteoporosis, bed rest is associated with an additional 4% loss of bone mineral density.

The period of acute pain usually lasts 4 to 6 weeks, but in some circumstances pain persists beyond 3 months. Narcotic pain medications may be continued until the patient can bear weight comfortably. In elderly patients, use of narcotics may be associated with as many functional problems as the underlying fracture. Nasal calcitonin and bisphosphonates, useful in the treatment of osteoporosis, also may be effective in decreasing fracture-related pain.

A limited contact orthosis, such as a tri-pad Jewett extension brace or Cash brace, is easy to fit, but compliance varies. In short, obese, elderly patients, body habitus limits brace effectiveness. Patients with concomitant shoulder problems have difficulty donning and doffing the brace. Physical therapy may aid the patient's recovery to mobility.

At least 150,000 compression fractures per year are refractory to nonoperative measures and require hospitalization, with protracted periods of bed rest and narcotics. Fractures less likely to improve with standard medical management include fractures of the thoracolumbar junction (T11-L2), fractures with burst patterns, wedge compression fractures with more than 30 degrees of sagittal angulation, fractures with a radiographic vacuum shadow in fractured body (ischemic necrosis of bone), and fractures with progressive collapse in office follow-up.

## TABLE 24-4 DETERMINANTS OF FRACTURE RISK IN OSTEOPOROSIS

Load-bearing capacity of bone
Material characteristics
   Microarchitecture/loss of trabeculae/microcracks
   Tissue density/mineralization
Structural characteristics
   Bone mass
   Bone geometry
Loads applied to bone
   Propensity to trauma/falls
   Severity of trauma/falls
   Activities of daily living

Vertebral body augmentation (VBA) procedures may be indicated in some patients with continuing vertebral collapse or intractable pain (Table 24-5). Vertebral augmentation with polymethyl methacrylate (PMMA) variably restores strength and stiffness to a fractured body. Strength reflects the ability of the vertebral body to bear load and may protect against future fracture of the treated segment. Stiffness limits micromotion within the compromised vertebral body and is ostensibly the source of symptom relief.

Kyphoplasty and vertebroplasty gain access to the vertebral body through a 1-cm incision. With vertebroplasty the vertebra is filled with liquid PMMA through an 11-gauge needle (Fig. 24-5). With kyphoplasty, a balloon tamp is used first to create a void in the bone and to attempt fracture reduction (see Fig. 24-1C) These procedures may be performed under general anesthesia or with local anesthesia and intravenous sedation. The patient is placed prone on a radiolucent table or frame and bolstered to allow partial postural reduction of the fracture. The crucial first step in either procedure is to obtain true anteroposterior and lateral images with fluoroscopy. Most typically, a transpedicular route to the vertebra is selected. In some thoracic cases, the narrow and straight pedicle precludes appropriate medialization, and an extrapedicular approach is required. Kyphoplasty usually is performed through a bilateral approach. Vertebroplasty may be performed unilaterally or bilaterally.

Beginning with an anteroposterior fluoroscopic view, an 11-gauge Jamshidi needle is positioned at the 10 o'clock or 2 o'clock position on the pedicular ring. In contrast to pedicle screws, the goal is not to proceed "straight down the barrel," but rather to medialize through the cylinder of the pedicle. The clinician starts lateral and aims medial. When in bone, the clinician verifies the trajectory on the lateral image. If

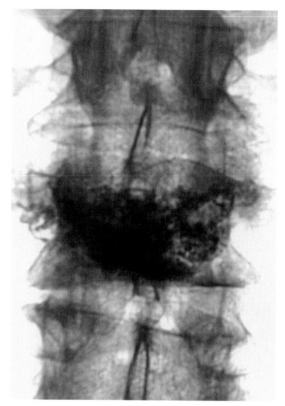

**Figure 24-5** Postoperative radiograph after a midlumbar vertebroplasty performed through a unipedicular approach with a curved needle.

the anteroposterior and lateral images do not show a clearly intrapedicular position, an en face or oblique view is useful. When the tip of the needle reaches the medial border of the pedicle on the anteroposterior view, it must be at or anterior to the junction of the pedicle and vertebral body on the lateral view.

Although there are several different systems and needles employed for vertebroplasty, most require advancement of the cannulae into the central portion of the vertebral body. PMMA is mixed and delivered under live fluoroscopy. In kyphoplasty, additional instruments are employed. The Jamshidi needle is replaced with a working cannula through which inflatable bone tamps are delivered. These balloons are inserted to within 4 mm of the anterior vertebral body cortex. When both balloons have been placed, they are inflated sequentially in 0.5-cc increments until one of the following end points:

- Realignment of vertebral end plates
- Maximal balloon pressure (>220 psi) without decay (i.e., loss of pressure)
- Maximal balloon volume—4 cc for 15/3 and 6 cc for 20/3
- Cortical wall contact

The void created by the inflatable bone tamp is filled with viscous PMMA. Sterile barium is added to the powder to increase its radiopacity. For vertebroplasty, the PMMA is injected into the body in a fairly liquid state to allow

## TABLE 24-5 INDICATIONS AND CONTRAINDICATIONS FOR VERTEBRAL BODY AUGMENTATION

Indications
  A painful vertebral body fracture from
    Primary osteoporosis
    Secondary osteoporosis
    Multiple myeloma
    Osteolytic metastasis
Contraindications
  Local spinal infection
  Burst fracture with retropulsed bone or neurologic symptoms
  Young patients
  Pregnancy
  Osteoblastic metastasis
  High-velocity (traumatic) fractures
  Primary spinal neoplasm
  Fractured pedicles or facets
  Allergy to devices or contrast medium
  Uncorrectable bleeding disorders
  Severe cardiopulmonary difficulties
  Technical feasibility problems
    Vertebra plana
    Level above T5

it to interdigitate between the crushed trabeculae of the fracture. For kyphoplasty, the PMMA is inserted when it reaches a toothpaste-like consistency. The balloons are removed, and the PMMA is implanted under continuous fluoroscopy. The wound may be closed with a suture or Steristrip. No braces or particular postoperative precautions are needed. Newer resorbable calcium phosphate and hydroxyapatite cements also are being tested.

There are few appealing treatment options for sacral insufficiency fractures. If there is a concomitant pubic ramus fracture, limited weight bearing on the affected side and walker ambulation are recommended. For bilateral fractures, a walker helps the patient decrease weight bearing through the fracture to a degree. There are no effective braces for these injuries. For fractures with significant displacement or neurologic compromise, operative reduction and stabilization may be required.

Osteoporotic burst fractures (senile burst fractures) are more common than previously thought. In my experience, fractures with more than 50% height loss usually have associated posterior cortical compromise. In many cases, this compromise takes the form of buckling of the cortex. If the canal occlusion is less than 33%, VBA procedures may be entertained in select cases. If comminution exists, VBA should not be undertaken because of the increased risk of cement extravasation. In patients with neurologic compromise, open surgery may be required.

Open surgery is indicated in osteoporotic patients only in the context of significant or progressive neurologic deficit or deformity. Operative intervention is associated with high morbidity and mortality in this frail patient population. Similarly, spinal instrumentation systems often fail in osteoporotic bone. Often, combined anterior and posterior surgeries are required to achieve adequate fixation. Screws can be augmented with PMMA to increase their pull-out strength.

## Results and Outcomes

Based on population-wide studies, it is becoming increasingly evident that any VCF can have significant functional and physiologic effects, such as:

- Acute and chronic pain
- Recurrent fracture
- Kyphotic deformity
- Gastrointestinal dysfunction
- Pulmonary dysfunction
- Functional decline
- Increased hospitalization rates
- Increased mortality

Acute VCFs are variably painful. Although some patients note only mild and transient symptoms, others require hospitalization. Although most patients report significant symptomatic improvement in the first 4 weeks, the period of acute pain can persist for months. When the acute pain subsides, chronic pain disorders can develop. Many of these disorders seem to arise from the change in the sagittal balance of the spine. Some patients report painful rubbing of the ribs on the ilium. The risk of developing chronic pain increases with the number of VCFs.

This pain is intensified with many typically daily activities, such as standing, sitting, or bending. In many patients, standing tolerance decreases to only a few minutes. Pain is relieved on lying down, but the increase in bed rest, just as in patients with acute fractures, serves only to accelerate bone loss.

Increased kyphosis and VCF are associated with decreased truncal strength and with greater back-related disability, annual number of bed days, and annual number of limited-activity days. This loss of strength and decrease in activity level increases the risk of additional fractures. Various studies have cited increased risks of additional spinal fractures from 5 to 25 times baseline. Similarly the risk of hip fracture increases five times in patients sustaining VCF. In one study of physical function, common tasks, such as walking, bending, dressing, carrying bags, climbing stairs, rising from supine position, and rising from seated position, were assessed. Only 13% of VCF patients were able to accomplish these activities without difficulty, 40% had difficulty, and 47% required assistance.

The deformity associated with each of these fracture types may have multiple physiologic implications. Taken together, the osteoporotic body habitus is characterized by loss of height and thoracic hyperkyphosis (the dowager's hump). Abdominal protuberance and loss of lumbar lordosis also may be noted. Many otherwise active, elderly patients complain bitterly about the cosmetic effects. Women sustaining osteoporotic vertebral compression fractures report many debilitating psychological effects, including poor body image and self-esteem, depression, and anxiety. Beyond the cosmetic effects, compression on the abdominal viscera by the rib cage or by loss of height through the lumbar spine leads to decreased appetite, early satiety, and weight loss. Similarly, thoracic hyperkyphosis leads to compression of the lungs, decreased pulmonary function, and an increased risk of pulmonary death.

The risk of neurologic deficit after VCF is not known. Although uncommon, deficits are not as rare as first thought. Tardy neurologic decline may occur 18 months from the initial injury. These late neurologic changes are thought to represent dysfunction of the spinal cord as it drapes over the apex of kyphosis. The 5-year survival after osteoporotic spinal fracture is significantly worse than for age-matched peers (61% versus 76%) and is comparable to, or slightly worse than, survival rates after hip fracture. Mortality risk increases with the number of fractures.

One of the goals of VBA procedures is to interrupt the cycle of decline seen in patients with VCF. There are no randomized trials yet comparing nonoperative management with VBA. Many case series have shown, however, that vertebroplasty and kyphoplasty procedures tend to be well tolerated and associated with 70% to 95% pain relief.

In 2001, Grados et al reported the first long-term outcomes of osteoporotic VCF treated by percutaneous vertebroplasty. On a 100-mm visual analogue scale, pain decreased significantly from a mean of 80 mm to 37 mm at 1 month. Results were stable over time. There were no severe treatment-related complications. The vertebral deformity did not progress in any of the injected vertebrae. A slight, but significant, increase in adjacent segment fracture risk was reported. Garfin et al noted that 95% of patients treated with either kyphoplasty or vertebroplasty could expect significant improvement in pain and functional status. Kyphoplasty conferred the additional advantage of 50% increase in vertebral height. Lieberman et al reported the use of kyphoplasty inflatable bone tamp in the treatment of symptomatic VCF in 70 consecutive procedures in 30 patients. There were no major technique-related complications. A mean 47% height restoration was encountered in 70% of the fractures. Bodily pain and physical function scores showed significant improvement.

Vertebroplasty and kyphoplasty are associated with the same types of complications. There are no unique complications reported from use of the balloon tamp or from attempted reduction. Complications can be categorized into medical, anesthesia, instrument placement, and PMMA problems. Failure to improve, in most cases, is due to inappropriate patient selection. In any spinal procedure, concordance between the history, physical examination, and imaging findings improves outcome. The more diffuse the patient's pain, the less likely the patient is to benefit from VBA. Placement of PMMA may increase the risk of adjacent segment fracture. The correction of proper weight-bearing axis with kyphoplasty may decrease the risk of additional fracture.

Medical and anesthesia problems are not unusual in this elderly patient population, but VBA procedures are not significantly physiologically taxing. Technical errors related to misplacement of the vertebroplasty or kyphoplasty instrumentation are more likely. Quality imaging and meticulous surgical technique with frequent evaluation of anteroposterior and lateral fluoroscopy decrease these risks. The most devastating complications of VBA procedures result from PMMA extravasation. In vertebroplasty, a 6% leak risk per level has been identified. Most of these leaks are asymptomatic. One potential benefit of kyphoplasty is the placement of more viscous cement into a cavity of known volume. High-quality, live image intensification during placement, additional radiopacifying agent, avoidance of high-risk fracture patients, and placement of viscous PMMA decrease these risks.

# SUGGESTED READING

Baba H, Maezawa Y, Kamitani K, et al. Osteoporotic vertebral collapse with late neurological complications. Paraplegia 1995;33: 281–289.

Cooper C. The crippling consequences of fractures and their impact on quality of life. Am J Med 1997;103:12S–19S.

Garfin SR, Yuan HA, Reiley MA. New technologies in spine: kyphoplasty and vertebroplasty for the treatment of painful osteoporotic compression fractures. Spine 2001;26:511–515.

Heggeness MH. Spine fracture with neurological deficit in osteoporosis. Osteoporos Int 1993;3:215–221.

Kado DM, Browner WS, Palermo L, et al. Vertebral fractures and mortality in older women: a prospective study. Arch Intern Med 1999;159:1215–1220.

Lieberman IH, Dudeney S, Reinhardt MK, Bell G. Initial outcome and efficacy of "kyphoplasty" in the treatment of painful osteoporotic vertebral compression fractures. Spine 2001;26:1631–1638.

Myers ER, Wilson SE. Biomechanics of osteoporosis and vertebral fracture. Spine 1997;22:255–315.

Nevitt MC, Ettinger B, Black DM, et al. The association of radiologically detected vertebral fractures with back pain and function: a prospective study. Ann Intern Med 1998;128:793–800.

O'Neill TW, Felsenberg D, Varlow J, et al. The prevalence of vertebral deformity in European men and women. The European Vertebral Osteoporosis Study. J Bone Miner Res 1998;11:1010–1018.

Schlaich C, Minne HW, Bruckner T, et al. Reduced pulmonary function in patients with spinal osteoporotic fractures. Osteoporos Int 1998;8:261–267.

# ANATOMY AND APPROACHES

# 25.1 ANTERIOR AND POSTERIOR CERVICAL APPROACHES

CHRISTOPHER M. BONO

## ANTERIOR (STANDARD) APPROACH TO THE CERVICAL SPINE (C3-7)

### Indications and Contraindications

The anterior approach can be used for a variety of pathologic conditions from C3-7, including:

- Anterior cervical discectomy
- Corpectomy
- Spinal cord decompression
- Bone grafting
- Instrumentation procedures

### Preoperative Planning

Preoperative evaluation should include examination of the carotid pulses (decreased or bruits) and thyroid gland (for thyromegaly, which can inhibit exposure). If previous anterior surgery was performed, the patient must be evaluated carefully for a recurrent laryngeal nerve palsy (using direct laryngoscopy) if the surgeon decides to approach the contralateral side. Appropriate imaging studies should confirm the exact location of the pathology to be approached.

### Technique

A small bump or roll can be placed between the scapulae to extend the neck slightly and drop the shoulders poste-

riorly. The head is rotated about 10 degrees to 15 degrees to the contralateral side. The medial border of the sterno-cleidomastoid (SCM) is palpated and marked. This represents the location of the longitudinal incision, if so desired, which is useful for multilevel, extensile approaches. If one-level or two-level surgery is planned, a transverse incision can be used and is centered over the desired vertebral level, which results in a more cosmetically acceptable scar. Surface landmarks are used to decide on the incision location, as follows:

- Hyoid bone—C3 body
- Thyroid cartilage—C4-5 disc space
- Cricoid cartilage—C6 body

After skin incision, the skin flaps are undermined, and the platysma is identified. It is divided in line with the incision. A plane deep to the platysma is developed to ensure adequate visualization of the medial fascial border of the SCM. The trachea is palpated medially through the overlying strap muscles, which include the sternohyoid and sternothyroid. Dissection, through an investing fascial layer, between the strap muscles and the SCM is developed bluntly.

Staying medial to the carotid sheath (by feeling the pulse), continue blunt dissection in a posteromedial direction toward the spine. The anterior aspect of the spine can be palpated through the alar and prevertebral fascia within this interval (Fig. 25.1-1). The trachea and esophagus are

217

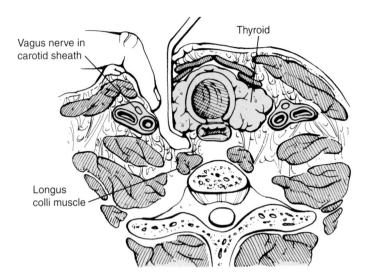

**Figure 25.1-1** Superficially, an interval between the sternocleidomastoid and midline strap muscles is developed. Deeper, dissection proceeds between the carotid sheath (laterally) and the trachea and esophagus (medially).

Vagus nerve in carotid sheath

Thyroid

Longus colli muscle

retracted gently to the contralateral side, allowing visualization of the alar fascia, which overlies the prevertebral fascia. These fascial layers are cut to expose the anterior surface of the spine. A peanut dissector now can be used to sweep the tissue from the midline to reveal the anterior longitudinal ligament, longus colli, and underlying disc spaces. Identification of the disc spaces in the arthritic spine may be impeded by large protruding osteophytes. In general, the disc spaces are located at peaks, whereas the midvertebral bodies are in the "valleys." The correct level can be confirmed with a lateral radiograph by marking the disc space with a spinal needle.

With the desired levels identified, the longus colli is elevated subperiosteally off the anterior cervical body and disc space; this is stopped laterally as soon as the vertebral body starts to turn posteriorly. The vertebral arteries can be injured with more posterolateral exposure. Next, a deep-bladed, self-retaining retractor can be inserted deep to the longus colli with toothed blades on the lateral side and smooth blades on the medial side.

Before closure of the subcutaneous layer and insertion of a drain, the wound is irrigated copiously with normal saline, and the esophagus is inspected for possible injury. Indigo carmine (or blue food coloring) can be infused orally into the esophagus to show subtle tears. The skin can be closed with a running 4-0 subcuticular stitch.

## Postoperative Care

After short procedures, the patient usually can be extubated safely in the operating room. After longer procedures, extubation may be delayed until airway swelling has resolved. The need and type of postoperative immobilization are determined by the stability of the spine. Prophylactic antibiotics are administered for 24 to 48 hours. Drains are removed when the output is less than 10 mL per 8-hour period.

## Complications

Dysphonia, from recurrent laryngeal nerve (RLN) or superior laryngeal nerve injury, occurs in about 4% to 5% of cases. The risk of RLN palsy is extremely low with surgery performed above C5. The RLN is thought to be at more risk in the following situations:

- Right-sided versus left-sided surgery (slight, probably insignificant)
- Exposure below C5 (significant)
- Revision surgery (10% of cases)

On the left side, the RLN is located more consistently within the carotid sheath and has less medial-lateral variability than on the right side. Although the left RLN descends in a fairly consistent manner to loop under the arch of the aorta, the right RLN does not extend as far distal before looping around the subclavian artery back toward the larynx. Despite these anatomic differences, a study showed no difference in the incidence of RLN palsy between right-sided and left-sided exposure.

Horner's syndrome can arise from injury to the sympathetic plexus, which lies on top of the longus colli muscle and is at most risk at C6. It is diagnosed clinically by the presence of:

- Ptosis (drooping eyelid)
- Meiosis (papillary constriction)
- Anhydrosis (dry eye)

Unrecognized esophageal tears can be a cause of late wound infection. The risk of infection after uncomplicated anterior cervical spine surgery is less than 1%.

# TRANSORAL (TRANSPHARYNGEAL) APPROACH TO THE UPPER CERVICAL SPINE

## Indications and Contraindications

Direct anterior exposure of the upper cervical spine can be achieved through a transoral approach. It is used most often to excise or débride infections and tumors (i.e., odontoidectomy). It allows access to the anterior aspects of C1-2 articulations, dens, and, with some extension, the anterior occipitocervical junction and upper body of C3. The approach is contraindicated in the presence of active oral infection or maxillomandibular pathology, which would inhibit adequate exposure.

## Preoperative Planning

Oral cavity and dental infection should be detected and treated preoperatively. The mouth should be examined for loose teeth and the integrity of the posterior oropharyngeal membranes. Jaw mobility should be assessed because it can be a limiting factor to visualization. Macroglossia, which occurs with some syndromic conditions, can make lingual retraction difficult and may necessitate midline division (the so-called tongue-splitting approach) for adequate exposure. Preoperative sagittal magnetic resonance imaging or computed tomography reconstructions can be used to determine the location of the hard palate and glossal muscles, which influence the extent of attainable exposure.

## Technique

The patient is positioned supine. Endotracheal intubation is preferred because nasotracheal intubation leaves the tube crossing the surgical field in front of the oropharynx. Slight Trendelenburg position can help prevent migration of irrigant and debris into the patient's airway during the procedure, in addition to an adequate seal around the endotracheal tube cuff balloon. Antibiotic prophylaxis should include gram-negative coverage.

A specially designed, rectangular, self-retaining retractor should be used to keep the mouth open and the tongue depressed inferiorly. The incision can be determined by landmarks and intraoperative radiographs. The C2-3 disc space is palpable near the inferior aspect of the oral cavity; the anterior C1 ring often can be palpated superiorly. If in doubt, a spinal needle can be inserted and a lateral radiograph obtained.

The four fascial layers (pharyngeal mucosa, pharyngeal constrictor muscles, buccopharyngeal fascia, and prevertebral fascia) are incised as one layer down to the bone of the vertebrae. Then the fascia is stripped subperiosteally laterally as a unit with a periosteal elevator until the lateral masses of the C1-2 joints are exposed. The soft palate can be retracted cranially to expose the anterior atlantooccipital membrane (the occipital insertion of the anterior longitudinal ligament, which stems from the superior C1 ring to the foramen magnum) and the apical ligament (which projects from the odontoid process to the foramen magnum). Inferior retraction of the tongue may give access to the C3 body and the C3-4 disc space. Exposure of these structures is provided better by other approaches, however.

After the bone work has been completed, the wound is irrigated copiously with saline-antibiotic solution. Closure should be watertight because this is thought to be a major factor in decreasing the incidence of postoperative infection using this approach.

## Postoperative Care

A nasogastric drain helps minimize the chances for aspiration after extubation. The patient routinely remains intubated for at least 24 hours until oral swelling has resolved. Early tracheostomy might be considered if prolonged intubation is likely.

## Complications

Transoral exposure crosses an inherently unsterile field. The infection risk is relatively high. Early reports, published before the routine use of perioperative antibiotics, documented infection rates of 66%. Larger contemporary series documented rates of 0% to 3%, similar to other cervical approaches. Specific antibiotic prophylaxis, multilayer closure, and avoidance of spinal implants are thought to be responsible for the lower infection rates.

Fracture or loosening of the teeth, laceration of the tongue, and injury to the gingiva are other potential complications. Aspiration of debris and secretions can occur if the endotracheal balloon cuff seal is lost during or after surgery. Early extubation (<24 hours) may lead to acute respiratory distress, necessitating emergent reintubation that may risk neurologic compromise in an unstable spine.

# ANTERIOR APPROACH TO THE CERVICOTHORACIC JUNCTION (C7-T3)

## Indications and Contraindications

Although most commonly used for tumors, the anterior approach to the cervicothoracic junction can be used for anterior corpectomy, discectomy, or osteotomy for fractures, herniated discs, infection, or deformities. Because the upper thoracic vertebrae are accessed with inferior retraction of the arch of the aorta, congenital anomalies of the great vessels may be a relative contraindication.

## Preoperative Planning

Lesions from T3 and above can be accessed readily, whereas T4 lesions may be approached better through a high thoracotomy. Sagittal magnetic resonance imaging can show the axial relationship of the manubrium, sternum, and clavicle to the upper thoracic and lower cervical vertebrae. An unusually high manubrium in relation to the spine can preclude adequate exposure of the desired levels, making a transsternal approach preferable.

## Technique

An L-shaped incision is made. The midline portion of the incision is made from midsternum to 1 cm above the sternal notch. The incision is carried laterally, usually to the left side, along a line about 1 cm proximal to the midpoint of the clavicle.

The sternum and clavicle are exposed by subperiosteal dissection along their anterior surfaces. The two heads of the SCM are visualized inserting deep to the bones. The tendons are released from their bone attachments, and their ends are tagged and retracted superiorly. Next, the sternohyoid and sternothyroid tendons are visualized, dissected, tagged, transected as far distally as possible, and reflected proximally. A small area of fatty tissue beneath the sternal notch is visualized and removed using a peanut dissector.

The medial third of the clavicle and a rectangular section of manubrium are resected carefully. The contralateral sternoclavicular joint should be left intact. Deep to the periosteal layer is the subclavian vein and the thymus. The spine is accessed proximally using the standard anterior retropharyngeal approach. The interval between the carotid sheath and the trachea/esophagus is continued carefully caudally by blunt dissection along the anterior surface of the spine. A narrow Deaver-type retractor is placed at the inferior aspect of the wound to retract the subclavian vein and arch of the aorta. At the completion of the procedure, the wound is irrigated, and the strap and SCM muscles are reapproximated to the remaining periosteal sleeve.

## Complications

The RLN is more at risk with right-sided approaches because it often crosses the operative field in the lower cervical spine. The thoracic duct is at greater risk with left-sided approaches. It lies lateral to the carotid sheath, deep to the subclavian artery and vein, and should be suture ligated proximally and distally to prevent chylothorax if injured.

# POSTERIOR APPROACH: OCCIPUT TO T1

## Indications and Contraindications

The posterior approach is extensile because it can be used to expose from the occiput to the sacrum. It is indicated for a variety of diagnoses and is useful for the following:

- Insertion of instrumentation and fusion
- Decompressive procedures, such as laminectomy or laminoplasty

Posterior surgery is contraindicated as a method of removing anterior neurocompressive pathology, such as midline herniated discs and abscesses.

## Preoperative Planning

A preoperative neurologic exam should be done just before surgery. An awake, fiberoptic intubation is recommended if the spine is unstable.

## Technique

A midline incision is made over the desired region. Dissection is carried through the subcutaneous tissue to the trapezius fascia. The fascia is incised, and dissection proceeds through the relatively avascular plane within the ligamentum nuchae. With the tips of the spinous processes exposed, dissection is taken laterally to maintain the interspinous ligaments. One of the spinous processes can be marked with a clamp to confirm intraoperative radiographic identification of the correct level. Subperiosteal dissection is carried over the spinous processes and laminae, elevating the paraspinal muscles off the bone. Care is taken to leave the facet capsule intact until, or if, exposure and decortication for fusion has been decided at that level.

In the occipitocervical region, the ring of C1 should not be exposed more than 1.5 cm from the midline for risk of

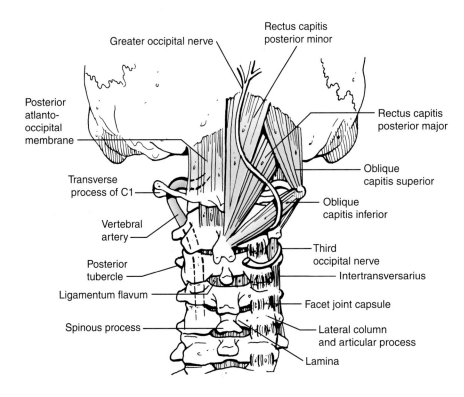

Greater occipital nerve
Rectus capitis posterior minor
Posterior atlanto-occipital membrane
Rectus capitis posterior major
Transverse process of C1
Oblique capitis superior
Vertebral artery
Oblique capitis inferior
Posterior tubercle
Third occipital nerve
Intertransversarius
Ligamentum flavum
Facet joint capsule
Spinous process
Lateral column and articular process
Lamina

**Figure 25.1-2** Dissection beyond 1.5 cm from the midline of the C1 ring risks injury to the vertebral artery. Lateral dissection or retraction at the level of the external occipital protuberance risks injury to the greater occipital nerve (sensation to the back of the head). Care must be taken to maintain instruments at the subperiosteal level.

injury to the vertebral artery (Fig. 25.1-2). Lateral dissection or retraction at the level of the external occipital protuberance risks injury to the greater occipital nerve (sensation to the back of the head). Care must be taken to maintain instruments at the subperiosteal level. The wound is irrigated with copious amounts of warmed normal saline solution. If desired, a medium-sized drain can be placed deep to the fascia layer. Closure of all layers (muscle, fascia, subcutaneous tissue, and skin) is routine.

## Postoperative Care

As with any surgery, postoperative immobilization is decided based on cervical stability. External methods may not be needed if rigid internal fixation was implanted. Prophylactic antibiotic coverage is continued for 24 to 48 hours after surgery. Drain outputs tend to be higher than after anterior cervical procedures. They are removed when outputs are less than 30 to 40 mL per 8-hour shift but should not remain more than 48 hours.

## SUGGESTED READING

Beutler WJ, Sweeney CA, Connolly PJ. Recurrent laryngeal nerve injury with anterior cervical spine surgery: risk with laterality of surgical approach. Spine 2001;26:1337–1342.
Ebraheim NA, Lu J, Yang H, et al. Vulnerability of the sympathetic trunk during the anterior approach to the lower cervical spine. Spine 2000;13:1603–1606.
Fang H, Ong G. Direct anterior approach to the upper cervical spine. J Bone Joint Surg 1962;44A:1588.
Hoppenfeld S, deBoer P. Surgical exposures in orthopaedics. Philadelphia: JB Lippincott, 1994.
Kurz L, Pursel S, Herkowitz H. Modified anterior approach to the cervicothoracic junction. Spine 1991;16:S542–S547.
Lu J, Ebraheim NA, Nadim Y, et al. Anterior approach to the cervical spine: surgical anatomy. Orthopedics 2000;23:841–845.
McAfee PC, Bohlman HH, Riley LH, et al. The anterior retropharyngeal approach to the upper part of the cervical spine. J Bone Joint Surg 1987;69A:1371–1383.
Merwin G, Post J, Sypert G. Transoral approach to the upper cervical spine. Laryngoscope 1991;101:780–784.
Netterville JL, Koriwchak MJ, Winkle M, et al. Vocal fold paralysis following the anterior approach to the cervical spine. Ann Otol Rhinol Laryngol 1996;105:85–91.
Succo G, Solini A, Crosetti E, et al. Enlarged approach to the anterior cervical spine. J Laryngol Otol 2001;115:994–997.

# 25.2 ANTERIOR THORACIC AND LUMBAR APPROACHES

**PAUL C. LIU ▪ HANSEN A. YUAN**

When an anterior approach to the thoracic or lumbar spine is required to address spinal pathology, the vertebral levels that require exposure determine the options for surgical access. The anterior approach should be considered for spinal pathology involving the anterior and middle columns of the spine in Denis' three-column model. The mechanical advantages achieved with anterior reconstruction of the load-bearing capabilities of the spine are significant. Indications for surgery via the anterior approach mostly fall into the following six categories:

- Trauma
- Infection
- Tumor
- Degenerative disc disease
- Iatrogenic causes
- Deformity

For the thoracic spine, we describe thoracotomy and thoracoscopy. For the lumbar spine, we describe retroperitoneal-flank incision, retroperitoneal-medial incision, transabdominal, and laparoscopic/endoscopic approaches.

## TRANSTHORACIC AND TRANSDIAPHRAGMATIC APPROACHES

The transthoracic approach provides exposure from T2-12. This approach provides the best exposure to the midthoracic vertebral bodies; the view at the cephalad and caudal extremes of the thoracic segments is more limited. The relatively narrow thoracic inlet and scapula limit the view in the cephalad direction. The diaphragm limits the view of the caudal vertebral bodies, unless the diaphragm is detached as part of the dissection (see later under approach to thoracolumbar junction). This approach can provide excellent anterior exposure of the thecal sac, multiple vertebral bodies are exposed easily, and instrumentation across multiple levels can be performed readily. Only the contralateral pedicles and posterior elements are inaccessible in this approach. The main disadvantage of this approach is the increased pulmonary and chest wall morbidity of thoracotomy compared with thoracoscopy or posterolateral, extrapulmonary approaches. Another drawback is that a posterior approach is required to address additional posterior spinal pathology and for placement of posterior instrumentation.

Although most procedures on the thoracic spine can be approached from the left or right side, many surgeons advocate the use of a left-sided approach because of the relative ease and safety of mobilizing and retracting on the aorta versus the vena cava or the azygos venous system. For upper thoracic lesions (T2-6), a right-sided thoracotomy is preferred because the left side of the upper thoracic spine is less accessible owing to the location of the aortic arch and great vessels. For lower thoracic and thoracolumbar lesions (T7-L2), a left-sided thoracotomy is preferred because it is technically easier to mobilize the aorta, and liver retraction is avoided. Within these generalizations, the side of the approach should allow maximal exposure of the pathology being treated.

## Operative Technique

### Transthoracic

After induction of endotracheal general anesthesia, the patient is placed in the full lateral decubitus position with the side to be operated in the up position. The thoracic spine now is oriented perpendicular to the floor to facilitate safer spinal cord decompression and hardware placement into vertebral bodies. For approaches to the upper thoracic to midthoracic spine (T2-8), the use of a double-lumen endotracheal tube allows for selective lung ventilation, maximizing lung deflation on the operated side to facilitate spine exposure. For lesions below T8, a double-lumen tube usually is not necessary. Fluoroscopy or plain radiographs are taken to mark the appropriate vertebral level and to plan the incision. The rib level may be identified by palpating and counting ribs from distal to proximal.

A curved skin incision is made from the anterior axillary line, below the angle of the scapula, to the border of the paraspinous muscles posteriorly for exposure of upper thoracic lesions. For midthoracic to lower thoracic lesions, the incision generally is made over the rib one to two levels above the vertebral level of interest. For thoracolumbar lesions, the incision is made over the 10th or 11th rib.

The latissimus dorsi, serratus anterior, and posterior muscles are divided in line with the skin incision (Fig. 25.2-1). For upper thoracic exposures, part of the trapezius and rhomboid muscles are divided, and the scapula is retracted anteriorly and superiorly to facilitate deep exposure. Subperiosteal dissection of the rib is performed, and care is taken to avoid injury to the neurovascular bundle in the subcostal groove on the inferior surface of the rib. The rib is resected from the costochondral junction anteriorly to the angle of the rib posteriorly, about 3 to 4 cm from the rib head. With intrapleural exposures, the chest is entered through the rib bed periosteum, the underlying endothoracic chest wall fascia, and the parietal pleura. The ribs are spread using a self-retaining thoracotomy retractor (i.e., Finochietto retractor). The lung is deflated, and deep retractors are placed to expose the vertebral bodies.

Unless grossly diseased, the vertebral bodies and discs are covered by a glistening parietal pleura. The intervertebral discs protrude prominently (the "mounds"), and the vertebral bodies between are relatively concave (the "valleys"). After appropriate levels are confirmed radiographi-

cally and anatomically by counting ribs, a pleural flap is elevated to expose the spine. The segmental vessels are ligated, if necessary, at the midpoint of the vertebral body. The anastomotic vascular arcade in the region of the proximal neural foramen should be preserved to decrease the risk of ischemic thoracic spinal cord complications. The vascular watershed area of the thoracic spinal cord is located between T5-9. The artery of Adamkiewicz, the largest of the thoracic radicular feeder arteries, usually is found on the left side at the level of T10, but this anatomy is variable. The sympathetic trunk lies at the level of the costovertebral articulation, lateral to the prominent rib head. The intended operation on the thoracic spine is carried out.

### Transdiaphragmatic

In the transdiaphragmatic approach to the thoracolumbar junction to expose the lower thoracic spine to the upper lumbar spine, the skin incision is made in the region of the 10th or 11th rib. This incision is carried more obliquely and ventrally, depending on the caudal exposure required. The 10th or 11th rib is exposed and resected, and the lower chest cavity is entered in a standard fashion. The costal cartilage is split longitudinally, allowing access to the preperitoneal fat layer that lies caudal to the diaphragm and is contiguous with the rostral aspect of the retroperitoneal space (Fig. 25.2-2). The costal cartilage is tagged with suture for repair during wound closure. The peritoneum is cleared from the undersurface of the diaphragm using a sponge stick, avoiding entry into the peritoneal cavity. Rents in the peritoneum should be repaired with absorbable suture. The diaphragm is kept under tension, and a circumferential incision is made along its peripheral attachment to the costal margin, leaving a generous 2-cm cuff of diaphragm muscle for later repair. The diaphragm muscle can be marked with suture to facilitate repair during closure. The spleen, kidney, and stomach are retracted medially using a broad, padded, malleable retractor. The left crus of the diaphragm is tagged with suture and cut at its attachment to the anterior longitudinal ligament at L1 and L2. The vertebral bodies of the thoracolumbar junction are visualized. The great vessels are protected carefully with malleable retractors. Segmental vessels are identified and ligated at the level of the midvertebral body. The psoas muscle is retracted posteriorly. Then the intended operation on the spine is carried out. A right-sided approach to the thoracolumbar junction may be required in unusual cases (e.g., tumorous involvement of the right-side L1 vertebral body and pedicle). The right-sided approach is similar to the left-sided approach except that care should be taken to retract the liver and great venous structures on the right side. After the spinal procedure is completed, the diaphragm should be reattached accurately to the cuff of diaphragm on the costal margin. The crus should be reattached to the anterior longitudinal ligament. The costal cartilage is repaired.

For wound closure, a chest tube is placed posteriorly in the chest cavity, directed superiorly toward the apex, and brought out below the incision. The lung is reinflated. The adjacent ribs are reapproximated and secured using heavy absorbable suture. The rib bed is reapproximated to reestablish a pleural seal. Superficial muscles and soft tissue are closed in anatomic layers.

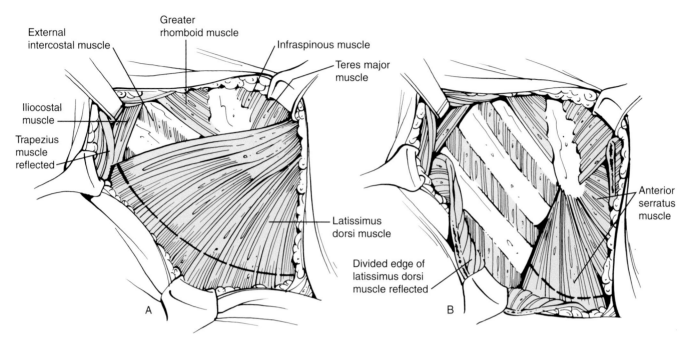

**Figure 25.2-1** The first step of the transthoracic approach is incision of the skin and subcutaneous fascia. This exposes the underlying muscles (**A**), which, for most exposures, is the latissimus dorsi. This muscle is divided in line with the incision to expose the underlying ribs and intercostal muscles (**B**).

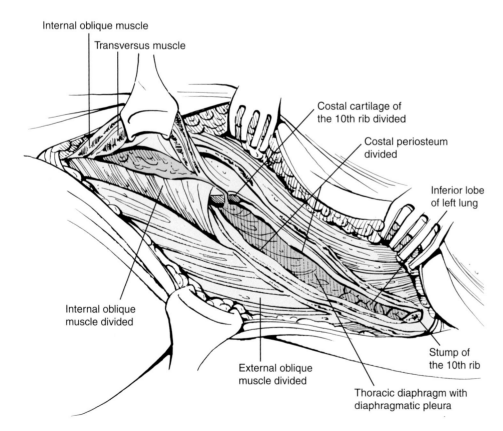

**Figure 25.2-2** The 10th rib has been resected. After resection of the costal cartilage, exposure of the thoracolumbar junction is afforded.

Pulmonary complications are most common with transthoracic approaches. Atelectasis, pneumonia, pleural effusions, and airway obstruction are possible complications. Chest wall discomfort is significant after thoracotomy, and 10% of patients experience chronic chest wall pain. Congestive heart failure and pulmonary edema can occur, related to excessive fluid replacement in susceptible patients.

Spinal cord injury is possible, especially during cases involving corrective osteotomy. Anterior spinal artery syndromes have been reported after scoliosis correction or circumferential spinal osteotomy.

### Thoracoabdominal

The thoracoabdominal approach adds significantly to the risk of surgery because two major body cavities are exposed. In addition to specific complications related to thoracotomy, injury to the spleen, kidney, or ureter may occur during surgical dissection or retraction. Ileus may develop postoperatively. Injury to the sympathetic chain may produce asymmetric warmth of the involved extremity, but this rarely is a problem for the patient. Careful closure of the peritoneum and diaphragm prevents herniation of visceral structures. Combined thoracoabdominal exposure should be reserved for patients with satisfactory cardiopulmonary reserves who are likely to tolerate the surgical risks.

Rapid mobilization and early involvement by physiatrists and physical therapists are important for these patients. Rapid mobilization prevents pulmonary complications and decreases the risk of postoperative thromboembolic complications.

# THORACOSCOPIC APPROACH TO THE SPINE

Video-assisted thoracoscopic exposure of the lateral thoracic spine was introduced by Regan in the early 1990s (Mack et al, 1993). Since then, the field of endoscopic spine surgery has been expanding at a rapid rate. The main benefit of these "minimal incision" techniques is to lessen the "approach-related" trauma associated with the classic open surgical approaches. Because endoscopy requires only small incisions, the level of postoperative pain and length of hospital stay are less than with traditional open procedures. Patients experience less chronic chest wall discomfort and improved cosmesis with the endoscopic technique.

The major disadvantage of video-assisted thoracoscopic surgery (VATS) is the steep learning curve. The basic anatomy and dissection techniques are familiar to most spine surgeons. Significant adaptation of thoracoscopic surgical techniques using longer tools, restricted access, and new methods of perceiving, visualizing, illuminating, and magnifying the operative site create distinct technical challenges, however. Refinement of surgical techniques and instruments has expanded the use of VATS in spine care to include many procedures that previously could be performed only by open approaches (Table 25.2-1).

A double-lumen tube to allow one-lung ventilation is required for VATS. This procedure is contraindicated in patients who cannot tolerate one-lung ventilation. Another contraindication to VATS is pleural adhesions. Extensive scarring from a previous operation at the site of spinal pathology also may preclude thoracoscopic techniques.

## Operative Technique

The thoracic spine can be approached from the right or the left side, depending on the location and eccentricity of the spinal lesion. Thoracoscopically, exposure from T1-2 to the T12-L1 interspace is possible. A right-sided approach is preferred when possible because more spinal surface area is available behind the azygos vein than behind the aorta. If exposure is needed from T10-12, a left-sided approach is preferred because the liver causes the right diaphragm to ride higher, limiting visibility to the spine.

After a right-sided or left-sided approach is chosen, the patient is positioned in the lateral decubitus position as described for a transthoracic approach. The surgeon should be prepared to convert to open thoracotomy if thoracoscopic methods fail. Video monitors are placed on both sides of the patient so that the surgeon and assistants can see the thoracoscopic image.

Specialized tools used for thoracoscopic surgery include the following:

- 1-cm rigid rod lens endoscope (0-degree and 30-degree angle field of view)
- FRED antifog solution
- Harmonic scalpel (high-frequency coagulator)
- Suction/irrigation apparatus
- Endoscopic fan retractor

Additionally, specialized instruments designed for operating on the thoracic spine, which is 14 to 30 cm from the surface of the skin, are required, including the following:

- Cobb elevator
- Rib dissector
- Rib cutter
- Pituitary rongeurs
- Graspers
- Nerve hooks
- Osteotomes
- Microscissors
- DeBakey type forceps
- Right-angle tissue forceps
- Peanut dissectors
- Bone graft impactors

Long drill bits with protective sleeves are required to remove bone. A robotic arm can hold the thoracoscope during surgery.

Usually three or four portals are required to operate in one area of the thoracic spine. The first portal is made in the sixth or seventh intercostal space in the anterior axillary line. The portals are created to minimize the risk of injury. First, the lung is deflated on the operated side. The skin incision is made directly over the intercostal entry sites. Blunt finger dissection directly on top of the rib prevents injury to the intercostal neurovascular bundle. A blunt puncture of the parietal pleura allows finger feel and dissection to ensure that the lung is not adherent at the portal site. Then a flexible trocar is introduced, and a 1-cm diame-

## TABLE 25.2-1  INDICATIONS FOR THORACOSCOPIC SURGERY OF THE SPINE

| Infection | Tumor | Degenerative | Deformity | Trauma | Other |
|---|---|---|---|---|---|
| Biopsy<br>Debridement<br>Spinal abscess, drainage | Biopsy<br>Excision (e.g., metastatic, dumbbell)<br>Corpectomy and grafting<br>Internal fixation | Excision of herniated disc<br>Fusion for discogenic pain | Anterior release for rigid scoliosis >75°<br>Anterior release and fusion for Scheuermann's kyphosis >90°<br>Anterior epiphysiodesis to prevent crank-shaft phenomenon<br>Anterior arthrodesis for congenital anomalies or neuromuscular deformities | Fracture repair<br>Decompression fusion<br>Internal fixation | Thoracoplasty<br>Rib excision for thoracic outlet syndrome |

From Zdeblick. TA, Endoscopic approaches to the anterior thoracic spine. In: Zdeblick. TA, Anterior approaches to the spine. St. Louis, Quality Medical Publishing, 1999:129.

ter rigid-rod endoscope with a 0-degree or 30-degree angled lens is inserted for visualization. A flexible trocar decreases the risk of postoperative portal pain compared with rigid trocars. Additional portals are placed strategically for retraction of lung tissue, for placement of working instruments, and for placement of implants. Portals are placed far enough apart to prevent "fencing" of the instruments, and the portal placement should triangulate over the area of the spine being worked on (Fig. 25.2-3).

In the case of thoracoscopic discectomy for illustration, important structures are noted as in a right-sided approach. The azygos vein and pulsatile aorta lie anteriorly. The second rib can be visualized in the apex of the lung. The "mounds" of the spine represent the intervertebral discs, and the "valleys" represent the vertebral bodies. The segmental vessels lie in the valleys. After confirmation of the appropriate spinal disc level using a marking needle and radiography, the pleura is incised longitudinally. If necessary, the segmental vessels may be ligated away from the neuroforamen with the harmonic scalpel. The sympathetic chain lies lateral to the prominent rib head. The rib head directs the surgeon to the disc space, and 2 cm of the rib head is removed by dissecting it free from the stout costovertebral and costotransverse ligaments. (The T9 rib head leads to the T8-9 disc space, and so on.) The superior portion of the pedicle can be removed with a high-speed drill or Kerrison rongeur. Stabilization of working instruments against the chest wall promotes safety. The lateral aspect of the thecal sac is visualized so that the disc herniation can be removed safely. Absolutely clear visualization must be maintained during decompression of the spinal cord. After discectomy, the rib head provides adequate bone for interbody fusion, with or without instrumentation.

For closure, the pleural flaps may be approximated if desired. A small chest tube is placed under direct vision in the posterior chest cavity directed toward the apex. Lung reinflation is observed to check for air leaks. Portals are removed, and the wounds are closed in layers to prevent air leak. The chest tube is connected to water seal or suction. A postoperative chest radiograph is taken to rule out pneumothorax and to check graft/hardware placement.

Potential intraoperative complications are related to the anatomy. Any structure of the mediastinum and thorax is at risk. Cardiac arrhythmias are prevented by avoiding use

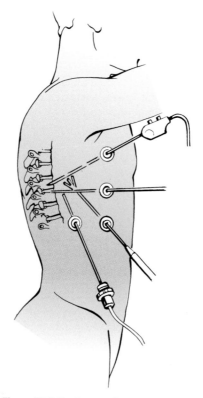

**Figure 25.2-3**  During thoracoscopic spine surgery, the portals should be placed far enough apart to prevent "fencing" of the instruments, while allowing triangulation over the operative area.

of monopolar cautery near the heart. Fan retractors can lacerate the lung if not used carefully. Neurologic complications and spinal cord injuries can occur. The surgeon always must be prepared to obtain hemostasis if a great vessel injury should occur: A 4 × 4 sponge stick and a thoracotomy tray should be immediately available. One must never "plunge" with any instruments to avoid catastrophic great vessel injury.

Potential postoperative complications include the following:

- Pneumothorax
- Hemothorax
- Chylothorax
- Atelectasis
- Pneumonia
- Neurologic injury
- Intercostal neuralgia
- Infection
- Spinal instability
- Fixation-related problems

Despite the use of the thoracoscopic technique, aggressive pulmonary physiotherapy is required to decrease the risk of serious pulmonary complications.

# RETROPERITONEAL APPROACH TO THE LUMBAR SPINE

## Flank Incision

The retroperitoneal approach is ideal for access to the midlumbar spine (L2-5). A left-sided approach is preferred because the thin-walled inferior vena cava usually does not tolerate the degree of manipulation that the aorta does. In addition, liver retraction is avoided with a left-sided approach. It provides broad exposure of the lumbar spine with less risk to the viscera and great vessels compared with the transperitoneal approach. This approach provides unilateral exposure of the lumbar spine. When bilateral exposure of the lumbar spine is required, a supine-position medial incision retroperitoneal approach or a supine-position transperitoneal approach is used.

### Operative Technique

The patient is positioned in a right lateral decubitus position with the left side tilted upward 60 degrees (Fig. 25.2-4). Beanbags provide support for the torso and hips. The break in the table should be used to widen the space between the iliac crest and ribs. The right leg is kept straight, and the left hip is flexed to relax the ipsilateral iliopsoas muscle to facilitate retraction. Intraoperative radiographs are used to localize the appropriate vertebral levels and to plan the location of the skin incision.

First, the latissimus dorsi and posterior inferior serratus are incised. The external oblique fascia is identified, and the muscle is opened in line with the skin incision to the lateral border of the rectus fascia. The internal oblique and transversus abdominis muscles are opened. Deeply the iliocostal muscle is divided partially posteriorly. The transver-

salis fascia is incised to enter the plane of the retroperitoneal space. Carefully the peritoneum is dissected free from the abdominal wall. Dissection of the medially located muscle layers and fascia is more difficult, and peritoneal tears can occur. Tears in the peritoneum are repaired. Posteriorly the peritoneum is dissected free from the inferior pole of the left kidney and from the posterior abdominal wall. A plane between the retroperitoneal organs (e.g., kidney and ureter) and the quadratus lumborum/psoas muscles is developed with blunt dissection. The retroperitoneal organs and peritoneal sac are retracted medially and toward the dependent side using a self-retaining, broad-based, table-mounted retraction system (Bookwalter or Omni self-retaining retractor system). Fluoroscopy or plain radiograph is used to confirm the appropriate spinal level. The psoas muscle is mobilized posteriorly using a Cobb elevator to expose the spine. Care is taken to avoid aggressively mobilizing, retracting, or even transecting the psoas muscle and to avoid damaging critical neural structures—the lumbosacral plexus within the psoas muscle, the genitofemoral nerve (sensation to the scrotum and inner thigh) on the ventral surface of the muscle, and the sympathetic trunk along the medial border of the muscle. Avoiding excessive use of monopolar cautery in this area is important to avoid injury to the sympathetic trunk. Segmental vessels are identified as the neural foramina are approached. If necessary, these vessels are ligated midway between the parent vessel and the foramen to minimize vascular compromise of the neuronal elements. After the segmental vessels are secured, the aorta and iliac vessels are mobilized with a Cobb elevator to expose the ventrolateral surface of the vertebral bodies. The intended operation on the spine is performed. When closing, all peritoneal and retroperitoneal contents are allowed to fall back into normal anatomic position. Abdominal muscle layers are closed anatomically. Skin is closed in the standard fashion.

If upper lumbar (L1-2) exposure is needed, the skin incision is curved proximally to the end of the 11th or 12th rib. After the retroperitoneum is entered, upper lumbar exposure is achieved by retracting the lower pole of the kidney medially and superiorly. After the ureter is mobilized, the left diaphragmatic crus, which extends to the second vertebral body, is taken down.

Vascular, bowel, and ureteral injuries all are possible with the retroperitoneal approach. In revision approaches to the retroperitoneum, preoperative ipsilateral ureteral stenting can help the surgeon identify and avoid ureter injury during dissection. Because one or more major anterior abdominal wall muscles are divided, wound dehiscence, herniation, and hematoma can occur. Unsightly bulging of the abdominal musculature can result postoperatively. The surgeon should be prepared for vascular anomaly, and instruments for dissection and repair of vascular structures always should be available when performing retroperitoneal or transperitoneal approaches. All bowel perforations must be oversewn, usually with the help of a general surgeon. Ureteral injury or delayed ureteral fibrosis can result from excessive manipulation or traction.

## Medial Incision

A medial incision can provide broad bilateral exposure to the midlumbar and lumbosacral regions. Because disc pa-

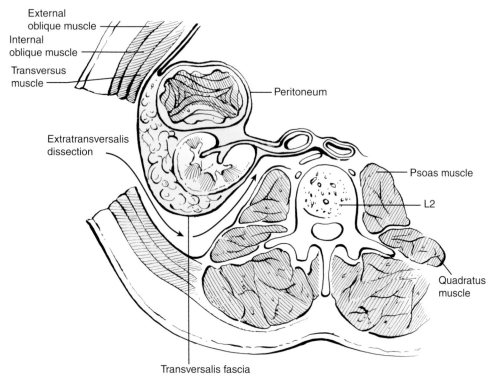

**Figure 25.2-4**   The plane of dissection during a retroperitoneal approach to the lumbar spine.

thology is found most commonly at L5-S1, L4-5, and L3-4 levels, this exposure commonly is required to perform anterior lumbar interbody fusion (ALIF). Insertion of an artificial disc implant (currently undergoing U.S. Food and Drug Administration clinical trials) requires a direct anterior disc exposure that can be provided by this approach. The muscles of the abdominal wall can be spared from transection with this approach. A medial incision also allows for conversion to a transperitoneal approach if necessary. A left-sided approach is described.

## Operative Technique

The patient is positioned supine with the sacrum elevated (either by a bolster or by gently angling the operating table to a Trendelenburg position) to displace the abdominal contents rostrally. Intraoperative fluoroscopy is used to visualize the appropriate lumbar segment in the anteroposterior and lateral projections. This fluoroscopic localization helps to confirm the location of the skin incision and to determine the angle of approach to a particular disc space on the lateral view. A pulse oximeter can be placed on the left great toe to monitor blood flow to the left lower extremity to adjust retractor tension when deep retractors are used to retract the great vessels during deep surgical dissection. A midline, left-sided paramedian, or Pfannenstiel incision can be used. A midline incision along the linea alba decreases the risk of rectus muscle denervation as the rectus muscle is approached medially and is retracted laterally. An incision above the umbilicus allows exposure of L4 and above; an incision below the umbilicus allows for exposure of L4 to S1. An approach to L5-S1 generally requires an incision to

extend to just above the superior aspect of the symphysis pubis. The rectus sheath is entered, and the left rectus muscle is retracted. The transversalis fascia is exposed, and the plane of retroperitoneal approach is entered. Electrocautery is used to cauterize deep epigastric vessels during blunt retroperitoneal dissection. The peritoneal sac is dissected from the abdominal wall using a sponge stick. The inferior part of the posterior rectus sheath is incised to allow better exposure of deeper structures. A table-mounted, self-retaining retractor system (Omni) is used. As the ventral spine is approached, the discs have a convex morphology, and the vertebral bodies have a concave morphology.

The L5-S1 disc space is generally approached below the aortic bifurcation. Injury to the superior hypogastric plexus, which lies directly anterior to the L5 vertebral body and L5-S1 disc space, produces retrograde ejaculation in male patients. The prevertebral tissues, including the superior hypogastric plexus, are displaced en bloc by blunt dissection over the disc space to decrease the risk of hypogastric plexus injury. Use of bipolar electrocautery or vascular clips in this area, instead of monopolar cautery, also reduces the risk of hypogastric plexus injury. The iliac vessels are retracted laterally to expose the L5-S1 disc space. The middle sacral artery and vein, if present, can be ligated using clips or cauterized using bipolar cautery. The intended procedure is performed on the L5-S1 disc.

Most often, the L4-5 and L3-4 disc spaces are approached by mobilizing the great vessels to the right. Lumbar segmental vessels are ligated. The iliolumbar vein must be isolated and doubly ligated to mobilize effectively the great venous structures to the right sufficiently to expose

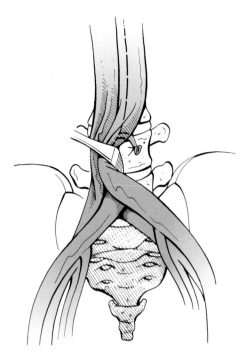

**Figure 25.2-5** The level of the bifurcation of the great vessels can vary, but it usually is located at or near the L5 vertebral body. Direct anterior exposure of the L4-5 disc space usually requires lateral retraction. Ligation of the iliolumbar vein facilitates this maneuver. Exposure of the L5-S1 disc space usually can be performed by working in between the bifurcation.

past the midline to the right side of the disc (Fig. 25.2-5). Lymphatic channels may be entered during this dissection with generally little clinical consequence. Atraumatic retractors are placed to expose the disc space, retracting vascular structures to the right. The intended operation is the performed on the L4-5 or L3-4 or both disc spaces. For closure, the retractors are removed, and the peritoneal sac is allowed to fall back into anatomic position. The abdominal wall fascia is closed securely to prevent hernia formation. The posterior rectus sheath can be left unrepaired. Subcutaneous tissue and skin are closed in layers. Concurrent to the retroperitoneal exposure, a second surgeon can harvest anterior iliac crest bone, if required, through a separate incision.

Retroperitoneal and transperitoneal approaches have similar potential complications. Vascular and bowel injuries are more likely to occur with transperitoneal approaches, whereas ureteral injury occurs more commonly with retroperitoneal approaches. Both approaches are associated with sterility in men secondary to retrograde ejaculation due to inadvertent injury to the superior hypogastric plexus.

# TRANSPERITONEAL APPROACH TO THE LUMBAR SPINE

The transperitoneal approach provides excellent bilateral exposure of the L5-S1 region. It also can be used for expo-

sure of L4-5, but this can be problematic because of the location of the aortic bifurcation. The location of the aortic bifurcation can be determined preoperatively by studying the vessel pattern anterior to the lower lumbar spine as seen on magnetic resonance imaging. L3-4 can be approached by mobilizing the great vessels to the right after ligation of segmental lumbar vessels and the ascending lumbar vein. The transperitoneal approach is contraindicated in the presence of spinal infection.

## Operative Technique

A bowel preparation is employed the day before surgery, and broad-spectrum antibiotics are used preoperatively. The patient is placed in the supine position with the sacrum angled and elevated upward on the operating room table. The Trendelenburg position allows the abdominal contents to shift into the upper abdomen. Skin incision caudal to the umbilicus provides exposure of L5-S1. A midline or transverse (Pfannenstiel's) incision may be used. Fluoroscopy is used to identify the level of the spinal lesion. A small incision of less than 6 cm can be used for exposure of one or two disc spaces, and this "mini-open" approach is adequate for ALIF procedures. The incision is carried down in the midline through the subcutaneous tissues, fascia, and peritoneum. After the abdominal contents are retracted rostrally with a table-mounted, self-retaining retractor, the posterior peritoneum is exposed. The pelvic portion of the colon and its mesentery are retracted to the left, and the ureters are identified and protected. The retroperitoneal space is entered by incising the posterior peritoneum in the midline and extending the peritoneal opening caudally past the aortic bifurcation by following the course of the right common iliac artery to its bifurcation at the external and internal iliac arteries. The right ureter is identified and avoided as it crosses over the right external iliac artery.

The L5 body, L5-S1 disc space, and sacral promontory are palpated easily and visualized below the aortic bifurcation. The prevertebral tissues, including the hypogastric plexus and the middle sacral artery, are identified and mobilized laterally. When a large left common iliac vein hinders access to the body of L5 and the sacral promontory, it must be mobilized properly and protected before the disc space is incised. The left iliac vein occasionally can appear as a flat, white, bloodless ribbon across the L5-S1 disc space. Retrograde ejaculation is one of the significant complications directly resulting from insult to the hypogastric plexus; monopolar cautery should be avoided to reduce risk of damage to the hypogastric plexus. Retractors are placed to expose the L5-S1 disc space (Fig. 25.2-6).

Using the transperitoneal approach for more proximal lumbar levels is possible with significant vascular dissection and mobilization; the retroperitoneal route usually is a more appropriate choice for accessing the upper lumbar and midlumbar spine. At the conclusion of the spinal procedure, the posterior peritoneum is closed with 3-0 polyglactin 910 (Vicryl) suture, the bowel and omentum are returned to their normal anatomic position, and the abdominal fascia and anterior peritoneum are closed with interrupted sutures. The subcutaneous tissue and skin are closed. Postoperatively an ileus is expected.

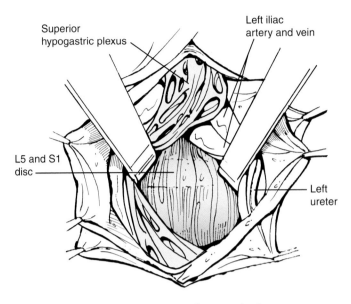

**Figure 25.2-6**   Using a transperitoneal approach, the prevertebral tissues, including the hypogastric plexus and the middle sacral artery, are identified and mobilized laterally. When a large left common iliac vein hinders access to the body of L5 and the sacral promontory, it must be mobilized properly and protected before the disc space is incised. The left iliac vein occasionally can appear as a flat, white, bloodless ribbon across the L5-S1 disc space.

# LAPAROSCOPIC/ENDOSCOPIC APPROACHES TO THE LUMBAR SPINE

Laparoscopic and endoscopic approaches lessen "approach-related" trauma compared with open approaches. A laparoscopic transperitoneal approach can be used to perform ALIF in the lower lumbar spine and lumbosacral junction. Laparoscopic techniques require additional equipment and special operating room setup and are associated with a steep learning curve. Laparoscopic ALIF can be used as a "standalone" procedure, or it can be combined with posterior spinal fusion with instrumentation using minimally invasive or open techniques. Similar to open techniques, injuries to deep anatomic structures potentially can occur.

## Laparoscopic Approach to L5-S1

Equipment is positioned in the room to allow the surgeon an optimal view of the C-arm monitor and the video monitor. The patient is placed supine on a radiolucent table in the Trendelenburg position to displace the abdominal contents rostrally out of the pelvis. Pillows are placed under the patient's hips to accentuate lordosis at the lumbosacral junction and beneath the knees to prevent hyperextension. A nasogastric tube and Foley catheter are placed to decompress the stomach and bladder.

The fluoroscope is used to verify midline. Generally, four incisions are used: Two paramedian incisions provide conduits for the working forceps; an umbilical incision provides access for the viewing camera; and the incision for the in-

terbody working channel and devices is centered over the midline suprapubic region and measures 2 to 3 cm in width (Fig. 25.2-7). The viewing camera is placed through the umbilical portal and is held by a robotic arm (AESOP; Computer Motion Inc, Goleta, CA). Sealing trocars are used to allow carbon dioxide insufflation (15 mL/min at 10 mm Hg pressure).

Deeply, adequate disc space exposure is crucial. The sacral promontory is identified by palpation and by fluoroscopy, and the midline is confirmed by fluoroscopy. The peritoneum is opened sharply. In male patients, unipolar cautery should be avoided, and a blunt Kittner dissector is used with a gentle sweeping motion to mobilize the presacral sympathetic plexus. This maneuver may help to decrease the incidence of retrograde ejaculation, which is a known complication associated with anterior approaches in the lumbosacral region. In female patients, unipolar cautery can be used to expose the anterior face of the vertebral body and disc space.

The first anatomic structures seen are the middle sacral artery and vein, which are ligated and divided. These vessels do not predict the midline of the vertebral body. The anterior curvature of the lumbosacral junction is palpated, as are the left and right lateral convexities in conjunction with fluoroscopy to help delineate the midline. The left iliac vein protrudes more anteriorly and may require more retraction. When the disc space is well exposed with protective retractors in place, ALIF with grafting can be performed. After completion of the ALIF, the peritoneum is closed using clip or running suture ligation. The abdominal wall incisions are closed with interrupted absorbable suture.

## Endoscopic Approach to the Upper Lumbar Spine

An endoscopic approach can be adapted for the retroperitoneal flank approach to the upper lumbar and midlumbar discs. The long flank incision is replaced by four smaller endoscopy incisions. The patient is placed in the fully lateral position with the appropriate disc space localized with a C-

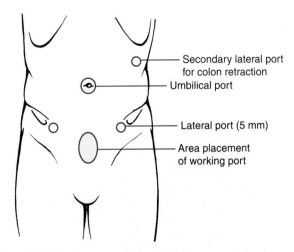

**Figure 25.2-7**   Location of portals for laparoscopic lumbar surgery.

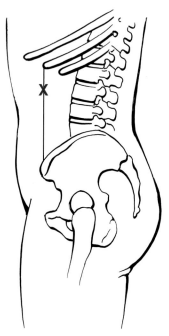

**Figure 25.2-8** The initial skin incision for endoscopic lumbar surgery. The anterior limit of the retroperitoneum is delineated by a line between the anterior tip of the 11th rib and the anterior superior iliac spine.

arm. The initial viewing portal is established directly over this disc space, and an optical trocar is inserted and used to dissect through the retroperitoneal space down to the level of the psoas muscle. The retroperitoneal space is dilated and maintained with carbon dioxide insufflation. Three additional working/visualization portals are established. The anterior limit of the retroperitoneaum is delineated by a line between the anterior tip of the 11th rib and the anterior superior iliac spine (Fig. 25.2-8). A marking needle is used to confirm the trajectory into the pathologic disc space. The disc space is reached by splitting the fibers of the psoas longitudinally or by retracting the psoas muscle posteriorly. Endoscopic curets and pituitary rongeurs are used to perform discectomy and scraping of the end plates.

A single lateral fusion cage is inserted with autograft harvested from the ipsilateral iliac crest. The final position of the cage is confirmed with the C-arm in anteroposterior and lateral projections. Hemostasis is obtained with cautery-tipped graspers or with the harmonic scalpel. The endoscopic instruments are removed, and the small fascial incisions are closed with absorbable stitch. Skin and subcutaneous tissue are closed in the usual manner.

A gasless retroperitoneal flank endoscopy can be performed by using a specialized retractor system with custom deep blades when the retroperitoneal cavity has been established by gas insufflation, balloon dissection, or manual dissection. A gasless retroperitoneal endoscopic approach to L5-S1 can be performed with the patient in a supine position. The retroperitoneal cavity is established via a midline infraumbilical incision and an endoscopic portal in the right or left flank. A specialized retractor system is used to expose the L5-S1 disc space.

## SUGGESTED READING

Bauer R, Kerschbaumer F, Poisel S. Atlas of spinal operations. New York: Thieme Medical Publishers, 1993.

Chedid MK, Green C. A review of the management of lumbar fractures with focus on surgical decision-making and techniques. Contemp Neurosurg 1999;21:1–5.

Dickman CA, Karahalios DJ. Thoracoscopic spinal surgery. Clin Neurol Surg 1996;43:392–422.

Frempong-Boadu AK, Fessler RG. Surgical exposure of the thoracic and lumbar Spine. Contemp Neurosurg 2000;22:1–7.

Johnson RM, Murphy MJ, Southwick WO. Surgical approaches to the spine. In: Rothman RH, Simeone FA, eds. The spine. Philadelphia: WB Saunders, 1999:1537–1571.

Kaneda K, Taneichi H, Abumi K, et al. Anterior decompression and stabilization with the Kaneda device for thoracolumbar burst fractures associated with neurological deficits. J Bone Joint Surg 1997; 79A:69.

Levine AM, Eismond J, Garfin SR, Zigler J. Spine trauma. Philadelphia: WB Saunders, 1998.

Mack MJ, Regan JJ, Bobecko WP, et al. Application of thoracoscopy for diseases of the spine. Ann Thorac Surg 1993;56:736.

Obenchain TG, Cloyd D. laparoscopic lumbar discectomy: description of transperitoneal and retroperitoneal techniques. Neurol Clin North Am 1996;7:77–85.

Rosenthal D, Paolucci V, Zdeblick A. Combined endoscopic retroperitoneal approach to the lumbar spine using microsurgical endoscopy. In: Zdeblick TA, ed. Anterior approaches to the spine. St. Louis: Quality Medical Publishing, 1999:219–241.

# 25.3 POSTERIOR THORACIC AND LUMBAR APPROACHES

**GREGORY C. WIGGINS ■ CARLO BELLABARBA ■ JENS R. CHAPMAN**

## INDICATIONS AND CONTRAINDICATIONS

### Midline

The midline approach is the most common exposure for lumbar pathology. It allows easy access to multiple levels for decompression, instrumentation, and arthrodesis. It is a versatile exposure through which many procedures can be performed, such as:

- Microdiscectomy
- Laminotomy/laminectomy/laminoplasty
- Facet fusion
- Intertransverse fusion
- Posterior lumbar interbody fusion
- Instrumentation

Absolute contraindications are rare. In some cases, an isolated anterior procedure without posterior exposure may be preferred. Previous midline surgery, such as laminectomy, may be considered a relative contraindication because reexposure increases the risk of durotomy, but a second midline approach often remains the best option for revision surgery.

### Lumbar Paramedian

A paramedian lumbar approach allows direct visualization of the facet joints and transverse processes without midline exposure or significant retraction of the paraspinal muscles. This approach is ideal for patients undergoing posterolateral fusions (with or without instrumentation) who do not need midline decompression. It is especially useful in avoiding the midline of patients with previous laminectomy who do not require revision decompression because direct access to the fusion bed is permitted without dissection around midline scar tissue. Finally, a paramedian approach is the ideal exposure for excision of far-lateral disc herniations.

### Posterolateral

Direct posterior thoracic spine approaches do not allow access to the anterior column; however, posterolateral approaches, such as costotransversectomy and lateral extracavitary exposures, can allow excellent visualization of the ipsilateral pedicle and thecal sac to the midline, while avoid-

ing a formal thoracotomy. Indications include tumor, trauma, degenerative conditions, and infections involving the ventral or ventrolateral aspect of the spinal column or thecal sac.

## TECHNIQUE

### Preoperative Planning

Preoperative imaging is essential to create a three-dimensional perspective of the pathologic lesion, including the important relationships between the bone, neural, and surrounding visceral structures. Computed tomography of the bone and magnetic resonance imaging in the axial, coronal, and sagittal planes help create the three-dimensional image in the surgeon's mind. With this image and the knowledge of normal anatomic relationships, the surgeon can rehearse the operation in his or her mind in a stepwise fashion, predicting areas of difficulty. This rehearsing also helps predict if a selected approach would give adequate exposure to address the pathology completely.

Preoperative radiographs also must be checked for abnormal anatomy. The number of non-rib-bearing lumbar vertebrae is noted. Lumbarized or sacralized distal segments are noted. The numbering of vertebrae on the plain films must coincide with the numbering on ancillary studies. Surgeons tend to start counting the lumbar vertebrae caudally, backward from the last mobile segment, whereas radiologists number starting at the first non-rib-bearing vertebrae. This difference may result in a discrepancy between the numbering of the surgeon and radiologist if a transitional vertebra is present. Additionally, preoperative radiographs can identify spina bifida occulta and bifid sacral areas that lack protective bone overlying the dura and neural elements.

### Positioning

All patients should receive standard perioperative antibiotics and deep venous thrombosis prophylaxis with thigh-high stockings and sequential compression devices. Provisions are made for electrophysiologic monitoring if deformity is to be corrected. With few exceptions, patients are placed in a prone position on an operative frame allowing the abdomen to hang free, diminishing the amount of epidural venous engorgement and reducing operative blood loss. For uninstrumented procedures, the patient may be placed on a Wilson frame to expand the interlaminar spaces. We prefer to use the Jackson table with the hips extended for instrumented lumbar procedures to prevent loss of lumbar lordosis. We do not place patients in the lateral decubitus or

---

The views expressed in this chapter are those of the authors and do not reflect the official policy or position of the U.S. Government, the Department of Defense, or the Department of the Air Force.

three-quarter prone position for posterior or posterolateral approaches. These positions can be disorienting and make it difficult for the surgeon and assistant to have adequate visualization.

The upper extremities are placed in a "90-90" position with the arms abducted not more than 90 degrees to avoid brachial plexus stretch injury. If the procedure involves the upper thoracic spine, the arms are tucked at the patient's side. The arms are padded adequately with special attention paid to the ulnar groove, avoiding peripheral compressive neuropathy. The head is placed in a neutral position, avoiding extension or pressure on the orbits. For longer procedures or procedures involving the cervicothoracic junction, the head is secured with three-point fixation.

The operative level is estimated by using posterior bone landmarks. The bone landmarks help orient the surgeon and limit the dissection necessary during the initial exposure. The patient is prepared and draped widely, allowing proximal or distal extension if necessary. The area also should include the iliac crest if bone graft is to be harvested. Intraoperative radiography and fluoroscopy are key to identifying definitively the appropriate operative level.

## Specific Techniques

Table 25.3-1 summarizes specific techniques.

### Midline Approach

The midline exposure in the thoracic and lumbar spine is similar, allowing for either unilateral or bilateral access to the posterior spinal canal at any vertebral level. The incision is marked in the midline and infiltrated with epinephrine to aid in hemostasis. We prefer a straight midline incision as opposed to transverse, "T," hockey-stick, or omega incisions because all the latter stray off midline, increasing the chance of skin necrosis or poor wound healing. The skin and subcutaneous tissues are incised with a scalpel. Weitlaner or cerebellar self-retaining retractors are placed. The muscle fascia is incised in the midline with electrocautery. It is important to adhere to the midline in a subperiosteal plane because dissection within the muscle needlessly increases bleeding. Although there are many ways to perform the subperiosteal dissection, we prefer to use electrocautery and either a periosteal elevator or a sturdy suction tip for retraction. In the presence of bone destruction by tumor, trauma, infection, or intrinsic bone disease, blunt dissection with a periosteal elevator may result in catastrophic neural injury. Difficulty also may occur in patients with previous laminectomy. Risks are minimized by identifying areas of normal anatomy above and below the laminectomy defect, which act as a guide to identifying the dural plane, then dissecting the scar off the dura.

During dissection, it is imperative to preserve the facet capsules. Injury to the facet capsule cephalad to a fusion can increase the risk of subsequent adjacent-level instability. It often is easier for the contralateral surgeon to perform the dissection lateral to the facet and along the transverse process in the lumbar spine or the ribs in the thoracic spine. With lateral dissection, it is important to identify and coagulate the arteries on the lateral aspect of the pars interarticu-

laris and the lateral aspect of the facet joint. As dissection is deepened, bigger self-retaining retractors are placed. We use angled Gelpi retractors because of their small radiographic profile and their small surface area, which minimizes muscle trauma and ischemia.

The midline approach in the lumbar spine allows harvesting of posterior iliac crest bone graft. The midline thoracodorsal fascia is reapproximated temporarily with towel clips. A plane is developed just superficial to the thoracodorsal fascia out to the posterior superior iliac spine, then along the iliac crest laterally. The thoracodorsal fascia inserts onto the iliac crest from above, and the fascia of the gluteus maximus and medius insert onto the iliac crest from below. The dissection is made on the curve of the iliac crest to minimize blood loss. Then the gluteus can be elevated subperiosteally off the posterior surface of the iliac crest allowing harvesting of corticocancellous bone graft. Alternatively a separate vertical incision is made overlying the iliac crest. An oblique incision along the crest should be avoided because this runs perpendicular to and endangers the superior cluneal nerves, resulting in diminished sensation over the posterior buttocks and the potential formation of painful neuromas.

### Paramedian Approach

Wiltse popularized a posterolateral paramedian approach to the lumbar spine. This approach may be performed with a midline or a paramedian skin incision. In either case, a fascial incision is placed approximately two to three fingerbreadths (approximately 3 to 4 cm) lateral to the midline. The key to this exposure is to identify the intermuscular plane between the multifidus and longissimus muscles. This provides an avascular plane that directly leads to the junction of the lateral aspect of the facet and the medial transverse process. There is frequently a small line of indentation in the fascia identifying this plane. After opening the fascia, the index finger is used to dissect through the muscle mass down to the facet joints and transverse processes. While palpating for the right plane, it is easy to mistake the facet for the tip of the transverse process because the transverse process is much deeper than expected. After placement of a self-retaining retractor, the transverse process and lateral pars interarticularis are stripped of muscular attachments.

### Far-Lateral Disc Exposure

Variations of the Wiltse exposure have been used to approach far-lateral disc herniations. Smaller unilateral paramedian skin and fascial incisions are made. Then the muscle-splitting dissection is performed and self-retaining retractor placed. By incising and reflecting the intertransversarii muscle, the offending far-lateral disc and exiting nerve root are visualized. Extreme care should be used when dissecting around the dorsal root ganglion to avoid postoperative neuropathy.

Another alternative technique for far-lateral discectomy is a transverse incision over the level of the far-lateral disc herniation. Dissection between the erector spinae and the ventral quadratus lumborum exposes the transverse process. At this point, it is imperative to use a table-mounted retractor to reflect the erector spinae muscles medially and

## TABLE 25.3-1  SPECIFIC TECHNIQUES

| Approach | Type | Indications | Contraindications | Advantages | Disadvantages |
|---|---|---|---|---|---|
| Midline | Laminectomy or discectomy | Access to posterior elements for neural decompression without significant ventral compression | Ventral neural compression | Simple and safe approach; dorsal instrumentation can be performed simultaneously | Spinal cord compression is typically ventral and not accessible via midline approaches; may destabilize if ventral pathology is present |
| | Transpedicular | Ventrolateral neural compression | Midline pathology requiring manipulation of spinal cord for exposure; ventral reconstruction or instrumentation | Less extensive surgery; some access to lateral vertebral body | Limited exposure; incomplete decompression; unable to reconstruct the anterior spine |
| Paramedian | Wiltse | Access to facet or intertransverse region while avoiding midline | Need for significant midline exposure | Less muscle retraction; direct exposure for fusion and pedicle screw placement | Unfamiliar approach; difficult to perform midline decompression |
| | Far-lateral | Access to far-lateral disc herniation | Significant component of disc in the canal | Access to the far-lateral disc without loss of stability | Unable to access compressive pathology within the canal |
| Posterolateral | Costotransversectomy | Ventrolateral pathology | Need for complete exposure to contralateral pedicle | Less blood loss than lateral extracavitary | Unable to place ventral instrumentation; less angle of exposure than lateral extracavitary |
| | Lateral extracavitary | Ventrolateral pathology | Need for complete exposure to contralateral pedicle | More lateral angle of exposure | More muscle dissection than costotransversectomy |

dorsally. The resulting angle of exposure is similar to that with the muscle-splitting approach.

## Costotransversectomy

Costotransversectomy is the basis for all other posterolateral approaches and is described first. A midline skin incision long enough to expose three levels above and three levels below the planned decompression is needed to allow for lateral muscle retraction. Usually this approach is supplemented with posterior instrumentation so that bilateral subperiosteal muscle takedown is performed out to the tip of the transverse processes. We do not advocate transverse section of the paraspinal muscles because this weakens them.

Thoracic pedicle screws are placed bilaterally usually two or three levels above and below the pathologic level before any decompression. A temporary rod is connected to the pedicle screws contralateral to the planned approach. This rod allows for temporary stabilization and avoids any movement that may jeopardize the spinal cord as the spine is progressively and often circumferentially destabilized. Dis-

secting from medial to lateral under the paraspinal muscles exposes 3 to 5 cm of each rib. By starting at the midline, the dissection can proceed deep to the trapezius and rhomboid muscles in the upper thoracic spine and directly onto the ribs.

A hemilaminectomy is performed. The transverse process is removed by incising the costotransverse ligaments, freeing the transverse process from the underlying rib. Usually the rib at the level of the lesion and one level below are removed for adequate exposure. The neurovascular bundle is protected as the ribs are dissected free with a Doyen dissector. The ribs are cut 3 to 5 cm lateral to the junction of the rib and the transverse process. The radiate ligament is incised, freeing the rib from the vertebral body. The freed rib is removed and saved for bone graft. The pleura is dissected bluntly off the anterolateral vertebral bodies.

The intercostal bundle is followed back to identify the neural foramen. The intercostal artery and nerve root at the pathologic level are identified, doubly ligated, and divided. This should not be done bilaterally to avoid spinal cord devascularization. It is important to ligate the nerve proximal to the dorsal root ganglion to avoid painful neuroma formation. After exposure, decompression can be performed anteriorly and posteriorly. The vertebral body can be reconstructed and bilateral posterior instrumentation placed as needed.

### Lateral Extracavitary Approach

The lateral extracavitary approach is an extension of costotransversectomy to allow farther lateral approach to the vertebral body. A midline, paramedian, or hockey-stick incision is made exposing at least three levels above and below the pathology. A subcutaneous flap is developed exposing the midline and lateral edge of the paraspinous muscles. The thoracodorsal fascia is incised in a "T" or paramedian manner. In the thoracic spine, the upper back musculature (trapezius, latissimus dorsi, and rhomboids) is flapped from the midline or split along their fibers to access the underlying dorsal rib cage lateral to the paraspinous muscles.

The erector spinae muscles are dissected from lateral to medial off the dorsal rib cage or the quadratus lumborum in the lumbar spine. If the erector spinae is extremely bulky, a vertical muscle-splitting incision eliminates excessive muscle retraction, but it provides a less ventral view of the dural sac. The paraspinal muscles are retracted to the contralateral side. If instrumentation is planned, the paraspinal muscles also are dissected off the midline structures (spinous process and lamina) to allow placement of posterior instrumentation.

In the thoracic spine, the medial 8 to 10 cm of one to three ribs are resected, and the procedure proceeds as with costotransversectomy described previously. In the lumbar spine, the nerve roots cannot be sacrificed owing to their contribution to lower extremity function. This fact along with the large bulk of the paraspinous muscles in the lumbar spine significantly complicates exposure below the L2 level.

## POSTOPERATIVE MANAGEMENT

As with any surgery that involves neural decompression, it is mandatory to perform a neurologic exam as the patient is waking up in the operating room, followed by a more complete exam after the effects of anesthesia have worn off. Patients are mobilized as quickly as possible to improve pulmonary toilet and to diminish the risk of deep venous thrombosis. The need for a postoperative orthosis is dictated

### TABLE 25.3-2 MORBIDITY OF POSTERIOR THORACIC AND LUMBAR APPROACHES

| | |
|---|---|
| Cardiovascular | Coagulopathy, deep venous thrombosis, myocardial infarction |
| Infectious disease | Sepsis, wound infection |
| Injury | Aorta, bladder, bowel, ureter, vena cava |
| Neurologic | Intercostal neuralgia, nerve root injury, spinal cord injury |
| Positioning | Blindness, brachial plexus, compartment syndrome |
| Pulmonary | Aspiration, hemothorax, pleural effusion, pneumonia, pneumothorax, pulmonary embolus |
| Technical | Incomplete decompression, wrong level surgery |
| Wound | Cerebrospinal fluid leak, dehiscence, incisional hernia, hematoma |

by the amount of instability due to the pathologic process and the amount of surgical destabilization. It is imperative after the posterolateral approaches to check a chest radiograph to evaluate for pneumothorax.

## COMPLICATIONS

Table 25.3-2 lists the potential morbidity associated with posterior thoracic and lumbar approaches. Many of these complications are similar to complications seen with any other surgical procedure and need no further explanation.

## SUGGESTED READING

Benzel EC. The lateral extracavitary approach to the spine using the three-quarter prone position. J Neurosurg 1989;71:837–841.

Fessler RG, Dietze DD, Millan MM, Peace D. Lateral parascapular extrapleural approach to the upper thoracic spine. J Neurosurg 1991;75:349–355.

Larson SJ, Holst R, Hemmy DC, Sances A. Lateral extracavitary approach to traumatic lesions of the thoracic and lumbar spine. J Neurosurg 1976;45:628–637.

Wiltse LL, Spencer CW. New uses and refinements of the paraspinal approach to the lumbar spine. Spine 1988;13:696–706.

# CERVICAL DECOMPRESSION

**JOHN M. RHEE**

26

In general, pathologic compression of neural structures in the cervical spine occurs in two main locations—centrally, where the spinal cord or exiting nerve root (or both) can be impinged, or in the foramen, where the exiting root can be impinged. Depending on whether the involved structure is the spinal cord or the nerve root, clinical symptoms consistent with myelopathy, radiculopathy, or both can result. Surgical management of these problems requires skill at identifying and decompressing the neural elements in these two regions. This chapter reviews the indications and techniques—anterior and posterior—for achieving cervical spine decompression.

## DECOMPRESSION FOR CERVICAL RADICULOPATHY

### Pathoanatomy

Cervical radiculopathy arises from compression of a cervical nerve root and manifests as a radiating pain from the neck into the upper extremity in the distribution of the affected root. The exact location and pattern of pain can vary widely, and a classic distribution of pain frequently is absent. Associated sensory, motor, or reflex disturbances may or may not be present.

Cervical root compression most commonly occurs in four ways:

- *First,* soft disc herniations, depending on the location, may impinge the exiting nerve root (Fig. 26-1A) as it leaves the spinal cord or as it traverses the neuroforamen (Fig. 26-1B).
- *Second,* chronic disc degeneration can result in the formation of degenerative osteophytes. Most commonly, these osteophytes arise from the uncinate regions of the posterolateral vertebral body (uncovertebral osteophytes) and compress the exiting nerve root as it enters the neuroforamen (Fig. 26-1C).
- *Third,* chronic disc degeneration can lead to disc height loss, which may result in loss of foraminal height. The loss of height, combined with superior migration of the superior facet joint, can lead to foraminal compression.
- *Fourth,* hypertrophy of the facet joints can cause forami-

nal encroachment, more commonly in the upper rather than the lower cervical spine.

A thorough understanding of these four mechanisms of nerve root compression, including the anatomic locations in which compression occurs, is crucial to performing safe and effective nerve root decompression.

## Indications for Anterior Versus Posterior Nerve Root Decompression

In general, nerve root compression arises most commonly from anterior structures, such as disc herniations and uncovertebral osteophytes. As a result, the anterior approach is preferred in most cases of cervical radiculopathy. The decision must be tempered, however, by an understanding of the advantages and disadvantages of each approach. A major advantage of anterior decompression is that it provides for direct access and removal of uncovertebral osteophytes and herniated discs without the need for neural retraction. In contrast, posterior cervical discectomy, with potentially good results in certain situations, requires manipulation of the nerve root and potentially the spinal cord. Although posterior foraminotomy can enlarge the foramen through partial resection of the facet joint, accessing and removing an uncovertebral spur from the posterior route can be difficult. It also is difficult to restore foraminal or disc height from a posterior approach, whereas an anterior bone graft can be placed readily to restore height.

Other advantages of the anterior approach include extremely low rates of infection or wound breakdown. If the incision is placed transversely in the creases (Langer's lines) of the neck, the incision heals with a virtually imperceptible scar. The anterior approach also requires little muscle dissection and tends to be associated with less perioperative incisional pain than the posterior approach, which requires subperiosteal dissection.

Anterior cervical decompressions traditionally are performed with an associated fusion. Doing the anterior fusion has several potential advantages. Fusion may help relieve associated neck pain, improve overall alignment of the neck, address instability, and protect the decompression from recurrent disease. Placement of structural bone graft in the

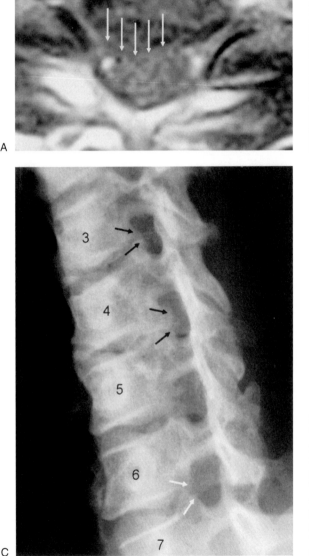

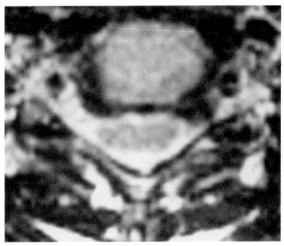

**Figure 26-1**   (**A**) Large posterolateral disc herniation. The disc compresses the thecal sac and the exiting nerve root. A disc in this location would be difficult to access safely from a posterior approach. (**B**) Foraminal disc herniation, left side. (**C**) Uncinate hypertrophy. The uncinate spurs arise from the superior and the inferior vertebral bodies at C3-4 and C4-5, leading to foraminal narrowing (*black arrows*). This is a common mechanism for foraminal stenosis in the cervical spine. At C6-7 (*white arrows*), there is no foraminal stenosis and no uncovertebral osteophytes.

anterior disc space also can restore foraminal height, providing indirect decompression of the nerve root. Regaining disc height additionally reduces infolding of the posterior longitudinal ligament and ligamentum flavum, which can relieve root compression.

The advantages of fusion performed in conjunction with anterior decompression come at a cost, including the potential for accelerated adjacent segment degeneration. Pseudarthrosis also remains a problem, particularly when multiple levels are performed. Other potential disadvantages to the anterior approach include speech and swallowing disturbances, which are encountered temporarily in virtually every patient postoperatively and encountered permanently in a small percentage. Airway obstruction also can occur,

particularly after multilevel anterior decompressions for myelopathy.

Posterior approaches to cervical spondylotic radiculopathy possess advantages to anterior decompression in selected circumstances. The keyhole foraminotomy procedure can be used to decompress the nerve root without significantly destabilizing the spine and can be considered in cases of foraminal disc herniation or stenosis. The key is to identify pathology on preoperative imaging studies (e.g., magnetic resonance imaging [MRI] or computed tomography-myelography) that is lateral enough to be accessible posteriorly without necessitating spinal cord retraction and that can be accessed through a laminoforaminotomy (see Fig. 26-1). Posterior discectomy can be performed after laminoforaminotomy for foraminal disc herniations and potentially can avoid the need for fusion. Posterior foraminotomy also can be effective for treating high cervical radiculopathies (e.g., C2-3 or C3-4) because, in contrast to the lower levels of the cervical spine, foraminal stenosis at these upper levels more commonly arises from facet overgrowth rather than uncovertebral hypertrophy. A major advantage of the posterior foraminotomy is that it can be performed with minimal patient morbidity. Because the procedure does not attempt to restore disc height at the diseased level, however, a disadvantage is the potential for deterioration of results with time if the degenerative process continues at that level. Although fusion is not routinely necessary with a posterior foraminotomy, if more than 50% of both facet joints are resected to decompress the nerve root adequately, posterior fusion with lateral mass plates or spinous process cables should be considered.

There are few, if any, absolute indications for decompressing the nerve root anteriorly or posteriorly. If a patient has had prior surgery from one approach, it may be advantageous to perform surgery from the opposite approach to avoid working through scar tissue. A common salvage procedure for patients with persistent radiculopathy after anterior cervical discectomy and fusion is posterior foraminotomy. Alternatively a revision anterior procedure can be performed with excellent results.

## Equipment

Several pieces of equipment are crucial to nerve root and spinal cord decompression, regardless of whether an anterior or posterior approach is used. A high-speed bur is useful for removing uncovertebral osteophytes and decorticating the end plates. A self-retaining cervical retractor set allows anterior surgery to be performed with minimal assistance, although care must be taken to ensure proper placement of retractors and avoidance of prolonged compression of vital neck structures, such as the esophagus, airway, and carotid vessels. Some form of disc space distraction also is helpful, such as vertebral body distraction pins or a small self-retaining vertebral body spreader. Microcurets are mandatory to remove osteophytes and disc herniations. Ideally, they should have a thin footplate to avoid intrusion into the canal. Finally, to perform a safe but complete and adequate neural decompression, high-quality illumination and magnification are essential. I prefer to use an operating microscope versus a headlight and loupes; the illumination and visualization are superior, and the view obtained by the assistant is equal to that of the operating surgeon.

# ANTERIOR NERVE ROOT DECOMPRESSION

## Positioning and Exposure for Anterior Surgery

The patient is positioned supine with the neck extended gently. A head halter or Gardner-Wells tong is optional but not routinely necessary. A doughnut pad is placed behind the occiput to prevent pressure necrosis. The shoulders are taped down gently to facilitate intraoperative radiographic visualization. Excessive force should be avoided when taping to prevent brachial plexus injury. If a patient has a short neck and a stocky body habitus, it may not be possible to visualize the lower cervical segments radiographically. In these situations, rather than taping the shoulders with excessive force throughout the entire case, it is advisable to tape the shoulders more loosely, then scrub out or have unscrubbed assistants briefly pull longitudinally on the arms while radiographs are being taken. The amount of preoperative cervical extension tolerated by the patient determines the limit of initial intraoperative positioning. In particular, excessive extension during positioning must be avoided in patients with myelopathy.

The surgical approach is described elsewhere in this text, but several points merit mentioning when performing anterior cervical decompressions. The skin incision can be placed obliquely anterior to the sternocleidomastoid or transversely in a major neck crease. An oblique incision can be extensile and may be used for multilevel surgery. In general, a transverse incision is preferred because it heals much more cosmetically and still provides access to multilevel pathology. A large incision placed in a crease heals more cosmetically than a small incision placed outside of a crease. The incision may extend from the anterior two thirds of the sternocleidomastoid to beyond the midline. Because the skin in the anterior neck tends to be highly mobile, multilevel access is possible with a transverse incision if the tissue planes beneath the platysma and in the interval medial to the sternocleidomastoid are undermined and spread. The omohyoid, if it impedes access, can be divided with minimal adverse consequences. Any crossing structures should be preserved if possible so that inadvertent injury to the superior or recurrent laryngeal nerves can be avoided. Crossing vessels can be ligated, but the surgeon must be certain that the structure in question is not a laryngeal nerve. After the appropriate levels have been localized, the longus colli should be subperiosteally dissected laterally such that the uncinates are visualized clearly. Exposure from uncinate to uncinate is necessary because the lateral limits of the decompression are determined relative to the position of the uncinates (Fig. 26-2). The retractor blades are placed beneath the elevated longus colli. It is preferable to place a toothed retractor blade under the longus colli on the side ipsilateral to the carotid sheath (lateral). A smooth blade is placed under the longus colli on the side epsilateral to the trachea and esophagus (medial).

## Technique for Anterior Cervical Discectomy

The disc is sharply incised with a No. 15 blade and removed with a combination of curets and pituitary rongeurs. Intervertebral body distraction pins can be placed to distract the disc space gently and allow for better posterior visualization. A key maneuver to facilitate disc space visualization and subsequent neural decompression is to remove the anterior portion of the inferior end plate of the superior vertebral body, particularly if the disc is severely degenerated and the disc space is narrow (Fig. 26-3A). This surface almost always is concave, and the anterior portion overhangs the disc space, preventing direct visualization into the posterior disc space if not removed. Removal can be done with either a

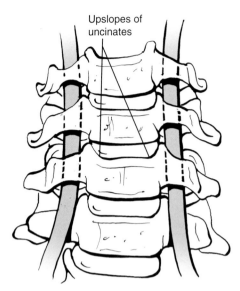

Upslopes of
uncinates

**Figure 26-2**   The longus colli should be elevated subperiosteally from uncinate to uncinate such that the upslope of each uncinate is identified clearly. Bipolar cautery is useful in doing this. The uncinates are the key anatomic landmarks for decompression. The vertebral artery is several millimeters lateral to the lateral border of the uncinate. If extreme lateral exposure is necessary, one can identify the lateral border of the uncinate by carefully placing a No. 4 Penfield dissector superiosteally around the lateral edge of the joint, protecting the vertebral artery.

Kerrison rongeur or a high-speed bur. Removing this portion often dramatically improves access to the posterior disc space and provides a line of sight that is parallel to the disc space (Fig. 26-3B); this is crucial to performing the decompression, especially when using a microscope. If a parallel view is not achieved, the surgeon may become disoriented and stray away from the disc space into the body of a vertebra. One way of maintaining a direct line of site is to fashion the end plates such that they are parallel to each other. In effect, the goal is to create a rectangular disc space by removing the concavities naturally present in each vertebral body. Doing so also facilitates optimal fit and contact between the end plate and graft or cage. A posterior lip can be left in place to prevent posterior impaction of the graft intraoperatively or subsequent posterior displacement, if it does not impede adequate decompression.

The end plates should be cleaned thoroughly of cartilaginous material and decorticated to reveal bleeding bony surfaces. Alternating use of the high-speed bur, curets, and pituitary rongeur allows the surgeon to reach the posterior disc space and the posterior longitudinal ligament. Often, in an acute disc herniation, there is a rent in the posterior longitudinal ligament readily seen under the microscope. By carefully probing the posterior longitudinal ligament with a microcuret, the extruded fragment can be gently "fished out" of the spinal canal. Depending on the location of the disc herniation, the exiting nerve root or spinal cord or both is visible. Gentle probing posterior to the posterior longitudinal ligament can be done until all loose fragments have been removed. The portion of the posterior longitudinal ligament contralateral to the side of the disc herniation does not routinely need to be removed. It is advisable, however, to take down enough posterior longitudinal ligament care-

fully on the side of the radiculopathy to confirm that the exiting nerve root is free.

## Technique for Anterior Foraminotomy

There is controversy as to whether a formal anterior foraminotomy is necessary to treat foraminal stenosis. Direct anterior foraminotomies have been considered unnecessary because of reports indicating resorption of uncinate spurs after fusion, with subsequent resolution of radiculopathy. I believe, however, that an anterior foraminal decompression is important in consistently relieving foraminal stenosis. Although foraminal height restoration is possible with anterior grafting, this does not increase the anterior-posterior dimension of the foramen, which often is narrowed by a posteriorly protruding uncinate osteophyte (see Fig. 26-1C). Although uncinate osteophytes may resorb over time, this process may take months and is completely dependent on achieving a solid arthrodesis, which does not happen in every case. Gratifying, immediate relief of radicular symptoms can be achieved with direct anterior foraminotomy, which is independent of achieving arthrodesis.

For two reasons, the key to performing a foraminotomy is intimate knowledge of uncinate anatomy:

■ *First,* orientation to the uncinates is essential because they represent the lateral borders of a safe zone for working in the disc space without injuring the vertebral artery (see Fig. 26-2).

■ *Second,* exposure and resection of the medial aspect of the uncinates is important because osteophytes responsible for radiculopathy most commonly arise from this region.

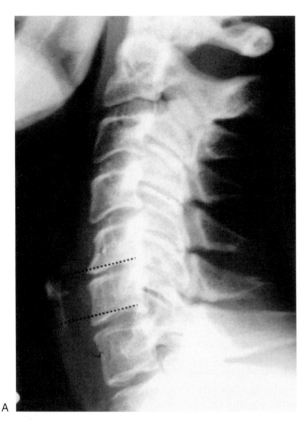
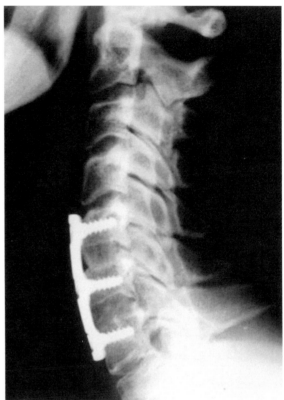

A                                                                                                                B

**Figure 26-3** (**A**) Spinal images of a 54-year-old woman with radiculopathy arising from C5-6 and C6-7 spondylosis. Severe disc degeneration at C5-6 impedes access to the posterior disc space, unless the inferior lip of C5 is resected (*dotted line*). A similar procedure should be considered at C6 to gain access to the posterior structures at C6-7 (*dotted line*). (**B**) Status-post two-level anterior cervical discectomy and fusion. The inferior lip at each level was resected, resulting in parallel disc spaces with parallel end plates. Doing so allowed visualization posteriorly for uncovertebral osteophyte resection and complete resolution of radiculopathy. The rectangular disc space created allowed intimate contact of the end plates with the bone graft. Because this patient did not have any central stenosis, it was not necessary to decompress the spinal cord. The posterior lips were left alone centrally at each level to protect against graft intrusion.

The foraminotomy should be attempted after the discectomy has been performed to the level of the posterior longitudinal ligament, and exposure of the uncinate has been achieved. The medial aspect of the posterior uncinate is thinned under direct visualization with a high-speed bur. Constant irrigation is performed to prevent thermal injury and to clear away bone debris. If visualization is adequate, continued thinning of the osteophyte can progress until only a thin shell of bone is left. A microcuret is used to resect the thinned osteophytes and the posterior longitudinal ligament medial to the uncinate. This move allows visualization of the exiting nerve root and the lateral edge of the dural sac and provides access to the foramen. Using microcurets and the bur, the foramen can be carved out gently and progressively to increase its anterior-posterior diameter and to resect the posteriorly protruding uncinate osteophytes. When entering the foramen, the curet should hug the posterior aspect of the uncinate to avoid nerve root injury. In addition, the exiting nerve root should be visualized during the maneuver. Blind placement of a curet into

the foramen is dangerous and should be avoided. Foraminotomy is complete when a micro-nerve hook or microcuret can be passed easily into the foramen anterior to the exiting root without resistance. Bone grafting and plating are performed if indicated.

If further lateral decompression of the foramen is necessary, it can be done by undercutting within the posterior one third of the disc space, which usually is dorsal to the location of the vertebral artery. In this manner, sufficient foraminal decompression can be achieved safely laterally at the level of the disc space while reducing potential risks of vertebral artery laceration. Because the vertebral artery typically lies in the anterior two thirds of the disc space, undercutting within the posterior one third usually does not put the artery at risk (Fig. 26-4). Going out further laterally in the anterior two thirds of the disc space can be dangerous, however. When curetting disc material in this area, vertebral artery laceration might occur if the curet strays lateral to the lateral border of the uncinate. This event is more likely to occur when the disc space is under distraction be-

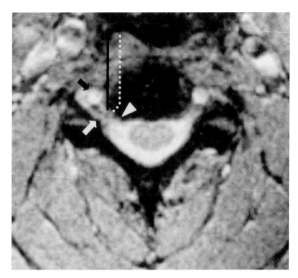

**Figure 26-4**  The vertebral artery (*black arrow*) typically lies in the anterior two thirds of the disc space. It is ventral to the usual location of nerve root compression (i.e., at the level of the posterior uncinate [*white arrowhead*]). The lateral border of the uncinate marks the lateral safe zone (*black line*). To decompress the nerve root laterally in the foramen (*white arrow*), while avoiding injury to the vertebral artery, the trajectory of decompression should course laterally in the posterior aspect of the disc space (*dotted line*).

cause this reduces the protective overhang between adjacent level uncinates (Fig. 26-5). In all cases, to minimize the incidence of vertebral artery complications, one should scrutinize preoperative MRI or computed tomography to rule out the presence of an anomalous vertebral artery

coursing medial to its usual position within the intertransverse foramen and lateral to the lateral border of the uncinate. If anomalies are suspected, angiography should be considered preoperatively.

# POSTERIOR LAMINOFORAMINOTOMY

## Positioning and Exposure for Posterior Surgery

As is the case when performing anterior decompression, the same neurologic and spinal cord monitoring considerations apply when positioning patients for posterior surgery. The amount of preoperative extension tolerated should be assessed, and consideration should be given to using awake fiberoptic intubation and spinal cord monitoring for patients with concomitant myelopathy. In addition to potential neurologic sequelae, excessive extension may make posterior foraminotomy technically more difficult to perform because of the increased overlap between adjacent laminae, which results with relative neck extension versus flexion (Fig. 26-6). Flexion of the neck is helpful if an isolated foraminotomy without fusion is being performed. If an associated fusion is necessary, however, excessive flexion during positioning may lead to undesirable kyphosis over the instrumented segments. In these situations, relative—although not excessive—extension is preferred, or the neck can be repositioned into lordosis after decompression.

During posterior cervical operations, improper positioning also can lead to excessive bleeding. The abdomen must be free of compression. Putting the patient into reverse Trendelenburg's position reduces venous pressure in the neck and bleeding. Although bleeding from posterior cervical operations is rarely of the magnitude to cause hemodynamic compromise, undue bleeding may hinder visualiza-

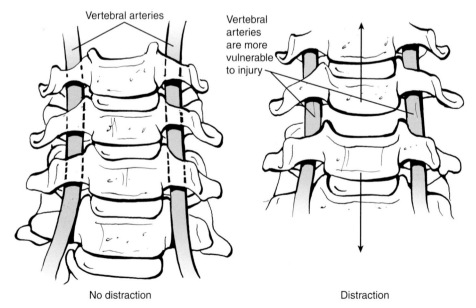

**Figure 26-5**  When the disc space is distracted, the protective overhang of the uncinates on the vertebral artery is reduced, making the artery more susceptible to laceration by a stray curet, bur, or other instrument. It is crucial to control carefully all instruments passed into the disc space during anterior cervical surgery.

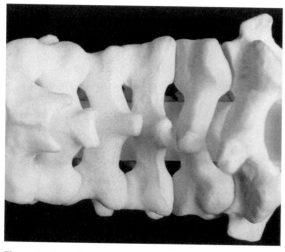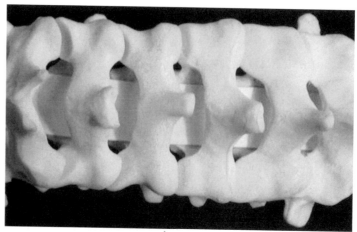

**Figure 26-6**    When the neck is in relative extension (**A**), there is increased overlap of the facets and laminae, leading to shingling of the laminae. In relative flexion (**B**), the facets and laminae overlap less.

tion during foraminotomies. Usually, if the patient is positioned properly, foraminal bleeding can be controlled readily with the brief application of absorbable gelatin sponge (Gelfoam) and cottonoids. In contrast, if the patient is not positioned properly and venous pressure is unduly high, foraminal bleeding may obscure safe visualization during foraminotomy despite attempts at hemostasis.

A Mayfield headrest is useful when positioning patients for prone cervical surgery. A horseshoe headrest is not recommended because of the possibility for pressure necrosis on the eyes and face. Two longitudinal bolsters are placed (one on each side of the body) spanning the chest and abdomen to allow the abdomen to hang free. The shoulders are taped down, with care being taken to avoid excessive traction. When positioning a patient into reverse Trendelenburg's position, care also must be taken to avoid the inadvertent application of traction on the neck and spinal cord. This traction can occur with the use of tongs (especially Mayfield) because the head is relatively fixed, whereas the body may slide caudally owing to gravity. This problem can be avoided by flexing the table at the knees (Fig. 26-7). A sling placed behind the buttocks with an upward-directed

vector also can be beneficial in this regard. Alternatively, seated, awake positioning for surgery has been described for performing posterior foraminotomies. Air embolism is a potential risk, however.

Posterior foraminotomy can be done in a minimally invasive fashion for nerve root decompression without fusion. Alternatively, it can be done in conjunction with a fusion, laminectomy, or laminoplasty. The amount of exposure necessary depends on the procedure being performed. Laminoforaminotomy alone can be done with unilateral muscle dissection and a small incision. Fusion, laminoplasty, or laminectomy requires bilateral exposure and a larger incision. The surgical approach is described elsewhere in this text. To limit muscle bleeding and perioperative neck pain, it is important to stay in the midline raphe during the approach to the spinous process, then maintain a strict subperiosteal plane as dissection proceeds laterally. It also is necessary to avoid injury to the facet capsules of uninvolved levels.

## Technique for Posterior Laminoforaminotomy

Cadaveric experiments suggest that up to 50% of the facet joint can be removed without risking iatrogenic instability when performing foraminotomies. Because the first priority should be to achieve satisfactory nerve root decompression, consideration should be given to concomitant fusion if more facet resection is necessary. In most cases, adequate neural decompression is possible, however, without sacrificing stability.

After careful positioning and exposure, a high-speed bur under constant irrigation is used to outline the margins of the foraminotomy. In most cases, the initial bur hole can be centered over the lamina-lateral mass junction (Fig. 26-8). The inferior facet of the level above (e.g., the C5 facet when performing a C5-6 foraminotomy) is not the offending structure narrowing the foramen but is an "obstacle" to access of the true culprit—the superior facet of the level below (e.g., the C6 facet). Because the inferior facet is "pro-

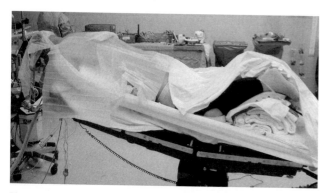

**Figure 26-7**    A properly positioned patient for posterior cervical surgery.

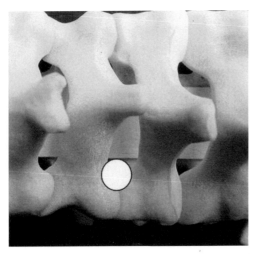

**Figure 26-8** Approximate area of bone resection during lamino-foraminotomy. The superior, not inferior, facet represents the posterior bone wall of the foramen. Because the nerve root in a sense is protected by the superior facet during drilling, removal of the inferior facet can be done with appropriate speed and aggressiveness. When the foramen has been entered by removing the circled portion of the facet joint, undercutting can be done laterally if necessary with a micro-Kerrison rongeur or curet.

tected" by the more anteriorly positioned superior facet, initial burring through the inferior facet can be quick and relatively aggressive. When the superior facet is reached, the pace of burring should proceed more slowly. Bleeding is common during foraminotomy, but can be controlled with Gelfoam and pledgets. Burring should continue until the anterior cortex of the superior facet has been reached. This landmark can be seen under the microscope as the bone changes color and takes on the gray-blue tinge of the nerve root and dura. When the superior facet has been thinned in this manner, a microcuret can be introduced over the nerve root to lift away the thinned bone. As the hole is enlarged, a micro-Kerrison rongeur is introduced to decompress the nerve root progressively. The bone at the lateral mass-lamina junction also should be removed to visualize the takeoff of the exiting root from the spinal cord. Decompression is judged complete when a nerve hook can be passed into the foramen without resistance beyond the lateral border of the pedicle. A fusion, laminectomy, or laminoplasty can be performed if necessary.

# DECOMPRESSION FOR CERVICAL MYELOPATHY

## Indications for Anterior Versus Posterior Decompression

Considerable debate exists regarding the optimal surgical approach for treating cervical myelopathy. Anterior and posterior approaches can improve neurologic function, and each has its advantages and disadvantages. Anterior decompression directly relieves spinal cord compression due to the most common impinging structures, such as her-

niated discs, spondylotic bars, and ossification of the posterior longitudinal ligament. Stenosis with kyphosis, which in some cases can contribute to compression because the cord is draped over the posterior vertebral body osteophytes, is approached better anteriorly. Posterior laminoplasty avoids fusion and its attendant graft-related complications and complications related to the anterior approach. It can be performed quickly and with minimal blood loss. Because the major offending structures impinging on the spinal cord tend to arise anteriorly, laminoplasty, in contrast to anterior decompression techniques, relies primarily on an indirect decompression as the cord floats away posteriorly. In most cases, the cervical spine should be relatively lordotic or at least neutral for the spinal cord to be able to drift posteriorly and the desired decompressive effect to be obtained with laminoplasty.

Despite the controversy, there are some general principles in selecting the appropriate approach. If myelopathy is arising from one or two levels, anterior decompression and fusion typically is preferred. If pathology exists at three levels, either anterior decompression or laminoplasty can be considered. If more than three levels are involved, laminoplasty is preferred because of its relative simplicity and lack of need for a long strut graft. In patients who are medically frail or have poor potential for healing a fusion (e.g., smokers, diabetics, steroid users), laminoplasty may be favored. Laminoplasty also may be preferable in severe cases of ossification of the posterior longitudinal ligament to avoid complications related to dural deficiencies and dural tears with an anterior approach. If a patient has a substantial amount of neck pain, a fusion should be considered, either anteriorly or posteriorly, in conjunction with laminectomy or laminoplasty.

If the neck is kyphotic, anterior surgery is recommended because laminoplasty cannot undrape the cord over a kyphos. The absence of lordosis is not an absolute contraindication to laminoplasty, however. In patients showing compressive lesions the presence of arising posteriorly, laminoplasty can achieve a direct decompressive effect despite kyphosis (Fig. 26-9). Also, in kyphotic patients with extremely tight cervical stenosis, laminoplasty can be considered as a first-stage operation. If the clinical circumstances indicate and postoperative imaging studies show persistent compression after laminoplasty, a staged anterior decompression and fusion of selected levels can be performed at a later date. In these situations, even if the cord drifted only a few millimeters posteriorly after laminoplasty and persistent anterior compression exists, the anterior decompression now may be less risky because of the amount of space gained. Fewer levels now may need anterior decompression. One of the unsolved complications of laminoplasty, however, remains segmental root level palsy (especially C5), which may arise in 5% to 12% of cases.

In general, performing a laminectomy that compromises the facet joints without fusion is not recommended because of the risk of instability and postlaminectomy kyphosis. Neurologic function may improve early on after laminectomy but can deteriorate over time if the neck becomes kyphotic. For this reason, laminoplasty is preferred to multilevel laminectomy. Studies have indicated superior out-

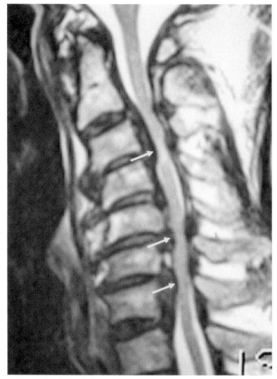
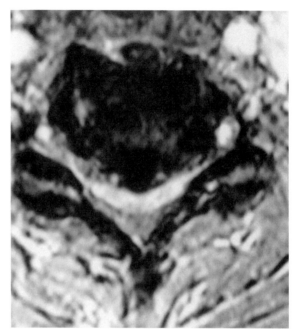

**Figure 26-9** (**A** and **B**) Spinal images of a 78-year-old man with severe insulin-dependent diabetes, chronic renal failure, stroke, and chronic obstructive pulmonary disease, who presented with a 1-year history of progressive myelopathy rendering him nonambulatory. Circumferential stenosis due to severe multilevel ossification of the posterior longitudinal ligament and congenital stenosis is noted at multiple levels (*arrows*) on the sagittal image (**A**). Cord signal change is evident at C3-4. Axial image (**B**) also shows circumferential stenosis. Despite his cervical kyphosis, a laminoplasty was performed because of his tenuous medical status and the presence of circumferential stenosis. Even if the cord fails to drift posteriorly completely, some degree of decompression is achieved by relieving the dorsal compression. A staged anterior decompression and fusion can be done after obtaining postoperative MRI, if necessary.

comes with laminoplasty over laminectomy, even with fusion.

## Positioning Myelopathic Patients

Proper positioning is especially crucial when operating on myelopathic patients, regardless of whether the surgery is performed anteriorly or posteriorly. Excessive extension during positioning must be avoided in these patients because extension diminishes the space available in the spinal canal and can cause cord compression intraoperatively. Awake, fiberoptic intubation should be considered to avoid excessive extension and potential spinal cord injury during intubation. Spinal cord monitoring is recommended when operating on patients with myelopathy and is optional when operating on nonmyelopathic patients. A baseline set of data should be obtained after intubation, then compared after positioning to ensure that the patient has been positioned safely.

## Technique for Anterior Cervical Corpectomy

The patient is positioned as described for anterior discectomy. Placement of Gardner-Wells tongs with mild traction

(5 to 10 lb) is recommended to stabilize the head and neck when doing corpectomies. The corpectomy is performed after the anterior exposure, discectomy, and foraminotomy (if necessary) as described earlier. Completing the discectomies first allows the surgeon to estimate the depth of the corpectomy. The width of the corpectomy required is the width of the spinal cord and should be estimated based on preoperative imaging studies. It rarely is necessary to extend lateral to the uncinates, and the uncinates are again a key surgical landmark. It is imperative to analyze carefully the course of the vertebral arteries on preoperative imaging studies to ensure that they do not traverse medial to their usual location.

When the limits of the corpectomy have been delineated, a large Leksell rongeur can be used to remove large portions of the vertebral body. This bone also is useful for subsequent grafting. Under direct visualization, a high-speed bur is used to remove bone until a thin shell of posterior cortex remains. Microcurets are used to flake off the remaining bone. When choosing a location to enter the spinal canal, it may be safer to find a plane laterally, where there is usually more room, then proceed centrally. Extreme caution must be observed when performing a corpectomy over regions with ossification of the posterior longitudinal ligament. If severe, the dura may be deficient or absent, and the surgeon should be prepared to place a dural patch and insert a lumbar drain. Instead of removing the entire ossification of the posterior longitudinal ligament, an alternative technique is the "floating method," in which the adherent ossification of the posterior longitudinal ligament fragment is detached laterally where it is not adherent to the dura, then allowed to float away anteriorly with the spinal cord. Fusion and plating are performed.

## Technique of Open-Door Laminoplasty

There are several methods for performing a laminoplasty:

- Open door
- French door (T-saw)
- Z-plasty

The open-door method is described here. The patient is positioned in the same manner as for posterior cervical foraminotomy. Overall neutral or slightly flexed alignment of the cervical spine facilitates opening of the laminoplasty by diminishing the shingling effect of the C2 lamina on the C3 lamina. If the neck is too extended, the overlap of the C2 lamina onto C3 prevents opening of C3, unless the inferior portion of C2 is removed. For a standard C3-7 laminoplasty, exposure should be performed from the inferior edge of the C2 lamina to the superior portion of T1. Some authors believe that the nuchal attachments onto the C2 spinous process should be preserved or, if necessary, removed with a piece of bone to facilitate later reattachment and prevention of postoperative kyphosis. The facet joints should be preserved—only the medial aspect of the joint needs to be exposed.

After exposure and confirmation of levels, the hinge side is created first using a high-speed bur. The hinge is located at the junction of the lamina with the lateral mass. Only the posterior cortex needs to be removed. To preserve the

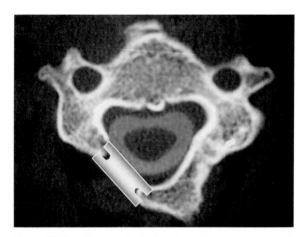

**Figure 26-11**  One method of maintaining an open-door laminoplasty. A clothespin-shaped graft is wedged between the lateral mass and the cut edge of the lamina. If the springiness of the hinge side has been maintained, excellent stability of the graft can be achieved, and additional fixation is not necessary.

"springiness" of the hinge, aggressive removal of bone from the hinge side should be avoided. The thickest portion of the lamina is always at the cephalad end. Because of the shingling effect, it is common for the cephalad portion of the lamina to be covered by the caudal portion of the lamina above. If the hinge fails to give, it almost always is due to inadequate posterior cortical bone removal at the cephalad portion of the lamina.

Next, the opening side is created, generally on the side of greatest compression or clinical symptoms. A high-speed bur is used to remove the posterior cortex at the junction of the lateral mass with the lamina. If burring is performed too medially, there may be a portion of the spinal cord that is not uncovered after opening the hinge. If burring occurs too laterally, the surgeon enters the lateral mass rather than the spinal canal and is not able to open the lamina. During

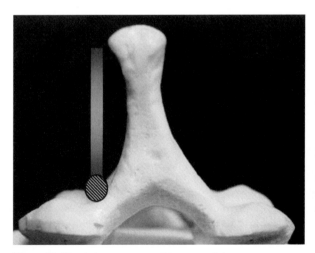 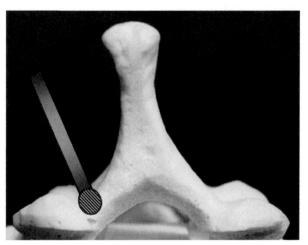

**Figure 26-10**  (**A**) During initial burring of the posterior cortex, the bur can be oriented vertically. If this course continues, however, the bur tends to carve the lateral mass rather than enter the spinal canal. (**B**) To enter the spinal canal, the bur subsequently should be oriented perpendicular to the lamina, at approximately a 45-degree angle.

the initial passes of the bur, it should be held vertically (Fig. 26-10). Subsequent burring should be done at approximately a 45-degree angle, however, so that the bur enters the canal rather than burrowing into the lateral mass. The bur is used to thin the lamina to a flake of anterior cortex. At this point, a microcuret or micro-Kerrison rongeur can be used to remove the remaining bone. Extreme care must be exercised to avoid spinal cord injury during this maneuver.

When the lamina at each level has been cut, the C2-3

and C7-T1 interspinous ligaments are resected. The surgeon then firmly, but gently, pushes on the spinous processes from the open side, creating greenstick fractures on the hinged side. After the laminoplasty is opened, dural pulsations can often be seen. Epidural bleeding, if encountered, can be controlled with gentle application of Gelfoam or bipolar cautery. If the hinge does not yield and the laminoplasty does not open, further burring may be necessary, usually of the cephalad portion of the lamina. If overlap of C2 on C3 prevents opening of C3, a dome osteotomy of the inferior portion of C2 may be necessary. A C2 dome osteotomy also may allow for greater posterior spinal cord drift in patients with cervical kyphosis. Ideally, each lamina should open with a "springy" sensation. Complete fractures on the hinge side should be avoided if possible, especially if allograft rib struts are used to keep the laminoplasty open, because the struts would not lock in as firmly. The rib struts typically are 12 to 14 mm in height and are fashioned with grooves that lock in to the lateral mass on one side and the cut edge of the lamina on the other (Fig. 26-11). The tension of the greenstick fracture keeps the struts in place, and typically no supplemental fixation is necessary. Three struts placed at C3, C5, and C7 are recommended. Alternatively, sutures, suture anchors, or miniplates can be used to keep the laminoplasty open (Fig. 26-12). Regardless of the method used, the objective is to keep the laminoplasty open until the greenstick fracture heals on the hinge side. Premature closure of the laminoplasty may result in inadequate spinal cord decompression.

## SUGGESTED READING

Bazaz R, Lee MJ, Yoo JU. Incidence of dysphagia after anterior cervical spine surgery: a prospective study. Spine 2000;27:2453–2458.

Curylo LJ, Mason HC, Bohlman HH, Yoo JU. Tortuous course of the vertebral artery and anterior cervical decompression: a cadaveric and clinical case study. Spine 2000;25:2860–2864.

Edwards CC, Heller JG, Murakami H. Corpectomy versus laminoplasty for multilevel cervical myelopathy: an independent matched-cohort analysis. Spine 2002;27:1168–1175.

Grieve JP, Kitchen ND, Moore AJ, Marsh HT. Results of posterior cervical foraminotomy for treatment of cervical spondylitic radiculopathy. Br J Neurosurg 2000;14:40–43.

Williams RW. Microcervical foraminotomy: a surgical alternative for intractable radicular pain. Spine 1983;8:708–716.

Yamaura I, Kurosa Y, Matuoka T, Shindo S. Anterior floating method for cervical myelopathy caused by ossification of the posterior longitudinal ligament. Clin Orthop1999;359:27–34.

Zdeblick TA, Bohlman HH. Cervical kyphosis and myelopathy: treatment by anterior corpectomy and strut-grafting. J Bone Joint Surg 1989;71A:170–182.

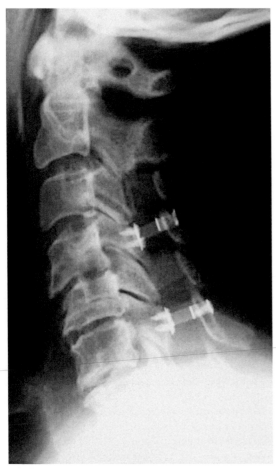

**Figure 26-12** Status-post open-door laminoplasty with rib struts at C3, C5, and C7 and mini-laminoplasty plates at C4 and C6. This degree of door stabilization typically is not necessary. Note the cut edge of the laminae seen en face and the widening of the spinal canal resulting from this procedure.

# THORACOLUMBAR DECOMPRESSION: ANTERIOR AND POSTERIOR

**FRANK M. PHILLIPS**
**MIKE H. SUN**

The primary goal of spinal decompressive surgery is to relieve compression of the neural elements without causing further iatrogenic neurologic injury. A secondary consideration to decompression is avoiding unnecessary destabilization of the spine. There are numerous thoracolumbar spine pathologies that may result in neural compression, including the following:

- Trauma
- Tumor
- Infection
- Deformity
- Degenerative conditions (e.g., spinal stenosis or herniated disc)

Several decompressive techniques are discussed in this chapter, each with unique advantages and disadvantages. In general, the choice of decompressive procedure and surgical approach is dictated by the location of the neural compressive pathology. Factors such as spinal stability and alignment, medical comorbidities, history of prior surgeries, and surgeon expertise all may play a role, however, in the selection of a particular approach to decompression.

To perform an effective decompression, the spine surgeon must have an intimate knowledge of spinal anatomy and biomechanics. The surgeon should minimize the removal of uninvolved structures during decompression that unnecessarily might compromise spinal stability. In situations in which decompression renders the spine unstable, the surgeon must be prepared to proceed to a stabilization procedure.

## ANTERIOR CORPECTOMY

### Background

Decompressive anterior corpectomy involves removal of the vertebral body and adjacent intervertebral discs to effect decompression of the neural elements. To perform a corpectomy, the spine is approached through the thoracic or abdominal cavity or via the retroperitoneal space, depending on the level of the offending pathology.

### Indications and Contraindications

Anterior corpectomy for decompression purposes usually is prescribed for the treatment of pathology located in the ventral spinal canal, most commonly the result of burst fracture, tumor, or infection. Corpectomy facilitates direct decompression of the anterior neural elements and avoids manipulation and retraction of neural tissue, as might be necessary to remove anterior compressive pathology through a posterior approach. Particularly above the level of the cauda equina, any manipulation of the spinal cord should be avoided to prevent iatrogenic injury. When considering corpectomy for decompression, the surgeon must consider the feasibility of postcorpectomy reconstruction of the spine to ensure stability.

Anterior corpectomy is not indicated when neural compression is caused by the posterior structures of the spine (i.e., from the lamina, facet joints, ligamentum flavum, or posterior abscess or tumor). The ability to perform an anterior approach and corpectomy also may be limited by prior abdominal or thoracic surgery. Resultant scarring can make dissection and exposure difficult. In the lower lumbar spine, anterior corpectomy and subsequent reconstruction is technically challenging because of the intimate anatomic relationships of the major vessels to the vertebral bodies.

### Technique

#### Preoperative Planning

Preoperative evaluation varies depending on the underlying pathology necessitating the corpectomy. The decision to proceed with an anterior corpectomy for decompression is usually the result of identifying neural compression arising anterior to the neural elements. A careful history and thorough neurologic examination are essential to define the patient's neurologic status. Laboratory studies may be helpful when considering a diagnosis of infection or tumor. In general, plain films are useful to determine spinal alignment, identify and classify vertebral fractures, and understand the extent of vertebral body destruction. The health of adjacent vertebrae, which may have implications for reconstruction strategies, also should be assessed. Computed tomography (CT)–myelography is valuable for identifying the extent of neural compressio n and determining whether bone or soft tissue is the offending pathology. The excellent bone visualization afforded by CT also allows for evaluation of the extent of bone disruption or destruction. Magnetic resonance imaging (MRI) allows for excellent soft tissue visualization and is helpful in evaluating marrow replacement processes, disc pathology, and visualization of the neural elements.

When considering anterior corpectomy, the patient must be medically fit to undergo a transthoracic, transabdominal, or retroperitoneal surgical approach. If an approach through the thoracic cavity is planned, the patient's pulmonary function should be evaluated preoperatively. If corpectomy is being performed to address a tumor, preoperative tumor embolization may help reduce surgical blood loss.

### Surgical Technique

The anatomic level of the pathology dictates the surgical approach to the vertebral body (Fig. 27-1). In general, anterior access to the T4-10 vertebral bodies requires a thoracotomy, whereas exposure of T11-S1 levels typically is accomplished through a retroperitoneal approach. Access to the lower lumbar spine also may be achieved via a transperitoneal anterior approach. Intraoperative radiographs are essential to identify the appropriate vertebral level. When the vertebral body is exposed, the segmental vessels at the level of the pathologic vertebra are ligated. The pedicle of the involved vertebra serves as an important landmark for orien-

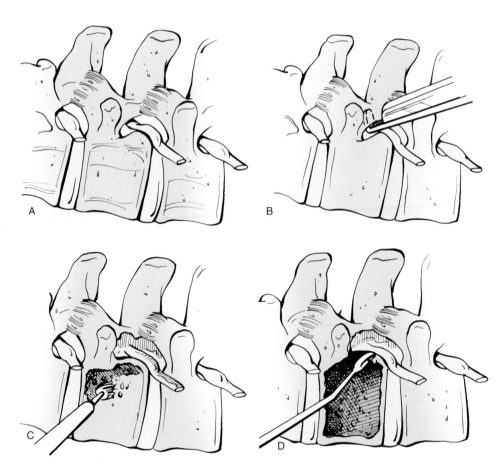

**Figure 27-1**    Technique of anterior thoracolumbar corpectomy. (**A**) Exposure of the involved vertebral level. The pedicle and associated exiting nerve root and foraminal vessels are identified. In the thoracic spine, resection of the rib head facilitates visualization of the pedicle. (**B**) The caudal portion of the pedicle is removed with a Kerrison rongeur. This allows for visualization of the neural elements and floor of the spinal canal. (**C**) After removal of the intervertebral discs cephalad and caudad to the involved vertebra, the vertebral body is removed with a Leksell rongeur and high-speed bur. The posterior vertebral body cortex is maintained to protect the neural elements until the final stage of decompression. (**D**) Using a reverse-angle curet, the remaining shell of the posterior vertebral body cortex is collapsed into the vertebral body defect (*arrow*), decompressing the neural elements.

tation with regard to the location of the spinal canal and should be identified. In the thoracic spine, the rib head may be excised to facilitate visualization of the underlying pedicle of the involved vertebra. Resection of the pedicle or part of the pedicle with a Kerrison rongeur allows visualization of the neural elements and identification of the spinal canal. During resection of the pedicle, the exiting nerve root and foraminal vessels that hug the caudal aspect of the pedicle should be protected. A discectomy at the disc above and below the involved vertebra is performed. This procedure may be facilitated by subperiosteal elevation of the disc from the end plates. An attempt should be made to perform as complete a discectomy as possible, including removal of contralateral (far-side) disc material, which helps facilitate complete corpectomy. During discectomy, care should be taken to preserve the integrity of the vertebral end plates.

Vertebral body removal may be initiated with osteotomes or rongeurs, which allow for collection of corpectomy bone that may be used for later bone grafting (e.g., with a burst fracture) or culture and biopsy (e.g., tumor or infection). During vertebral body removal, the posterior vertebral body cortex is maintained to protect the neural elements until the final stages. The corpectomy is completed from ventral to dorsal with a high-speed bur until a thin shelf of posterior vertebral cortex remains. The remaining thin cortical shelf can be collapsed into the corpectomy defect using reverse-angle curets with minimal pressure exerted on the adjacent neural elements. The decompression should be continued across the entire width of the vertebral body until the far-side pedicle can be palpated, to ensure complete decompression. Unless a total corpectomy is indicated, such as for a primary bone malignancy, the far-side lateral vertebral body wall may be maintained.

After completion of the corpectomy, the surgeon proceeds with reconstruction of the anterior column. This reconstruction usually involves placement of a strut spanning the corpectomy defect, which may be stabilized by spinal instrumentation.

### Postoperative Management

Postoperative antibiotics usually are administered for 48 hours or until drains are removed. If the anterior approach was accomplished through a thoracotomy, a chest tube often is placed, and this needs to be managed postoperatively. Attention should be directed toward pulmonary toilet after thoracotomy. Patients may sit and ambulate at a graduated pace as comfort and strength permit after surgery. Based on the stability of the postcorpectomy reconstruction, a brace may be required. In cancer patients, adjuvant radiation therapy should be delayed at least 3 weeks to allow soft tissue healing and initial fusion healing.

## POSTERIOR DECOMPRESSION

The posterior approach is the "workhorse" approach to decompressing the neural elements. In most cases in which degenerative pathology gives rise to neural compression, the posterior approach provides effective decompression. When indicated, posterior decompression can be combined with posterior instrumentation.

## LAMINECTOMY

### Indications and Contraindications

Laminectomy is indicated to address symptomatic compression of the neural elements originating from the posterior elements of the spine. Specific indications for decompressive laminectomy include:

- Spinal stenosis (degenerative or congenital)
- Tumors involving the posterior bone elements
- Fractures of the posterior bone elements
- Large herniated lumbar discs, particularly when centrally located
- Epidural hematoma or abscess

With the exception of herniated lumbar discs, if compressive pathology is located anterior to the neural elements, laminectomy is less successful in effecting decompression than direct anterior decompression. In the presence of kyphosis, posterior decompression (laminectomy) also may be less effective. Laminectomy has not been shown to be effective in the treatment of axial low back pain.

### Technique

#### Preoperative Planning

Plain radiographs indicate bone integrity, the presence of disc degeneration, and spinal alignment and stability. In addition, if short pedicles are seen, congenital spinal stenosis might be suspected. Radiographs remain the primary imaging modality on which a diagnosis of spinal instability or deformity necessitating arthrodesis surgery is based. When considering surgery, CT-myelography and MRI may be considered complementary studies. CT-myelography provides detailed bone anatomy and delineates the extent and location of neural compressive pathologies. MRI with its excellent soft tissue detail allows direct visualization of the neural elements and further assessment of neural compression.

#### Surgical Technique

After anesthesia is administered, the patient is placed in a prone position. A kneeling position (hips and knees flexed) helps increase the interlaminar spaces, which is helpful during lumbar decompression. This position reduces lumbar lordosis, however, which should be considered during instrumented fusions. The abdomen should be free of compression to reduce epidural bleeding. All bone prominences should be well padded. Standard posterior midline exposure of the spine is performed. The facet joints and pars interarticularis should be visualized clearly so that these structures can be preserved to maintain spinal stability. Before bone decompression, the anatomic level should be confirmed with radiographs. The spinous process and interspinous ligaments are removed as necessary. The laminae are removed in piecemeal fashion with a 45-degree Kerrison rongeur, starting in the midline, where a space beneath the lamina typically exists even in the presence of severe spinal stenosis. In areas of thick bone where large instruments may cause injury to the underlying neural structures, the lamina may be thinned using a Leksell rongeur or a high-speed bur before bone removal. If severe stenosis exists, working from less severely involved levels toward the most severely stenotic areas reduces the likelihood of iatrogenic neural injury.

The pedicle serves as a useful landmark to guide the extent of decompression. Identifying the pedicle from within the spinal canal helps facilitate locating the neural foramina and the takeoff and path of the exiting nerve roots. Bone ledges adjacent to the pedicles should be removed to decompress the lateral recess. When the shoulder of the nerve root is decompressed adequately, the neural foramen must be inspected meticulously for stenosis. When performing foraminotomy, the exiting nerve root should be visualized and protected. To minimize the risk of cutting across the nerve root, the Kerrison rongeur should be advanced into the foramen parallel to the exiting nerve root. The foramen is decompressed by undercutting the facet joint. Adequacy of the foraminal decompression may be assessed visually and by palpation of the foramen with an angled instrument, such as a Penfield elevator. At least 50% of the facet joint and the pars interarticularis should be preserved to avoid creating iatrogenic instability (particularly if not performing a concomitant arthrodesis). Discectomy in the presence of a laminectomy may result in instability. If decompression renders the spine unstable, the surgeon should be prepared to proceed with arthrodesis.

### Postoperative Management

A deep drain may be required, and perioperative antibiotics are administered. Early postoperative ambulation and resumption of usual activities are encouraged. If concomitant arthrodesis is performed, postoperative rehabilitation and activity level usually are dictated more strongly by the type and extent of arthrodesis procedure performed. Back strengthening and rehabilitative exercises may be recommended postoperatively.

# LAMINOTOMY WITH DISCECTOMY

## Indications and Contraindications

Laminotomy with discectomy is performed most often for the treatment of radiculopathy caused by lumbar disc herniation. Indications for discectomy include radiculopathy not responsive to a reasonable period of nonoperative care or profound or progressive motor deficit with concordant disc pathology identified on imaging studies. Laminotomy with foraminotomy may be used to treat isolated foraminal bone stenosis. Multilevel laminotomies have been described to treat degenerative spinal stenosis.

## Technique

### Preoperative Planning

When sciatica symptoms persist, MRI is the imaging modality of choice because it details the extent and location of the disc herniation. Gadolinium enhancement may be useful in helping to differentiate scar tissue from a recurrent or retained herniated disc in a patient who has had previous spinal surgery. In cases in which isolated lateral recess stenosis or hard disc (ossification or calcification of a prolapsed disc) is the suspected pathology, CT-myelography may offer more information with regard to the bone architecture.

### Surgical Technique

Patient positioning is as described for laminectomy. Before skin incision, a localizing radiograph should be obtained to allow for precise placement of a small incision, limiting soft tissue dissection required to access the spine. Magnification provided by the operating microscope or loupes is helpful when performing discectomy. The paraspinal muscles are elevated from only the side of the spine on which the disc herniation is present. The interlaminar window, bordered superiorly by the inferior edge of the lamina of the cranial vertebra, laterally by the facet joint and pars interarticularis of the caudal vertebra, inferiorly by the leading edge of the lamina of the caudal vertebra, and medially by the spinous process, should be identified carefully (Fig. 27-2). The spinal canal is entered through the interlaminar window after the ligamentum flavum is elevated or removed, allowing for visualization of the underlying neural elements. We prefer initially detaching the ligamentum flavum from its attachment to the cranial edge of the caudal lamina. A small amount of bone resection may be required to visualize the neural structures and to access the intervertebral disc. The involved nerve root is identified and retracted gently, allowing for visualization of the underlying offending disc. Retraction on the nerve root should be released frequently to prevent iatrogenic nerve root injury. If the disc is contained,

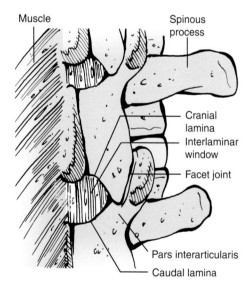

**Figure 27-2** Interlaminar window. The interlaminar window provides access to the spinal canal for performing a discectomy. The interlaminar window is bordered superiorly by the inferior edge of the lamina of the cranial vertebra, laterally by the facet joint and pars interarticularis of the caudal vertebra, inferiorly by the leading edge of the lamina of the caudal vertebra, and medially by the spinous process.

the anulus and posterior longitudinal ligament are incised with a sharp knife directed away from the neural elements. The offending disc fragment and any loose fragments within the disc space are removed with a pituitary rongeur. After the disc fragment is removed, the nerve root should be tension-free as it traverses into the neural foramina.

When treating a foraminal or extraforaminal (so-called far-lateral) disc herniation, the paramedian muscle splitting approach advocated by Wiltse is favored by many spine surgeons. With this approach, the erector spinae muscle is split bluntly longitudinally approximately 5 cm lateral to the posterior midline. The appropriate level transverse processes are identified. The intertransverse ligaments and fascia are incised, and the intertransverse membrane is opened bluntly so that the extraforaminal nerve root is visualized. The nerve is traced medially at 45 degrees toward the foramen. The nerve root may be retracted, and the underlying disc is identified. The offending disc fragments may be removed safely.

### Postoperative Management

Laminotomy with discectomy usually is performed as an outpatient procedure or with an overnight hospital stay. Patients are encouraged to resume usual activities in the early postoperative period, and patients may ambulate as soon as comfort permits after surgery.

# TRANSPEDICULAR DECOMPRESSION

## Indications and Contraindications

The transpedicular approach uses a posterior approach to the spine to access pathology anterior to the neural elements, such as may occur with tumors or burst fractures. With this approach, the vertebral body or intervertebral disc or both are accessed lateral to the spinal cord or cauda equina so that any neural retraction is minimized. This approach is useful to relieve thoracic spinal cord compression arising from involvement of the anterior vertebral elements in patients who are unable to tolerate the risk or morbidity of a thoracotomy. It also can be used in the lower lumbar region.

## Technique

### Preoperative Planning

Preoperative imaging and planning are similar to that required for any other decompressive procedure. After transpedicular decompression, spinal stability usually is compromised, so the surgeon must be prepared to reconstruct the spinal column. The surgical team must be prepared to manage substantial blood loss that can occur during transpedicular decompression.

### Surgical Technique

With the patient placed in a prone position, a standard posterior midline incision is used to expose the spinous process, lamina, and facet joints. After laminectomy, the pedicle is identified at the junction of the transverse process and the superior articular process. The pedicle may be entered with a rongeur or high-speed drill. While initially preserving the inferior-medial pedicle wall to serve as a protective barrier during the decompression, the remainder of the pedicle is removed. Combinations of straight and angled curets are placed through the base of the pedicle to remove cancellous bone from the vertebral body to create room for subsequent fragment reduction. Then the inferior-medial pedicle cortex can be removed. As the dura is protected with a curved elevator, the retropulsed bone fragments or tumor tissue either are pushed anteriorly with an impactor or reverse-angle curet or are removed carefully. In view of the destabilizing nature of a transpedicular decompression, posterior instrumentation is recommended.

### Postoperative Management

Postoperative management is similar to that prescribed after laminectomy and fusion procedures.

# COMPLICATIONS

## Dural Tear

Dural tearing during decompressive procedures is common, particularly in revision cases in which peridural scarring may be abundant. When noted intraoperatively, incidental durotomies should be repaired primarily if possible. The repair may be reinforced with fibrin sealant. Occasionally, subarachnoid drainage may be required to help promote sealing of the tear. Clear drainage from the wound postoperatively may indicate a dural tear. This tear may be confirmed by the presence of $\beta_2$-transferrin in the wound drainage or by visualization of a cerebrospinal fluid collection on MRI. Treatment options include epidural blood patches or placement of a subarachnoid drain to promote sealing of the leak. If cerebrospinal fluid leakage persists, surgical repair or "patching" of the dural tear may be required. Unrecognized dural tears may result in pseudomeningoceles or cerebrospinal fluid fistulas.

## Vascular Injury

In posterior spinal surgery, vascular injuries are associated more commonly with discectomy (L4-L5 > L5-S1). Injury to major abdominal vessels typically is the result of forceful use of a pituitary rongeur with penetration through the anterior anulus fibrosus. The mortality rate from arterial injury and venous injury has been reported to be 78% and 89%, respectively. A vascular injury should be suspected in any patient undergoing discectomy who develops hypotension or abdominal distention. This possibility must be surgically explored immediately and repaired. If a vascular injury is unrecognized, the patient may develop an aneurysm or arteriovenous fistula, which may manifest with high cardiac output and abdominal bruit.

When performing anterior decompressive spinal surgery, the major vessels must be well visualized and retracted to prevent vascular injury. The segmental vessels at the corpectomy site must be securely ligated.

## Infection

Wound infection after decompression surgeries has been reported to occur in less than 5% of patients, with a higher incidence in patients with instrumentation. Irrigation, débridement, and antibiotics are the mainstay of treatment for infection after noninstrumented spinal surgery. For wound infection in the presence of spinal instrumentation, a combination of serial irrigation, débridement, systemic antibiotics, and antibiotic-impregnated beads have been shown to be effective treatment. When instrumentation is required to maintain spinal stability, the surgeon should attempt to retain the instrumentation.

## Iatrogenic Instability

The decision as to what constitutes "instability" as a result of surgical interruption of the various motion segment stabilizers is imprecise, but results of biomechanical studies may provide some objectivity to this determination. The extent of bone resection performed can assist in making an intraoperative decision as to whether to proceed with arthrodesis after laminectomy. Experimental division of the interspinous ligament alone does not increase sagittal motion; however, removal of greater than 50% of the facets at a level or complete unilateral facetectomy results in significant instability. Destruction of the facet capsule and articular cartilage significantly destabilizes the motion segment. In addition, the intact pars interarticularis plays an important role in maintaining stability and should not be disrupted inadvertently during decompression. If iatrogenic instability is created, the surgeon should be prepared to proceed with arthrodesis.

## Neurologic Injuries

Nerve injury during spinal decompressive surgery may be the result of excessive retraction, contusion, laceration, or electrocauterization of the neural structures. The incidence of neurologic complication after all lumbar spine surgery has been estimated to be 0.2%. The risk is higher in complex cases in which instrumentation is required and deformity correction is performed. Excessive neural retraction can be avoided by ensuring adequate exposure and by gentle and mindful handling of the nerve roots and spinal cord. To minimize the risk of cutting across a nerve root, decompression should be performed parallel rather than perpendicular to the nerve root. In addition, the surgeon should visualize the nerve root to avoid accidental nerve injury.

A thorough preoperative evaluation of the patient's particular spinal anatomy is crucial in avoiding neural injury. Preoperative imaging studies may reveal spina bifida occulta, a laminectomy defect, anomalous nerve roots, and peridural scarring, which, if unrecognized, may increase risk of neural injury. These findings mandate a more cautious surgical exposure and decompression.

Anterior decompression of the lumbar spine may result in damage to the lumbar sympathetic plexus, causing retrograde ejaculation (0 to 2%) and transient lower extremity sympathectomy (10%) To reduce the risk of these complications, blunt dissections should be employed anterior to L4, L5, S1, and bipolar electrocautery only should be used.

## SUGGESTED READING

Bohlman HH, Kirkpatrick JS. Anterior decompression for late pain and paralysis after fractures of the thoracolumbar spine. Clin Orthop 1994;330:24–29.

Garfin SR, Herkowitz HN, Mirkovic S. Spinal stenosis. Instr Course Lect 2000;49:361–371.

Garfin SR, Herkowitz HN, Mirkovic S. Spinal stenosis. J Bone Joint Surg 1999;81A:572–582.

Hansraj KK, Cammisa FP, O'Leary PF. Decompressive surgery for typical lumbar spinal stenosis. Clin Orthop 2001;384:10–17.

Hansraj KK, O'Leary PF, Cammisa FP, et al. Decompression, fusion, and instrumentation surgery for complex lumbar spinal stenosis. Clin Orthop 2001;384:18–25.

Harrington KD. Metastatic tumors of the spine: diagnosis and treatment. J Am Acad Orthop Surg 1993;1:76–86.

Hodgson A, Stock F. Anterior spine fusion for the treatment of tuberculosis of the spine. J Bone Joint Surg 1960;42A:295.

Riley LH III, Frassica DA, Kostuik JP, Frassica FJ. Metastatic disease to the spine: diagnosis and treatment. Instr Course Lect 2000;49: 471–476.

Spivak JM. Degenerative lumbar spinal stenosis. J Bone Joint Surg 1998;80A:1053–1064.

# SPINAL INSTRU-MENTATION

## CHRISTOPHER M. BONO

Various types of spinal instrumentation are available to the contemporary spine surgeon. The primary intention of spinal instrumentation is to stabilize the *mechanically unstable* spine. Gross instability can be secondary to trauma, neoplasm, infection, inflammatory disease, or iatrogenic removal of anterior or posterior spinal elements. More subtle forms of mechanical instability can occur with degenerative processes, such as cervical or lumbar spondylolisthesis. Spinal instrumentation is used to maintain alignment and restore stability until solid bone fusion occurs. Although still considered controversial, the use of spinal instrumentation, in particular lumbar pedicle screws and anterior cervical plates, in the treatment of *mechanically stable* processes, such as discogenic disease, leads to higher fusion rates. More recently, a variety of spinal implants have been developed to aid in reconstruction of the anterior column.

## IMPLANT MATERIALS

Most spinal instrumentation is composed of metal, most commonly stainless steel or titanium. Stainless steel is strong, is ductile, and is resistant to notch failure. It is ideal for long corrective constructs, as used for idiopathic scoliosis. Its high strength enables large corrective forces to be delivered to the bone. Ductility allows rods to be bent into the desired shape without having to be "overbent." Low notch sensitivity means that a nick or impression made on the rod surface during contouring would not increase the chances that it would fail at the notch under cyclic loading. The disadvantages of steel implants are that they are ferromagnetic, making postoperative magnetic resonance imaging (MRI) difficult to interpret because of artifact. There also are possible risks of implant migration, especially for broken wires or hooks that are near or within the spinal canal.

Titanium implants have become more popular. Titanium is not as strong as steel, but this has potential advantages for spinal fusion. Because the elastic modulus is closer to that of bone (compared with steel), titanium implants allow more load sharing of the fusion mass, which may encourage healing and remodeling. A titanium pedicle screw may have less tendency to loosen because of a better elastic modulus match with bone. These risks remain theoretical, however,

with no study showing better fusion rates or lower loosening rates with titanium versus stainless steel implants. Titanium has greater notch sensitivity than stainless steel. In addition, titanium tends to have "memory" because of lower ductility. Although it still can be contoured, titanium rods need to be overbent to achieve the desired shape. For these reasons, many surgeons still prefer to use stainless steel systems for deformity correction. The major advantage of titanium is that it is compatible with MRI. Interbody and corpectomy cages, for the most part, are constructed from titanium for these and other reasons.

Many nonmetallic materials are being used in the fabrication of spinal implants. Carbon fiber interbody cages have been developed. Implanted from either a posterior or an anterior approach, carbon fiber implants are radiolucent, facilitating unobstructed radiographic assessment of the fusion. They also may allow more load sharing by the surrounding bone and fusion mass. Bioresorbable implants, made of such materials as polylactic acid, show future promise as temporary stabilization devices that disappear over time. Resorbable anterior cervical and lumbar plates have been used successfully in the spine. The stability provided by these implants is questionable, however, because their effect on fusion rate is unclear.

## GOALS OF INSTRUMENTATION

The various forms of spinal instrumentation are used to achieve one or more of the following goals:

- Stabilization
- Deformity correction
- Reconstruction/replacement
- Facilitate/enhance fusion (discussed in Chapter 33)

### Stabilization

Spinal instrumentation is used most often to provide stability. An illustrative example of this use is posterior segmental instrumentation of an unstable thoracolumbar fracture-dislocation. In this case, the traumatic injury created mechanical instability by disruption of the stabilizing ligaments in addition to bone fractures. After open reduction and alignment, the instrumentation provides long-lasting, durable stability to the destabilized segments. Spinal stabilization can be achieved with the use of anterior or posterior implants.

## Deformity Correction

Spinal deformity can result from a variety of disorders. Some disorders cause rapidly progressing deformities. These usually are associated with infectious diseases, such as vertebral body osteomyelitis. If treated early, these typically kyphotic deformities usually are quite mobile and easily correctable.

Many other processes produce slowly progressing deformities. Idiopathic scoliosis results in coronal and sagittal deformities that occur over years. The diagnosis usually is not made until the deformity becomes cosmetically visible.

Another example is the hyperkyphotic deformity of the thoracic or cervical spine associated with ankylosing spondylitis. In these cases, the abnormal spinal curvature becomes relatively *fixed*. To correct fixed deformities, instrumentation can be used to impart large corrective forces to the spine.

## Reconstruction and Replacement

Reconstruction refers to "rebuilding" or replacing a part or parts of the spinal column. One of the most common forms is *anterior column reconstruction*. Anterior column reconstruction is necessary when the anterior aspects of the spine (vertebral body or intervertebral discs or both) are missing or incompetent. The vertebral bodies can be eroded or destroyed by infection or tumor (Fig. 28-1A). Highly comminuted burst fractures can result in anterior column insuffi-

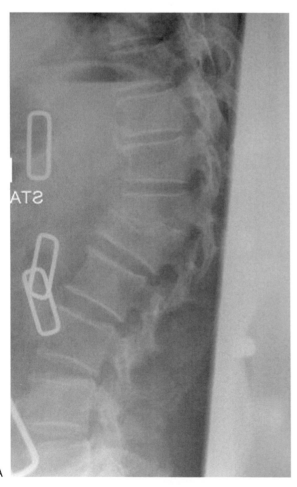

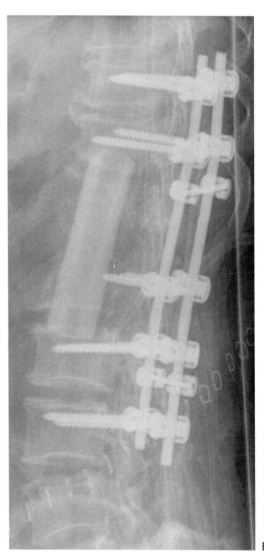

A                                                                                                      B

**Figure 28-1**  (**A**) Granulomatous infection led to a progressive kyphotic gibbus, intractable pain, and neurologic compromise. (**B**) Anterior corpectomy of T12 and L1 was followed by allograft strut interposition to reconstruct the anterior column. Posterior instrumented fusion was performed in a second stage.

ciency. Removal of the vertebral body during surgery necessitates anterior column reconstruction.

Ideally, one would be able to reconstruct a long segment of the spine using an implant that is anatomically and biomechanically similar to the normal spine. The reconstruction would allow segmental motion just as normal vertebral bodies and discs do. Current methods necessitate fusion across the reconstructed segments, however. These requirements define the twofold purpose of anterior column reconstruction. First, the implant or device must fill the missing gap between the vertebrae. In doing so, it must sustain the large compressive loads placed on the anterior spine. Second, it must provide a conduit for fusion. The ultimate goal of anterior column reconstruction is to restore and maintain desired height, while enabling solid arthrodesis between the bridged vertebral segments.

Some implant/devices can fulfill both of these purposes. A solid piece of iliac crest autograft can be osteotomized

from the anterior pelvis. The size of the piece is determined by the size of the spinal defect to be bridged. The bone is tamped into place, interposed between the upper and lower vertebral bodies. In this example, the graft is the load-bearing structure and the conduit for fusion. With time, the graft becomes fully incorporated and replaced by live bone via creeping substitution.

Allograft bone also can be used to provide structural support and a fusion conduit (Fig. 28-1B). It must be kept in mind, however, that the rate of allograft incorporation is much slower. For longer defects (anything more than a disc space), incorporation may not extend much past the contacting ends of the strut. Creeping substitution after allograft interposition occurs slowly and incompletely. Regardless, allograft struts provide an effective and durable method of anterior column reconstruction.

Titanium mesh cages can be used to reconstruct the anterior column. These are hollow tubes that can be cut to

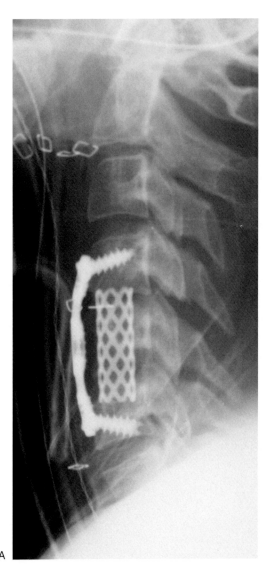
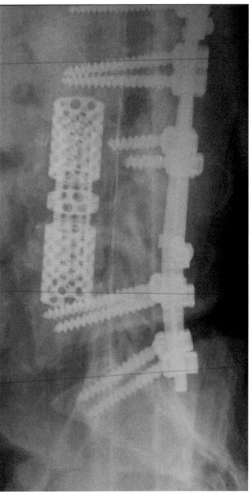

**Figure 28-2**  Titanium mesh cages can be filled with morcellized, cancellous autograft. They can be used to reconstruct the anterior column after cervical (**A**), thoracic, or lumbar (**B**) corpectomy.

custom fit a defect. The porosity of the mesh facilitates peripheral bone and vascular ingrowth. The cages can be filled with morcellized bone graft. The advantage of a cage is that the healthy bone removed during a procedure, such as a corpectomy of a burst fracture, can be reused to pack the cage. Additional morcellized autograft can be removed from the iliac crest through a limited incision and without the large defect created by structural iliac crest harvesting. With this method, the titanium cage is the weight-bearing device providing structural anterior column support, whereas the morcellized bone graft is the conduit for bone fusion (Fig. 28-2). The increased surface of the bone graft also may hasten incorporation, which does not rely on creeping substitution.

In rare circumstances, a vertebral body spacer can be placed without the intention of fusing the segments. This procedure most often is indicated in cases of metastatic tumor in which the patient's expected life span is short. Polymethyl methacrylate cement commonly is used in this way. In a soft doughy state, the cement can be molded to custom fit the vertebral defect. When hardened, the cement interdigitates with the exposed end plates and surrounding bone to maintain its position. Kirschner wires or Steinmann pins inserted into the end plates can be used to span the defect before cement insertion to reinforce the construct. With this method of anterior column reconstruction, immediate stability is provided, despite the lack of ability for eventual fusion.

# THORACIC AND LUMBAR POSTERIOR INSTRUMENTATION

## Posterior Segmental Fixation

The term *segmental fixation* implies that bone anchors (i.e., screws, hooks, or wires) are placed at each site (or many) along the construct. This contrasts with *nonsegmental* fixation, which attaches to the spine at only two sites (one upper, one lower). A classic example of nonsegmental fixation is a Harrington distraction rod. By using an up-going hook cranially and a down-going hook caudally, distraction is applied and maintained. Harrington rods first were used to correct scoliotic deformities (Fig. 28-3). Later on, with the addition of compressive rods (down-going hooks cranially and up-going hooks caudally), Harrington instrumentation and its variations were used to treat a variety of pathologies. Although a revolutionary step in the world of spinal instrumentation, nonsegmental fixation rarely is used by contemporary spine surgeons except for the stabilization of a single motion segment.

Pedicle screws offer superior biomechanical stability compared with other segmental constructs. They offer excellent longitudinal (compression-distraction), torsional, and sagittal stability. Hooks are reliant on longitudinal compressive and distractive forces for their purchase. Although they offer excellent sagittal stability, they have inferior torsional stability compared with pedicle screws. Wire constructs can be effective in correcting deformities by pulling the vertebra to the rod. They offer good sagittal plane stability; however, they cannot be used to provide compression or

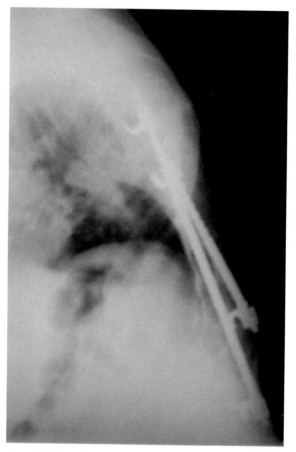

**Figure 28-3**    Harrington rods rely on distractive forces delivered at only two points. This is a classic example of nonsegmental fixation.

prevent longitudinal collapse of a spinal segment. Torsional stability also is limited.

## Pedicle Screws

Pedicle screws are a useful method of segmental fixation of the spine. They can be inserted into virtually any level of the thoracic and lumbar spine, provided that the screw can be accommodated by the pedicle. Preoperative measurement of the transverse diameter determines the maximal diameter of the screw that may be inserted. The screw should be undersized in relation to the pedicle diameter. In general, 6-mm or 7-mm screws usually can be accommodated in the lower lumbar spine. The upper lumbar pedicles (L1 and L2) usually are smaller than the lower thoracic pedicles (T10, T11, T12) and may accept only a 5-mm screw. The smallest transverse pedicle diameters are found in the midthoracic region (T4-7, approximately). Counterintuitively the upper thoracic pedicles (T1-3) usually are larger than their midthoracic counterparts.

Conceptually, pedicle screws provide three-column stability, being anchored to the anterior and posterior vertebral bodies and the pedicle. This is in contrast to segmental hook systems, which are anchored only to posterior elements (laminae, pedicle, or transverse process). Because of this ability, pedicle screw constructs can be used to deliver large corrective forces to the spinal column, which are particularly useful in the treatment of scoliosis, kyphosis, and other deformities. Pedicle screw constructs are ideal for stabilizing spinal fractures and dislocations (Fig. 28-4). In contrast to hook or wire constructs, pedicle screws can be used to stabilize laminectomized vertebrae.

**Advantages and Disadvantages.**   Pedicle screws offer superior biomechanical stability in normal bone. Disadvantages are that insertion is more technically demanding than hooks or wires, and fixation in osteoporotic bone is difficult.

**Lumbar Pedicle Screw Insertion.**   The starting point for lumbar pedicle screw insertion is at the intersection of two imaginary lines (Fig. 28-5), as follows:

- A transverse line dividing the transverse process into upper and lower halves
- A vertical line that is just lateral to the midpoint of the facet joint

Alternatively a more lateral starting point can be used,

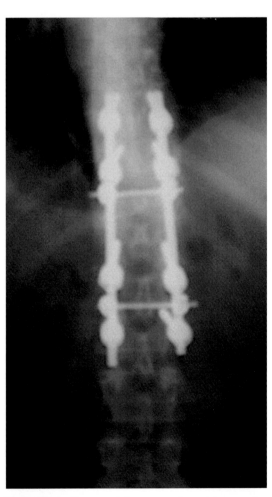

**Figure 28-4**  Segmental fixation, such as this example of pedicle screws stabilization of a thoracolumbar burst fracture, uses multiple points of fixation.

located at the junction of the transverse process and the facet joint. When using this portal, however, the screw must be angled more acutely medial. The starting portal can be created using a sharp awl, drill bit, or a small (3-mm) bur tip.

Next, a pedicle finder is inserted. Each pedicle screw system has its own pedicle finder in the set; a small (3-mm) curet also can be used. The instrument is advanced into the cancellous bone of the pedicle, using tactile feedback to ensure that the cortex is not penetrated. If resistance is felt, the orientation of the pedicle finder should be reconfirmed by visualization of bone landmarks or an intraoperative radiograph. Many surgeons use fluoroscopy to guide pedicle screw insertion.

The amount of medial angulation depends on the vertebral level. At L5, the pedicle usually is angled about 20 degrees medially. With each cranial level, the medial angulation decreases so that the L2 pedicle is angled only about 10 degrees medially. Although these numbers are useful guidelines, orientation of the pedicle is assessed best using preoperative computed tomography or MRI.

The pedicle probe should be advanced into the cancellous bone of the vertebral body. The length of the screw can be measured using this device, which usually has graduated markings for this purpose. Then the probe is removed. A pedicle feeler can be inserted to "sound" the walls of the pedicle to detect cortical perforations. The hole is tapped, and the screw is inserted. Final screw position can be confirmed by radiograph.

Additional methods have been developed to confirm cortical integrity and screw positioning. Electrical impedance measurement by directly stimulating the screw with a specially designed probe can be helpful. Low impedance suggests that the screw has penetrated the pedicle borders. Other investigators have developed methods of electrically testing the pedicle hole before screw insertion. The use of image guidance may increase the accuracy of pedicle screw insertion, particularly in cases of abnormal or anomalous anatomy. The use of either image guidance or intraoperative fluoroscopy usually is needed in revision cases if the anatomic landmarks are unclear.

**Thoracic Pedicle Screw Insertion.**   Although the basic principles of screw insertion are the same, the landmarks for thoracic pedicle screws are slightly different than in the lumbar spine. The starting portal is located at the junction of the transverse process and the inferior articular process. In contrast to the lumbar spine, it is aligned with the superior border of the transverse process (Fig. 28-6).

Thoracic pedicles are medially angulated between 0 and 10 degrees. They also can be quite small, in particular at the T4-7 levels. Although 5-mm screws may fit in the lower thoracic spine, smaller diameter screws may be safer to insert at more cranial levels. As in the lumbar spine, preoperative planning using axial computed tomography or MRI is crucial.

An alternative insertion method involves considering the thoracic pedicle and adjacent rib together as the "effective pedicle width." In this method, the screw is inserted more laterally, intentionally perforating the lateral pedicle cortex, but still being contained by the adjacent cortex of the rib.

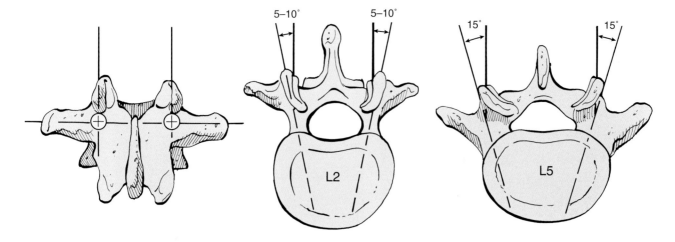

**Figure 28-5**  Entry site and screw orientation for lumbar pedicle screws.

This method necessitates more medial angulation to avoid lateral vertebral body perforation.

### Thoracic and Lumbar Hooks

Although they offer only posterior column support, hooks remain an effective and versatile method of stabilizing the spine. Hooks can be anchored onto the laminae, pedicles, or transverse processes. Hooks can be placed to create "claws," which act as independently stable fixation regions at the cranial or caudal aspects of a construct (Fig. 28-7). Although Harrington rods rely on distraction (or compression) across the entire construct, segmental hook fixation with claws can be used to deliver varying amounts of compression/distraction precisely at individual vertebral levels. This feature is particularly helpful to enable three-dimensional correction of scoliosis.

**Advantages and Disadvantages.** For most surgeons, hook placement is easier and quicker than pedicle screw insertion. Disadvantages are that hooks are an intracanal, space-occupying device that have the potential for neural compression.

**Lamina Hooks.** Lamina hooks are the workhorse of segmental hook fixation. They can be inserted as down-going or up-going hooks. For *up-going hook placement,* the ligamentum flavum is released from the inferior border of the lamina using a small, sharp curet. Next, a Kerrison rongeur is used to remove a small amount of the lamina to create a rectangular notch. Careful attention to avoid intrusion into the spinal canal must be paid to avoid neurologic injury. A trial hook can be used to ensure that the final implant will seat properly. When inserting the hook, the tip of the implant should be walked along the bone, keeping contact

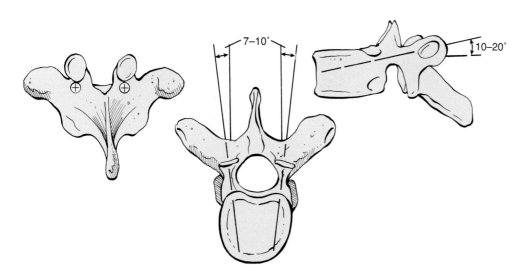

**Figure 28-6**  Entry site and screw orientation for thoracic pedicle screws.

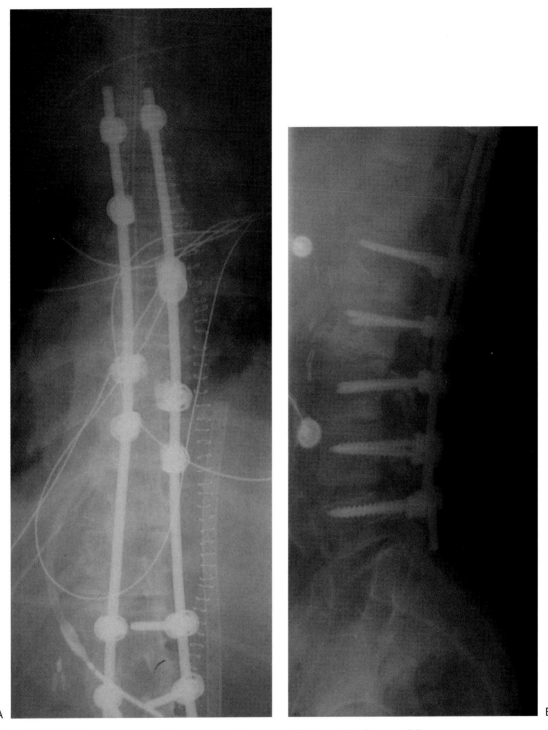

**Figure 28-7**    Hook constructs are effective means of segmental fixation. (**A**) They can deliver strong distractive and compressive forces simultaneously to correct spinal deformities. (**B**) Although some surgeons still use hooks in the lumbar spine, most prefer to anchor long constructs with multiple pedicle screws in the lumbar vertebrae.

with the undersurface of the lamina at all times. Gentle tapping of the end of the hook inserter facilitates final seating of the implant.

For *down-going hook placement,* the ligamentum flavum is released from the superior aspect of the laminae. Because of the shingle-like overlap of the upper lamina over the lower lamina, more bone removal is necessary than for up-going hooks, which are interposed between the laminae. A small portion of the inferior border of the cranial lamina is removed to gain access to the interlaminar space. Then a rectangular notch can be cut into the superior aspect of the lower lamina. The hook trial is placed, walking it along the bone surface. The final implant is tamped into place. Hooks are often loose and wobbly until the construct is assembled and tightened; they can be dislodged easily.

### Pedicle Hooks.

**Pedicle Hooks.** Although pedicle hooks provide the strongest anchoring point, they can be placed only in an up-going fashion. The facet joint inferior to the pedicle (e.g., T6-7 joint for a T6 pedicle hook) is exposed. The articular capsule is removed with a curet. A hook trial is inserted into the facet joint, walking it along the anterior surface of the inferior articular process of the upper vertebrae. The hook trial is advanced until the U-shaped end straddles the inferior surface of the pedicle. Then the final implant is tamped into place.

### Sublaminar Wiring

To place sublaminar wires in the thoracic and lumbar spine, the spinous processes and interspinous ligaments are removed. The bone can be salvaged for use as autograft. This maneuver allows full exposure of the posterior border of the laminae. Next, the interlaminar space is identified. The ligamentum flavum is released from the undersurface of the laminae but not removed. A flat, angled instrument, such as a Woodson elevator, is used to release the remaining soft tissues underneath the laminae within the midline. Although this maneuver is "blind," it is crucial to keep the instrument in contact with the surface of the bone at all times to protect the underlying neural structures. After a midline tract has been created, the blunt end of a looped wire is passed from caudad to cranial. If braided cables are used, the malleable leader is used to pass the wire. When the loop is visualized at the superior aspect of the lamina, a small nerve hook can be used to pull the wire through. After all wires have been placed, rods are cut and contoured. The wires are tensioned to the rods in sequential fashion depending on the surgical indication.

**Advantages and Disadvantages.** Sublaminar wires are easy to place. Wire constructs are the least expensive method of posterior segmental spinal fixation. They also may have biomechanical advantages over pedicle screws in osteoporotic bone (because the anterior aspect of the laminae are least affected by bone density losses). Disadvantages are that wire passage can injure the neural elements, and multiplanar stability is limited.

# THORACIC AND LUMBAR ANTERIOR INSTRUMENTATION

The evolution of anterior thoracic and lumbar instrumentation finds its roots in scoliosis surgery. In the 1960s, Dwyer developed anterior vertebral body screws that were connected by a tensioned wire. In later systems, the tensioned wire was replaced by a rod that could be locked rigidly to the screws. This change allowed better rotational control and correction. As the applications for anterior instrumen-

tation were broadened to include stabilization of fractures, anterior plates were developed. Plates were fixed to the lateral aspect of the vertebral body by coronally oriented vertebral body screws. Initial plate designs allowed only static interlocking. Later, plates with oval holes and compression devices allowed the graft/strut to be compressed and "locked in" after insertion. Subsequent revisitation to the rod/screw concept resulted in development of the Kaneda system. This is a cross-linked, double-rod system that includes a vertebral body staple through which the screws are inserted (to act as a washer). Cadaver biomechanical studies have shown the Kaneda system to be among the strongest constructs for anterior spinal stabilization.

## Anterior Vertebral Body Screw Insertion

Exposure of the lateral aspect of the vertebral body should be performed. The segmental artery, located in the mid aspect of the vertebral body, should be ligated and subperiosteally reflected to avoid injury during hardware insertion.

If a single-rod system is used, the screw is centered longitudinally and transversely within the vertebral body. Optimal orientation of the screw is parallel to the adjacent end plates in the coronal plane (Fig. 28-8). After a starting hole is created with an awl or small bur, a bicortical hole is drilled. Penetration of the far cortex must proceed carefully so as not to injure major visceral or vascular structures. In some cases, circumferential subperiosteal exposure of the vertebral body enables one to palpate the contralateral side of the bone. The hole is tapped, and the screw is inserted.

If a plate or double-rod system is used, two screws are inserted into each vertebral body. The first screw is inserted within the posterior aspect of the vertebral body, angled slightly anterior to avoid the spinal canal. It is crucial to place the screw parallel to the end plates to facilitate fixation to the rod or plate.

With most modern plate systems, the posterior screw is actually a bolt. The bolts are placed first into the cranial and caudal vertebral bodies. The plate is attached to the bolt with a locking nut. The anterior screw hole is drilled through the plate. The use of a guide is helpful in directing the screw about 15 degrees posterior, creating a triangular construct to improve bony purchase. The bolt-plate-nut complex creates a fixed-angle device.

With a Kaneda-type, double-rod system, a staple washer is tamped into the mid-vertebral body. The screws are inserted into the bone through the staple. The vertebrae can be distracted or compressed through the screws before, during, and after strut or cage insertion. The rods are inserted into holes in the screw heads and secured. Cross-linking greatly enhances the mechanical stability of the system.

## Advantages

The advantage of anterior plates is that they are relatively low profile. Smaller plates have been designed for use in the upper thoracic vertebrae. The advantage of single-rod systems is ease of application, especially when stabilizing multiple vertebral levels for scoliosis. The advantage of

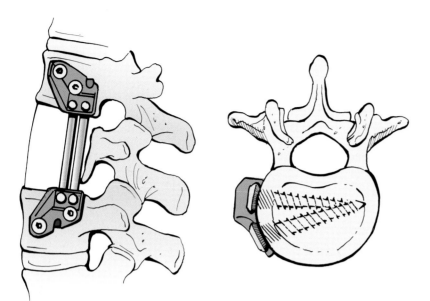

**Figure 28-8**  Diagram depicting optimal placement of anterior vertebral body screws. In this example, the screws are offset in the longitudinal plane to avoid crowding.

Kaneda-type, double-rod systems is superior biomechanical stability.

### Disadvantages

The disadvantage of anterior plates is that they generally provide less stability than double-rod systems. Because they commonly are used to stabilize spinal fractures, this becomes an issue. The disadvantage of the double-rod systems is bulkiness, which limits their use to the lower thoracic and upper lumbar spine. Although single-rod designs are useful in correcting scoliotic deformities, they remain a relatively weak fixation method.

## CERVICAL INSTRUMENTATION

Anterior cervical instrumentation is limited primarily to plating methods. These can be used to stabilize a single motion segment, such as after a discectomy and bone grafting procedure, or multiple segments, such as after corpectomy and strut placement. The goal of anterior plating is to provide immediate stability to the operated segments until bone fusion occurs.

More options are available for posterior cervical instrumentation. Historically, wires were the first method of fixation. These can be placed beneath the laminae, beneath the spinous processes, across the facet, or through the bone of the occiput. More recently, screws have become a popular method of posterior cervical fixation. Screws can be placed within the lateral mass, into the pedicle, or across a joint.

### Occipital-Cervical Fixation

Earlier methods of craniocervical fixation and fusion relied on use of structural iliac crest bone graft. Wide strips of bicortical graft are harvested. Occipital wires are passed between the inner and outer diploë of the cranium through holes created using a sharp towel clamp. Sublaminar wires are placed at C1, C2, or both, in a similar manner as described earlier. Wires are passed through drill holes within the upper and lower portions of the graft. Tightening of the wires to the graft provides stabilization and a fusion conduit. Additional morcellized bone graft can be placed along the decorticated posterior elements of the occiput and cervical laminae. In cases of instability, a halo fixator should be placed. Techniques of more rigid internal fixation of the occipitocervical junction can obviate the need for postoperative halo immobilization. They allow better correction of deformities, and device contouring enables more precise control of head position. Optionally, occipital and sublaminar cervical wires also can be fixed to rods or a Luque rectangle so that stability does not depend entirely on the integrity of the bone graft strips.

Plates and screws can be used to stabilize this region. The location of occipital screws should be considered. The central region centered at the external occipital protuberance has the thickest dimensions. Unicortical screws placed in this area have equivalent pull-out strength as more laterally placed bicortical screws. Many fixation systems take advantage of this fact by enabling screw placement within this central region.

Reconstruction plates, Y-plates, and other specially designed implants can be used to stabilize the craniocervical junction. With the rising popularity of lateral mass screw-rod fixation, hybrid plate-rod systems have been developed (Fig. 28-9). These designs incorporate the advantages of lower profile plating at the occiput (less soft tissue prominence and irritation) and polyaxial screws in the lower cervical spine. These systems are ideal for extended multilevel occipitocervical fusions. Regardless of the method of fixation, the amount and quality of graft and adequate decortication of the bone surfaces are crucial in achieving solid fusion.

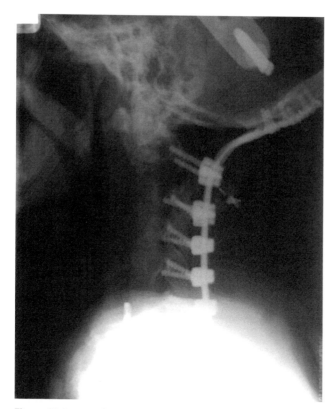

**Figure 28-9**  Newer methods of occipitocervical fixation use a rod-plate system. The plate portion allows low-profile fixation to the occiput. The rod portion enables the use of polyaxial lateral mass screws in the cervical spine.

not be considered rigid fixation because supplemental halo immobilization may be required.

Transarticular C1-2 screws provide rigid stabilization of the atlantoaxial junction. They are placed from posterior-inferior to anterior-superior. The starting point is just superior and lateral to the medial border of the C2-3 facet capsule. The screw is angled cranially, placed through the pedicle of C2, to cross the articular surfaces of the lateral C1-2 facet joints. This technique is highly technically demanding and relies on high-quality intraoperative fluoroscopy. The vertebral artery, located within the vertebral foramen, is in danger of lateral cortical violation. Medial penetration risks the spinal cord within the spinal canal. Although transarticular screws provide excellent stabilization, they are not by themselves a fusion method. A posterior Gallie fusion with wiring should be performed to effect posterior atlantoaxial fusion. If the laminae have been removed for neural decompression, morcellized bone graft can be packed into the C1-2 facet joint with care to protect the exiting C2 nerve root.

Another technically demanding option is insertion of pedicle screws into C1. These can be attached to C2 pedicle screws with a rod. Polyaxial screws are ideal for this application. The starting point for a C1 pedicle screw is approximately 2 cm from the midline, aligned parallel to the sagittal plane. In contrast to C1-2 transarticular screws, the starting point for C2 pedicle screws is more superior and along the lateral aspect of the C2 lateral mass (Fig. 28-10). The screw is angled medially to enter the C2 body. The vertebral artery

## Atlantoaxial Fixation

Instability of C1 on C2 can be the result of incompetence of the transverse (dens to C2) and alar (dens to cranium) ligaments. This incompetence can occur from trauma, inflammatory disease, or congenital/developmental disorders. Atlantoaxial instability also may result from odontoid fractures, nonunions, or os odontoideum. Fusion of C1 to C2 is the usual surgical treatment. Stabilization of the atlantoaxial joint facilitates solid fusion.

Wiring techniques are useful. Sublaminar wires are passed beneath the posterior C1 ring. These wires then can be looped underneath the C2 spinous process. Alternatively a C2 sublaminar wire can be used. A tricortical or bicortical block of iliac crest can be placed between or over the decorticated C1 and C2 surfaces. In the Gallie technique, a notch is cut into the inferior portion of the graft so that it straddles the superior portion of the C2 spinous process. Cranially, it lies over the C1 ring. This method is the least stable method of atlantoaxial fixation. Stability relies on the integrity of the bone graft. Postoperative halo immobilization is often useful.

With a Brooks technique, a block graft is interposed between the C1 and C2 laminae. Care must be taken not to avoid intrusion of the graft into the spinal canal. Sublaminar C1 and C2 wires are tensioned to compress the graft in place. Although more stable than Gallie wiring, it should

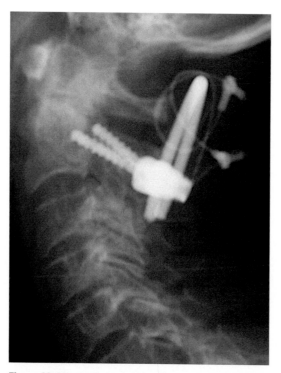

**Figure 28-10**  In this example of C1-2 fusion, pedicle screws were placed into C2 through a posterior approach. Sublaminar wires secured C1 to a U-shaped rod connected to the pedicle screws and piece of bicortical iliac crest bone graft.

(lateral) and the spinal canal (medially) are at risk with screw misplacement.

## Posterior Subaxial Cervical Spinal Fixation

### Interspinous Process Wiring

A hole is created at the base of the spinous process of the upper vertebra. This hole can be started with a small bur and completed with a sharp towel clip. A wire or cable is passed carefully through the hole. It then is passed below the caudad spinous process and tensioned. This method is not possible if a laminectomy is performed.

### Lateral Mass Screws

Various methods for lateral mass screw placement have been advocated, with plate and rod techniques available today. To orient the screw head as flush to the plate as possible, the initial technique, popularized by Roy-Camille, placed the screw perpendicular to the longitudinal axis, an-

gled laterally about 10 degrees. In efforts to stay farther away from the vertebral artery (transverse foramen), An recommended starting the screw more inferior and medial, angling it cranially about 15 degrees and laterally about 30 degrees. To place a longer screw in more bone, Magerl advocated aligning the screw parallel with the facet joint, angling it laterally by 25 degrees.

When using a lateral mass plate, the screw must be placed through the plate. The disadvantage is that the location and orientation of the screw are determined by the distance between the holes in the plate. The advantage of screw-rod constructs is that the screws can be placed at each level first, allowing placement to be determined by the patient's anatomy. The screws are connected rigidly to a rod (Fig. 28-11). Rod contouring can be challenging.

### Cervical Pedicle Screws

To gain greater bone purchase, a cervical pedicle screw can be used. Screws should be small in diameter because cervical pedicles are narrow. Placement is highly technically de-

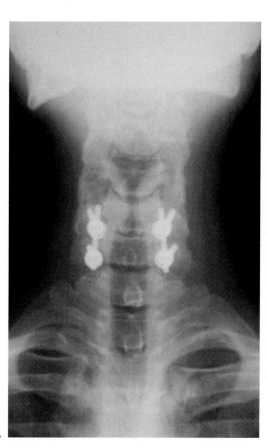
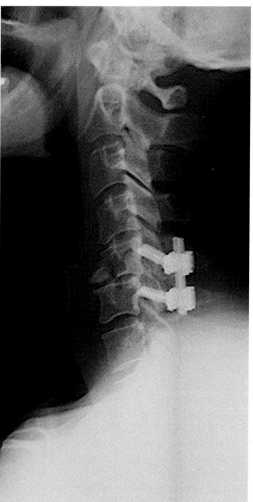

A

B

**Figure 28-11** Lateral mass screws can provide rigid fixation to the subaxial spine. (**A**) Note the lateral angulation of the screws on the anteroposterior view. (**B**) On the lateral view, the screws approximate the plane of the facet joints.

manding and risks injury to the spinal cord and the vertebral artery. Intraoperative fluoroscopy is not as useful as with C2 pedicle screw placement so that in most cases insertion is guided primarily by anatomic landmarks and tactile feel. The pedicle at C2 is dimensionally larger than the pedicles at C3-7.

## Anterior Cervical Plating

Anterior cervical plates can be used to stabilize a variety of spinal pathology. Its use as an adjunct after discectomy and fusion for degenerative conditions has become increasingly popular, with advantages of higher fusion rates and possible protection from anterior graft extrusion. Plates can be used after single-level or multilevel discectomies. In these cases, screws can be inserted into each of the stabilized vertebral bodies. After corpectomy, a spanning plate is used. It is fixed to the cranial and caudal levels. Although a one-level or two-level corpectomy might be sufficiently stabilized with anterior plating alone, posterior fixation should be considered after three or more levels have been spanned.

Screws are inserted into the mid aspect of the vertebral body (Fig. 28-12). Screws are angled toward the midline about 10 degrees to 15 degrees. This angling triangulates contralateral screws to improve bone purchase and avoids lateral penetration that can endanger the vertebral artery.

Bicortical screws have higher pull-out strength than unicortical screws. In most cases, however, unicortical screws are preferred because they avoid intrusion into the spinal canal. Although bicortical purchase can maintain length of the spanned segments, fixed-angle unicortical screws may be a safer option to achieve the same goal. These implants have screws that lock into the plate at the desired angle. This locking minimizes the chances of postoperative subsidence of the interbody graft or device into the vertebral bodies. Although this may be desired in some cases, this feature places greater stresses on the plate, which can lead to fatigue failure. Most plating systems are not fixed-angle devices. Almost all have locking mechanisms, however, by which screw back-out from the plate is prevented.

Some surgeons prefer to allow the graft to settle into the vertebral bodies over time. It is believed that this settling may aid incorporation and fusion. Short plates can be placed at the cranial and caudal vertebrae after multilevel corpectomies to act as antikick plates. It is intended that the plates would help prevent anterior kick-out of the graft, while being nonspanning fixation, to allow vertical settling. Alternatively, dynamic plates have been devised that allow subsidence to occur, while still providing additional stability.

# SPECIAL TECHNIQUES

## Odontoid Screw Fixation

Direct osteosynthesis of odontoid fractures can be effected by placement of one or two lag screws from the base of the C2 body into the tip of the dens. One or two screws provide adequate stability. The advantage of this technique is that it is motion sparing because there is no fusion involved.

A standard anterior retropharyngeal approach to the cervical spine is performed at the C5-6 level. This approach facilitates the proper trajectory. After exposure of the anterior aspect of the spine, the surgeon's finger is swept cranially to palpate the C2-3 disc space. A small starting hole can be created at the inferior lip of the C2 body with a pituitary rongeur. The drill bit is advanced carefully into the C2 body. After crossing the fracture site (which should be noted by tactile feel and imaging), the drill bit is advanced to the tip of the odontoid process. Proper trajectory is crucial and must be confirmed on anteroposterior and lateral images. The drill and screw should be contained within bone on all views. If a single-screw technique is used, the screw is centered within the odontoid. A supplemental Kirschner wire should be inserted to prevent rotation of the fragment during screw insertion. Cannulated screw systems can be helpful in optimizing screw position before drilling.

## Translaminar Lumbar Facet Screws

Posterior stabilization of a single lumbar motion segment can be provided by translaminar facet screws. These can be placed through an open incision or percutaneously, using cannulated devices. The screw is placed from the junction of the spinous process and the contralateral lamina, through the ipsilateral lamina, and across the articular surfaces of the facet joint. One of the more useful applications for translaminar screws is supplemental fixation after anterior lumbar interbody fusion.

# SUGGESTED READING

Chen IH. Biomechanical evaluation of subcortical versus bicortical screw purchase in anterior cervical plating. Acta Neurochir (Wien) 1996;138:167–173.

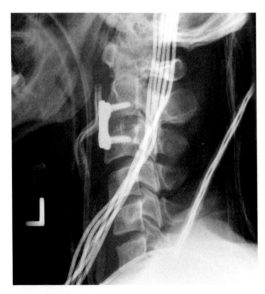

**Figure 28-12** Radiograph of an anterior cervical plate placed after discectomy and fusion. Placement of anterior vertebral body screws into C2 requires adequate proximal exposure, which can be difficult to obtain.

Delloye C, Simon P, Nyssen-Behets C, et al. Perforation of cortical bone allografts improve their incorporation. Clin Orthop 2002;396: 240–247.

Hitchon PW, Goel VK, Rogge T, et al. Biomechanical studies on two anterior thoracolumbar implants in cadaveric spines. Spine 1999; 24:213–218.

Jenkins JD, Coric D, Branch CL. A clinical comparison of one and two-screw odontoid fixation. J Neurosurg 1998;89:366–370.

Liljenqvist U, Hackenberg L, Link T, et al. Pullout strength of pedicle screws versus pedicle and laminar hooks in the thoracic spine. Acta Orthop Belg 2001;67:157–163.

McAfee PC, Werner RW, Glisson RR. A biomechanical analysis of spinal instrumentation systems in thoracolumbar fractures: Comparison of traditional Harrington distraction instrumentation with segmental spinal instrumentation. Spine 1985;10:204–217.

Richter M, Schmidt R, Claes L, et al. Posterior atlantoaxial fixation: biomechanical in vitro comparison of six different techniques. Spine 2002;27:1724–1732.

Skinner R, Maybee J, Transfeldt E, et al. Experimental pullout testing and comparison of variables in transpedicular screw fixation: A biomechanical study. Spine 1990;15:195–201.

# COMPLICATIONS

**CHOLL W. KIM**

Although the incidence of complications related to spinal surgery has been reduced, complications can be serious and potentially life-threatening. The complications can be categorized by the period of time during which they occur relative to the surgical procedure, as follows:

- *Intraoperative,* which occur in the operating room
- *Perioperative (early postoperative),* which occur within a few days after surgery, usually during hospitalization
- *Delayed postoperative,* which occur weeks to years after surgery

Intraoperative complications may be related to the following:

- Patient positioning
- Technical aspects of surgical exposure
- Insertion of spinal instrumentation
- Harvesting of autograft bone

Perioperative complications include the following:

- Superficial wound infections
- Deep venous thrombosis
- Pulmonary embolism
- Urinary retention
- Malnutrition

Postoperative complications include the following:

- Late postoperative instability
- Infection
- Deformity
- Pseudarthrosis
- Adjacent segment disease
- Epidural fibrosis
- Arachnoiditis

## INTRAOPERATIVE COMPLICATIONS

### Positioning

The potential for complications begins with positioning on the operating table. Care must be taken to ensure that the airway is protected when the patient is transferred from a stretcher to the operating table, especially if the patient is being turned from a supine to a prone position. In the prone position, the face must be padded evenly to avoid pressure ulceration. Direct pressure on the eye must be avoided to prevent catastrophic retinal artery occlusion and loss of vision. Direct pressure applied to the scalp has been associated with alopecia, usually reversible, but occasionally permanent.

Meticulous padding of vulnerable areas, such as the elbows, hips, and knees, helps prevent injuries to the ulnar, lateral femoral cutaneous, and common peroneal nerves. The brachial plexus can be at risk in the lateral decubitus or prone position. An axillary roll (which is placed 5 to 10 cm distal to the axilla) and avoidance of excessive abduction of the shoulder can help reduce the incidence of postoperative brachial plexopathy.

Systemic venous return must be considered during patient positioning. The abdomen should remain free to prevent vena cava compression. Decreased venous return can lead to loss of cardiac preload and subsequent hypotension. Batson showed that obstruction of caval flow can produce increased venous pressure around the epidural sinusoids of the spine, which may lead to increased blood loss.

### Surgical Exposure

#### Cervical Spine

Injuries to vascular and visceral structures during anterior surgery on the cervical spine may occur. Meticulous atraumatic dissection and careful placement of deep retractors can minimize these complications. The recurrent laryngeal nerve runs between the esophagus and the trachea. When deep retractors are placed, the recurrent laryngeal nerve can be pinched between the retractor and the endotracheal cuff (Fig. 29-1). Some authors believe that it is important to deflate the endotracheal cuff to lower pressure of the recurrent laryngeal nerve. Releasing the endotracheal cuff and reinflating the cuff at a lower tension decreases the pressure on the recurrent laryngeal nerve and decreases the incidence of postoperative vocal cord paralysis. The airway must be maintained clear of secretions, however, to avoid retrograde flow or aspiration into the lungs.

The vertebral artery is at risk from anterior and posterior approaches. It is at particular risk during placement of C1-2 transarticular screws. Most vertebral artery lacerations

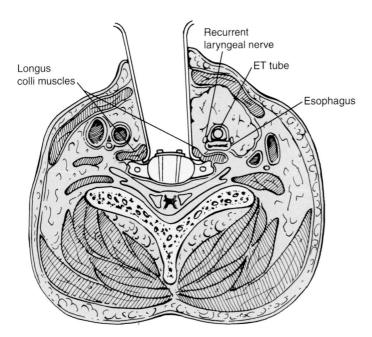

**Figure 29-1**  Cross-sectional anatomy of the cervical spine during anterior cervical spine surgery. The retractors are shown under the longus colli muscles. The recurrent laryngeal nerve lies between the retractor blade and the trachea. ET, endotracheal. (From Apfelbaum RI, Kriskovich MD, Haller JR. On the incidence, cause, and prevention of recurrent laryngeal nerve palsies during anterior cervical spine surgery. Spine 2000;25:2906–2912.)

can be treated by packing with thrombin-soaked absorbable gelatin sponges. In rare cases, ligation may be required for hemostasis. Although most patients tolerate unilateral vertebral artery ablation, a small percentage have symptomatic vertebrobasilar symptoms, such as syncope, nystagmus, dizziness, or Wallenberg syndrome (ipsilateral loss of temperature and pain sensation of the face and contralateral loss in the extremities and trunk, dysphagia, dysarthria, and nystagmus). If possible, repair of an injured vertebral artery might be considered.

Injury to the esophagus is associated with a high incidence of deep infection. Palpation of the nasogastric tube can help identify the location of the esophagus. Subperiosteal elevation of the longus colli muscles from the anterolateral vertebral bodies with placement of deep retractors under the elevated muscle edge can help prevent injury. The most frequently occurring symptoms are neck pain, odynophagia, dysphagia, and hoarseness. Cervical osteomyelitis or cervical abscess develops in about half of patients. Clinical findings include fever, cervical tenderness and induration, weight loss, tachycardia, crepitus from emphysema, and hematemesis. A combination of endoscopy and a swallow study is regarded by most authors to have the highest diagnostic yield.

Management of esophageal perforation is surgical. Nonoperative management, including observation, intravenous nutrition, feeding tube or gastrostomy, appropriate antibiotic coverage, and aspiration precautions, should be reserved for small perforations in patients otherwise too sick to undergo surgery. The literature indicates high morbidity and mortality with nonoperative management of all but the smallest of perforations, especially with tears of the lower esophagus. Consultation with a thoracic or esophageal surgical specialist is recommended in all cases. The esophagus should be examined carefully after any anterior cervical spinal operation before closure. Any esophageal injury noted in the operating room should be repaired by an experienced surgeon. The repair can be augmented, if necessary, with a muscle flap, such as a proximally based sternocleidomastoid rotational flap. This augmentation is of particular utility in cases of delayed diagnosis and of large defects that are not amenable to primary repair.

### Thoracic and Lumbar Spine

Anterior thoracic and lumbar surgery can be complicated by pneumothorax, hemothorax, and chylothorax. Massive hemothorax may occur from profuse vertebral body bleeding. This condition may require surgical tamponade of venous sinuses in the vertebral body with bone wax or ligation of the respective segmental arteries.

The presence of a thoracic fracture also should alert the physician to the possibility of a thoracic duct injury. The thoracic duct has a winding course along the spine. In the lower thoracic spine, it lies anterior and slightly to the right of the spine between the aorta and azygos vein and behind the esophagus. In the upper spine, it crosses over to the left side, behind the aortic arch. Iatrogenic chyle leaks have been reported after spinal surgery. Most leaks are clinically insignificant and heal spontaneously. If a chylothorax is suspected postoperatively, diagnostic thoracentesis and tube thoracostomy should be done. Oral intake should be discontinued because even low-fat clear liquids markedly increase chyle flow. Traditionally, continued chylous chest drainage for more than 6 weeks is an indication for open surgical intervention. Some authors recommend surgical treatment within 2 weeks to prevent ongoing protein and lymphocyte losses and to minimize the risk of infection.

Trauma or severe stenosis may make the spinal cord more sensitive to the effects of mild ischemia. Anterior procedures of the spine often require mobilization or ligation of the segmental vessels over numerous levels. In most cases, ligation of multiple ipsilateral segmental arteries can be performed without neurologic compromise. In some cases, especially in the setting of congenital deformity correction, segmental artery disruption may lead to neurologic compromise.

The anterior lumbar spine can be approached via the retroperitoneal or, less commonly, the transperitoneal approach. If the location of the pathology does not necessitate one side or the other, a left-sided approach is preferred because the aorta is easier to mobilize than the thin-walled vena cava. The left common iliac vein is the vessel most at risk during left-sided retroperitoneal and transperitoneal exposures. Regardless of approach, instrumentation should be placed on the lateral side of the vertebral body and should not contact the great vessels. The ureters and great vessels are at risk in retroperitoneal dissections, especially in the revision setting. Consideration should be given to preoperative ureteral stenting before revision procedures. Injury to the sympathetic plexus overlying the anterior aspect of the lower lumbar and upper sacral vertebrae may lead to retrograde ejaculation in men.

Vascular complications during posterior lumbar spinal surgery are uncommon. Vascular injury may occur during discectomy if the anterior longitudinal ligament is violated. The pituitary rongeur is the most frequent culprit (Fig. 29-2). Unless acute hypotension occurs intraoperatively, these injuries initially may go unnoticed. Late abdominal rigidity, abdominal pain, tachycardia, and anemia should alert the physician to the possibility of this complication.

## Dural Injury

Cerebrospinal fluid (CSF) leaks can lead to positional headache, wound complications, meningitis, arachnoiditis, and pseudomeningocele. Postoperatively, persistent CSF leaks lead to clear drainage from the wound or a subcutaneous fluid collection. Severe headache exacerbated by upright posture may be noted. Large volumes of fluid can be seen because the choroid plexus produces more than 20 mL of CSF hourly. If it is unclear whether drainage is CSF, testing for $\beta_2$-transferrin can be useful. A pseudomeningocele may develop if a dural tear occurs and is not repaired in a watertight fashion. A pseudomeningocele may occur days to months postoperatively.

The first step in repair is complete exposure of the dural rent. The goal is a watertight repair that is tension-free. Usually this repair can be accomplished with 6-0 polypropylene suture placed in a running locking stitch. A Valsalva maneuver to 40 torr may be simulated by the anesthesiologist after repair to assess for residual leak. If leakage occurs after repair, augmentation with additional suture, gelatin sponge, autogenous fat, or fibrin glue is advised. More complex tears may require grafting with fascia lata or with commercially available dural patches. Meticulous watertight fascial closure is as important as the dural repair itself because the healing of the fascial barrier is important in preventing durocutaneous fistulas. Most surgeons avoid the use of wound drains in the presence of a dural tear because negative pressure may encourage a persistent leak.

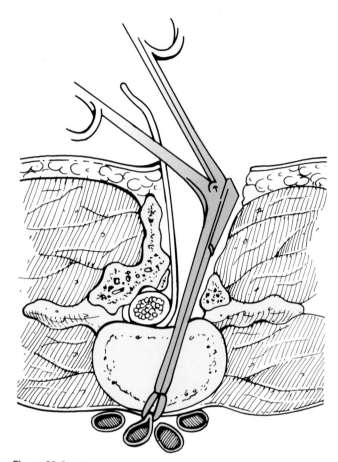

**Figure 29-2** The pituitary rongeur may injure anterior vessels during discectomy, particularly if the anterior longitudinal ligament is disrupted. (From Garfin SR. Complications of spine surgery. Baltimore: Williams & Wilkins, 1989.)

## Instrumentation

Complications related to spinal instrumentation may result. Systems employing rods and hooks can fail from hook pullout, hook-rod disengagement, or rod fracture. Hook pullout occurs commonly if used in osteoporotic bone or at the apex of a kyphotic segment.

The advent of pedicle screw fixation has improved the reliability and versatility of spinal fixation; however, the potential complications can be significant. A short screw or a screw placed too lateral can have suboptimal fixation. A medially and inferiorly placed screw may violate the canal or foramen and cause a dural tear or neurologic injury. A screw that is excessively long may violate the anterior aspect of the vertebral body with potentially life-threatening perforation of the great vessels. Similarly, excessive compression of the reconstructed segments can lead to foraminal encroachment (Fig. 29-3). In experienced hands, the rate of complications is low. In a large series, only 0.2% of screw fixations needed reoperation for nerve root irritation and 0.5% of screws were fractured at follow-up.

## Bone Graft Harvest

Autogenous bone graft remains the gold standard for achieving arthrodesis. Significant complications can occur

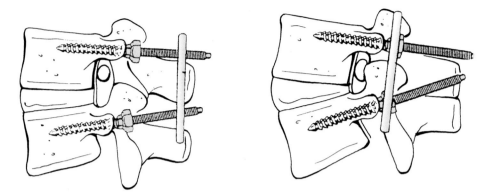

**Figure 29-3** Foraminal encroachment of the nerve root by hyperextension with pedicle screw instrumentation. (From Richardson WJ. Complications in spinal surgery. Curr Opin Orthop 1993; 4:155–159.)

with its harvest. The most common complication is persistent pain at the donor site. Often this pain is more bothersome and lasts longer than the pain associated with the principal procedure. Although there is no accepted method to avoid donor site pain, most authors agree that limited muscle dissection and periosteal stripping is helpful.

Another common complication of iliac crest bone graft harvesting is injury to the lateral femoral cutaneous nerve leading to meralgia paresthetica. The lateral femoral cutaneous nerve is a sensory branch of the lumbar plexus that supplies the lateral aspect of the thigh. It emerges from the lateral border of the psoas muscle and crosses the anterior border of the iliacus muscle to reach the anterior superior iliac spine. It passes into the thigh usually inferior to the

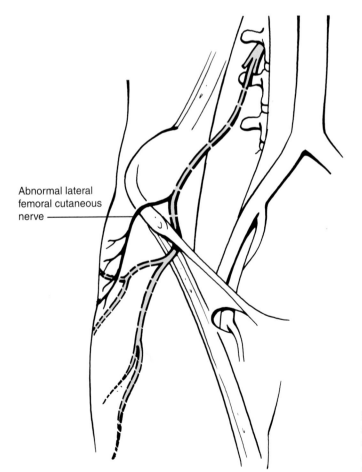

Abnormal lateral femoral cutaneous nerve —

**Figure 29-4** Anteroposterior view of the right hemipelvis showing an anomalous course of the lateral femoral cutaneous nerve, which may be 2 cm lateral to the anterior superior iliac spine. (From Garfin SR. Complications of spine surgery. Baltimore: Williams & Wilkins, 1989.)

inguinal ligament and medial to the anterior superior iliac spine. Retraction of the iliacus muscle may traumatize the nerve, particularly if an inner table graft is taken. Some patients have an anomalous anatomy path in which the nerve may be located as far lateral as 2 cm from the anterior superior iliac spine, above the inguinal ligament (Fig. 29-4). Careful visualization of this potential variant is required during dissection.

The superior gluteal artery and nerve are at risk during posterior iliac crest harvesting. The superior gluteal artery branches off the internal iliac artery and enters the gluteal region through the most superior aspect of the sciatic notch. These structures may be injured during subperiosteal dissection with elevators or inadvertent penetration by a toothed retractor. If the artery is transected, it tends to retract into the pelvis. Hemostasis may require further bone resection to expose the stump, embolization, or anterior exploration and ligation.

Pelvic fractures may occur on the side of bone graft harvesting and are likely due to a stress riser created in the ilium at graft acquisition. This phenomenon is most likely to occur in older osteoporotic patients with long lumbosacral fusions. Protected weight bearing typically is adequate for resolution of symptoms.

# PERIOPERATIVE (EARLY POSTOPERATIVE) COMPLICATIONS

## Infection

The postoperative infection rate in the spine is 2% to 3%. Simple lumbar discectomy has less than a 1% infection rate, whereas combined fusion and instrumentation is associated with rates of 4% to 8%. Risk factors include the following:

- Increased age
- Obesity
- Diabetes
- Smoking
- Immunosuppression
- Duration of preoperative hospitalization
- Spinal dysraphism
- Myelodysplasia
- Revision surgery
- Operative time
- Use of instrumentation, bone graft, or methyl methacrylate

The use of perioperative antibiotic prophylaxis to prevent infection is widespread. Patients with instrumented fusions have a decreased infection rate with the use of prophylaxis compared with patients having surgery without prophylaxis. Commonly the antibiotic dose is administered before the incision and for 24 hours postoperatively, although some surgeons prefer to administer antibiotics until suction drains or catheters are removed. The choice of antibiotic is guided by consideration of multiple factors, including host immunocompetence; the bacterial flora common in the region; and procedure type, cost, and side-effect profile. Most commonly a cephalosporin is used. With increasing concerns regarding the development of bacterial resistance, drugs such as vancomycin should be discouraged and re-

served only for patients at increased risk of methicillin-resistant staphylococci infections; this includes patients with lymphopenia, recent or current hospitalization, postoperative wound drainage, and alcohol abuse.

Early, superficial wound infections may be treated with antibiotics and local wound care. Nonresponsive superficial infections require early surgical intervention. The débridement should proceed in a systematic fashion. Each layer is débrided and cultured before advancing deeper with the dissection. In most cases, the infection tracks to the bone or hardware, and deep débridement should be performed.

Although solidly fixed instrumentation typically is left in place in the early postoperative period, all other foreign bodies, such as bone wax and collagen sponges, must be removed. Hematomas should be evacuated. Adherent bone graft may be retained, whereas loose and necrotic graft is removed. Susequent bone grafting may be performed at a later débridement after the infection is controlled better. Primary wound closure over drains, often with retention sutures to prevent dehiscence, is favored. Depending on the amount of devitalized tissue, routine serial débridements often are required. Complex wound infections may require musculocutaneous flaps. Postoperatively, antibiotic therapy is required for at least 10 to 14 days for superficial infections. Six weeks of parenteral antibiotic treatment is recommended in cases of bone involvement, deep infection, or retained foreign bodies (e.g., metal, graft).

## Malnutrition

Nutritional status after surgery is known to have significant effects on morbidity and mortality. The degree of malnutrition is related to the number of spinal levels treated. Prospective studies have shown that patients undergoing six-level fusions require at least 6 weeks to recover, whereas patients undergoing 13-level fusions require at least 12 weeks. Perioperative malnutrition is especially problematic in patients undergoing staged anterior and posterior procedures. There is often little or no enteral intake between stages. Combined with the catabolic state after major surgery, patients often have deleterious malnutrition leading to higher rates of postoperative complications, such as wound infection, sepsis, and pneumonia. Total parenteral nutrition between stages of anterior and posterior procedures may lower rates of pneumonia, urinary tract infections, and wound complications.

## Urinary Retention

Urinary retention often is ignored after spinal surgery. The incidence of urinary retention can be 38%, however. Advanced age and preoperative use of β-blockers are risk factors for this problem. Patients undergoing lumbar laminectomy are at higher risk than patients undergoing simple discectomy or cervical spinal surgery. Prolonged bladder catheterization leads to a higher risk of urinary retention, possibly by mechanical irritation of the trigone, which serves to straighten and shorten the bladder neck. When the patient can stand, the catheter is removed. Straight catheterization is performed every 6 hours for urinary retention.

# LATE POSTOPERATIVE COMPLICATIONS

## Pseudarthrosis

Pseudarthrosis is a complication of instrumented and non-instrumented fusions. Rates of pseudarthrosis after posterior spinal fusion vary widely in the literature from 0% to 50%. The most common sequela of pseudarthrosis is pain. Diagnosis can be challenging. Instrumentation often obscures radiographic evaluation, and back pain often persists even in patients with a solid fusion. Screw fracture or lucency around screws suggests fusion failure.

The rate of pseudarthrosis increases with the number of attempted fusion levels. Tobacco use, advanced age, malnutrition, and use of nonsteroidal antiinflammatory drugs have been associated with decreased rates of fusion. If patients stop smoking for at least 6 months after lumbar fusion surgery, the rate of nonunion may be comparable to that of nonsmokers.

## Adjacent Segment Degeneration

Adjacent segment degeneration refers to the accelerated degeneration that occurs above and below the level of a fusion. Instrumented fusions seem to be more prone to this phenomenon than fusions without instrumentation. The cause of adjacent segment disease is unclear. Possible causes include direct impingement of instrumentation on the facet joints or denervation of the surrounding tissues, especially the facet capsule, leading to neuropathic destruction of the facet. The facet joint adjacent to the fusion site should be protected. One should avoid ending a fusion at a region of stenosis, spondylolisthesis, or posterior column deficiency.

## Failed Back Surgery Syndrome

### Epidural Fibrosis

The failed back surgery syndrome loosely describes a subset of patients who have poor clinical outcomes after lumbar procedures. It is likely that some of these cases are a result of epidural scarring. With the advent of magnetic resonance imaging (MRI), exuberant epidural fibrosis is recognized after spinal surgery.

Clinical reports have produced contradictory evidence concerning the importance of epidural fibrosis. Several studies have failed to show a correlation between epidural scarring and clinical outcome. A large multicenter, randomized, double-blind, prospective clinical trial showed, however, that the presence of epidural scar increases the likelihood of a poor outcome after lumbar surgery. In a study of 197 patients undergoing contrast-enhanced MRI after single-level laminotomy and discectomy, patients with extensive peridural scar were 3.2 times more likely to have recurrent radicular pain that patients with less extensive scarring. These findings suggest that epidural scar formation increases the likelihood of a poor outcome after lumbar disc surgery.

Numerous methods to prevent scar formation have been studied. Barriers such as absorbable gelatin sponge (Gelfoam), gelatin films, collagen sponges, and cellulose sponges have been shown to be ineffective in preventing epidural scar formation. Fat grafts, polyglactin 910 (Vicryl) meshes, and fibrin glue have moderate inhibitory effects on scar formation but do not affect clinical outcomes. More contemporary barriers include viscous carboxymethylcellulose, carbohydrate polymer sheets, collagen sealant, and silicone tubing. These barriers have been shown to decrease scar formation in animal models.

## Arachnoiditis

Arachnoiditis refers to a pathologic inflammation of the pia-arachnoid membrane surrounding the spinal cord, cauda equina, or nerve roots. It is an intradural process. There is a continuum of involvement, ranging from mild membrane thickening to dense scarring that can block CSF flow. Patients show a wide constellation of pain and neurologic symptoms. The causes of arachnoiditis are variable. Oil-based intrathecal contrast media used for myelography and meningeal infections were the main causes of this disease until more recently. Failed back surgery syndrome, marked by persistent pain, numbness, and weakness after spinal surgery, is thought to be due in part to arachnoiditis. Arachnoiditis is more frequent in patients who have had extensive procedures, repeated procedures, postoperative spinal infections, or intraoperative dural tears.

Delamarter et al described the MRI characteristics of arachnoiditis using a three-group classification system. Group 1 showed conglomerations of adherent nerve roots residing centrally within the thecal sac. Group 2 showed nerve roots adherent peripherally to the meninges, giving rise to an "empty sac" appearance. Group 3 showed a soft tissue mass replacing the subarachnoid space. MRI resulted in accurate diagnosis and had excellent correlation with computed tomography–myelography and plain film myelographic findings.

The mainstay of treatment is oral medications (antiinflammatory, nerve stabilizing, and narcotic) combined with activity modification and physical therapy. Intrathecal infusion of morphine, transcutaneous nerve stimulation, and dorsal column stimulators have produced variable results. Surgery involving extensive microsurgical dissection and lysis of fibrotic tissue produces good short-term results in selected patients, but these results diminish greatly with time, and surgery rarely is indicated. Given the challenges of treatment, concentrated effort at avoiding this problem is warranted.

# SUMMARY

The complications of spinal surgery are numerous and challenging. Complications may occur during various periods of surgical treatment. Intraoperatively, meticulous technique guided by known potential risks of each procedure is essential. Perioperatively, wound care, pulmonary toilet, bladder care, and nutrition must be diligent. Postoperatively, pseudarthrosis, adjacent segment disease, kyphosis, epidural fibrosis, and arachnoiditis may develop months to years after surgery. Regular follow-up and prompt recognition of potential complications provide a better opportunity for effective treatment.

# SUGGESTED READING

Apfelbaum RI, Kriskovich MD, Haller JR. On the incidence, cause, and prevention of recurrent laryngeal nerve palsies during anterior cervical spine surgery. Spine 2000;25:2906–2912.

Boulis NM, Mian FS, Rodriguez D, et al. Urinary retention following routine neurosurgical spine procedures. Surg Neurol 2001;55:23–28.

Brown CW, Orme TJ, Richardson HD. The rate of pseudarthrosis (surgical nonunion) in patients who are smokers and patients who are nonsmokers: a comparison study. Spine 1986;11:942–943.

Delamarter RB, Ross JS, Masaryk TJ, et al. Diagnosis of lumbar arachnoiditis by magnetic resonance imaging. Spine 1990;15:304–310.

Farcy JP, Weidenbaum M, Glassman SD. Sagittal index in management of thoracolumbar burst fractures. Spine 1990;15:958–965.

Garfin SR. Complications of spine surgery. Baltimore: Willimas & Wilkins, 1989.

Geisler FH. Prevention of peridural fibrosis: current methodologies. Neurol Res 1999;21:S9–S22.

Glassman SD, Anagnost SC, Parker A, et al. The effect of cigarette smoking and smoking cessation on spinal fusion. Spine 2000;25:2608–2615.

Jacofsky DJ, Currier BL, Kim CW, et al. Complications in the treatment of spinal trauma. Philadelphia: WB Saunders, 2003.

Lenke LG, Bridwell KH, Blanke K, et al. Prospective analysis of nutritional status normalization after spinal reconstructive surgery. Spine 1995;20:1359–1367.

Richardson WJ. Complications in spinal surgery. Curr Opin Orthop 1993;4:155–159.

Ross JS, Obuchowski N, Modic MT. MR evaluation of epidural fibrosis: proposed grading system with intra- and inter-observer variability. Neurol Res 1999;21:S23–S26.

# MICROINNER-VATION: PAIN GENERATORS

## F. TODD WETZEL

## OVERVIEW

This chapter reviews the pertinent anatomy and physiology of nociceptive spinal anatomy. Many parts of the spinal column are pain sensitive, are richly innervated, and are potential pain generators. These parts of the spinal column include the following:

- Anterior and posterior longitudinal ligaments
- Vertebral body
- Synovium of the articular facets
- Nerve roots
- Muscle
- Supporting soft tissues

The intervertebral disc itself also is richly innervated.

## NOCICEPTORS

Nerve receptors that respond primarily to noxious stimulation are termed *nociceptors*. Nociceptive nerve fibers are classified with respect to three characteristics:

- Presence and degree of myelination (e.g., unmyelinated C fiber versus myelinated A fiber)
- Type of stimulation that provokes nerve fiber response
- Type of response

To be a potential source of pain, any given anatomic structure must have nociceptive innervation. In general, the skin, mucous membranes, and periosteum may be considered the most "peripherally" innervated tissues. Innervation is concentrated within these "coverings." There are various receptors in these structures. Some are specific for a single stimulus type (e.g., heat or pressure), whereas others are polymodal.

The presence of free nerve endings (i.e., receptors) usually suggests a nociceptive function for that fiber. Two nerve fiber types in particular seem to be important for pain transmission: nonmyelinated C fibers and a specific subset of myelinated A fibers known as *thinly myelinated A delta fibers*. The relative amounts of myelin influence the speed of nociceptive pain transmission. The cell bodies of these afferent fibers are located within the dorsal root ganglion of each spinal nerve root or within the gasserian ganglia of the trigeminal nerves (centrally, cranial nerves). The neurons themselves are bipolar, with axons extending from the cell bodies to the innervated structure (afferent) and another extending to the spinal cord or brainstem.

In the spinal cord (Fig. 30-1), the central fibers of the primary nociceptive afferents (A delta and C) terminate in the superficial regions of the dorsal aspect of the spinal cord. Pain information first is "integrated" within the dorsal root entry zone. The *dorsal root entry zone* is defined as the proximal aspect of the dorsal nerve root and its corresponding superficial layers within the dorsal horn of the spinal cord. From there, secondary fibers proceed to the thalamus via the spinothalamic tract. Physiologically the A delta fibers are faster conducting (because they are partially myelinated) and transmit sharp, localized pain; the unmyelinated C fibers are slower and transmit poorly localized, dull, burning, or aching sensations.

Receptor type varies with location. A fiber mechanical/heat nociceptors are present in high density within the skin of the hand. Mechanically insensitive afferent fibers have a high mechanical threshold and are more prevalent within highly mobile diarthrodial joints with synovial capsules, such as the knee.

The location of the innervated structure influences the character of the pain that is transmitted. Deeper structures, such as muscle, ligament, and the intervertebral disc, produce pain sensations that are diffuse and poorly localized, whereas cutaneous nociception usually is sharp and easily localized. Deep pain also can be associated with autonomic nervous responses. These often are produced by stimuli that are not tissue damaging.

### Nociceptive Innervation of Neural Tissue

Nerves themselves can be a source of pain. The pia mater covering the spinal cord and nerve roots has copious unmyelinated fiber nociceptive innervation. Little is known about the physiology of the primary afferent fibers innervating the meninges (Fig. 30-2). Janig and Koltzenburg suggested that pain fibers in the ventral root may serve as the primary afferent fibers that innervate the root or sheath itself. These fibers have no resting neural discharge and seem to be maximally activated by noxious stimuli.

This concept may help explain the phenomenon of pain-

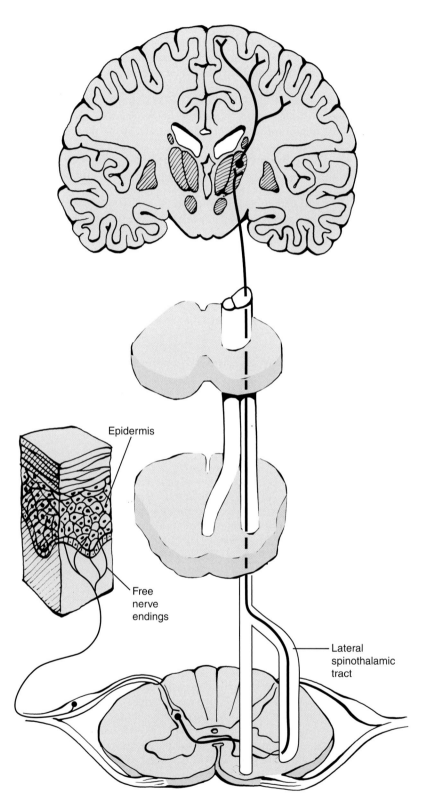

Epidermis

Free
nerve
endings

Lateral
spinothalamic
tract

**Figure 30-1**    Pathways for nociception, which
begin with the pain receptor (free nerve ending)
and end in the brain, where pain actually is per-
ceived.

ful radiculopathy from a herniated disc. Assuming that
these fibers are relatively mechanically insensitive,
compression of a noninflamed, normal nerve may not produce radicular pain, whereas it causes neural deficit.
Compression of an inflamed nerve root is more likely, how-

ever, to produce typical referred neuropathic pain, in addition to corresponding dermatomal anesthesia or motor deficit. This phenomenon has been shown elegantly in animal
studies.

Pain associated with nerve root compression or damage

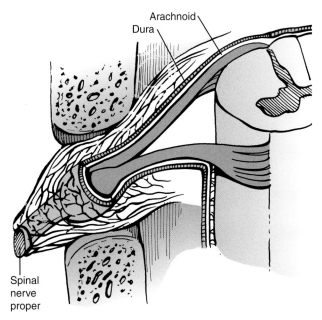

**Figure 30-2** The dura, becoming confluent with the perineurium of the spinal nerve proper within the neural foramen, is richly innervated and may be a source of pain itself.

is associated with referral along the peripheral distribution of fibers in the root. Although dermatomal maps are accurate and clinically useful, the exact cutaneous afferent distributions of spinal nerves are not defined precisely in humans, with considerable variability within and among individuals. This has been referred to as *normal pain,* which is thought to be mediated via the nociceptive innervation of the nerve root sheath resulting in the perception of sciatica.

Normal pain is distinct from so-called *neuropathic pain.* This pain classically is related to nerve root or spinal cord injury. Clinically, neuropathic pain may result in different sensations. It can be spontaneous and not associated with tissue damage. Neuropathic pain may result in *allodynia,* in which a normally benign stimulation produces pain; *hyperalgesia,* in which an exaggerated painful sensation follows a noxious stimulation; or *hyperpathia,* which is characterized by abnormal pain from an area where fibers have reset to a lower threshold for detection of any sensation. Referral of pain and allodynic tenderness with skin stimulation without deep tissue damage is relatively common.

*Wind-up* is a normal mechanism in which successive painful stimuli lead to greater than usual pain sensation. This mechanism is physiologically mediated by C fiber nociceptors. If peripherally activated by stimuli that are no more than 3 seconds apart, the pain intensity increases with each successive stimulus. This increase in intensity is thought to be due to an increased response of spinal dorsal horn neurons to repeated C fiber input.

Wind-up may play an important role in pain transmission in patients with autonomic dysfunction. In these patients, the sensation of mechanical allodynia is mediated by activation of tactile A beta low-threshold mechanoreceptors (not C fibers), whose activation normally is followed by tactile sensations. Repeated A beta stimuli produce burning pain sensations of increasing intensity when stimuli are presented at intervals of 3 seconds or less. This situation clearly is pathologic because the lower threshold mechanoreceptors are providing direct input to the central mechanism via an underlying wind-up mechanism, which normally is mediated by C fiber nociceptor input.

In assessing neuropathic pain syndromes clinically, it is important to realize that acute and chronic pain may coexist. Normal pain due to a reversible source, such as inflammation or injury, may coexist with neuropathic pain. A classic example is persistent radiculopathy after lumbar disc excision. Although residual compression to a nerve root should be ruled out as a source of the failed surgery, coexistent nerve damage may be producing symptoms of allodynia or hyperpathia, which may not respond to revision decompression. Allodynia and hyperpathia should be differentiated from normal motion segment pain from activation of periosteal nociceptors in the facets and normal sciatic pain due to activation of nociceptors within the affected neural sheath. Normal pain is that which is produced through nonpathologic nociceptive mechanisms.

## Nociceptors within Specific Structures

This section considers the microinnervation of the spinal column, specifically the lumbar discs, facets, and supporting ligaments.

### Intervertebral Disc

Disc degeneration is a normal component of aging. Disc degeneration per se does not cause discogenic pain. The pathophysiology of discogenic pain is incompletely understood. The interplay of the underlying anatomy and physiology of disc innervation and the degenerative cascade appear to be key components (Fig. 30-3).

In the normal intervertebral disc, sensory nerves do not penetrate more deeply than the outer one third of the anulus, shown as an association between ingrowth of nerves expressing substance P and discal degeneration. The extent of this neoneuralization was greatest at the intervertebral disc level where the patients experienced pain. Coppes et al noted that disc degeneration is associated with centripetal growth of nerve fibers into the disc. This finding provides a potential morphologic basis for discogenic pain.

Malinsky noted five types of free nerve endings within the outer anulus that he described based on anatomic organization (e.g., simple versus loops). He also found encapsulated and partially encapsulated nerve endings on the superficial anulus. These studies agree with clinical work that identifies the disc as a source of back pain. In these studies, stimulation of the posterior anulus produced back pain in most subjects. One theory of disc degeneration hypothesizes that peripheral tears of the anulus lead to acceleration of dehydration and fraying of the nucleus. This theory has been tested in a sheep model, wherein peripheral tears in the anulus were observed to contain vascular ingrowth. Nociceptors may accompany this vascular ingrowth and, in the degenerated disc, may account for the presence of an afferent sensory nerve supply in the inner anulus. This does

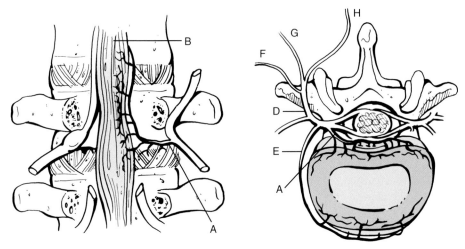

**Figure 30-3** (*Left*) The innervation of the disc and facet joints is complex. Branches of the sinuvertebral nerve (A) innervate the posterior longitudinal ligament (B). Usually the nerve root overlies these branches. (*Right*) The sinuvertebral nerve (A) also innervates the dorsal portion of the disc. Branches from the ventral ramus (E) supply the ventral disc and anterior longitudinal ligament. Only the outer 50% of the anulus is richly innervated in the normal disc. The dorsal ramus (D) divides into lateral (F), intermediate (G), and medial (H) branches. The medial branches innervate the facet joint and are the target of radiofrequency rhizotomy.

not appear to be the case in the normal (i.e., undegenerated) disc (Fig. 30-4).

The posterior longitudinal ligament also has been shown to be a potential pain generator. Central stimulation of the posterior longitudinal ligament produces central back pain

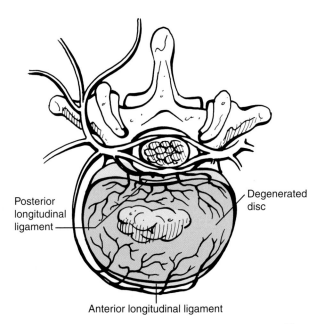

Posterior longitudinal ligament

Degenerated disc

Anterior longitudinal ligament

**Figure 30-4** In the degenerated disc, nociceptive nerve fibers can penetrate more deeply (>50%). These fibers may be accompanied by buds of vascular ingrowth. In the degenerated disc, this may account for the presence of an afferent sensory nerve supply within the inner anulus. This does not appear to be the case in the "normal" (i.e., undegenerated) disc.

with right or left stimulation producing right-sided or left-sided pain. The posterior longitudinal ligament is connected intimately with the posterior aspect of the anulus fibrosus; the microinnervation is similar in this structure. The main afferent pathway involves the nerve to the vertebral body (sinuvertebral nerve). This nerve also may be implicated in the pathophysiology of spinal compression fractures.

The sinuvertebral nerve is the primary afferent pathway formed by the ventral ramus and autonomic root from the gray-ramus communicans. This nerve innervates the ventral aspect of the dural sac, posterior longitudinal ligament, anulus, and blood vessels of the vertebral body. The branches of the sinuvertebral nerve go only to structures in the spinal canal. Transverse and descending branches supply the posterior longitudinal ligament in intervertebral discs at the level of nerve entry, with an ascending branch to the next rostral level, overlapping the innervation of the sinuvertebral nerve at that level. The anterior longitudinal ligament is supplied by the gray-rami communicans or from the sympathetics.

Inflammatory pathways also may be a significant mechanism of discogenic low back pain. Burke et al compared levels of interleukin-6, interleukin-8, and prostaglandin $E_2$ in disc tissue from patients undergoing discectomy for sciatica versus patients undergoing fusion for discogenic low back pain. There were significant differences in the production of interleukin-6 and interleukin-8 in the sciatica and in the low back pain groups, with high levels of proinflammatory mediator found in disc tissue from patients undergoing fusion. This finding suggests that production of these mediators within the nucleus may be a factor in the development of a painful disc. These mediators may stimulate the nociceptive pathways that have penetrated the anulus as part of the degenerative cascade.

## Posterior Elements

The facet joint is richly innervated with encapsulated, unencapsulated, and free nerve endings (Fig. 30-5). As a rule, free nerve endings may be pain receptors or temperature sensitive, whereas encapsulated nerve endings usually are pressure or position sensitive. The medial branch of the posterior primary ramus is the primary afferent pathway from the capsule. The capsule can undergo extensive stretch during normal physiologic loads.

Work by Ashton et al has shown the presence in the capsule of substance P, calcitonin gene-related peptide, and vasoactive intestinal peptides, which are known mediators of inflammation. The facet joint can serve as a pain generator. Does it serve as a clinically relevant pain generator? A question arises as to the exact mechanism of pain generation: Does capsular deformation or bone impingement result in pain? Classically the literature suggests that synovial folds lack innervation. This has been shown not to be the case, however, with several works reporting nerve endings on blood vessels and fat cells in synovial folds in the human. Whether or not these nerve endings are sensitive is questionable. In several studies, human tissue did not show immunoreactivity to substance P. On the basis of the relative neuropeptide immunoreactivity, it has been suggested that the sensory nerves are involved in regulation of blood flow and not nociception. Clinically the association of posterior element pain with facet degeneration has been well described.

Mooney and Robertson reproduced "typical" low back pain by injection of hypertonic saline into the facet joint capsules. The clinical significance of this study is not clear, however. The most reproducible diagnostic technique to identify so-called facet-mediated pain remains the intracapsular extraradicular facet block. In a prospective study of

109 patients with back pain, Lilius et al found no difference in rates of pain relief in the group that received a standard steroid/local anesthetic injection from the group that received a saline injection. In a larger study (n = 454), Jackson et al attempted to identify the clinical characteristics of patients responsive to facet injections but could not do so.

Under specific circumstances, notably the so-called whiplash syndrome, facet-mediated pain may play a more readily definable role. A percutaneous radiofrequency rhizotomy or neurotomy has been described as a potential treatment for facet-mediated pain via interruption of the medial branch of the posterior primary ramus. In a prospective study, patients with chronic facet-mediated neck pain secondary to whiplash syndrome identified by facet blockade were randomized to one of two groups. One group was treated with radiofrequency rhizotomy (which ablates the nociceptive innervation of the facet) versus a sham procedure. Greater pain relief (statistically significant) was observed in the experimental versus control group. Pain relief was not permanent in the rhizotomy group, however.

### Muscle Pain

Although the most common diagnosis for low back pain is "sprain or strain," scientific evidence for a muscular origin for low back pain is lacking. Whether or not there is primary persistent muscle pain that occurs in the absence of an underlying structural disease is not clear.

Muscle is well innervated with small-diameter afferents; however, nociceptors are in the relative minority. Mence studied muscle units in the triceps and the tendocalcaneus of cats, and found a variety of fibers, including low-threshold, pressure-sensitive, nociceptive, contraction-sensitive, and thermosensitive fibers. Quantitatively the nociceptors accounted for approximately 38% of the fibers.

There are four groups of sensory fibers in muscles. Group I and group II are related to proprioception; group III and group IV are afferents. Group III are A delta fibers signaling pain, temperature, and touch, whereas group IV are C fibers signaling itching as well.

Substances that increase discharge from fibers include bradykinin, prostaglandin $E_2$, and serotonin. Authors have speculated that an increased discharge rate on the basis of muscle inflammation with consequent expression of these mediators could account for the spontaneous pain in tissue inflammation. The clinical significance of this speculation is unclear, however.

## SUMMARY

Many structures in the spinal column are capable of initiating or conducting painful impulses. Many of the neuropathic pain impulses are mediated via the dorsal root ganglion. The large-diameter cells in the ganglion give rise to large myelinated A beta fibers, whereas small-diameter cells give rise to unmyelinated C fibers and finely myelinated A delta fibers. The dorsal root ganglion also has been shown to contain inflammatory peptides and may serve as a modulator of disc-related nociception. Additionally, virtually all

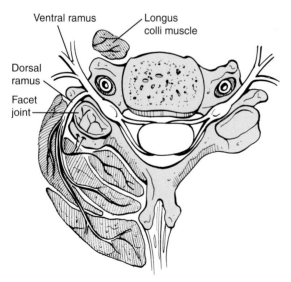

**Figure 30-5**  Branches from the dorsal ramus supply the muscles of the paraspinal muscles of the cervical spine and the facet joint. This may help explain the common occurrence of muscle soreness and pain in patients with facet degeneration, despite a lack of structural injury to the muscle itself.

of the structural elements in the spine (intervertebral disc, supporting spinal ligaments, especially the posterior longitudinal ligament, facet capsules, and muscles) may be sources of pain generation. The interplay of the various elements is complex, and the ability of various structures (e.g., muscle) to cause pain in the absence of a more global problem with the motion segment is unclear.

# SUGGESTED READING

Asbury AK, Fields HL. Pain due to peripheral nerve damage: an hypothesis. Neurology 1984;34:1587–1590.

Ashton IK, Ashton BA, Gibson SJ, et al. Morphological basis for low back pain: the demonstration of nerve fibers and neuropiptides in the lumbar facet joint capsule and not in the ligamentum flavum. J Orthop Res 1992;10:72–78.

Bogduk N, Tynan W, Wilson AS. The nerve supply to the human lumbar intervertebral discs. J Anat 1981;132:39–56.

Burke JG, Watson RW, McCormack D, et al. Intervertebral discs which cause low back pain secrete high levels of proinflammatory mediators. J Bone Joint Surg 2002;84B:196–201.

Coppes MH, Marani E, Thomeer RT, Groen GJ. Innervation of "painful" lumbar discs. Spine 1997;22:2342–2349.

Jackson RP, Jacobs RR, Montesano PX. Facet joint injection in low back pain: a prospective statistical study. Spine 1988;13:966–971.

Janig W, Koltzenburg M. Receptive properties of pial afferents. Pain 1991;4:77–85.

Lillius G, Laasonen EM, Myllymen P, et al. Lumbar facet syndrome: a randomized clinical trial. J Bone Joint Surg 1989;71B:681–684.

Lord SM, Baensley L, Wallis BJ. Percutaneous radiofrequency neurotomy for chronic cervical zygapophyseal joint pain. N Eng J Med 1996;335:1721–1726.

Malinsky J. The ontogenic development of nerve terminations in the intervertebral discs. Acta Anatomica 1973;38:96–113.

Mense S. Nervous outflow from skeletal muscle following chemical nerve stimulation. J Physiol 1977;267:75–88.

Mooney V, Robertson J. The facet syndrome. Clin Orthop Rel Res 1976;115:149–156.

# SPINAL BIOMECHANICS

**THOMAS R. HAHER**
**ANTONIO VALDEVIT**
**STEVEN CARUSO**

The interaction of hard and soft tissue in the maintenance of stability and performance of kinematic tasks renders the human body one of the most complex machines known. Within its structure, the multijoint nature of the human spine possesses its own unique set of biomechanical challenges. A thorough understanding of the physical forces that govern the static and the dynamic properties of this anatomic structure is crucial. In this chapter, a basic and elemental definition of mechanical concepts and terms is presented as an initial step to understanding spinal biomechanics.

## OVERVIEW OF MECHANICS

The study of the deformation and flow of materials under load has evolved from being an aspect of pure materials science to its own specific discipline of biophysics called *rheology.* Commonly used "engineering terms," such as *elasticity, plasticity, viscosity,* and *strength,* although usually used to describe the properties of pure plastics or metals, can be applied to the characteristics of the materials that compose the human spine. These properties determine the relationships between the individual components of the spine, including ligament, bone, and disc. These terms can be used to describe and forecast the interaction of implanted devices within the spine. Combined with information concerning the biologic processes and the details of tissue physiology, an understanding of the influence of the local mechanical environment on fusion healing, disc degeneration, and scoliosis progression can be achieved.

Mechanically the spine can be considered a composite structure. Similar to a skyscraper, the behavior of the construction as a whole is determined by the interaction of its individual parts and materials. Steel, glass, and concrete each have their own mechanical properties (e.g., elasticity, plasticity, ductility). When used in combination, however, the properties of the new construction are determined by the relative interplay between the different materials. The spinal column is a composite structure of bone, ligament, and intervertebral disc. Although the material properties of these individual tissues can be defined easily, prediction of the interaction between the tissues is much more complex and has been the focus of countless biomechanical investigations.

The mechanical conditions of the spine can be altered through surgical intervention. The orthopaedic spine surgeon is obliged to possess an understanding of basic biomechanics.

## MECHANICAL DEFINITIONS

The following terms are defined:

- Force
- Stress
- Strain

The definition of the most basic unit, *force,* stems from Sir Isaac Newton, the father of modern mechanics. A force is proportional to the *acceleration* of an object. The constant of proportionality is the *mass* of the object. Formally, this famous equation is expressed as $F = m \times a$, and its unit bears the name of its discoverer. A *newton* is defined as the force required to accelerate a 1-kg mass at 1 meter per second squared. Mathematically, this is written $1\ N = 1\ kg \times 1\ m/s^2$.

*Stress* is defined as the force ($F$) per unit area ($A$), where the area is expressed in square meters. The expression for stress is $\sigma = F / A$ and possesses units of $N/m^2$ or pascals (Pa). Because of the great magnitudes, the typical unit expressed for most materials concerning the spine is the megapascal (MPa), which is equivalent to $10^6$ Pa.

*Strain* is defined as the change in length ($L$) of a material under a particular force (or load). It is the ratio of the new length over the original length and is expressed as $\epsilon = (L_{final} - L_{initial}) / L_{initial} = \Delta L / L_{initial}$. Because the denominator and the numerator have units of length, strain is a dimensionless parameter and has no units.

### Pure Material Properties

The following terms relate to "pure" material properties:

- Elasticity
- Plasticity
- Viscoelasticity

*Material properties* are intrinsic to the substance (i.e., material) of which an object is composed. These properties are independent of geometry and are independent of each other; they include elasticity, plasticity, and viscoelasticity.

Perhaps the best way to understand *elasticity* is by examining a spring. When a spring (or other elastic material, such as bone, which has some springlike properties) is loaded, a specific amount of deformation is achieved. The deformation is proportional to the load applied. When the load is removed, the spring returns to the original geometry. This ideally elastic spring is said to recover fully from deformation. Up to a specific load, any elastic material would deform under an applied force (F) and return to its original geometry on removal of that force. For an elastic material, the plot of applied forces and resulting deformation would be linear. The value of the slope within this linear region defines the *stiffness* of the elastic material. The stiffness is designated by *K* and by definition possesses units of force/deformation (N/m). This quantity often is expressed in units of N/mm to express the quantity more easily because biologic samples such as bone typically do not deform to any great extent (Fig. 31-1).

The *plasticity* of a material describes its characteristics beyond the elastic region. *Plastic deformation* results in a permanent change in the geometry of the specimen on removal of the deforming force. Plastic deformation is, by definition, permanent deformation without return to original dimensions. The plastic region of a material still may possess a linear region; however, it "recoils" to a point beyond the elastic region. The plastic region may be long, as the case is for steel or titanium, or it may be short, as is the case for brittle materials, such as ceramic. The *yield point* represents the transition from the elastic to the plastic regions (Fig. 31-2). This is the "point of no return" for the material. Any additional deformation beyond the yield point is permanent.

The net change in deformation may be computed using the stress versus strain (or the load versus deformation) curve of a material. In the elastic region of the curve, removal of the applied load results in nonpermanent change in the geometric dimensions of the material. When the iden-

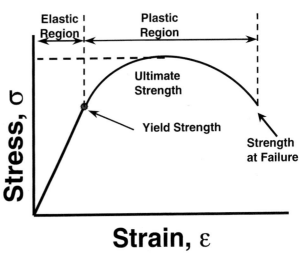

**Figure 31-2**  Stress versus strain curve illustrating the elastic and plastic regions of a material under static loading conditions.

tical process is repeated in the plastic portion of the curve, however, a permanent change in deformation results. If a line is drawn from the point of load release, parallel to the slope of the elastic curve, it intersects the x-axis of strain (or deformation). This value is the *permanent deformation* for the applied load (Fig. 31-3).

All biologic materials display *viscoelasticity*. Although the manifestation of this characteristic may be dramatic, as in soft tissues (e.g., muscle, tendons, and ligaments), viscoelasticity in harder materials (e.g., bone and cartilage) is more subtle.

To understand viscoelasticity, one first must understand viscosity. Shear and flow are resisted by viscosity. Viscosity is time dependent in nature (Fig. 31-4). In the case of an instantaneous load application, a viscoelastic material displays an initial exponential rise in deformation until a steady state of deformation is obtained. This equilibrium is achieved when the internal viscous and material forces are sufficient to resist the collapse of the applied load. The viscous component of the force resistance is termed *creep* and is common to all viscoelastic materials. The comparable effect is observed when instantaneous deformation is applied and maintained. In this case, the viscoelastic properties balance and minimize the internal forces. The initial stresses decay exponentially to an equilibrium level on application of an instantaneous and constant strain. This phenomenon is termed *stress relaxation* and, similar to creep, is common to all viscoelastic materials. The resulting deformation displayed by the material is related to the force magnitude and the rate of force application (Fig. 31-5). The deformation rate of a viscoelastic material is directly proportional to the force magnitude applied. In contrast to nonviscoelastic materials, no elastic return to the original geometry results when the applied load is removed.

## Impure Material/Structural Properties

The following terms relate to "impure" material/structural properties:

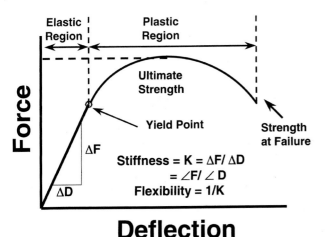

**Figure 31-1**  Characteristics of the load versus deformation curve under static loading conditions. (The terms "deflection" and "deformation" may be used interchangeably.)

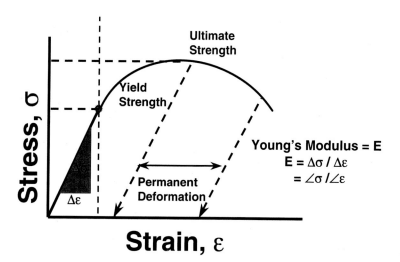

**Figure 31-3** Characteristics of the stress versus strain curve under static loading conditions. Note the similarities to the load versus deformation curve in Figure 31-1. Permanent deformation results at load levels beyond the yield point.

- Strength
- Ductility
- Fatigue

At this point, a clarification of structural versus material properties would be useful. The substance of which an object is composed determines material properties, such as elasticity and plasticity. These properties are independent of the geometry. The structural properties of an object are determined by its shape or geometry. The steel used to create a piece of sheet metal has the same material properties as the steel used to create an I-beam. The I-beam, for its intended use to span long segments and act as a weight-bearing structure, is much stronger, however. Strength (and ductility and fatigability) is determined partially by the material in addition to the geometry or dimensions into which it is formed. A biologic structure, such as bone, also has material and structural properties. Bone has a specific elastic modulus, stiffness, and other material properties. The geometry that the bone assumes, such as a hollow tube (long bone), influences the strength of the bone. A purely structural property is bending or torsional resistance. It is determined only by the geometry of an object.

*Strength* defines the point at which a material would fail. It is related to the magnitude of force (or stress) required to cause a structural (rather than material) failure in the material. Strength is the force beyond which "catastrophic failure" occurs. It is beyond the yield point of the material. The *ultimate tensile strength* describes the maximal tensile force or stress that a structure can sustain before catastrophic failure.

Materials for spinal implants are selected to be stiff, ductile, strong, and lightweight. These characteristics are not interdependent and are defined uniquely by the characteristics of the material. In the load-deflection (or stress-strain) curve, the stiffness (or modulus in the stress-strain curve) is defined as the slope of the linear region in the elastic portion of the curve (Fig. 31-6). It is common practice to perform a linear regression of the load (or stress) versus deformation (or strain) to compute the stiffness (or modulus). It also is important to examine the regression coefficient, $r^2$. This value ideally would be equal to unity (or 1) if the result were a perfectly straight line.

For nonbiologic tissues, this value is usually greater than 0.95. It is influenced by the linearity of the curve and the

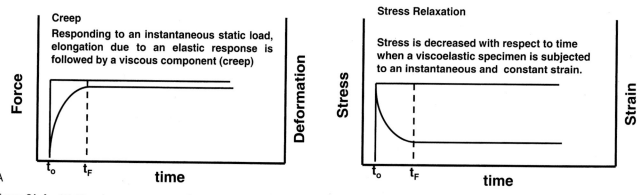

**Figure 31-4** (**A**) Visual representation of creep resulting from an instantaneous application of a constant load. (**B**) Visual representation of stress relaxation resulting from an instantaneous application of a constant strain. The stress values follow an exponential decrease until equilibrium is achieved.

Strain Rate Dependent Properties
Viscoelastic materials such as soft tissues exhibit higher
loads to fracture with less elongation when stretched faster.

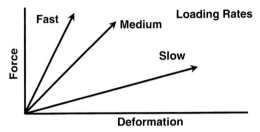

**Figure 31-5** In viscoelastic materials, the maximal force achieved and the material stiffness are affected by the rate of applied loading.

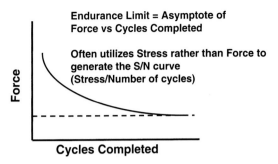

**Figure 31-7** Typical load versus cycles to failure curve. At some applied load no failure will occur, regardless of the number of cycles.

number of data points taken during the test. Too few data points decrease the $r^2$ value despite a linear trend. This is an important point to note, especially in the case of biologic tissues, in which viscoelasticity and loading rate can influence dramatically the profile of the load-deformation (or stress-strain) curve. In such cases, too few data points may lead erroneously to a seemingly linear curve and inaccurate computation of stiffness or the elastic modulus.

As strength is defined as the magnitude of the load required for failure, *ductility* represents the amount of plastic deformation obtained before failure (i.e., the total deformation between the yield point and the *failure point* of the material or implant). Consideration of this property is vital in the design of spinal implants. If a device *yields* but possesses sufficient ductility such that it does not *fail* under continued loading (and if this amount of deformation does not cause pain clinically), the likelihood of clinical implant failure is low. In contradistinction, if the implant possesses minimal ductility and it mechanically yields under physiologic loads, failure is likely.

Optimizing these properties is the focus of spinal implant design. In the case of operative scoliosis correction, rods should be stiff to maintain curve correction and to provide sufficient spinal stability. The rods also must be strong so as to prevent failure of the implant or construct under cyclic physiologic (fatigue) loading. Finally, the rods must be ductile so that the surgeon can contour the rods to the desired shape to achieve curve correction. If the rod was not ductile,

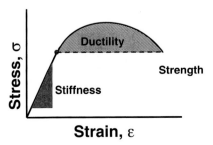

**Figure 31-6** Ideal implants display a sufficiently high stiffness property in addition to a large region of ductility to prevent catastrophic failure.

bending it would lead to potential breaking points that eventually would lead to implant failure.

All materials possess a *fatigue* limit. The fatigue limit is the number of cycles that a material can sustain *without failure*. This property is *load dependent*. Higher magnitude loads result in decreased number of cycles to failure. It also is *mode dependent*. The number of cycles to failure for a given material may be different in different loading directions. Bone is strongest under compressive loads, but it is weakest, and usually fails, under torsion or bending loads.

Materials also display a characteristic *endurance limit* (Fig. 31-7). This is the load magnitude below which failure would not occur regardless of the number of cycles applied to the material. This property is crucial when considering the design and selection of material for an implant. The endurance limit of the final design should be well above the anticipated maximal physiologic loads.

## Pure Structural Properties

The *moment of inertia* is related to the cross-sectional area of a structure and is a fundamental geometric property of the structure. The moment of inertia describes the spatial distribution of material within a structure with respect to a particular axis of rotation or bending. The equation is expressed as $I = \Sigma\ m_i r_i^2$—the sum of each elemental mass ($m_i$) that is located at a distance ($r_i$) from the neutral or selected axis. For most geometric structures, with a central axis of symmetry, such as a round rod or rectangular plate, moments of inertia can be calculated using simple equations.

Moment of inertia is a *structural property* only and is not related to the material used. One of the most useful applications of this property is calculation of resistance to bending for various structures. A large increase in the bending resistance of a rod can be achieved by small increases in the rod's diameter (Fig. 31-8). For cylindrical objects with a neutral axis through their center, the moment of inertia is proportional to the fourth power of the rod radius ($r$). The equation defining this relationship is:

$$I = (\pi\ /\ 4)\ r^4$$

The moment of inertia for a 4-mm solid rod is 12.56 mm$^4$, whereas for a 7-mm rod it is 118 mm$^4$. In other words,

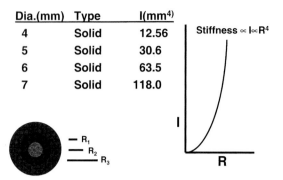

| Dia.(mm) | Type | I(mm⁴) |
|---|---|---|
| 4 | Solid | 12.56 |
| 5 | Solid | 30.6 |
| 6 | Solid | 63.5 |
| 7 | Solid | 118.0 |

Stiffness $\propto$ I$\propto$R⁴

**Figure 31-8** The moment of inertia for a cylindrical rod is proportional to the fourth power of the radius. Small increases in radii can manifest large increases in the moment of inertia and the resulting stiffness of the rod and construct.

the moment of inertia for a 7-mm rod is 10 times that of a 4-mm rod.

The bending stiffness for rectangular objects is related to the height cubed. To a lesser degree, increases in the height of the object (or thickness) result in exponential increases in the bending resistance. Using an equation, this can be expressed as:

$$I = b\,h^3 / 12$$

The base (*b*) refers to the length of the plate, whereas the height (*h*) refers to the thickness.

# MECHANICS OF THE INSTRUMENTED SPINE: EFFECT OF THE MOMENT OF INERTIA ON SPINAL MECHANICS

Increasing rod diameter to achieve a greater moment of inertia creates a stiffer rod. The overall effects of spinal implants must be considered in concert with the mechanical properties of the spinal column itself, however. Although the spine is a composite structure by itself, it becomes more so with the introduction of instrumentation. Using the example of the rod, the resulting stiffness is a combination of spinal column stiffness and the rod. This stiffness is highly influenced by the location of the implant within the spine and the dimensions and materials properties.

# BIOMECHANICAL ETIOLOGY OF SCOLIOSIS

The etiology of idiopathic adolescent scoliosis is by definition unknown. Although various underlying genetic, neurologic, muscular, and skeletal mechanisms have been suggested, none seem to be solely responsible for development of this disorder. More recently, a biomechanical explanation of the initiation of scoliosis has been suggested. This explanation is grounded in considering the spine as a buckling column.

The vertebral bodies are arranged in a long, relatively thin (compared with the dimensions of the entire body) column. Under compressive loading, such a structure would fail primarily through "buckling." Euler computed that the critical buckling load is defined by:

$$F_{cr} = E\,I\,\pi^2 / L$$

(Critical buckling load = constant / column length) where *L* is the length of the column, and *E* and *I* are material and property constants (Fig. 31-9). It is the load at which buckling is initiated, and it is inversely proportional to column length. It follows that the longer the column, the less force required to achieve buckling.

Euler's formula is applicable only to columns consisting of homogeneous material. The human spinal column is not such a structure. It is composed of discs and bone among a complex of muscles and ligaments. The natural curvature of the spine (cervical lordosis, thoracic kyphosis, and lumbar lordosis) resides in an already buckled, or "prebuckled," condition. Although Euler considered buckling to be catastrophic for a structure, this is not the case for the human spinal column.

Scoliosis may be considered pathologic buckling that occurs over time. It does not lead to catastrophic failure immediately. Scoliotic buckling results in disharmony of the normal spinal curvature, producing abnormal coronal buckling. The critical buckling force to produce a scoliotic curve may be used to predict what loads (from the head, trunk, and extremities) might lead to a progressive scoliotic curve (Fig. 31-10). The critique of such theoretical calculations is that they do not take into account the osteologic and ligamentous responses to these forces, which would be crucial in the growing adolescent spine.

Spinal motion is *coupled*. Motion in one of the three orthogonal planes induces motion in one or both of the other planes (Fig. 31-11). When the lumbar spine undergoes rotation, lateral bending also occurs. This relationship is commutative, in that lateral bending of the spine induces rotation. In reverse, derotation of the spine should correct coronal deformity. This correction is maximized by resection of other structures, such as the costovertebral joints in

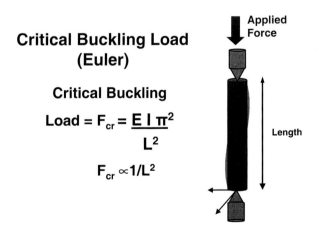

## Critical Buckling Load (Euler)

**Critical Buckling**

Load = $F_{cr}$ = $\dfrac{E\,I\,\pi^2}{L^2}$

$F_{cr} \propto 1/L^2$

Applied Force

Length

**Figure 31-9** Euler's formula for the force transmitted through a long cylindrical column supported and loaded by a single point. The critical buckling load for a column is inversely proportional to the square of the column length.

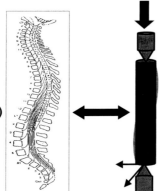

- Non-homogeneous structure
- Pre-Buckled
- Buckling (Failure) occurs slowly

- Homogeneous structure
- Straight
- Buckling (Failure) occurs almost instantaneously

**Figure 31-10**   The human spine is a prebuckled nonhomogeneous structure in which pathologic buckling occurs gradually.

the thoracic spine that propagate rotation. The resultant coupled motion decreases the scoliotic curvature. Conversely, the rotation of the spine leads to rib cage deformity.

## AXIS OF ROTATION

The axis of rotation for a given plane is the point about which all other parts rotate. In the spine, the axis is not located at a single point, but because of the intricacy of the three-joint structure, it moves within a complex pattern (or collection) of points. To preserve the relative position of the neural elements, the axis of rotation in the transverse plane is located within the spinal canal (Fig. 31-12). Although considerable work has been done in attempting to locate the locus of the axis of rotation during flexion/extension and lateral bending, the definitive answer remains elusive because in vitro investigation can only simulate in vivo motion, with one vertebra moving in relation to an adjacent fixed vertebra. Physiologically, both vertebrae are moving relative to a global reference frame and relative to each other (Fig. 31-13). The local reference frame is in motion. With that said, it generally is believed that the sagittal axis of rotation is located within the center of the intervertebral disc (Fig. 31-14).

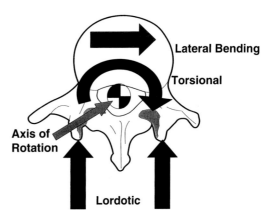

**Figure 31-12**   Instantaneous axis of rotation during motion of a single vertebral body in relation to a fixed location.

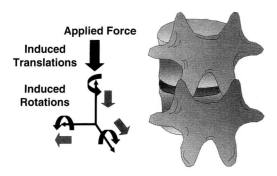

**Figure 31-11**   Force direction generated by proper instrumentation and implantation can be used to control spinal deformity in various planes.

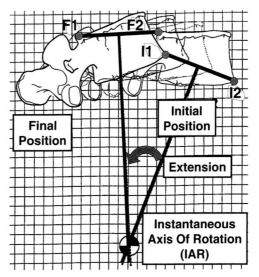

**Figure 31-13**   The instantaneous axis of rotation (IAR) in vivo is influenced by the relationship of one vertebra with another and the orientation of both vertebrae in relation to a global reference frame.

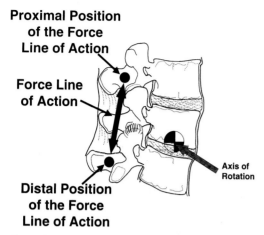

**Figure 31-14** During flexion/extension movements, the estimated axis of rotation is located within the center of the intervertebral disc.

# FUTURE DIRECTIONS

The future of spinal biomechanics may lie in the generation of geometrically scalable anatomic models complete with soft tissues. Although this undertaking may yield new insight, the focus should remain on the influence of physiologic loading. From a practical perspective, such complex loading conditions would be enormously difficult to simulate in an in vitro setting. Even if computationally possible, experimental verification would be nearly impossible, with the task remaining an academic exercise.

# SUGGESTED READING

Adams MA, Freeman BJ, Morrison HP, et al. Mechanical initiation of intervertebral disc degeneration. Spine 2000;25:1625–1636.

Azegami H, Murachi S, Kitoh, et al. Etiology of idiopathic scoliosis: computational study. Clin Orthop 1998;357:229–236.

Bastian L, Lange U, Knop C, et al. Evaluation of the mobility of adjacent segments after posterior thoracolumbar fixation: a biomechanical study. Eur Spine J 2001;10:295–300.

Belmont PJ Jr, Polly DW Jr, Cunningham BW, Klemme WR. The effects of hook pattern and kyphotic angulation on mechanical strength and apical rod strain in a long-segment posterior construct using a synthetic model. Spine 2001;26:627–635.

Cripton PA, Jain GM, Wittenberg RH, Nolte LP. Load-sharing characteristics of stabilized lumbar spine segments. Spine 2000; 25170–25179.

Haher TR, O'Brien M, Felmly WT, et al. Instantaneous axis of rotation as a function of the three columns of the spine. Spine 1992;17: S149–S154.

Kazarian LE. Creep characteristics of the human spinal column. Orthop Clin North Am 1975;6:3–18.

Lucas LL, Cooke FW, Friis EA. A primer of biomechanics. New York: Springer, 1999.

# SPINAL ORTHOSES

**MICHAEL J. VIVES**
**KENNETH G. SWAN, Jr.**

## ORTHOTICS

Orthotics (from the Greek *ortho,* meaning "straight") have played an integral role in the management of spinal pathology for thousands of years. Smith, in his 1908 article, "The Most Ancient Splints," described brace use in ancient Egypt more than 2500 years ago. Much of the early literature focused on treatment of spinal deformities, including Pare's metal jacket, popular in the late 16th century, and Andre's iron cross cervical brace, featured in the early 18th century. Today, spinal bracing continues to be a mainstay of treating deformity and acute and chronic spinal injuries.

*Orthotics* are defined as external devices applied to restrict motion in a particular segment. As such, they can be categorized broadly based on the region they are employed to immobilize, as follows:

- Cervical orthoses
- Cervicothoracic orthoses (CTOs)
- Thoracolumbosacral orthoses (TLSOs)
- Lumbosacral orthoses (LSOs)
- Sacroiliac orthoses

This chapter focuses on the biomechanics, laboratory studies, and clinical utility of commonly used, commercially available spinal orthoses.

## BIOMECHANICS AND BIOMATERIALS

Many of the advances in spinal bracing have developed as a result of better understanding of spinal biomechanics. Conceptually the spine can be thought of as a series of semirigid segments interconnected by viscoelastic linkages. Spinal kinematics involves motion in 6 degrees of freedom, with rotation about three axes and translation along the three coordinates. For clinical considerations, testing (particularly involving normal subjects) generally has been confined to three planes of motion:

- Flexion/extension
- Axial rotation
- Lateral bending

The efficacy of an orthosis to limit spinal motion can be evaluated by a variety of methods. Standard radiography, typically using flexion/extension views, has been employed. Cineradiography evaluates motion using fluoroscopy with movie film. Goniometry uses external devices attached to the subject to measure spinal motion. Goniometry has been shown to correlate fairly well with radiographic techniques and avoids exposing subjects to radiation. This advantage is offset, however, by some decreased accuracy and lack of information on motion at any particular segment.

Because bracing attempts to control the position of the spine through the application of external forces, orthotic design must account for regional variations of the surrounding anatomy. These variations include the vital soft tissue structures of the anterior neck, the rigid thoracic ribcage, and the bony pelvis at the base of the lumbar spine. The surrounding soft tissue envelope has a substantial effect on the ability of an externally applied force to control spinal movement. Pressure measurements on the soft tissues may be an objective way to assess the fit of a spinal orthosis. The role of soft tissue pressure measurement as an index of applied corrective force for the deformity bracing is unclear. The intervening soft tissue envelope is also an area of potential complication with problems ranging from skin breakdown, local pain, decreased vital capacity, and increased lower extremity venous pressure.

Along with improved understanding of the biomechanics of spinal bracing, improvements in the materials available for brace manufacture have led to dramatic advancements in design. During the 18th century, braces generally were constructed of leather, iron, and wood. German developments in the 19th and early 20th centuries led to many new brace designs, with paper cellulose and glue being added to wooden or iron frames. Newer composite materials, polymer resins, and thermoplastics have led to a proliferation of commercially available orthoses that are lightweight and comfortable without sacrificing the stability afforded by the heavier, more cumbersome designs of the past. Commonly used materials in the fabrication of orthoses are listed in Table 32-1.

## CERVICAL ORTHOSES

Cervical orthoses can be divided into two broad categories—soft and hard. Hard orthoses are subdivided further

### TABLE 32-1 COMMONLY USED MATERIALS IN THE FABRICATION OF ORTHOSES*

Ionomer (Thermovac Surlyn)
Polypropylene (Oliphin)
Polycarbonate (Lexan)
Polyethylene (Vitrathene)
Polyethylene foam (Plastazote, Aliplast)
PVS (Kydex)
Resins (Epoxy, Polyester)

---

*Common product names in parentheses.
From Botte MJ, Garfin SR, Bergmann K, et al. Spinal orthoses for traumatic and degenerative disease. In: Herkowitz HN, Garfin SR, Balderston RA, et al, eds. The spine, 4th ed. Vol 2. Philadelphia: WB Saunders, 1999:1097–1124.

into cervical and cervicothoracic braces. Soft collars provide little immobilization but are used often in the treatment of whiplash-type injuries, for which they may provide comfort and proprioceptive feedback to help "remind" a patient to restrict motion voluntarily. The use of soft cervical collars in the management of cervical myelopathy is favored by some authors and questioned by others.

Rigid cervical orthoses and CTOs come in several forms. All forms must be able to accommodate the vital soft tissue structures in the neck and provide rigid immobilization of the mobile cervical spine. This generally is accomplished by firm seatings about the base of the skull and upper thorax

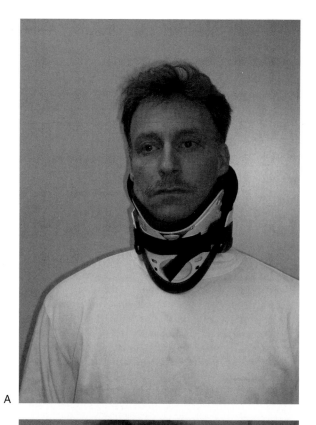

A

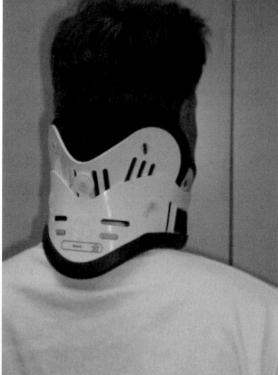

B

**Figure 32-2** Miami "J" cervical orthosis. (**A**) Frontal view. (**B**) Posterior view. Design includes anterior and posterior shells with a soft lining that can be changed for hygiene purposes.

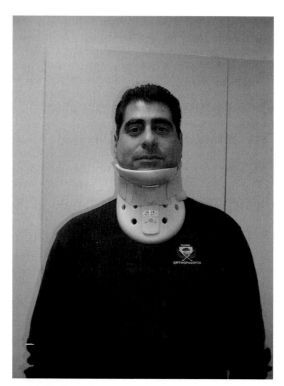

**Figure 32-1** Philadelphia collar. Design includes anterior and posterior shells, which are fastened with Velcro straps. The anterior hole is for a tracheostomy tube.

connected by a rigid column. Most rigid cervical orthoses include an anterior opening to accommodate a tracheostomy tube. Examples of cervical orthoses include the Philadelphia collar (Fig. 32-1), the Miami "J" collar (Fig. 32-2), and the Aspen cervical orthosis (Fig. 32-3).

The classic study evaluating the effectiveness of various orthoses in immobilizing the cervical spine was performed by Johnson et al. The methods of this study often have been emulated and its results frequently quoted since its publication in 1977. The authors evaluated the soft collar, Philadelphia collar, four-poster orthosis, sternooccipitomandibular immobilizer (SOMI), and a CTO. They used radiographs and overhead photographs taken at the extremes of motion in flexion/extension, rotation, and lateral bending. They quantified sagittal plane motion for each brace at every level of the cervical spine. As others had shown, Johnson et al found that a soft collar offered no restriction of motion in any plane. They found that increasing the length of the orthosis (extending it onto the thorax) and increasing the rigidity of the connection improved the flexion control, but lateral bending and total flexion and extension were less controlled. They also showed increased motion between the occiput and C1 in all the braces compared with the unbraced state. This "snaking" or paradoxical motion subsequently has been described throughout the cervical and thoracolumbar spine.

A more recent study compared five commonly used cervical orthoses in terms of their efficacy in restricting cervical motion. Radiographic and goniometer measurements found the NecLoc (Jerome Medical, Moorestown, NJ) orthosis to be superior to the Miami J, Philadelphia, Aspen, and Stifneck (Laerdal, Armonk, NY) orthoses in terms of flexion/extension, rotation, and lateral bending. The Miami J collar also was found to be significantly superior to the Philadelphia and Aspen orthoses in extension and combined flexion/extension.

Known complications of cervical orthoses include skin breakdown over bone prominences, such as the occiput, mandible, and sternum. Skin breakdown is especially prevalent in multitrauma patients with prolonged recumbency and in patients with altered sensorium. One study reported orthosis-related decubiti in 38% of patients with associated severe closed head injuries. Plaisier et al compared the skin pressure associated with the use of the Stifneck, Philadelphia, Miami J, and Aspen/Newport collars in supine patients. They found that the Miami J and the Aspen collar produced the lowest chin and occiput pressures, both being below the mean capillary closing pressure. Increased intracranial pressure as a consequence of rigid cervical orthotic immobilization has been described. Hunt et al studied the effects of rigid collar placement on intracranial pressure in head-injured patients. They found that rigid collars cause a small but significant increase in intracranial pressure, which may have deleterious effects in patients with severe head injuries and preexisting intracranial hypertension. Hunt et al recommended early removal of rigid collars from head-injured patients when cervical spine injury has been ruled out.

Methods for immobilizing the cervical spine of patients in the field also have been studied extensively, including use of a cervical collar, a short board or sandbag technique, or a combination of collar and short board. Cline compared the Hare extrication collar, the Philadelphia collar, and their immobilization protocol, which consists of a short board with forehead and chin straps. They concluded that the short board with straps provided the best immobilization and that the addition of a Philadelphia collar did not provide additional benefit. Podolsky et al used goniometry to evaluate the immobilization provided by a soft collar, hard collar, Philadelphia collar, Hare extrication device, and their sandbag technique (which uses a board plus forehead tape). They found that the sandbag technique provided the most effective immobilization, but that the addition of a Philadelphia collar provided additional benefit.

## CERVICOTHORACIC ORTHOSES

CTOs generally consist of occiput and chin supports attached to anterior or posterior (or both) thoracic plates. Examples include the SOMI (Fig. 32-4), the Minerva brace (Fig. 32-5), and the Yale brace (Fig. 32-6). Compared with cervical orthoses, CTOs improve control in all planes of motion. This improved rigidity comes at the expense of patient comfort, however. Some earlier authors distinguished between the two/four-poster designs and designs with more extensive connections between the head and thoracic components. The more recent, standardized classification system categorizes the poster braces as CTOs, however, along

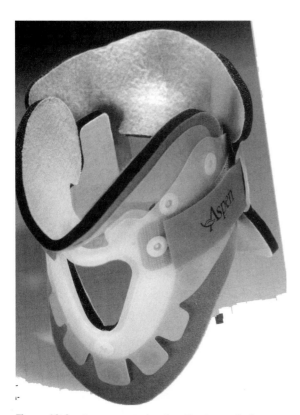

**Figure 32-3**  Aspen cervical collar. Design includes patented tabs that allow the collar to conform better to the patient when tightened.

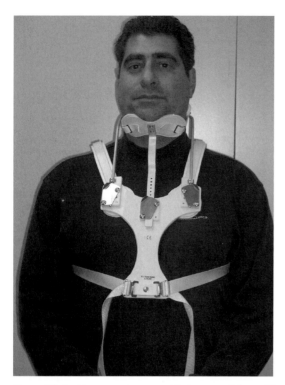

**Figure 32-4** Sternooccipitomandibular immobilizer. The three uprights that extend from the mandibular and occipital rests all connect on the anterior thoracic plate.

with the other designs. The traditional four-poster brace was shown to limit 79% of overall cervical flexion/extension and to limit midcervical flexion to a comparable degree as the more rigid CTOs. Because of their heavy design and high resting pressures on the chin and occiput, these braces are used less commonly today.

The SOMI (see Fig. 32-4) uses metal uprights to connect occipital and mandibular rests to a sternal plate that is secured to the thorax by padded metal "over-the-shoulder" straps and additional circumferential straps that cross in the back. Because there is no posterior thoracic plate, the occipital rests are supported by uprights from the sternal piece; this results in adequate control of flexion but deficient control of extension throughout the cervical spine. These braces generally are associated with fair patient comfort but also show high resting pressures at the chin and occiput.

The original Minerva brace consisted of a heavy, custom plaster jacket that created difficulties in maintaining patient hygiene and obtaining radiographs. As a result of the difficulties encountered in managing patients with this device, the halo came into popular use. Later the thermoplastic Minerva body jacket was developed, which preserved the noninvasive nature of the original concept. Its lightweight, bivalved, Polyform shell allowed improved patient comfort and hygiene and interfered less with follow-up radiographs. Donning this brace is complex, often requiring an orthotist for proper application. More recently a prefabricated version of the Minerva body jacket has been developed, the Minerva CTO (see Fig. 32-5). Its design features a forehead

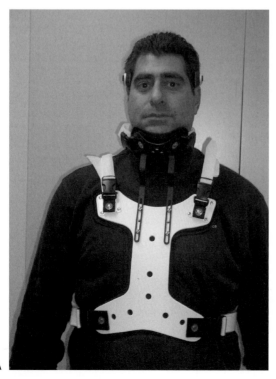
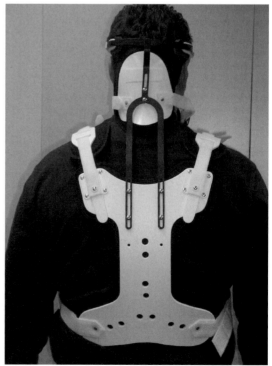

A                                                                                          B

**Figure 32-5** Minerva cervicothoracic orthosis. (**A**) Frontal view. (**B**) Posterior view. The padded, U-shaped hand band is attached to a large occipital flare that has a rigid connection to the posterior thoracic plate.

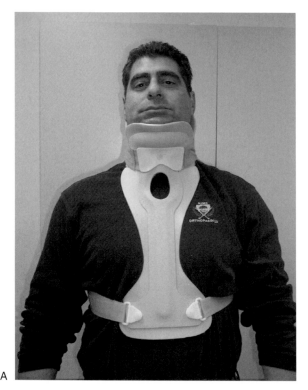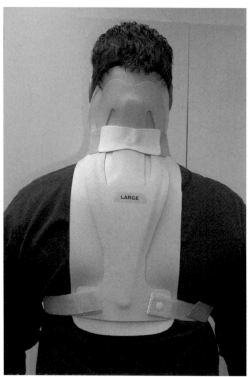

A                                                                                                    B

**Figure 32-6** Yale brace. (**A**) Frontal view. (**B**) Posterior view. Note the similarities of the head-rest to a Philadelphia collar, from which the early version originally was adapted.

band attached to a large occipital flare. Sharpe et al showed that this orthosis limits overall sagittal plane motion by 79%, axial rotation by 88%, and lateral bending by 51%.

The Yale brace (see Fig. 32-6) originally was designed as a modified Philadelphia collar with custom-molded anterior and posterior polypropylene thoracic extensions. The modern version is prefabricated and usually made of Kydex. Although lighter and less cumbersome than most of the other CTOs, the Yale brace has similar efficacy in controlling motion. In Johnson's study, the Yale brace restricted 87% of overall flexion-extension, 75% of axial rotation, and 61% of lateral bending. Although the CTOs have been shown to be fairly effective at limiting motion of the cervical spine, they should not be expected to immobilize rigidly below the C7-T1 level despite their thoracic components.

## HALO VEST

It generally is agreed that the halo vest provides the most rigid immobilization of the cervical spine of all the currently used orthoses. Originally inspired by a device used by Bloom to treat facial fractures in pilots with overlying burns during World War II, modified versions were used by Nickel and Perry to immobilize patients with polio who had undergone posterior cervical fusion. The early halo devices consisted of a circumferential stainless steel ring with four pins for skull fixation. The ring was attached to a plaster jacket by

upright posts. Numerous improvements have been made to the various components of the halo vest, but the overall design principles remain the same. A ring is fixed to the skull with multiple pins. The ring is attached to a vest by four connecting rods (Fig. 32-7). Newer rings are made of composite materials, which have the beneficial properties of light weight, radiolucency, and compatibility with magnetic resonance imaging (MRI). There does not seem to be a difference in fixation strength between newer radiolucent graphite rings and the early titanium ones. Rings that are open posteriorly or have crown-type designs have been developed. These designs allow for ease in placement because the head of the patient does not need to be passed through the ring. Additionally, because the patient is not lying on the back of the ring, there is less risk of cervical spine fracture displacement through ring manipulation.

The initial halo vest was fashioned from heavy plaster of Paris. With the development of plastic technology, newer lightweight, easily applied vests of various sizes based on chest circumference have been developed. Adjustable straps and supports help customize the fit. The connecting rods have been anodized to prevent seizing of the metal during tightening. The connecting rods in many designs are made of carbon fiber for their radiographic lucency and for compatibility with MRI. Torque wrenches are included in the application sets to prevent overtightening of the bolts that connect the rods to the vest and the ring. Mirza et al found that most commercially available vests provide comparable immobilization. Factors that they showed to decrease mo-

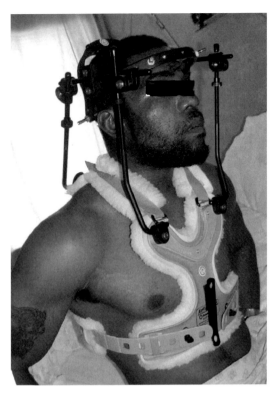

**Figure 32-7** The halo vest (Bremer). This crown-type design allows easier placement in the supine position.

tion included increasing vest snugness, decreasing the deformability of the vest, and appropriate fit and application.

Technologic advances also have been made in the field of halo pin materials and pin design. The current popular pin composition is stainless steel. Different pin tip designs have been studied to determine which may provide the greatest resistance to shear frequently encountered at the pin-bone interface. Interest has arisen regarding a bullet-type tip, which may be able to withstand higher shear forces. Some systems have torque wrenches that break off at a set torque. These wrenches are made to be low profile, allowing for ease of usage in cramped areas, such as the posterior aspect of the skull while the patient is supine.

## Halo Application Principles

Because many of the complications of halo fixation are related to inappropriate site selection or technique, a thorough understanding of pin insertion principles is essential. Many years of clinical data have fine-tuned the optimal location of halo pin placement. To minimize pin complications but maximize the rigidity of the halo-vest frame, two anterior and two posterior pins usually are placed. The standard position of the two anterior pins is 1 cm superior to the orbital rim, over the lateral two thirds of the orbit, being sure to be below the level of the greatest circumference of the skull (Fig. 32-8). This is considered the safe zone. In a cadaver study, it was found that the skull thickness in this region averaged approximately 2 mm for the outer cortical

table and 3 mm for the intercalvarial space or inner diploë. Pins placed too medial may damage the supraorbital or supratrochlear nerves. Also, the frontal sinus has a varied position in the midline. The outer table of the frontal sinus is thin, which can lead to perforation with medial pin placement. Laterally placed anterior pins have been proposed over the temporalis fossa to avoid unsightly scarring over the anterior forehead. At this location, however, the zygomaticotemporal nerve, which provides sensation to the area over the temple, may be injured. By entering through the temporalis muscle, the pin often causes irritation during mandibular motion. Additionally, in cadaver studies, the skull was found to have a thin outer and inner table with minimal cancellous diploë in this region.

Placement of posterior pins is less critical than for anterior pin location. There are no neuromuscular structures at risk, and the skull has a near-uniform thickness, with the thickest section being straight posterior. Direct posterior pin placement is avoided because the patient would lie on this pin in the supine position. The pins usually are placed diagonally opposite to the anterior pins, approximately 1 cm superior to the upper helix of the ear. Care must be taken to avoid any contact between the ring/pin and ear, while remaining inferior enough below the equator of the skull to prevent superior pin migration.

Because skull shapes differ, placing pins perpendicular to the tangent of the skull may be difficult. Because the halo is not a static unidirectional device, shear forces act at each of the pin sites. A biomechanical study looked at the transverse shear forces to failure of pins placed in decremental angles from 90 degrees, 75 degrees, and 60 degrees. The load to deformity and failure was substantially higher for pins inserted perpendicular compared with 60 degrees. To avoid the complication of pin loosening, it is imperative to place these pins perpendicular to the skull to provide the most strength at the pin-bone interface.

The initial pin-insertion torque recommendations of 6 in.-lb were based on empirical observations. Cadaver studies have shown, however, that 10 in.-lb of pressure barely penetrates the outer table. Biomechanical testing has shown that 8 in.-lb is more favorable compared with 6 in.-lb in adults. Clinical trials have borne this out with reduced pin site loosening and infection.

Application of the halo apparatus proceeds in a stepwise fashion (Table 32-2). With the cervical spine protected by manual traction, the patient's trunk can be elevated 30 degrees for vest placement. The posterior portion of the vest is applied and connected to the halo, followed by the anterior portion. Alternative methods include logrolling the patient, although it may be difficult to maintain cervical alignment. In rare instances of a stable fracture pattern or after surgical internal fixation, the patient can be instructed to sit upright, and the vest can be applied. All the locking bolts are tightened to 28 in.-lb of torque preset on the screwdriver. When all the bolts are tightened, cervical spine alignment should be confirmed radiographically.

When the halo is placed, the pins should be retightened 24 to 48 hours after placement. Studies have documented an immediate 2 to 4 in.-lb decrease in pin fixation purchase after vest placement. A commonly used pin care regimen

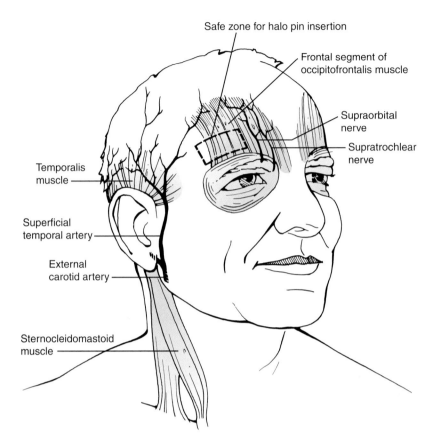

Safe zone for halo pin insertion

Frontal segment of
occipitofrontalis muscle

Supraorbital
nerve

Supratrochlear
nerve

Temporalis
muscle

Superficial
temporal artery

External
carotid artery

Sternocleidomastoid
muscle

**Figure 32-8** Diagram of the safe zone for placement of anterior halo fixator pins.

## TABLE 32-2 PROCEDURE SUMMARY FOR APPLICATION OF THE HALO SKELETAL FIXATOR

1. Determine ring or crown size (hold ring or crown over head to visualize size)
2. Determine vest size (from chest circumference measurement)
3. Identify pin site locations
4. Shave hair at posterior pin sites
5. Prepare pin sites with povidone-iodine solution
6. Apply local anesthesia
7. Advance sterile pins to level of skin
8. Have patient close eyes
9. Tighten pins at 2 in./lb increments in diagonal fashion
10. Tighten pins to 8 in./lb torque
11. Apply lock nuts to pins
12. Maintain cervical traction and raise patient trunk to 30°
13. Apply posterior portion of vest
14. Apply anterior portion of vest
15. Connect anterior and posterior portions of vest
16. Apply upright posts and attach ring to vest
17. Recheck fittings, screws, and nuts
18. Tape vest-removing tools to vest
19. Obtain cervical spine radiographs

Modified from Botte MJ, Garfin SR, Byrne TP, et al. The halo skeletal fixator: principles of application and maintenance. Clin Orthop 1989; 239:12–18.

consists of daily cleansing with dilute hydrogen peroxide (50/50 with water) on a cotton swab. Patients should have follow-up examinations at predetermined intervals to confirm lack of halo-vest complications. At this time, radiographs are taken to confirm adequacy of cervical immobilization.

## Biomechanical Analysis

Although the halo is the most rigid external orthosis for immobilization of the cervical spine, some motion and force transmission to the cervical elements does occur. In early studies, the halo device was found to permit only 4% of flexion/extension, 4% of lateral bending, and 1% of rotational motion of the normal native cervical spine. Follow-up studies have shown that such significant immobilization was not accurate, however. One study showed 51 degrees of motion with halo immobilization. Segmentally the greatest motion is observed at the occiput-C1 level (11.5 degrees). The lowest is at C2-3 (6.7 degrees). When flexion was observed at one segment of the spine, extension was observed at another level—a phenomenon called *snaking*. Motion of the cervical spine was observed with patient position changes from supine to prone or from supine to sitting. There was no increased motion at the level of injury, however. In contrast, a clinical series reported greater than 3 degrees of angulation and 1 mm of translation at the fracture site in 77% of the patients.

Studies also have examined the directional force generated by the halo device. Maximal forces seem to be exerted in the medial-lateral plane. In daily activities, however, it was observed that anterior-posterior and vertical forces were much larger. This observation was confirmed by Lind and Sihlbom, who noted no horizontal motion in the halo device. They reported significant differences in distractive forces between the supine and upright positions that can be attributed to the added weight of the head. Distractive forces were most increased with deep breathing, shoulder shrugging, and arm elevation, although no patient experienced any discomfort. These high distractive forces were most elevated in patients with tight-fitting vests. It was concluded that the halo vest can be elevated by the sternum and the scapulae. It was recommended that there be at least 30 mm of space between the sternum and the vest to prevent gross motion of the vest with daily activities. Patients also should be cautioned regarding exercises that involve twisting and bending because these tend to transmit undesirable forces to the cervical spine.

## Complications

Although clinical studies have shown the efficacy of the halo device, complications with its use are frequent. Awareness of the most commonly seen complications can help minimize their severity and avoid catastrophic sequelae.

Pin loosening has been identified as one of the most common problems with the halo device. In two large studies, pin loosening was observed in 36% and 60% of patients. This problem was confirmed experimentally in a biomechanical study in three patients. There was an 83% decrease in torque pressure measured at the time of halo removal. The mechanism of pin loosening is thought to be via bone resorption at the pin tip. If there is no sign of infection, the pins may be retightened to 8 in.-lb of torque as long as resistance is met on the first few turns of the pin. If no resistance is met, a new pin must be placed in an adjacent position. The old pin should be kept in place until the new pin has been placed rigidly to keep the correct orientation of the ring on the skull.

Halo pin infection rates have been documented to be approximately 20%. If drainage and erythema continue at a pin site even with aggressive pin care, bacterial cultures should be obtained, and appropriate oral antibiotics should be started. If cellulitis persists or an abscess forms, the pin should be removed and placed in another position. The patient may require incision and drainage of the abscess with parenteral antibiotics.

Skull and dural penetration by a halo pin are rare complications often related to patient falls. If a patient reports trauma to himself or herself or to the halo, radiographs must be taken tangential to the skull to determine whether pin perforation of the inner table has occurred. Clinically the patient may present with a headache, malaise, or visual disturbances if symptomatic pin penetration has occurred. Clear cerebrospinal fluid leakage from the pin site is a definitive sign that dural puncture has occurred. In these circumstances, a new pin should be placed in another region, and

the old pin should be removed. Elevation of the head decreases intracerebral pressure and facilitates closure of the dural tear. These tears usually heal in 4 to 5 days. If the tear does not heal or an infection is suspected (subdural abscess), formal surgical intervention may be necessary.

Patients may report difficulty with swallowing during halo immobilization. Deglutition dysfunction leading to aspiration has been reported. Many instances of swallowing difficulty are a result of the cervical spine's being immobilized in the extended position. Efforts to flex the cervical spine while maintaining cervical reduction may assist in dysphagia resolution.

Pressure sores have been reported in 4% to 11% of patients during halo immobilization. These sores frequently develop underneath the vest or cast vest secondary to pressure against prominent bone surfaces or are due to insufficient padding or incorrect sizing of the vest. Principles of pressure sore prevention include frequent turning, adequate vest padding, and routine skin inspections. Pressure sores are more prevalent in patient populations using a cast vest, rather than the padded prefabricated plastic vest; this is especially important in patients with neurologic deficits, who may not have adequate sensation over the trunk. Alternative strategies to halo immobilization, such as rigid internal fixation, should be considered in these patients. Pressure sore treatment may require split-thickness skin grafting and rotational muscle flaps for coverage.

## Pediatric Halo Considerations

Halo immobilization has been successful in the treatment of children and infants after unstable cervical injuries and congenital abnormalities. The recommended pin torque pressure in children is 2 to 5 in.-lb owing to the pediatric skull's being thinner and softer. In infants (<3 years old), a multiple, low torque pin system is recommended to achieve maximal stability.

Twelve pins can be inserted at 2 in.-lb of torque pressure under general anesthesia. Halo pins should be placed under the largest diameter of the skull, with care to avoid the frontal sinus and temporal regions. A computed tomography scan of the head may be beneficial to identify the location of suture line and bone fragments (in congenital cases) before placement of the halo. In the presence of open suture lines and fontanelles, vigilant care must be taken to ensure that equal pressure is being placed on the skull through the halo pins symmetrically to prevent skull deformity.

Owing to sizing, a custom-made ring and vest often are required. When the halo is placed, the vest is applied in normal fashion and connected to the halo. Children require the same pin care that adults require. A study has found that children have a higher rate of pin loosening. It is recommended that children with halo fixators have close supervision.

## Gardner-Wells Tongs

Although rarely used today as definitive treatment, patients with unstable cervical injuries may require initial stabilization or reduction using cervical skeletal traction. Gardner-

Wells tongs consist of two pins attached to a bow-shaped frame, through which traction may be applied. The neutral position for tong placement is at a level 1 cm posterior to the external auditory canal and 1 cm above the pinna. Depending on the injury pattern, tongs may be placed slightly anterior to impart an extension moment or slightly posterior to impart a flexion moment to the spine. Stainless steel tongs, rather than MRI-compatible graphite tongs, should be used when high weight reduction is being attempted. Radiographs should be obtained after the initial 10 to 15 lb of weight application to rule out occult occipitocervical injuries, which can be overdistracted easily. Neurologic status must be monitored for change during and after application of traction. If definitive treatment is delayed, patients may benefit from use of rotating beds while traction is maintained.

## THORACOLUMBAR AND SACRAL ORTHOSES

Sacroiliac orthoses, LSOs, and TLSOs are available in flexible and rigid variations. The flexible versions have a design similar to their rigid counterparts but provide only minimal immobilization. Sacroiliac orthoses generally encircle the pelvis, spanning the tops of the iliac crests to the trochanters. These may provide relief in traumatic postpartum separation of the sacroiliac joints. LSOs extend from the pelvis to the xiphoid anteriorly and the inferior angle of the scapula posteriorly. TLSOs extend higher, generally to the midscapular level.

Flexible LSOs and TLSOs are prescribed by some physicians for the treatment of low back pain. These corset-style devices are adjustable by means of laces, hooks, or Velcro straps. Some authors have reported that these orthoses decrease the myoelectric activity of the paraspinal muscles and increase intraabdominal pressure, possibly resulting in decreased loads on the intervertebral discs. Others have reported increased myoelectric activity, as measured through surface electrodes on the paraspinal muscles, when certain tasks are performed in braced subjects. Less controversy surrounds the effect on the abdominal muscles, with several authors reporting decreased measured myoelectric activity with brace wear. Clinical studies are conflicting regarding the role of lumbar supports for prevention and treatment of low back pain. Jellema et al performed a systematic review of the literature to assess this issue. They reviewed 13 studies, most of which they determined were low-quality research. Regardless, they determined that based on the liter-

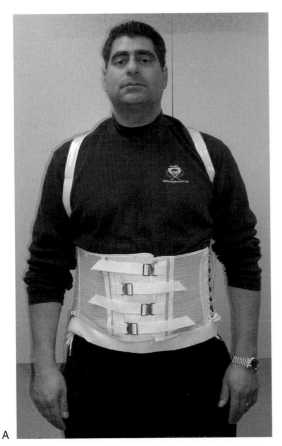 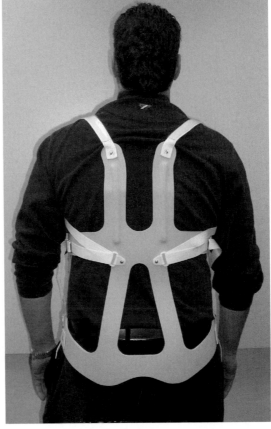

A                                                                                          B

**Figure 32-9**   Knight-Taylor orthosis. (**A**) Frontal view. (**B**) Posterior view. Control of thoracic sagittal plane motion is achieved through axillary straps attached to posterior thoracic uprights.

ature, there is no strong evidence to support the use of lumbar supports for prevention or treatment of low back pain.

Most conventional TLSOs are more effective in controlling motion in the sagittal plane than in controlling rotation or lateral bending. The Jewett hyperextension brace is an example of a non-custom-molded TLSO brace. It applies three-point fixation to the torso through anterior pads on the symphysis pubis and sternum and a posterior pad midway between the anterior pads. This arrangement of forces places the spine in slight extension. Similar to cervical collars, this brace is best in controlling motion in the flexion/extension plane and is less effective in controlling lateral bending and rotation. The Knight-Taylor brace (Fig. 32-9) is another commonly prescribed TLSO and can be prefabricated or custom molded. It has a corset-style front for abdominal compression and lateral and posterior uprights attached to over-the-shoulder straps for thoracic control. Prefabricated TLSOs often consist of the now common clamshell brace that can be ordered to measurements and usually are fabricated out of 1/8-inch to 3/16-inch, low-density polyethylene. Prefabricated "customizable" TLSOs also are commercially available with apron-style fronts that can be adjusted with Velcro straps and telescoping sternal pads (Fig. 32-10). These braces provide good control in all three planes, but the major restriction is in the flexion/extension plane. For optimal control in all three planes between T5 and L4, a fully custom-molded TLSO (Fig. 32-11) should be used. These often are formed from high-temperature thermoplastic that is custom-fitted from a plastic shell formed from the patient. When immobilization proximal to T5 is required, a cervical extension should be included. If immobilization distal to L4 is needed, a thigh cuff should be added to the orthosis to control pelvic rotation.

Compared with cervical orthoses, few studies have been performed to evaluate scientifically the ability of external orthoses to immobilize the thoracolumbosacral spine. Norton and Brown reported the earliest data on motion restriction with lumbar external supports. They evaluated three rigid LSOs, one flexible LSO, and a TLSO. Kirschner wires were inserted into the spinous processes of volunteers. The angles between the wires were measured to determine the amount of motion, and radiographic evaluation was performed. They reported increased motion across the lumbosacral junction in all of the braces. Increased motion at L4-5 also was noted while the subjects were sitting. Compared with the unbraced state, all of the braces resulted in some flexion at L4-5 and L5-S1 while standing. Lumsden and Morris reported similar findings when they studied lumbosacral rotational motion in subjects wearing either a chairback brace or LSO corset. Volunteers had Steinmann pins placed in their posterior superior iliac spines. Motion was determined by radiographs and measurement of pin rotation. In each case, the investigators found the braces increased motion at the lumbosacral level. Fidler and Plasmans used radiographs to compare the effect on lumbosacral motion of a corset, a brace, and a plaster jacket with and without a thigh cuff. They found the custom-molded plaster jacket to provide the best immobilization

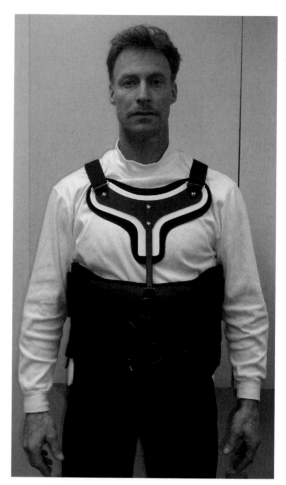

**Figure 32-10** Prefabricated "customizable" thoracolumbosacral orthosis. This particular design (Orthomerica) has an apron-style front with an adjustable sternal pad to help customize the fit.

at the L1-3 level. To improve immobilization at the L4-S1 levels, they recommended adding a thigh cuff to the orthosis.

Indications for TLSOs are less well defined than for cervical orthoses. As mentioned previously, bracing for compression fractures of the thoracolumbar spine is not tolerated well by elderly patients. Treatment in these patients usually consists of early mobilization and close follow-up. A soft binder or corset may provide support and symptomatic relief. In younger patients, however, anterior column fractures often are the result of greater energy than their osteoporotic counterparts, and a more cautious approach often is favored. These patients commonly are treated with a rigid Jewett or Knight-Taylor brace. The need for rigid bracing of these fractures is still a matter of debate, however. A study retrospectively reviewed the outcome of 129 young patients with mild compression fractures who were treated with or without a Jewett hyperextension brace. They found that one-column fractures of the thoracolumbar spine with 30% compression can be treated safely without bracing, instead prescribing early ambulation, hyperexten-

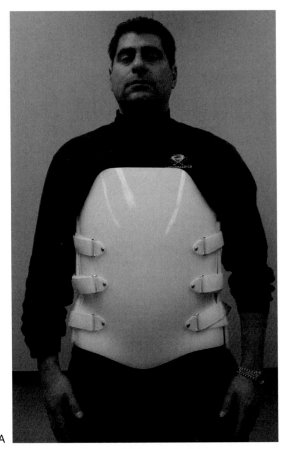
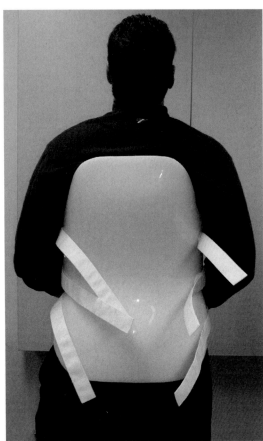

**Figure 32-11**    Custom molded thoracolumbosacral orthosis. (**A**) Frontal view. (**B**) Posterior view. This bivalve design is made from a plaster cast of the patient.

sion exercises, and close follow-up. Burst fractures constitute another entity in the spectrum of thoracolumbar injuries. Historically, neurologically intact patients with burst fractures were treated with bed rest for 4 to 12 weeks, followed by progressive mobilization. Today, controversy exists as to which injuries require surgical stabilization and which can be treated with bracing and early mobilization. Most would agree that any neurologic deficit is an indication for operative management. Canal compromise of 50% or more, kyphotic deformity of greater than 30 degrees, and posterior column involvement are other indications for aggressive intervention. The final determination often remains a case-by-case, multifactorial judgment call, however, on the part of the treating surgeon. Chow et al retrospectively studied functional outcomes in 24 patients treated with hyperextension body casts or Jewett hyperextension braces for thoracolumbar burst fractures. None of these patients had posterior column fractures, significant kyphosis, or neurologic deficit. Patients initially were treated with bed rest and logroll precautions until the predictable ileus and abdominal distention resolved 2 to 3 days later. At that point, patients were casted or braced and progressively mobilized. Patients were followed for a minimum of 1 year. The investigators concluded that hyperextension casting or bracing with early mobilization reduces hospital time, avoids costs and risks

of surgery, and allows patients a relatively early return to work. Additionally the authors mentioned that patients treated nonoperatively tended to experience moderate back pain for 1 year after the injury and that this pain eventually diminished over time.

LSOs (Fig. 32-12) often are prescribed for treatment after arthrodesis for degenerative conditions. As discussed earlier, several studies show little or no immobilizing effect from wearing LSOs and possibly an increase in L4-5 and L5-S1 motion after application of these orthoses. The point continues to be debated. Postlumbar fusion bracing is believed by some to help relieve pain and decrease the risk of pseudarthrosis and fixation failure and is prescribed by some surgeons for 12 weeks postoperatively. Others believe that LSOs do little to immobilize the lumbar spine, and rigid operative fixation is enough to produce good patient outcomes.

## SUMMARY

Spinal orthoses continue to be prescribed commonly for the management of traumatic and degenerative conditions. Many different types are commercially available, and the scientific evidence to document their effectiveness is vari-

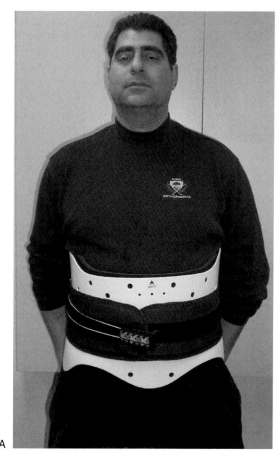
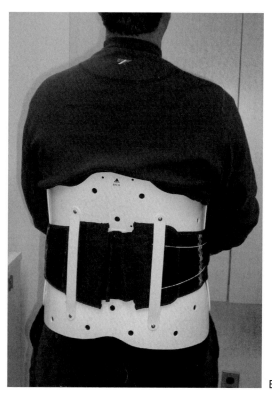

A      B

**Figure 32-12** Prefabricated lumbosacral orthosis. (**A**) Frontal view. (**B**) Posterior view. This design (Calfornia Compression Jacket, Orthomerica) has a patented "rip cord" used to help adjust the snugness of the fit.

able. Despite the potential for complications, the halo remains the gold standard for external cervical immobilization. A thorough appreciation of the biomechanics of spinal orthoses and their potential complications can help maximize their utility and minimize associated morbidity.

## ACKNOWLEDGMENT

The orthotics pictured in the figures were supplied by Precision Orthotics and Prosthetics, Linden, NJ. The models wearing the braces are Paul Goodman, CO, and David Sussman, CPO, both of Precision Orthotics and Prosthetics. We greatly appreciate their contribution to this chapter.

## SUGGESTED READING

Askins V, Eismont FJ. Efficacy of five cervical orthoses in restricting cervical motion: a comparison study. Spine 1997;22:1193–1198.

Botte MJ, Garfin SR, Byrne TP, et al. The halo skeletal fixator: principles of application and maintenance. Clin Orthop 1989;239: 12–18.

Fidler MW, Plasmans CMT. The effect of four types of support on the segmental mobility of the lumbosacral spine. J Bone Joint Surg Am 1983;65:943–947.

Garfin SR, Botte MJ, Centeno RS, et al. Osteology as it affects halo pin placement. Spine 1985;10:696–698.

Garfin SR, Botte MJ, Waters RL, et al. Complications in the use of halo fixation device. J Bone Joint Surg Am 1986;68:320–325.

Hartman JT, Palumbo F, Hill JB. Cineradiography of the braced normal cervical spine. Clin Orthop 1975;109:97–102.

Johnson RM, Hart DL, Simmons EF, et al. Cervical orthoses: a study comparing their effectiveness in restricting cervical motion in normal subjects. J Bone Joint Surg 1977;59A:332–339.

Mirza SK, Moquin RR, Anderson PA, et al. Stabilizing properties of the halo apparatus. Spine 1997;22:727–733.

Mubarak SJ, Camp JF, Vultich W, et al. Halo application in the infant. J Pediat Orthop 1989;9:612–614.

White AA, Panjabi, MM. Physical properties and functional biomechanics of the spine. In: White AA, Panjabi MM, eds. Clinical Biomechanics of the Spine, 2nd ed. Philadelphia: JB Lippincott, 1990.

# SPINAL FUSION

33

# 33.1 BIOLOGY OF SPINAL FUSION

## JOHN LOUIS-UGBO ■ SCOTT D. BODEN

There has been a steady increase in the rate of spinal fusion surgery since the 1990s. Currently, about 250,000 spinal fusion procedures are carried out each year in the United States, and nearly all of these require bone graft material. The most common reason for performing a spinal arthrodesis is to treat either instability (excessive motion) of a spine segment or a deformity that is at risk for progression. Most fusions are performed to treat degenerative disorders, and the most common region is the lumbar spine. Posterolateral lumbar fusion, the most commonly performed spinal arthrodesis, has been associated with the highest likelihood of failure (nonunion), ranging from 5% to 44% of patients with single-level fusion and more frequently when multiple levels are attempted. The successful repair of these pseudarthroses is even more challenging, with failures occurring in 35% to 51% of revision attempts. Nonunion often prevents the resolution of the clinical symptoms and usually results in greater medical costs and morbidity and the need for more surgeries.

Several strategies exist to augment healing or to replace autogenous bone graft in the spine (Table 33.1-1). Mechanical enhancement of spinal fusions using rigid internal fixation with hooks or screws and rods or plates has increased the successful fusion rate by approximately 10%; however, it has failed to eliminate nonunion in 10% to 15% of patients. Biophysical stimulation by either direct-current pulsed electromagnetic fields or low-intensity ultrasound has been shown to be a viable strategy for the enhancement of spinal fusion healing. Also, a variety of potential bone graft alternatives now are available. These alternatives include the following:

■ Different formulations of demineralized bone matrix, currently used as bone graft extenders only and not as a bone graft enhancer or substitute
■ Various ceramics, such as natural coral (calcium carbonate), coralline hydroxyapatite, or composites such as hydroxyapatite-tricalcium phosphate, which are used as bone graft extenders when mixed with autogenous bone graft but are unlikely to serve as stand-alone bone graft substitutes
■ Bone marrow cell-matrix interactions

A successful spinal arthrodesis requires the incorporation of bone graft material into the recipient site. The precise biologic, physiologic, and molecular mechanisms operating during this healing process are not understood fully. Successful fusion depends on a complex process influenced by the type of graft material used and on many local (biologic), biomechanical, systemic, and external factors affecting the healing response (Tables 33.1-2 and 33.1-3).

## BIOLOGY OF SPINAL FUSION AND GRAFT INCORPORATION

The healing of a spinal fusion is a multifactorial process, which makes it difficult to study in the clinical setting. The lack of reliable noninvasive techniques for assessing the success or failure of an arthrodesis limits prospective clinical studies. An animal model is a practical solution for studying individual factors involved in this complex process. A reliable spinal fusion animal model should mimic the inci-

297

## TABLE 33.1-1 ENHANCEMENT OF SPINAL FUSION

Mechanical
    Internal fixation (e.g., screws, hooks, rods, plates)
    External—braces
Biologic enhancement
    Bone graft materials
        Autogenous bone grafts
            Cancellous and morcellized
            Cortical
            Corticocancellous
            Vascularized and nonvascularized cortical
        Allogeneic bone grafts
            Fresh
            Frozen
            Freeze-dried
        Cell-based autogenous grafts
            Unfractionated fresh bone marrow
            Mesenchymal stem cells
            Genetically modified cells
            Differentiated osteoblasts and chondrocytes
    Bone graft extenders
        Mineralized bone matrices
            Ceramics (calcium phosphate, tricalcium phosphate, calcium sulfate)
            Collagen
            Composite grafts (e.g., collargraft)
        Bioactive glass
        Synthetic polymers
        Demineralized bone matrix
    Growth factors and cytokines
        Transforming growth factor-$\beta$
        Bone morphogenetic proteins
        $\alpha$ and $\beta$ fibroblast growth factors
        Platelet-derived growth factor
        Insulin-like growth factors
        Growth differentiation factors
    Gene-based therapy
        Ex vivo and in vivo
Biophysical
    Electrical stimulation
    Ultrasound stimulation

## TABLE 33.1-2 FACTORS AFFECTING SPINAL FUSION HEALING

Bone graft related
    Graft source
    Type of graft (cortical or cancellous)
    Quantity of graft
    Preparation or handling technique of graft material
    Morcellization of graft
Preparation of fusion site
Peculiarities of blood supply of soft tissues and fusion bed
Irradiation of fusion site
Previous surgery
Local bone disease (infection, tumor, marrow infiltrative disease)
Bone homeostasis (age-related factors)
Biomechanical
    Stability of fusion segment
    Loading and impaction of fusion segment
    Specific type of fusion
        Posterolateral intertransverse process
        Anterior interbody
        Anterior-posterior combined
    Location of fusion along the spine (cervical, thoracic, lumbosacral)
    Number of levels fused
    Efficacy of spinal immobilization (internal or external)
Systemic factors
    Systemic metabolic bone disease (e.g., osteoporosis, diabetes mellitus)
    Hormonal (growth hormone, anabolic hormones)
    Nutritional status
    Drugs (NSAIDs, dexamethasone, chemotherapeutic agents, bisphosphonates, corticosteroids)
    Infections
    Cigarette smoking and nicotine
    Severe trauma
Others
    Psychosocial factors
    Presence of central nervous system injury
    Primary diagnosis (e.g., myotonic dystrophy)
    Physical barriers (e.g., bulky instrumentation, presence of polymethyl methacrylate)

NSAIDs, nonsteroidal antiinflammatory drugs.

dence of nonunion and the surgical procedure seen in humans. Also, it should allow for the rapid observation of several subjects over a short time and allow for the valid extrapolation of data and results.

Despite detailed knowledge about the biology of fracture healing, far less is understood about the precise molecular mechanisms that control bone graft incorporation in a spinal fusion. Boden et al described the lumbar intertransverse fusion healing process in rabbits using autogenous iliac crest as a graft material. Mechanically solid fusions were observed by the 4th postoperative week with an overall nonunion rate of 30% to 40% (similar to what occurs in humans). Radiographic analysis also showed progressive remodeling of bone graft material with time, usually by 10 to 12 weeks, but as in humans, radiographs were accurate in assessing success or failure to attain solid fusion only 70% of the time. Vascular injection studies have shown that the

## TABLE 33.1-3 EFFECTS OF TOBACCO SMOKE AND NICOTINE ON BONE METABOLISM AND HEALING

Induces calcitonin resistance
Increases bone resorption at fracture ends
Interferes with osteoblastic function and bone metabolism
Delays revascularization and inhibits bone formation
Induces bone graft necrosis
Negative effect on intervertebral disc metabolism
Negative effect on gene expression in the fusion mass

**TABLE 33.1-4  STAGES OF SPINAL FUSION HEALING AS PROPOSED BY BODEN ET AL (1995) (HISTOLOGIC STAGES OF SPINAL FUSION)**

| | |
|---|---|
| Stage 1: early (inflammatory) phase, weeks 1–3 | No solid fusions observed. Hematoma surrounds the graft material. Influx of inflammatory cells. Neovascularization and formation of fibrovascular stroma. Recruitment of pluripotential cells from marrow cavity and transplanted autograft bone. Primary membranous ossification and osteoid seams appear over transverse process (corticocancellous ratio >1.4). Minimal endochondral ossification seen between graft fragments |
| Stage 2: middle (reparative) phase, weeks 4 and 5 | Solidification of fusion and remodeling occurs over transverse processes. Increased revascularization, resorption of necrotic tissue and graft fragments, and differentiation of osteoblastic and chondroblastic cells. Membranous bone extends toward central zone of fusion mass. Cartilaginous interface zone centrally. Endochondral ossification unites upper and lower halves of the fusion |
| Stage 3: late (remodeling) phase, weeks 6–10 | Solid fusion. No cartilage present. Corticocancellous ratio <1. Remodeling proceeds. Extension of trabecular bone from peripheral cortical rim toward center of fusion. Increased secondary spongiosa and bone marrow formation. Progressive resorption of graft material in the center of fusion mass |

primary blood supply to the fusion mass originates from the decorticated transverse processes. The failure to achieve spinal fusion in the absence of decortication emphasizes the importance of extensive decortication of the posterolateral spine elements (lateral facet, pars interarticularis, transverse process) in providing bone marrow, vascularization, and osteoprogenitor cells to the fusion mass.

Qualitative and quantitative analysis of histologic sections revealed three distinct, reproducible temporal phases of spinal fusion healing (inflammatory, reparative, and remodeling) (Table 33.1-4). These phases occurred in sequence but in a delayed fashion in the central zone of the fusion mass compared with the outer transverse process zones (Fig. 33.1-1). Maturation of the spinal fusion was most advanced at the ends of the fusion mass near the transverse processes ("outer" zone). Intramembranous bone formation was the predominant mechanism of healing over the decorticated transverse processes. A similar histologic progression occurred in the "central" zone, but was delayed in time. This site was characterized by a period of endochon-

dral bone formation during weeks 3 and 4, when cartilage formed and was converted to bone. This central "lag effect" may explain why many nonunions occur in the central zone of a fusion mass. Remodeling in the central zone equilibrated with the transverse process zones by week 10.

At a molecular level, bone formation is the end product of a cascade of cellular events believed to be controlled by various growth factors, including bone morphogenetic proteins (BMPs), transforming growth factor-$\beta$, fibroblast growth factor, platelet-derived growth factor, and insulin-like growth factor-1. A unique temporal and spatial pattern of osteoblast-related gene expression was observed in a reverse-transcriptase polymerase chain reaction analysis of RNA from the different zones of the fusion mass (Table 33.1-5). A lag effect in gene expression that correlated with the previously observed lag effect in the histologic healing sequence was noted in the central zone compared with the outer zones of the fusion. As with osteocalcin expression, the peak expression of all genes measured was seen in the central zone 1 to 2 weeks later than the peak in the outer

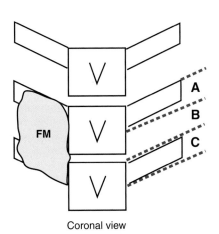

Coronal view

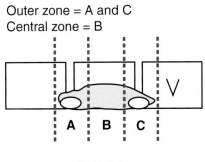

Outer zone = A and C
Central zone = B

Sagittal view

**Figure 33.1-1**  Schematic diagram of lumbar fusion mass divided into thirds in the coronal and sagittal views and their relationship to the vertebral bodies (*V*). The two outer zones (*A* and *C*) are distinguished from the single central zone (*B*). FM, fusion mass.

## TABLE 33.1-5 BONE MORPHOGENETIC PROTEIN GENE EXPRESSION AND BONE PROTEIN EXPRESSION DURING SPINAL FUSION HEALING

| | |
|---|---|
| Stage 1: early (inflammatory) phase, weeks 1–3 | Characterized by increased gene expression in outer zones. Increased expression of BMP-6 and BMP-4 mRNA in week 1. Increased alkaline phosphatase levels. Increased type I and type II collagen. Increased osteopontin and osteonectin mRNA. Peak expression of BMP-2 mRNA occurs in week 3 |
| Stage 2: middle (reparative) phase, weeks 4 and 5 | Characterized by increased activity in central zone. Peak expression of osteopontin, osteonectin, and osteocalcin. Second increase in BMP-6 mRNA level in central zone. Increased BMP-4 and BMP-2 mRNA in central zone. |
| Stage 3: late (remodeling) phase, weeks 6–10 | Return of gene expression to baseline levels. Persistent BMP-6 mRNA expression |

BMP, bone morphogenetic protein.
Data from Morone MA, Boden SD, Martin G, Hair G, Titus L. Gene expression during autograft lumbar spine fusion and the effect of BMP-2. Clin Orthop 1998;351:252–265.

zone (Fig. 33.1-2). This finding is consistent with the peripheral-to-central healing pattern observed histologically for fusions using autogenous bone graft. Laboratory indicators of bone formation are listed in Table 33.1-6.

Expression of the mRNA of several BMPs also was studied (Fig. 33.1-3). In the peripheral zones, BMP-2 mRNA expression was increased during weeks 2 through 6, with peak expression in weeks 3 and 4 (40-fold increase). BMP-

## TABLE 33.1-6 INDICATORS OF MESENCHYMAL CELL DIFFERENTIATION BY BONE MORPHOGENETIC PROTEINS

Increased mRNA expression
Increased osteocalcin, osteopontin, and osteonectin
Increased alkaline phosphatase
Increased collagen types I and II synthesis
Increased intracellular SMAD
Increased cartilage proteoglycan synthesis
Increased PTH-dependent cAMP production

cAMP, cyclic adenosine monophosphate; PTH, parathyroid hormone; SMAD, mammalian analogue of SMA gene.

6 in the outer zones had a first peak (54-fold) on day 2 and a second peak (100-fold) during week 5, whereas BMP-6 in the central zone showed an initial peak (34-fold) on day 2, but did not show the later peak. These findings suggest specific time patterns of expression and probably unique roles for each of the various BMPs during spinal fusion. It seems that BMP-6 is unique in that its mRNA levels showed the earliest peak and greatest relative increase of the BMPs studied. BMP-6 may play an initiating role in intramembranous bone formation. It also is an early marker for solid spinal fusion. The lower level of BMP-6 expression in the central zone of the fusion mass is correlated with the delayed timing and smaller amount of bone formation in the central zone of the fusion. The predilection for nonunion in the central zone also is apparent at a molecular biologic level.

The addition of rhBMP-2 to autogenous graft is associated with earlier peaks and higher levels of osteoblast-related gene expression in the central zone of the fusion mass, eliminating the central lag effect and perhaps decreasing the number of potential nonunions. The presence of nicotine significantly changes the gene expression associated with bone healing. The effect of nicotine on cytokine expression is seen mostly in the inner zone of the fusion mass. Table 33.1-5 summarizes molecular events occurring during the fusion process.

The mechanism and timing of bone healing may vary considerably depending on the region of the spine under consideration. The three primary locations are the anterior interbody, the intertransverse process, and the interlaminar-facet joint region. The incorporation process also differs for cortical and cancellous bone grafts. Specific descriptions of integration of various types of bone grafts and substitutes are provided in subsequent sections. For biosynthetic materials, new bone formation occurs by creeping substitution, and the resorbing cell is the foreign body giant cell, not the osteoclast. Also, two physical factors determine the incidence and speed of union between bone grafts and the adjacent host bone more than the characteristics of the grafts themselves:

- Stability of the construct
- Contact between host bone and the graft

## BIOLOGIC FACTORS AFFECTING SPINAL FUSION

A successful spinal fusion results in the elimination of movement across an intervertebral motion segment after bone union. Studies examining the clinical and radiographic success of spinal fusions with autograft have reported highly variable results. This variability may be due to many factors, including the following (see Table 33.1-2):

- Location and type of fusion
- Stringency of fusion outcome criteria
- Patient selection
- Severity of underlying pathology
- Use and type of internal fixation
- Technical preparation of the fusion bed
- Technical retrieval and preparation of the bone graft material

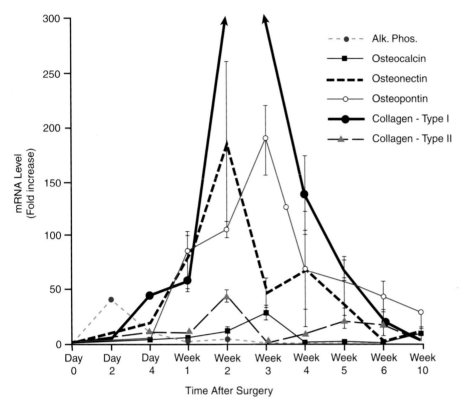

**Figure 33.1-2**   Osteoblast-related gene expression in the outer zone of the spinal fusion mass at specific times after surgery. The values of mRNA levels are given as fold increases over the level present in iliac crest bone (day 0). A reproducible sequence of gene expression was seen that was paralleled in the central zone (not shown) but delayed by 1 to 3 weeks.

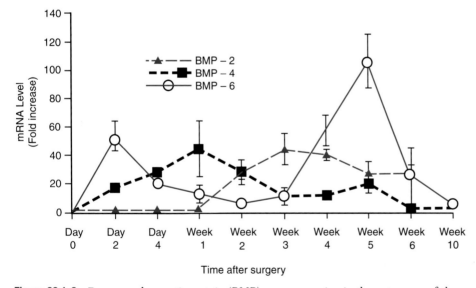

**Figure 33.1-3**   Bone morphogenetic protein (BMP) gene expression in the outer zone of the spinal fusion mass at specific times after surgery. The values of mRNA levels are given as fold increases over the level present in iliac crest bone (day 0). A reproducible sequence of gene expression was seen with BMP-6 mRNA peaking earliest on day 2, followed by BMP-4 mRNA, BMP-2 mRNA, and a second peak of BMP-6 mRNA.

Posterolateral lumbar fusion, the most commonly performed spinal arthrodesis, has been associated with the highest likelihood of failure (pseudarthrosis), ranging from 5% to 44%.

Mechanical loading (as in interbody fusion) tends to increase the fusion rate, whereas tensile forces as experienced during the consolidation of interlaminar or intertransverse process fusion may decrease it. It is believed that compressive forces acting on the interbody graft stimulate the ingrowth of vascular buds and proliferating mesenchymal cells from the cancellous host bone into the bone graft.

Higher fusion rates are associated with the use of internal fixation secondary to decreased motion in the fusion segments. The level of fusion (L4-5 versus L5-S1), the number of segments fused, the patient's weight and activity level, and external bracing after surgery may influence the outcome of the fusion. Implant loosening may cause increased nonunion. Instrumented fusion masses tend to be more rigid, narrower, and more compact than masses with uninstrumented fusions. Patients with disease conditions (e.g., muscular dystrophy, spinal muscular atrophy) that are associated with little voluntary motion often have higher than average fusion rates because of decreased spinal segment motion. Intraarticular preparation of the lumbar facet joints for arthrodesis may result in a 25% increase in sagittal plane mobility producing tensile strain and ultimately nonunion, and exclusion of the same may predispose to a less rigid fusion.

Numerous local and biologic factors can affect the healing of a spinal fusion. The spinal fusion process is affected greatly by the adequacy of local blood supply, the efficacy of the inflammatory response, and the availability of osteoprogenitor cells. Scarring of the fusion bed from multiple fusion attempts, excessive trauma to the fusion area, and presence of a local tumor or bone disease may replace normal marrow, structurally weakening the recipient bone and fusion mass. The health of the host bone bed is crucial in the process of osteoinduction because new osteoprogenitor cells are recruited by induction of residual mesenchymal cells in marrow reticulum, endosteum, periosteum, and connective tissue. Healthy soft tissue adjacent to a fusion process provides a source for diffusible growth factors and nutrition for migrating osteoprogenitor cells, but is less critical than having adequate decorticated host bone. Perioperative irradiation of the fusion area, especially in the first few weeks of fusion, may increase the nonunion rate because of its direct cytotoxic effects on the proliferating and differentiating cells and alteration of neoangiogenesis. Inadequate decortication and insufficient quantity of bone graft can predispose to nonunion. The larger the surface area decorticated for fusion, the greater the availability of potential osteogenic cells and the larger the contact area exposed to support a bone bridge large enough to carry a mechanical load. Also, physical barriers (e.g., bulky instrumentation or the presence of polymethyl methacrylate) can result in inadequate surface area for decortication or osseointegration of the fusion mass.

Several systemic factors influence the outcome of spinal fusion. There are no specific data concerning gender and delayed healing. Older age (of the patient) has been associated with a decrease in recruitment of bioactive growth factors and of pluripotential stem cells during the spinal fusion healing. Osteoporosis may affect the spinal fusion rate adversely. Possible factors implicated in the process include the following:

- Apparent decrease in bone mass
- Alterations in bone marrow quality
- Decrease in the osteogenic stem cells and vascularity
- Structurally weak bones, which provide inadequate stabilization through internal fixation

Hormonal disorders (e.g., diabetes mellitus and hyperthyroidism) can affect the rate of spinal fusion adversely. Corticosteroids have a negative effect on bone healing because they decrease osteoblast differentiation from mesenchymal cells, increase bone resorption, and decrease the rate of synthesis of major components of bone matrix necessary for bone healing. Nutritional disorders, including deficiencies in protein, iron, calcium, and phosphorus, have been associated with delayed callus formation and fusion consolidation. Systemic diseases, such as sickle cell anemia, thalassemia major, and diabetes, may reduce the osteogenic potential of bone marrow by overgrowth of hematopoietic cells at the expense of osteoprogenitor cells.

Drugs that delay or inhibit bone healing include the following:

- *Cytotoxic drugs* (e.g., doxorubicin [Adriamycin] and methotrexate) used in the immediate postoperative period inhibit bone formation and healing.
- *Nonsteroidal antiinflammatory drugs* (e.g., ibuprofen and ketorolac) may inhibit the healing of a spinal fusion possibly by suppressing the inflammatory response involved in the early stages of the healing process.
- Other drugs, including *antibiotics* (e.g., ciprofloxacin) and *anticoagulants* (e.g., heparin sodium and warfarin [Coumadin]) administered preoperatively and postoperatively have been associated with delayed bone healing.

Cigarette smoking and nicotine have been associated with delayed union and nonunion in spinal fusion (see Table 33.1-3). Smoking interferes with bone homeostasis and repair. Nicotine inhibits expression of a wide range of cytokines, including cytokines associated with neovascularization and osteoblast differentiation.

# BIOPHYSICAL ENHANCEMENT OF SPINAL FUSION

The biophysical arsenal for augmenting spinal fusion healing includes the exogenous induction of biophysical forces, such as electromagnetic fields, low-intensity ultrasound, and use of direct electrical stimulation. The scientific basis for these biophysical interventions is that they serve as surrogates for the regulatory signals normally arising through functional loading of the skeleton (Wolff's law) but are absent during the spinal healing process.

## Electrical Stimulation

The modern era of electrical stimulation for use in bone healing gained attention in the 1950s, when Yasuda published reports on the piezoelectric effects of bone. He showed new bone formation in the vicinity of a cathode (negative electrode) when low current was applied to a rabbit femur over 3 weeks. Electrical stimulation for clinical use has three distinct forms:

- Constant direct-current stimulation (invasive)
- Time-varying inductive coupling produced by a magnetic field (noninvasive)
- Capacitative coupling (noninvasive)

All these techniques produce electrical fields of about 10 mV/cm, which are comparable to endogenously produced electrical fields.

Direct current electrical stimulation (DCES) uses an implantable device in which the metallic lead or cathode is placed in direct contact with the decorticated transverse process and bone graft. The anode is implanted in the subcutaneous layer. The effective stimulation distance is approximately 5 to 8 mm from the cathode, and the area of stimulation may be adjusted by coiling the cathode wire to increase surface area. The implantable battery delivers a constant direct current for 6 to 9 months. Pulsed electromagnetic field (PEMF) stimulation requires a noninvasive external coil that delivers electromagnetic energy when driven by an electrical current. The coils usually are worn by the patient in a brace for 6 to 8 hours per day for 3 to 6 months. Capacitively coupled electrical field stimulation (CCEFS) uses an external pair of capacitive plates that produce electrical fields when an electrical current is applied. The capacitive plates usually are worn continuously for 9 months or until fusion occurs. PEMFs are generated by a time-varying current applied to metallic coils at a certain duration and intensity.

## Mechanism of Action

The precise mechanism by which DCES, PEMFs, and CCEFS stimulate osteogenesis is unknown. The molecular mechanism of action has been hypothesized to occur as a result of direct interaction between induced electrical fields and the target cell or alternatively by affecting the metabolism of drugs and endogenous factors. DCES is capable of triggering mitosis and recruitment of osteogenic cells in culture. The chemical changes in the local environment of bone cells in proximity to the active cathode are thought to trigger physiologic changes that lead to an osteogenic response. In vivo studies have shown that direct electrical currents stimulate osteogenesis through proliferation and recruitment of bone cells. It also may affect the activity of bone and cartilage directly through the activation of cyclic adenosine monophosphate within the stimulated cell, triggering an intracellular second messenger system.

The density of the current at the site of the fracture is an important variable. Electrically induced osteogenesis has been noted to occur within specific windows of electrical current parameters. In 1981, Brighton et al studied the relationship between charge, current density, and amount of new bone formation in the medullary canal of the intact rabbit tibia using a stainless steel wire cathode. They showed that a constant current of 20 $\mu$A resulted in the greatest amount of bone formation, with no signs of necro-

sis. There was no dose-dependent increase in bone formation when the current was increased to 40 $\mu$A, but some cellular necrosis was noted. A constant current of 80 $\mu$A was destructive, resulting in cellular necrosis. Titanium cathodes are believed to provide a more even distribution and delivery of the current to the surrounding tissue. Several studies have reported conflicting results with regards to what current would cause optimal bone formation or bone necrosis.

PEMFs have been found to be less effective in stimulating osteogenesis than constant DCES; however, a direct comparison of relative efficacy is difficult because comparative studies have not been performed. In contrast to the effects of DCES, PEMFs seem to affect differentiated bone cells instead of precursor cells. It has been shown that PEMFs may affect cellular functions, such as protein synthesis and bone matrix synthesis, through accelerated bone formation by osteoblasts and inhibition of osteoclastic bone resorption and macrocellular events, including vascularization and tissue calcification. With PEMF stimulation, the induced electrical field rather than magnetic flux is responsible for augmenting bone healing.

## Uses in Spinal Fusion

Electrical stimulation has been an established mode of therapy in the treatment of nonunion in long bones, and more recent studies have shown increased fusion rates for lumbar spinal fusion supplemented with electrical stimulation. There is evidence in the literature to support its use for selected indications, as follows:

- Multilevel fusion
- Reoperation for pseudarthrosis
- Presence of osteoporosis, smoking, or significant vascular disease

In 1974, Dwyer et al reported the first clinical studies on the efficacy of electrical stimulation on lumbar spinal fusion. They used implantable DCES successfully in the treatment of anterior and posterior spinal fusions and nonunited spinal fractures with fusion success rates of 92% and 85%.

## Animal Studies

Direct current stimulation has shown efficacy in a dog facet fusion model, in a pig posterior fusion model developed by Nerubay et al, and in a rabbit posterolateral lumbar fusion model (Table 33.1-7). Bozic et al found that coralline hydroxyapatite and direct current stimulation can be used together to increase the fusion rate and stiffness in a dose-dependent manner in a rabbit model. Two animal posterior fusion studies performed by Kahanovitz et al used PEMFs, with the electromagnetic devices placed externally. The first study investigated a bone-healing signal for a three-level posterior fusion in a dog model. The second study evaluated the effect of a newer fracture-healing signal on facet fusions in a dog model. Both of these studies failed to show any significant increase in fusion rates. Glazer et al, using a rabbit model to assess the efficacy of PEMFs, showed a decrease in the nonunion rate from 40% to 20%, but this was not statistically significant.

## TABLE 33.1-7 EFFECTS OF PULSED ELECTROMAGNETIC FIELDS (PEMF) AND DIRECT CURRENT ELECTRICAL STIMULATION (DCES) ON ANTERIOR AND POSTERIOR SPINAL FUSION MODELS

| Author, Year of Study | Modality | Effects | Model | Type of Fusion |
|---|---|---|---|---|
| Nerubay et al, 1986 | DCES | Increased fusion rate | Pig | Posterior |
| Kahanovitz and Arnoczky, 1990 | DCES | 100% fusion at 12 wk | Dog | Posterior facet fusion |
| Kahanovitz et al, 1984 | PEMF | No effect | Dog | Posterior fusion |
| Kahanovitz et al, 1994 | PEMF | No effect | Dog | Posterior fusion |
| Guizzardi et al, 1994 | PEMF | Enhanced callus formation | Rat | Posterior fusion |
| Glazer et al, 1997 | PEMF | Increased fusion and stiffness of fusion mass | Rabbit | Posterior lumbar intertransverse |
| Bozic et al, 1999 | DCES | Dose-dependent increased fusion rate | Rabbit | Posterior lumbar intertransverse |
| France et al, 2001 | DCES | Dose-dependent increased fusion rate and stiffness of fusion mass | Rabbit | Posterior lumbar intertransverse |
| Toth et al, 2000 | DCES | Increased fusion rate in spine fusion cages | Sheep | Interbody cage |

## Clinical Studies

Table 33.1-8 summarizes the published clinical studies on the efficacy of electrical stimulation in spinal fusion. It is apparent from clinical trials and experimental studies that DCES is a potential adjunct to spinal fusion surgery when it is applied to lumbosacral fusion or pseudarthrosis repair.

Kane reported the first multicenter, prospective, randomized trial in which results showed a significantly higher fusion rate in patient groups in which fusion was difficult to achieve. Several studies in instrumented and uninstrumented patients further support the use of electrical stimulation as an adjunct to interbody and posterolateral spinal fusion. Randomized, double-blind, prospective clinical

## TABLE 33.1-8 FUSION SUCCESS RATES FOR PREVIOUSLY PUBLISHED OR PRESENTED CLINICAL DATA SUPPORTING THE USE OF PULSED ELECTROMAGNETIC FIELDS (PEMF) AND DIRECT CURRENT ELECTRICAL STIMULATION (DCES) WHEN USED IN EITHER ANTERIOR OR POSTERIOR SPINAL FUSIONS

| Author, Year of Study | Modality | Fusion Rates (Stimulation Group) | Fusion Type |
|---|---|---|---|
| Dwyer et al, 1974 | DCES | 92% | Anterior/posterior fusion |
| Dwyer et al, 1975 | DCES | 85% | Nonunited spinal fractures |
| Kane et al, 1988 | DCES | 91%, 81%, 93% | 3 different groups—posterior fusion |
| Meril et al, 1994 | DCES | 93% | Anterior/posterior fusion |
| Rogozinski and Rogozinski, 1996 | DCES | 96% | |
| Kucharzyk et al, 1999 | DCES | 95.6% | PLIF |
| Tejano et al, 1996 | DCES | 91.5% | Posterior fusion (80% for pseudarthrosis revision) |
| Pettine et al, 1995 | DCES | 89–96% (high-risk patients) | |
| Mooney et al, 1985 | PEMF | 77% | Anterior interbody pseudarthrosis |
| Mooney et al, 1990 | PEMF | 92% | Anterior/posterior fusion interbody fusion |
| Lee et al, 1989 | PEMF | 67% | Pseudarthrosis |
| Simmons et al, 1989 | PEMF | 77% | Pseudarthrosis |
| Linovitz et al, 2000 | PEMF | 64% | Pseudarthrosis |
| Goodwin et al, 1999 | CCEFS | 85% | Pseudarthrosis |
| Linovitz et al, 2002 | PEMF | 64% fusion rate (more fusions in women) | Multiple indications |

PLIF, posterior lumbar interbody fusion.

trials of PEMFs and capacitatively coupled electrical stimulation, reported by Mooney and by Goodwin et al, and single-coil electromagnetic stimulation results reported by Linovitz et al have shown a significant beneficial effect (see Table 33.1-8) on certain types of lumbar fusion procedures. Other published clinical trials and animal experiments collectively have yielded mixed results, however (see Tables 33.1-7 and 33.1-8). Goodwin et al reported the results of the first randomized, double-blind, prospective trial of capacitatively coupled electrical stimulation as an adjunct to lumbar spinal fusion surgery. Stimulated patients were found to have a fusion success rate of 84.7% versus 64.9% for control patients, a statistically significant difference.

## Ultrasound Stimulation of Spinal Fusion

Ultrasound is acoustic radiation at frequencies beyond the limit of human hearing. It has been used as a physical signal in the detection or alteration of biologic effects for many years. Low ultrasonic intensities (milliwatts per square centimeter) are applied for diagnostic purposes to avoid excessive heating of the tissues; ultrasonic intensities of 1 to 3 $W/cm^2$ commonly are used to treat joint stiffness, pain, and muscle spasm and to improve muscular mobility. Ultrasound also has some beneficial effects on wound and tendon healing. A broad spectrum of experiments performed at the basic science and clinical levels have provided substantial evidence that low-intensity ultrasound can accelerate osteogenesis and augment the fracture-healing process.

### Mechanism of Action

The specific mechanism of action by which ultrasound accelerates bone healing is largely unknown. Low-intensity pulsed ultrasound is a noninvasive form of mechanical energy transmitted transcutaneously as high-frequency acoustical pressure waves around the cells. The mechanical stimulation inherent to ultrasound translates into a biologic response. Several biologic mechanisms (direct and indirect) have been proposed to explain the influence of ultrasound on the acceleration of the fracture-repair process. Ultrasound influences several stages of the healing process, including signal transduction (second-messenger activity of chondroblasts and osteoblasts), gene expression, blood flow, tissue modeling and remodeling, and mechanical attributes of the callus. In vivo studies have shown that ultrasound helps to initiate the healing process, increase callus formation and the biomechanical strength of fracture callus, and encourage clinical and radiographic healing. It also increases aggrecan mRNA, osteopontin mRNA, bone mineral density, and blood flow. Data from various in vitro studies suggest that ultrasound may induce conformational changes in the cell membrane, altering ionic permeability (increased calcium incorporation) and second messenger activity. Changes in second messenger activity conceivably could lead to downstream alterations in gene expression, resulting in an acceleration of the fracture-repair process

by upregulating cartilage-specific and bone-specific genes and others. Ultrasound also stimulates angiogenesis, chondrogenesis, and cartilage hypertrophy, resulting in an earlier onset of endochondral formation and leading to an increase in stiffness and strength of the fracture site.

### Animal Studies in Spinal Fusion

The study by Glazer et al was the first to assess the benefits of ultrasound in spinal fusion. Their findings indicated that ultrasound increased the rates of fusion, stiffness, and load to failure, suggesting an influence on the healing of trabecular and cortical bone. Histologic assessment confirmed that there was increased bone formation in the fusion masses that had been exposed to ultrasound. Although these results are preliminary, they suggest that the low-level mechanical signal may influence cellular processes in the axial and the appendicular skeletons. Aynaci et al evaluated the effects of ultrasound on posterolateral intertransverse process fusion by using muscle-pediculated bone graft in a rabbit model. Historically, this type of graft has a higher fusion rate. The investigators showed a statistically significant increase in fusion rate in 85% of the stimulated animals compared with 55% in the control group. There was increased bone formation radiologically and histologically in the fusions exposed to ultrasound. Based on several studies that have been done at nonspinal sites, it is hoped that in the near future definite clinical trials of ultrasound in spinal fusion in humans will be done in increasing numbers.

## SUGGESTED READING

Aynaci O, Onder C, Piskin A, Ozoran Y. The effect of ultrasound on the healing of muscle-pediculated bone graft in spinal fusion. Spine 2002;27:1531–1535.

Boden SD, Schimandle JH, Hutton WC, Chen MI. 1995 Volvo Award in Basic Sciences. The use of an osteoinductive growth factor for lumbar spinal fusion: Part I. the biology of spinal fusion. Spine 1995;20:2626–2632.

Bouchard JA, Koka A, Bensusan JS, et al. Effects of irradiation on posterior spinal fusions: a rabbit model. Spine 1994;19:1836–1841.

Glazer PA, Heilmann MR, Lotz JC, Bradford DS. Use of ultrasound in spinal arthrodesis. A rabbit model. Spine 1998;23:1142–1148.

Linovitz RJ, Pathria M, Bernhardt M, et al. Combined magnetic fields accelerate and increase spine fusion: a double-blind, randomized, placebo controlled study. Spine 2002;27:1383–1389.

Morone MA, Boden SD, Martin G, et al. Gene expression during autograft lumbar spine fusion and the effect of BMP-2. Clin Orthop 1998;351:252–265.

Nerubay J, Margant B, Bubis JJ, et al. Stimulation of bone formation by electrical current on spinal fusion. Spine 1986;11:167–169.

Sandhu HS, Grewal HS, Parvataneni H. Bone grafting for spinal fusion. Orthop Clin North Am 1999;30:685–698.

Toribatake Y, Hutton WC, Boden SD, Morone MA. Revascularization of the fusion mass in a posterolateral intertransverse process fusion. Spine 1998;23:1149–1154.

Yasuda I. Fundamental aspects of fracture treatment. J Kyoto Med Soc 1953;4:395.

Zdeblick TA. A prospective, randomized study of lumbar fusion: preliminary results. Spine 1993;18:983–991.

# 33.2 BONE GRAFTING AND FUSION

**JOHN LOUIS-UGBO ■ SCOTT D. BODEN**

## PROPERTIES OF GRAFT MATERIALS

A bone graft material is any implanted material that, alone or in combination with other materials, promotes a bone-healing response by providing:

- Osteogenicity
- Osteoconductivity
- Osteoinductivity

Graft materials placed in the spinal fusion bed participate in the fusion process in several ways, which depend on the properties of the graft materials. Some important properties of an ideal bone graft or substitute are listed in Table 33.2-1.

A graft's osteogenic potential is derived from its cellular content. Osteogenic graft materials contain viable cells that are capable of forming bone (i.e., differentiated osteogenic precursor cells) or have the potential to differentiate into bone-forming cells (inducible osteogenic precursor cells). Surface cells on cortical, and more so cancellous, grafts that are handled properly can survive and produce new bone. This early bone formed by viable graft cells often is

crucial in bone formation during the first 4 to 8 weeks after surgery. This potential to produce bone is characteristic only of fresh autogenous bone and marrow cells.

*Osteoinduction* is the process by which some graft-derived factors stimulate recruitment from the surrounding bed of undetermined mesenchymal-type cells, which then differentiate into cartilage-forming and bone-forming cells. The concept of osteoinduction first was introduced by Urist et al. The osteoinductivity of mineralized grafts is minimal, but the osteoinductive capacity of demineralized bone matrix (DBM) (Grafton, Osteotech, Eatontown, NJ) has been well characterized. Bone matrix contains several bone-forming cytokines, including bone morphogenetic proteins (Tables 33.2-2 and 33.2-3). These cytokines are capable of inducing or influencing the differentiation of mesenchymal cells into bone-forming cells. In addition to DBM and the above-mentioned factors, autogenous and allograft bone are known to possess osteoinductive properties.

*Osteoconduction* is the physical property of a graft material that allows the ingrowth of sprouting capillaries, perivascular tissue, and infiltration of osteoprogenitor cells from the recipient bed into the structure of a graft during the process of graft incorporation known as *creeping substitution*. A purely osteoconductive graft material transfers neither osteogenic cells nor inductive stimuli, but it acts as a nonviable scaffold or trellis that supports the healing process. Osteoconduction may result from active bone formation and osteoinduction (e.g., in a fresh corticocancellous autograft), or it may occur passively, without the active participation of the graft, as is the case with most cortical allografts. Osteoconduction often is determined by the structure of the graft, the vascular supply from the surrounding soft tissue, and the mechanical environment of the graft and surrounding structures. Osteoconductive materials include the following:

- Autogenous and allograft bone
- Bone matrix
- Collagen
- Calcium phosphate ceramics

In addition, graft materials can be used as a graft:

- *Extender* (a material that allows the use of less autogenous bone graft with the same end result or one that allows a given amount of autogenous bone to be stretched over a greater area with the same success rate)
- *Enhancer* (a device that when added to autogenous bone graft increases the successful healing rate of autogenous bone graft, using either the usual amount of graft or a smaller amount of bone graft)
- *Substitute* (a material that may be used entirely in place of autogenous bone graft to achieve the same or a better fusion success rate)

## TABLE 33.2-1 PROPERTIES OF GRAFT MATERIALS

| Properties | Description |
|---|---|
| Osteogenic | Contain cells capable of directly forming bone |
| Osteoinductive | Ability to induce differentiation of pluripotential cells from surrounding tissue to an osteoblastic phenotype |
| Osteoconductive | Ability to support growth of bone over its surface |
| Osteointegrative | Ability to bond chemically to the surface of bone without an intervening layer of fibrous tissue |
| Biocompatible | Elicit minimal or no immunologic reaction |
| Mechanically stable | Allow loading and impaction early to induce bone formation |
| Bioresorbable | Undergo remodelling |
| Modular | Ideal bone-graft substitute should be available in block form and as granular (easy to use) |
| Others | Cost-effective<br>Readily available<br>Structurally similar to bone |

## TABLE 33.2-2 FUNCTIONS OF GROWTH FACTORS

| Growth Factor | Functions |
| --- | --- |
| Insulin-like growth factors I and II | Stimulate osteoblastic and chondrocyte proliferation<br>Stimulate osteoblast chemotaxis<br>Stimulate osteoclast proliferation<br>Increase type I collagen expression<br>Mediate effects of systemic hormones and mechanical stresses on bone<br>Stimulate bone formation and fracture repair |
| Transforming growth factor-β | Stimulates cells of mesenchymal origin and inhibits cells of ectodermal origin<br>Stimulates osteoblastic proliferation<br>Stimulates periosteal cells to undergo endochondral ossification<br>Stimulates expression of differentiation markers in bone cells<br>Inhibits osteocalcin and alkaline phosphatase synthesis<br>Inhibits the osteoinductive activity of bone morphogenetic proteins and osteoblast differentiation<br>Inhibits immune system |
| Bone morphogenetic proteins | Initiate mesenchymal cell differentiation into osteoblasts and chondrocytes<br>In vivo and in vitro induction of cartilage and bone formation<br>Prenatal and postnatal skeletal development and limb morphogenesis<br>Mediate expression of other growth factors in bone formation<br>Stimulate expression of differentiation markers in bone cells<br>Convert stromal bone marrow and muscle cells to osteoblasts<br>Play a role in early fracture repair, periodontal regeneration, and ectopic bone formation<br>Regulate general tissue morphogenesis and growth |
| Growth and differentiation factors | Involved in skeletal morphogenesis<br>Play a role in fracture repair and ectopic bone formation |
| Basic and acidic fibroblast growth factor | Promote growth and differentiation of cartilage and bone cells<br>Promote growth and differentiation of epithelial cells and myocytes<br>Stimulate expression of differentiation markers in bone cells<br>Accelerate bone repair, fracture healing, and callus remodeling<br>Initiate normal embryonic limb bud formation<br>Angiogenesis and mesenchymal cell mitogenesis<br>Involved in peripheral and central nervous systems development<br>Play a role in granulation tissue formation and wound healing |
| Platelet-derived growth factor | Stimulates bone formation and bone resorption<br>Mitogenic for osteoblasts<br>Increases cell replication and collagen and noncollagen protein synthesis<br>Important for normal healing of wounds and fractures |

## TABLE 33.2-3 INDICATORS OF MESENCHYMAL CELL DIFFERENTIATION BY BONE MORPHOGENETIC PROTEINS

Increase mRNA expression
Increase osteocalcin, osteopontin, and osteonectin
Increase alkaline phosphatase
Increase collagen type I and II synthesis
Increase intracellular SMADs
Increase cartilage proteoglycan synthesis
Increase PTH-dependent cAMP production

cAMP, cyclic adenosine monophosphate; PTH, parathyroid hormone; SMADs, mammalian analogue of *C. elegans* gene, SMA

# AUTOGENOUS BONE GRAFT

Fresh autogenous bone graft by definition is bone taken from one part of an individual and transplanted to another anatomic site in the same individual. It is the most successful bone graft or the gold standard for grafting material in patients undergoing spinal fusion. Autogenous bone graft has osteogenic properties (numerous differentiated and undetermined stromal cells within the cavity lining), osteoinductive properties (noncollagenous bone matrix proteins, including growth factors), and osteoconductive properties (hydroxyapatite and collagen). Other advantages of autogenous grafts include the following:

- They are histocompatible.
- They are completely osteointegrative
- They do not pose the risk of donor-associated disease transmission or immune rejection.

Autogenous bone graft has major disadvantages in several clinical situations. These disadvantages include insufficient amount of graft material available for use, especially in multisegmental fusion, in revision surgery in which prior bone harvests have been undertaken, in children (who have limited donor sites), and when treating large osseous defects. Significant donor site morbidity has been reported in 25% to 40% of patients resulting in unsatisfactory outcome for spinal fusion (Table 33.2-4). Harvest of a posterior iliac crest bone graft is associated with a significantly lower risk of postoperative complications compared with the anterior iliac crest. Also the use of a separate incision to procure the bone graft may be associated with some complications.

## Autograft Bone Graft Harvest for Spinal Fusion

The most commonly used site for harvesting bone graft is the posterior iliac crest because it provides a large quantity of cancellous and corticocancellous bone. In general, one posterior iliac crest provides enough bone for a two-level intertransverse fusion or a three-level fusion if there is local bone available from spinous processes. The anterior ilium, fibula, and rarely proximal tibia also are used in decreasing order. Many techniques may be used to obtain iliac bone (Table 33.2-5 and Figs. 33.2-1 through 33.2-4), and, depending on the application for which it is used, the shape and substance of the bone graft can differ. Strut grafts used for anterior interbody fusion must have some capacity to bear the mechanical compressive loads applied to the intervertebral location. These grafts require cortical integrity and

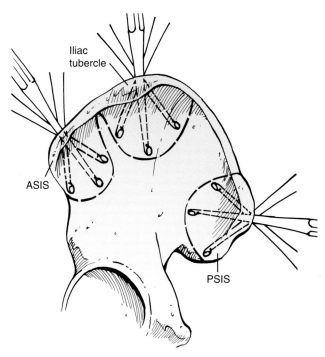

**Figure 33.2-1** Curettage technique for harvesting of cancellous bone grafts. ASIS, anterior superior iliac spine; PSIS, posterior superior iliac spine.

## TABLE 33.2-4 DONOR SITE MORBIDITY IN AUTOGRAFT HARVEST

| Donor Site | Complications (Features) | Reported Incidence (%) |
|---|---|---|
| Iliac donor site | Donor site pain (i.e., persistent pain ≥3 mo duration) | 2.8–49 |
| | Nerve injury—lateral femoral cutaneous, superior cluneal, ilioinguinal, iliohypogastric, superior gluteal, sciatic, and femoral nerves | <10 |
| | Vascular injury (superior gluteal artery injury and arteriovenous fistula, pseudoaneurysm) | <1 |
| | Fractures of the ilium (avulsion of ASIS) | <1 |
| | Pelvic instability (disruption of the pelvic ring) | <1 |
| | Violation of the sacroiliac joint (arthritis) | Unknown |
| | Abdominal hernia | <1 |
| | Peritoneal perforation | 1% |
| | Excessive bleeding and hematoma | Unknown |
| | Gait disturbance (abductor weakness) | <1 |
| | Infection (superficial and deep) | 1 |
| | Cosmetic deformity (unsightly scars) | Unknown |
| | Ureteral injury | Rare |
| | Others: increased hospital stay, increased blood loss, and additional cost | Unknown |
| Fibular donor site | Nerve injury (peroneal nerves in proximal third) | 4.9–11.8% |
| | Vascular injury (peroneal vessels in mid third of fibula) | Unknown |
| | Compartment syndrome | 10% |
| | Weakness of extensor hallucis longus muscle | 1.6% |
| | Ankle pain and instability (harvesting the distal 10 cm of fibula) | |
| | Others: footdrop, skin necrosis, infection, longer surgical time | |

ASIS, anterior superior iliac spine.

## TABLE 33.2-5  TYPES OF AUTOGRAFT AND HARVEST TECHNIQUES

| Type of Autograft | Special Harvesting Techniques | Probable Harvest Sites |
| --- | --- | --- |
| Cancellous bone grafts | Trephine curettage | ASIS<br>Iliac tubercle<br>PSIS<br>Proximal tibia |
| | Trapdoor technique<br>Splitting technique (Wolf and Kawamoto) | Iliac tubercle (3 cm posterior to ASIS)<br>Middle of iliac crest |
| Corticocancellous bone grafts<br>(unicortical and cancellous) | | Outer table of the posterior ilium (limit to 4 cm from PSIS)<br>Inner table of anterior ilium |
| | Corticocancellous acetabular reamer system | Acetabulum |
| Bicortical bone grafts | Subcrestal window technique | Below iliac crest |
| Tricortical bone grafts | | Anterior ilium (3 cm posterior to ASIS) |
| Nonvascularized or vascularized strut graft | | Fibula (middle third)<br>Iliac crest<br>Rib |

ASIS, anterior superior iliac spine; PSIS, posterior superior iliac spine.

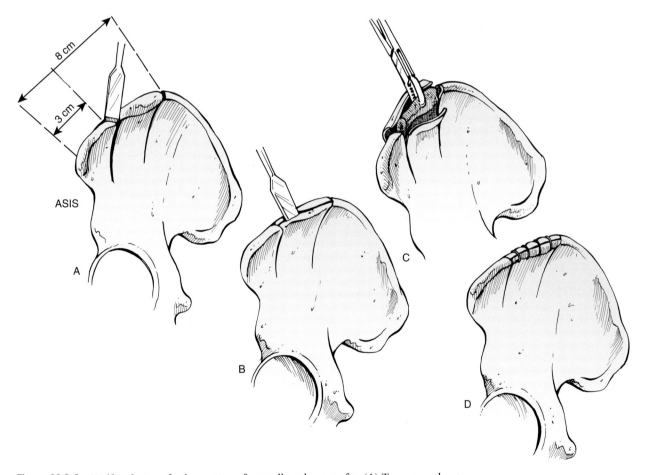

**Figure 33.2-2** Wolf technique for harvesting of cancellous bone grafts. (**A**) Two coronal cuts are made through the ilium. (**B**) Two oblique cuts are made, starting at the middle of the iliac crest. (**C**) Harvesting of the cancellous bone. (**D**) The inner and outer cortices of the iliac crest are fixed together with wires or sutures. ASIS, anterior superior iliac spine.

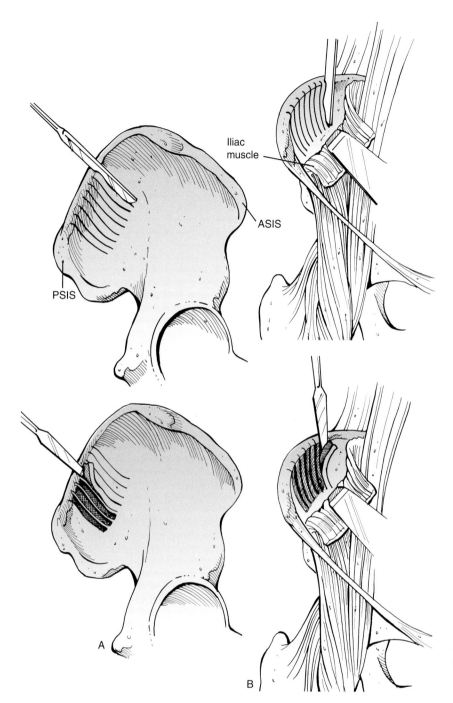

**Figure 33.2-3** Techniques for harvesting of corticocancellous bone grafts from the outer table of the posterior ilium (**A**) and from the inner table of the anterior ilium (**B**). ASIS, anterior superior iliac spine; PSIS, posterior superior iliac spine.

can be fashioned as tricortical blocks (cortices include the inner and outer iliac tables and the iliac crest) or as bicortical blocks or dowels (cortices include the inner and outer iliac tables only). Autografts used in nonloaded or tensile environments, such as the posterior and posterolateral (intertransverse process) spine, do not require cortical integrity. These grafts can be prepared as corticocancellous strips, morcellized fragments, or even particulate corticocancellous or cancellous-only bone.

*Cancellous bone grafts* contain a greater proportion of osteoconductive, osteoinductive, and osteogenic properties compared with the more mechanically supportive cortical

bone. Cancellous autograft initially has little structural integrity when placed on the fusion bed, until vascularization and interconnection of the graft fragments occur. Some osteoblasts and osteocytes of the graft survive and are capable of producing early bone. The porous nature of cancellous bone permits more rapid ingrowth of new blood vessels, which allow for the influx of osteoblast precursors. Bone formation and resorption usually occur concomitantly, with osteoblasts depositing bone on the surfaces of the preexisting trabeculae, whereas osteoclasts gradually resorb the dead trabeculae (creeping substitution). Eventually, all grafted cancellous tissue is resorbed and replaced by host

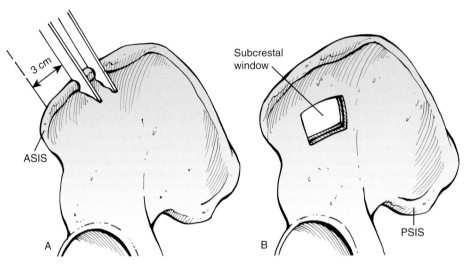

**Figure 33.2-4**  (**A**) Harvesting of a tricortical bone graft. (**B**) Subcrestal-window technique. ASIS, anterior superior iliac spine; PSIS, posterior superior iliac spine.

bone and marrow. As the spine is subjected to stress, it begins to remodel and form a mature fusion mass. This process typically is complete within 10 weeks in the rabbit model and within 6 to 12 months in humans.

*Cortical (strut) grafts* commonly are used in situations in which structural support is needed early. Structurally, they are dense, more compact than cancellous bone, and resistant to vascular ingrowth and remodeling. This structure slows the incorporation of the graft into the host spine. Cortical bone has less osteogenic potential, with fewer than 5% of cortical bone cells surviving transplantation. The blood vessels and cells of the host invade the cortical bone graft through preexisting haversian canal systems. At the peripheral margin of the cortical graft, intense osteoclastic tunneling and resorption occur to remove nonviable bone. Bone formation occurs only after resorption of dead lamellar bone. The graft ultimately loses about a third of its initial strength before consolidation begins. This resorptive phase can last for many months or years. Initially the cortical bone graft becomes incorporated in the spine only at its two vertebral body-graft interfaces. Cortical grafts almost never are remodeled completely and contain a combination of nonviable and living bone.

*Minced or morcellized cortical bone graft* does not have the same robust biologic activity as cancellous bone, although it may be helpful in extending the volume of graft material.

*Autogenous corticocancellous bone* is the most common graft material used for the fusion of spinal segments. The cancellous component of autograft contains greater osteogenic potential because of the large number of surviving cells in marrow, a trabecular environment favoring vascular ingrowth, and the accessibility of osteoinductive proteins. The cortical component contains greater mechanical strength and is useful for structural support.

*Free vascularized cortical grafts* of autogenous fibula, ribs, or iliac crest are preferred in situations in which avascular graft healing is poor, such as in areas of radiation-induced fibrosis or when radiation or chemotherapy or both are to be given preoperatively. The vascularized graft remains viable through its arterial supply and does not undergo significant cell necrosis. It unites directly with the host site without needing to be revascularized and replaced by creeping substitution. The graft is a ready source of osteogenic cells and precursors. Vascularized bone grafts are superior to nonvascularized bone grafts in terms of their osteogenic potential, vascularity, less resorption, good mechanical strength, and early bone union. After the initial 6 months, however, no difference in biomechanical strength is observed. The disadvantages of vascularized bone graft include donor site morbidity, increased surgical time, and a greater use of resources. The usefulness of a vascularized graft is determined by the extent to which the length of the soft tissue pedicle allows adaptation to the host site. Nonvascularized cortical grafts are less favorable, especially when the bridging defect is greater than 12 cm and in the treatment of stress-related fractures.

## Clinical Uses of Autograft in Spinal Fusions

Many published reports regarding the clinical and radiographic success of autografted spinal fusions have reported highly variable results. In addition to the influence of the type of autograft used, other variables that may affect a successful fusion outcome include:

- Location and type of fusion
- Stringency of fusion outcome criteria
- Patient selection
- Underlying pathology
- Use and type of internal fixation
- Preparation of the fusion bed
- Method of retrieval and preparation of the bone graft material

Differences in demographic data for specific disease conditions, follow-up periods, and rates of response complicate the comparison of published data on spinal fusion outcomes.

The regional differences of the spinal column seem to have a significant influence on the healing potential. The anterior or middle column of the spine is primarily cancellous bone with a larger surface area and experiences compressive mechanical loading. Load bearing and impaction of the graft early in the fusion process affords for stability and encourages early integration of the fusion mass. The posterior column of the spine has a greater combination of cortical bone, however, and a submuscular healing environment frequently under tensile stresses. The use of autograft in posterolateral lumbar fusion has been associated with the highest likelihood of failure (pseudarthrosis), ranging from 5% to 44%. Although the use of spinal instumentation has reduced this rate of nonunion in certain reports, the incidence still remains unacceptably high. Fusion rates using autograft in the posterior cervical and thoracic location are generally better compared with the posterolateral lumbar location. Posterior cervical fusions using iliac crest autograft have been successful in 88% to 100% of patients. Also, anterior cervical plate fixation combined with tricortical autograft produces fusion rates exceeding 97%. Autogenous tricortical iliac crest wedges and bicortical iliac dowels (used in anterior lumbar interbody fusion, used in revision surgery for pseudarthroses secondary to failed posterior fusion, and used to accompany posterior fusion surgery in patients who are at high risk for failure) are associated with favorable fusion rates but can undergo graft collapse; however, the presence of internal fixation lessens the likelihood of graft subsidence. Discectomy, decortication, and placement of the interbody graft are accomplished through anterior, laparoscopic, transperitoneal, or retroperitoneal approaches; posterior, interlaminar approaches; or far lateral, transforaminal approaches. The use of threaded interbody cages containing morcellized autograft has produced good fusion rates. Because of the morbidity associated with harvest of autogenous bone graft, the use of allograft and newer bone graft alternatives is becoming increasingly important in spinal fusion.

# ALLOGRAFT

By definition, allogeneic tissue is transplanted from one member of a species to another member of the same species or more commonly from one patient to another. Allograft bone products are the most common substitutes for autogenous bone grafts. Advantages of allografts include the following:

- Availability in virtually unlimited quantities
- Various formulations
- Avoidance of donor site morbidity associated with autograft

These materials are highly osteoconductive, weakly osteoinductive (if demineralized), and not osteogenic because the cells do not survive transplantation. For these reasons, concerns exist regarding the ability of allograft bone to produce a successful spinal fusion consistently. A decision to use allograft for spinal surgery depends on the underlying

disease condition, the region of spine where the graft is placed, the surgical goals, the types of graft available, the state of the host bed, and the preferences of the patient and surgeon.

Although allograft bone is versatile and used widely in spinal surgery, major concerns exist among surgeons and the public regarding the potential effects of different processing methods on allograft function and the risk of disease transmission. The principal pathogens involved are human immunodeficiency virus and hepatitis viruses B and C. The risk of disease transmission is determined by the rigor of screening procedures for donors and tissue; the only cases of disease transmission in musculoskeletal allografts from the method of graft preparation to date have involved frozen, unprocessed grafts. After meticulous screening of the sociomedical history of the donor and thorough laboratory testing, allograft bone is harvested under sterile conditions, usually within 24 hours of death, and is processed immediately thereafter.

Allografts are available as fresh, frozen, and freeze dried. The grafts are processed and preserved in ways that affect the osteoinductivity, osteoconductivity, and immunogenicity of the material. With fresh allografts, no preservation is required; this elicits an intense immune reaction and rejection, however, and it has a greater potential for disease transfer. Fresh allografts are not used in spinal fusion. Most allografts used are either frozen or freeze dried. Frozen allograft is maintained at a temperature of $-70°C$ and has a shelf life of 5 years. Deep frozen bone retains its material properties and can be implanted immediately after thawing. Freeze-drying significantly reduces the immunogenicity, alters the material properties of allograft cortical bone, and necessitates reconstitution (rehydration) of the graft before implantation. The mechanical strength of freeze-dried implants can be reduced by 50% compared with frozen grafts. The use of terminal gamma irradiation, gas, or ethylene oxide sterilization of allograft cortical bone may affect the biologic properties (osteoinduction) or biomechanical properties. Cancellous bone seems to be less affected by sterilization. Heating and autoclaving destroys the matrix proteins and is not commonly used.

## Allograft Incorporation

Allograft material is available as iliac bicortical and tricortical strips, patellar tricortical strips, cancellous cortical dowels, fibular struts, femoral cross sections, and ribs. Morcellated allograft rarely is used alone in spinal applications. When allograft is implanted, there is a programmed sequence of events at the site of the graft, including hemorrhage, inflammation, revascularization of the tissue, and creeping substitution and remodeling of the graft with locally derived tissue. Cancellous and structural grafts show significant differences in the histology of incorporation. Cancellous grafts show more rapid and complete revascularization than structural grafts. Cancellous bone remodels completely with time, whereas cortical bone remains a mixture of necrotic and viable bone. The process of creeping substitution also differs significantly between these forms of allograft, with new bone formation occurring appositionally followed by resorption in cancellous bone, whereas the process is reversed in cortical allografts. The most crucial factor in allograft incorporation is the host recipient bed because union occurs at the allograft-host junction. Other factors affecting allograft incorporation include the immune response and graft host stability. Allograft incorporation often is limited by fractures of the graft, infection, and nonunion. Structural allograft bone lacks the ability to remodel and depends on internal fixation devices for clinical function.

## Use of Allograft Bone in Spinal Fusion

An animal study comparing the use of allograft with autograft in anterior interbody and posterior spinal fusions in a dog model showed a slower fusion rate, greater graft resorption, and increased infection rate in the dogs in which allograft was used alone. This study has led many to use allograft as a graft extender rather than a graft substitute for autogenous bone. Although many animal studies have been done to evaluate allograft use in spinal applications, few well-controlled, prospectively designed clinical studies have been done. Allografts are used most successfully as structural grafts for anterior interbody fusions (cervical, anteroposterior lumbar). Morcellized allografts have not produced the same fusion rates for posterior laminar and transverse process fusion procedures as have structural allografts for the interbody applications. The larger surface area and the compressive forces in the intervertebral location may be the reason that allografts, being less osteoinductive, are more commonly successful for anterior fusions than for posterior fusions.

The clinical use of allograft with or without autograft for posterior lumbar fusion in adults has produced mixed results. An et al examined a prospective series of patients undergoing posterolateral lumbar fusion who were implanted with autograft alone, a mixture of autograft and freeze-dried allograft, fresh-frozen allograft alone, and freeze-dried allograft alone. These investigators observed that the sites implanted with autograft alone had the highest fusion rates, whereas the sites implanted with freeze-dried allograft alone had the lowest rates. Of grafts, 50% of the fresh-frozen grafts and 100% of the freeze-dried grafts had undergone complete resorption. In the anterior lumbar spine, cortical allografts (femoral rings) commonly are used for structural support in combination with autogenous bone graft, with pseudarthrosis being rare. When used in instrumented thoracic spinal fusions, the results are favorable.

The most favorable data for allograft use in human spinal fusion have been reported for interbody fusion in the cervical spine. Similar fusion rates to autogenous graft are presented for one-level fusion, but the union rate drastically decreases in multilevel fusion procedures. In 1976, Brown et al compared the use of frozen allograft with autograft and found that 32 patients treated with frozen allograft for single-level arthrodesis fused equally as well with an equal frequency of graft collapse as 29 patients implanted with autograft. They noticed a higher rate of graft collapse in multilevel fusions implanted with allograft. Zdeblick and Ducker observed a comparative fusion rate for freeze-dried tricortical allograft and autograft for Smith-Robinson-type cervical fusions in 87 patients undergoing single-level fusion. In patients undergoing two-level fusions, the rate de-

creased dramatically for allograft compared with autograft, and there was a higher incidence of graft subsidence.

The most suitable indication for nonstructural (morcellized) allografts seems to be in adolescent patients undergoing scoliosis correction and fusion. Allograft is successful in these patients for several reasons, as follows:

- Adolescent patients heal bone more easily.
- The posterior thoracic spine is mechanically stable, especially with fixation, and has large bone surface area for decortication that is a good source of blood supply and cells.

At present, the use of machine-threaded structural allograft bone dowels and allograft interbody cages harvested from midshaft of diaphyseal bone are gaining increasing popularity for anterior lumbar fusion because of their dual roles of bone graft material and fixation device. They allow for disc space distraction, placing the anulus under tension. The stretched anulus is desirable because it functions as a circumferential tension band, allowing impaction of the graft material. The threaded design allows fixation and prevents graft migration, and the hollow space (medullary canal) in the center of the graft permits inclusion of morcellized particles of autogenous bone from the iliac crest. Clinical outcome data using these allografts are limited. Femoral ring structural allografts have been used successfully in anterior lumbar interbody fusion. They maintain disc height and help correct deformity when combined with posterior instrumentation. Kozak et al reported a series of 45 patients with femoral ring allografts for anterior lumbar fusion with a 97% fusion rate based on flexion/extension films at 6- to 12-month follow-up. Aurori et al reported on 208 patients who underwent posterior spinal fusion for scoliosis with Harrington rod instrumentation. In this study, 114 patients were treated with iliac crest autograft, and 94 patients were treated with allograft. The investigators reported pseudarthrosis rates of 4.4% and 5.3%. The difference was not statistically different, but the amount of intraoperative blood loss and operating room time was increased significantly in patients who received autograft.

# DEMINERALIZED BONE MATRIX

DBM is a less immunogenic form of allograft bone that is produced by the acid decalcification of cortical bone. The osteoinductive capacity of DBM, initially shown by Urist, now has been well established. Clinically, DBM has been used with good results to augment autogenous bone grafts for fracture healing and tibial and femoral nonunions. The components of the bone matrix that remain behind after demineralization include:

- Noncollagenous proteins
- Bone osteoinductive growth factors, the most significant of which is bone morphogenetic protein
- Type I collagen

Bone morphogenetic proteins comprise only 0.1% by weight of all bone proteins and are abundant in diaphyseal cortical bone. The demineralization of bone allows these osteoinductive growth factors contained within the matrix to become locally accessible.

DBM provides no structural strength, and its primary use should be in a structurally stable environment. Although DBM primarily functions as an osteoinductive agent, the osteoconductivity also is important, and this can vary depending on its final configuration. The absolute amount of osteoinductive growth factors in DBM is extremely low. The source and processing of DBM have a direct effect on its osteoinductive capacity. Storage of bone at room temperature for more than 24 hours before processing, sterilization by ethylene oxide under certain conditions, and 2.5 mrad of gamma irradiation all substantially reduce osteoinductive and osteoconductive capacity of DBM.

## Incorporation of Demineralized Bone Matrix

Implantation of allogeneic DBM is followed by platelet aggregation, hematoma formation, and inflammation within 18 hours. Thereafter, fibroblast-like mesenchymal cells are attracted to and establish close contact with the implanted matrix. Interactions between DBM and mesenchymal cells result in cellular differentiation into chondrocytes around day 5 after implantation. Chondrocytes produce cartilage matrix, which is mineralized. By days 10 to 12, vascular invasion accompanied by osteoblastic cells is observed, multinuclear cells appear, and chondrocytes begin to degenerate. New bone is formed apposed to the surface of the mineralized cartilage. Remodeling and replacement of these composite structures with new host bone ensue. With time, all the implanted DBM is resorbed and replaced with host bone suitable for the environment in which it finds itself.

Different forms of DBM now are available for preclinical and clinical use, but their osteoinductivity is variable. Grafton DBM may be used intraoperatively to augment internal fixation or as an adjunct to other graft substitutes. The osteoinductive nature of Grafton has been shown in standard and more challenging animal models, and preclinical studies have shown positive performance when used alone and as an extender of autograft. Other bone-processing facilities also now are providing DBM composites using alternate carrier preparations. No clinical data are available for either of these materials.

## Animal Studies Using Demineralized Bone Matrix for Spinal Fusion

Many well-controlled studies in validated models of posterolateral spinal fusion have shown that certain formulations of DBM can function as viable bone graft alternatives (enhancer or extender). Experimental studies using DBM alone or in combination with autogenous bone marrow, autograft, or graft substitutes have reported spinal fusion rates comparable to autograft alone in rats, rabbits, and dogs. It also has been shown that DBM composites produce more rapid spinal fusion and stiffer fusion masses than autograft alone. Lindholm et al, in a rabbit model of posterior thoracic spinous process fusion, showed that DBM combined with bone marrow cells showed more rapid bone formation than DBM alone. The rates were identical in both test groups (86%) after 20 weeks. Morone and Boden, using a previ-

ously validated rabbit model of lumbar posterolateral intertransverse process arthrodesis, showed the efficacy of DBM gel (Osteotech, Eatontown, NJ) as an autograft extender. DBM gel did not increase the fusion rate when added to a standard amount of autograft. The addition of DBM gel to less than the standard amount of autograft (3:1 ratio) resulted, however, in fusion rates (70% and 60%) comparable to autograft alone. Other formulations of DBM have produced successful spinal fusions when used as standalone substitutes. Martin et al studied two new fiber-based formulations of Grafton DBM (Matrix DBM and putty DBM) in a rabbit posterolateral spinal fusion. These newer fiber-containing formulations showed better handling characteristics compared with DBM gel. When used as standalone graft substitutes, the putty and Matrix forms of grafton DBM also produced better fusion rates (83% and 100%) compared with the gel form (58%) and autograft (73%). They concluded that these two new formulations could function as graft extenders, graft enhancers, and potentially osteoconductive graft substitutes. The lower rate of fusion with DBM alone compared with autograft was even more pronounced when DBM was evaluated in the highly challenging nonhuman primate model of posterolateral lumbar intertransverse fusion. Grafton Matrix has exhibited the ability to improve healing when delivered with autograft bone in rhesus monkey posterolateral lumbar spinal fusions.

Bioceramics, such as biocoral and hydroxyapatite, have been used in comparison with and in combination with DBM in animal models of spinal fusion with varying results. Boden et al showed that DBM alone and biocoral alone produced lower fusion rates compared with autograft in a rabbit posterolateral fusion model. The addition of bovine-derived bone growth factor extract to DBM, to autograft, and to natural coral resulted in 100% fusion, however, with increase in fusion stiffness. Also, Ragni et al showed that porous hydroxyapatite blocks alone or in combination with DBM had similar radiographic fusion scores to autograft alone or autograft with DBM and bone marrow at 2 months. The variable efficacy of DBM in animal spine studies probably stems from a combination of problems with the models used and variability in the preparation of the DBM. The combination of growth factors with suitable osteoinductive and osteoconductive carriers, such as DBM, seems to be an especially potent promoter of spinal fusion in lower and higher order animals. Although the results in animal studies are encouraging, care must be taken when extrapolating results from small animal models to humans because of the increased difficulty of initiating osteoinduction in primates.

Although several preclinical studies using animal models have been performed, prospective clinical outcome data related to the use of DBM are lacking. There are a few retrospective clinical studies in which reported results show potential benefit with DBM (Grafton) in posterolateral lumbar fusions. Sassard et al retrospectively reviewed patients who underwent instrumented posterolateral lumbar spinal fusion with local bone graft and Grafton gel and compared them with an age-matched, gender-matched, and procedure-matched group of patients undergoing instrumented fusions with autograft. Using a bone mineralization rating scale, they did not find radiographic differences between the groups based on films taken 3, 6, 12, and 24 months after surgery. The fusion rates in the autograft with Grafton group and the autograft-only group were only 60% and 56% less than has been reported in other studies of instrumented posterior fusion. Based largely on preclinical data, it is speculated that these processed DBM products may be efficacious as bone graft extenders but not as bone graft substitutes for posterior spinal fusion procedures.

## SUGGESTED READING

An HS, Simpson JM, Glover JM, Stephany J. Comparison between allograft plus demineralized bone matrix versus autograft in anterior cervical fusion: a prospective multicenter study. Spine 1995;20: 2211–2216.

Boden SD, Schimandle JH, Hutton WC. 1995 Volvo Award in Basic Sciences. The use of an osteoinductive growth factor for lumbar spinal fusion: Part II. study of dose, carrier, and species. Spine 1995;20:2633–2644.

Lindholm TS, Urist MR. A quantitative analysis of new bone formation by induction in composite grafts of bone marrow and bone matrix. Clin Orthop 1980;288–300.

Martin G, Boden SD, Morone MA, Titus L. New formulations of demineralized bone matrix as a more effective graft alternative in experimental posterolateral lumbar spine arthrodesis. Spine 1999;24: 637–645.

Ragni P, Lindholm S. Interaction of allogeneic demineralized bone matrix and porous hydroxyapatite bioceramics in lumbar interbody fusion in rabbits. Clin Orthop 1991;272:292–299.

Zdeblick T, Ducker T. The use of freeze-dried allograft bone for anterior cervical fusions. Spine 1991;16:729.

# 33.3 BONE GRAFT SUBSTITUTES

## JOHN LOUIS-UGBO ■ SCOTT D. BODEN

## CELL-BASED SUBSTITUTES

Cell-based therapies for regeneration of bone comprise cells with osteogenic potential being transferred directly to the site requiring augmentation. Cell-based approaches do not depend on the host local osteoprogenitors; they are particularly attractive for patients in whom the host tissue bed has been compromised by irradiation, chemotherapy, severe trauma, tobacco use, osteoporosis, and metabolic derangements. So far, four different cell types have been used for bone regeneration, as follows:

- Unfractionated bone marrow
- Purified, cultured expanded mesenchymal stem cells (MSCs)
- Differentiated osteoblasts and chondrocytes
- Genetically modified cells that express bone morphogenetic protein (BMP)

To date, only bone marrow combined with osteoconductive or osteoinductive composites has received appreciable attention in its application in the augmentation of spinal fusion.

### Bone Marrow Use in Spinal Fusion

Bone marrow contains osteoprogenitor cells and has been used clinically as an adjunct to some graft materials for spinal fusion. The original observations of Goujon led to the initial interest in the osteogenic capabilities of bone marrow. The ability of bone marrow graft to perform its function as a graft depends on the presence of MSCs. The number of the stem cells in the marrow is limited. Marrow contains stem cells on the order of 1 per 50,000 nucleated

cells in young individuals and 1 per 2 million in the elderly. Stem cell concentration techniques, including centrifugation and ex vivo cell culture, can increase their number fivefold.

Autologous marrow is harvested from the posterior wing of the ilium in aliquots of 2 mL to reach total volumes of 5 to 10 mL and injected directly into the fusion site. Transplanted bone marrow tends to diffuse away from fusion site when used alone for augmentation. To prevent this diffusion, advances have been made in the delivery of the marrow. The marrow may be supplemented with a carrier, such as allograft, demineralized bone matrix, collagen, or ceramic, to stimulate bone healing. Bone formed by marrow graft has the same biomechanical properties as cancellous bone graft. The first clinical experience with the use of marrow cells in humans to stimulate fracture repair was reported in a 31-year-old patient with an infected nonunion of the tibia by Connolly and Shindell in 1986. Preclinical investigations and a few clinical studies have confirmed the efficacy of bone marrow as a graft substitute. Bone marrow in spinal fusion often is used clinically in combination with autograft and allograft bone or in composites of ceramic or other bone extenders. The use of bone marrow as a stand-alone material in spinal fusion or with ceramics has produced variable results. Also, Boden et al, in a posterolateral fusion model, observed no fusions when using bone marrow as a stand-alone graft substitute or in combination with coralline hydroxyapatite.

Some setbacks to the widespread application of bone marrow in bone healing include the following:

- Added morbidity of bone marrow harvest
- Difficulty in obtaining enough bone marrow with the requisite number of osteoprogenitor cells

- Aging or disease that is accompanied by a reduction in healthy bone marrow cells, especially the osteogenic precursors, which represent approximately 0.001% of the nucleated cells in healthy adult marrow

Techniques capable of selecting, expanding, and administering the progenitor cell fraction would be of great clinical benefit.

## Mesenchymal Stem Cell Use in Spinal Fusion

MSCs are known to have the capacity for extensive replication and can differentiate into several tissue types, including bone, cartilage, tendon, muscle, fat, and marrow stroma. Several investigators have described techniques for the isolation of adult human and animal MSCs from bone marrow and periosteum. Isolation of MSCs generally is done through density gradient centrifugation and cell culturing techniques. Using culture systems, MSCs from a small marrow aspirate can be expanded in number more than 1 billion-fold. This remarkable expansion makes MSCs a clinically useful source of osteoprogenitor cells for fusion procedures. Cui et al examined the effects of a cloned osteoprogenitor cell, D1-BAG, which was cloned from Balb/c mouse bone marrow stroma and transduced with a traceable gene encoding β-galactosidase, and mixed marrow stromal cells from marrow blowouts in posterior spinal fusion in athymic rats. The cloned cells showed an earlier osteogenic process with a larger amount of bone formation than mixed stromal cells. Successful spinal fusion at 6 and 9 weeks was observed in eight of eight (100%) animals receiving DI-BAG cells, four of eight (50%) in mixed marrow stromal cells, and none of eight (0%) in control animals. The investigators also noted that osteogenesis with D1-BAG cells occurred without a cartilaginous phase, in contrast to the process of endochondral ossification that was seen with mixed marrow cells. They concluded that cloned osteoprogenitor cells may serve as a substitute for bone autograft.

# BIOSYNTHETIC GRAFT MATERIALS

## Ceramics

Ceramic matrices include inorganic, ionically bonded preparations that mimic the mineral phase of bone. Biosynthetic ceramics have been used solely as osteoconductive bone graft substitutes. The calcium phosphates, particularly hydroxyapatite (HA) and tricalcium phosphate (TCP), or a combination of the two, are the most commonly used ceramics in orthopaedic surgery. As osteoconductive materials, HA and TCP tend to function best as bone graft extenders or carriers for an osteoinductive bone growth factor rather than as stand-alone bone graft substitutes in nonstructural clinical applications.

Advantages of ceramics include the following:

- They are biodegradable.
- They are biocompatible.
- They have little or no risk for disease transmission.
- They are available in unlimited quantities.

- They have no added risk of donor site complications that accompany the use of autograft.

Optimal remodeling of the fusion mass depends on the biodegradability of the ceramic. The various calcium phosphate composites differ with regard to their bioresorbability properties. A nonresorbable graft material may hinder remodeling, prolong the strength deficiency of new bone, and leave permanent stress risers in the fusion mass.

Disadvantages of ceramic use include the following:

- They are brittle and have little tensile strength and must be shielded until bone ingrowth has occurred.
- Persistent dense radiographic imagery makes it difficult to evaluate bone incorporation in the clinical setting.
- The unnatural pathways that are characteristic of intact ceramic matrices do not favor the normal process of bone ingrowth and remodeling that occurs after bone transplants.

Ceramics are produced commercially as porous implants, nonporous dense implants, or granular particles with pores. The optimal osteoconductive pore size for ceramics seems to be between 150 and 500 μm. The chemical composition, porosity, and surface area of the ceramic affects its rate of bioresorption. The larger the surface area, the greater the resorption; also a greater porosity enhances interface activity and bone ingrowth. The material density of the matrix and porosity of the ceramic could result in greater mechanical strength and resistance to degradation and promote long-lasting stability. TCP undergoes biologic resorption 10 to 20 times faster than HA. Within the body, TCP is converted partially to HA, which is degraded more slowly because the foreign body giant cell that specifically resorbs HA stops after resorbing 2 to 10 μm of HA. Large amounts of HA may remain in the body for more than 10 years.

Natural ceramic derived from sea coral has better interconnective porosity, is composed of 97% calcium carbonate in the form of aragonite, and is structurally similar to cancellous bone. Coral is extremely biocompatible. It has yielded promising results when used to replace or augment autogenous bone graft or as part of a composite with an osteoinductive protein. An alternative formulation is coralline HA, which converts much of the calcium carbonate to HA. Calcium sulfate (plaster of Paris) also has been used as a synthetic graft material in bone voids, although with limited documented success in posterolateral spine fusion.

### Integration of Ceramics

Immediately after implantation of coralline implants, fibrovascular tissue begins to invade the porosity. Typically a blood clot initially forms in the porosity. The blood clot must resolve to allow regenerating tissues to proliferate. This process takes 3 weeks for most implants with clinically relevant sizes, averaging about 2 to 3 mm/wk. Macrophages may play a significant role in this early stage of fibrovascular ingrowth; however, inflammatory cells are rare or only transiently evident. Ceramic implants are osteoconductive when they are placed next to bone. Bone grows into the implants only if the implant is in direct apposition to bone, the tissue of the host bed is conducive to bone formation, and the interface between bone and implant are stable. Bone formation within the implant initially occurs directly against the surface of the implant. Rarely are chondroblasts seen within the porosity. This process is more akin to membranous bone formation than to osteochondral bone formation. After osseous ingrowth, the mechanical properties of coralline implants are improved significantly as a result of the overlay of host bone.

## Animal Studies

Numerous animal studies have shown conflicting results regarding the ability of these synthetic biomaterials alone and in conjunction with demineralized bone matrix, extracted osteoinductive growth factors, and osteogenic bone marrow to heal osseous defects and spinal fusions Anterior interbody fusion in the thoracic spine of dogs was analyzed by Emery et al using tricortical iliac crest autograft, HA ceramic, calcium carbonate, and a composite of HA and TCP (60%/40%). All fusions were performed using spinal instrumentation. Autograft was the most effective graft material in this study, despite the use of internal fixation with calcium carbonate ceramic. While comparing the efficacy of 50/50 HA/TCP ceramic composites of varying porosity (30%, 50%, and 70% porosity) and autograft in a goat anterior cervical spine fusion model, Toth et al showed that the ceramic implants performed equal to or better than autograft iliac crest bone. The more porous implants had a higher union rate early on, but also had a higher incidence of graft fracture. Overall fusion rates were 67% for the ceramic implants and 50% for autograft. The goats used in this study had excessive head movement after surgery, and these low fusion rates put into question the ability of this model to be extrapolated to human anterior cervical fusions.

In the posterolateral lumbar environment, HA/calcium carbonate ceramic derived from coral was used in combination with platelet-rich plasma concentrate (growth factor gel) in a spinal fusion model in sheep. The results indicated increased osteoblastic activity deep in the graft. In a previously validated rabbit model, Boden et al evaluated the efficacy of coralline HA as a bone graft substitute for lumbar spine fusion when used with bone marrow, autogenous bone graft, or an osteoinductive bone protein extract. They observed that coralline HA with bone marrow could not function as a stand-alone graft substitute. When combined in a 1:1 ratio with autogenous iliac crest bone graft, coralline HA functioned as a graft extender. Also, coralline HA served as an excellent carrier for a bovine-derived osteoinductive growth factor extract with its bovine collagen composite functioning as a complete bone graft substitute in the posterolateral spine. These results were substantiated further by Baramki et al in a sheep lumbar spinal arthrodesis model. Other authors have found similar results in fusion rate when comparing different ceramics in spinal fusion.

Composites of HA/TCP proved to be a suitable carrier for rhBMP-2 in the posterolateral spinal fusion model in rhesus monkeys. Even in the presence of a laminectomy defect, there was no evidence of bone induction outside the confines of the ceramic carrier. The ability of different ceramic composites to induce spinal arthrodesis has been compared with that of autograft alone in a rabbit interbody fusion, in a sheep posterior spinal fusion, and in a dog poste-

rior spinal fusion, with varying results. Bozic et al showed a dose-dependent electrical stimulation enhancement of posterolateral spinal fusion in rabbits using HA/bone marrow aspirate.

## Human Trials

Many clinical studies have been published reporting the benefits of ceramics in spinal fusions for patients with scoliosis. Passuti et al advocated the use of ceramics as extenders for autogenous bone graft for long segment fusions in corrective deformity surgery. They used blocks of HA/TCP with or without autogenous bone graft for facet joint fusions in 12 adolescent patients with severe scoliosis who underwent internal fixation and fusion. All patients were followed clinically and radiographically for an average of 15 months postoperatively. Passuti's series achieved 100% fusion, with biopsy specimens from two patients showing histologic bony ingrowth into the pores of the ceramic. Delecrin et al, in a prospective randomized study, assessed the clinical and radiologic efficacy of a synthetic ceramic in scoliosis surgery. Fifty-eight patients with idiopathic scoliosis underwent posterior arthrodesis using autograft bone alone or in combination with porous biphasic HA/TCP composite. Radiographic incorporation of ceramic was evident in 12 months.

The best human clinical experience with ceramic materials in spinal fusion exists for anterior interbody fusion of the cervical spine. Successful fusion rates in the anterior and posterior cervical spine approach 100% in most series reported. The ultimate role of ceramic implants in spinal fusion procedures remains to be defined. Calcium phosphate biomaterials with appropriate three-dimensional geometry are able to bind and concentrate endogenous BMPs in circulation, may become osteoinductive (capable of osteogenesis), and can be effective carriers of bone cell seeds.

## Composite Grafts

No single bone substitute provides all the essential features of osteogenesis, osteoinduction, and osteoconduction as autogenous bone graft can. Composite grafts incorporate all the favorable properties of the various materials and have been used with success clinically in spinal fusion procedures. Ceramic composites consist of osteoconductive ceramic combined with an osteoinductive agent, such as demineralized bone matrix, autograft bone, extracted bone matrix proteins, or rhBMP-2. The ceramic implant maintains soft tissue position and provides an osteoconductive matrix, and the proteins stimulate osteoinduction. Composite grafts offer potential for the design of bone graft substitutes that are specific for the structural and biologic demands of the host, and it is likely that different composites would be used for anterior interbody arthrodesis than for long-instrumented posterior fusion.

Collargraft (Zimmer, Warsaw, IN; Collagen Corporation, Palo Alto, CA) is a commercially synthesized composite of suspended, deantigenated bovine fibrillar collagen and porous calcium phosphate ceramic (65% HA and 35% TCP). The composite is not osteoinductive; however, the addition of autogenous bone marrow provides osteoprogenitor stem cells and a limited amount of growth factors. Collargraft currently is available in paste form or as soft strips. Collargraft can deliver antibiotics and antineoplastic agents locally to treat bone disorders. It lacks structural integrity, however, and as a result tends to migrate to ectopic sites if adequate hemostasis is not maintained. Cornell et al compared Collargraft plus autogenous marrow versus cancellous iliac bone grafts in acute long bone fractures and found no significant functional or radiographic differences. Animal studies have documented various healing properties of composite grafts.

The use of Collargraft in animal spinal fusion has produced unconvincing results. Walsh et al showed that the use of Collargraft composite as a bone graft substitute or expander for autologous bone graft in a posterolateral spinal fusion model in sheep produced robust fusion masses, with greater mineral densities compared with the use of autogenous bone graft alone. Both study groups had similar mechanical properties, however. The use of Collargraft or Collargraft prototypes in previous preclinical spinal fusion studies resulted in mixed outcomes.

Ceramic composites, which consist of the osteoconductive ceramic combined with an osteoinductive agent such as demineralized bone matrix, bone marrow, extracted bone matrix proteins, or osteogenic growth factors such as recombinant BMP, have been investigated. Boden et al used a nonhuman primate lumbar intertransverse process arthrodesis model to evaluate rhBMP-2 in an HA/TCP carrier as a composite bone graft substitute. Twenty-one adult rhesus monkeys underwent a laminectomy and fusion with either autogenous iliac crest bone or 60/40 HA/TCP blocks saturated with a solution containing 0, 6, 9, or 12 mg of rhBMP-2. Fusion was not achieved in any of the monkeys treated with autogenous iliac crest bone graft. The monkeys treated with the HA/TCP blocks with rhBMP-2 achieved complete fusion. When the ceramic blocks were loaded with rhBMP-2, there was a dose-dependent increase in the amount and quality of bone throughout the ceramic carrier based on qualitative assessment. The HA/TCP composite proved to be a suitable carrier for rhBMP-2 in this posterolateral spinal fusion model in rhesus monkeys. Even in the presence of a laminectomy defect, there was no evidence of bone induction outside the confines of the ceramic carrier.

Fischgrund et al evaluated the use of rhBMP-2 with various types of carrier media and the effect of rhBMP-2 as an adjunct to autogenous iliac crest bone graft in a dog spinal fusion model. All fusion sites were assigned randomly to one of six fusion methods: autogenous bone graft (ABG) alone, ABG + rhBMP-2, ABG + collagen (Helistat) "sandwich" + rhBMP-2, ABG + collagen (Helistat) morsels + rhBMP-2, ABG + polylactic/glycolic acid sponge sandwich + rhBMP-2, and ABG + open-pore polylactic acid morsels + rhBMP-2. The results indicated that the addition of rhBMP-2 significantly increased bone graft volume on computed tomography scan, but no significant difference in carrier media for rhBMP-2 could be determined. Polylactic/

glycolic acid sites were associated with a greater incidence of voids within the fusion mass. Muschler et al studied the fusions in a dog posterior spinal fusion model using autograft, collagen/ceramic composite, collagen/ceramic/autograft composite, and no graft material. Autograft bone alone was the most effective graft material tested and had a statistically superior union score. Ceramic composites when used alone produced fusions equivalent to when no graft materials were used. The addition of demineralized bone protein extract to the composite significantly improved the union score, however, which was comparable to that obtained using composite plus autograft bone.

Boden et al compared efficacy of fusion using coralline HA alone or with bone marrow, autogenous bone graft, or 500 μg of bovine-derived osteoinductive bone protein extract for single-level posterolateral lumbar spinal fusions in a rabbit fusion model. Coralline HA alone or with bone marrow produced no solid fusions. When combined with an equal amount of autogenous iliac crest bone, fusion appeared in 50%. When combined with the osteoinductive growth factor extract, the coralline HA resulted in stronger and stiffer solid fusion in 100%. These data indicated that coralline HA with bone marrow was not an acceptable bone graft substitute for posterolateral spinal fusion in this model. When combined with autogenous iliac crest bone graft, coralline HA served as a graft extender, yielding results comparable to those obtained with autograft alone. Coralline HA served as an excellent carrier for the bovine osteoinductive bone protein extract, yielding superior results to those obtained with autograft or bone marrow.

# SUGGESTED READING

Baramki HG, Steffen T, Lander P, et al. The efficacy of interconnected porous hydroxyapatite in achieving posterolateral lumbar fusion in sheep. Spine 2000;25:1053–1060.

Boden SD. Spine 1999;24:1179–1185.

Connolly JF, Shindell R. Percutaneous marrow injection for an ununited tibia. Nebr Med J 1986;71:105–107.

Cui. Spine 2001;26:2305–2310.

Delecrin J, Takahashi S, Gouin F, Passuti N. A synthetic porous ceramic as a bone graft substitute in the surgical management of scoliosis: a prospective, randomized study. Spine 2000;25:563–569.

Emery SE, Fuller DA, Stevenson S. Ceramic anterior spinal fusion: biologic and biomechanical comparison in a canine model. Spine 1996;22:2713–2719.

Fischgrund JS, James SB, Chabot MC, et al. Augmentation of autograft using rhBMP-2 and different carrier media in the canine spinal fusion model. J Spinal Disord 1997 Dec;10(6):467–472.

Lynch KL, Ladwig DA, Skrade DA, Flatley TJ. Evaluation of collagen/ceramic bone graft substitutes in dogs with spinal fusion. Trans Soc Biomater 1990;13:196.

Muschler GF, Negami S, Hyodo A, et al. Evaluation of collagen ceramic composite graft materials in a spinal fusion model. Clin Orthop 1996;250–260.

Walsh WR, Loefler A, Arm DM. Growth factor gel and a resorbable porous ceramic for use in spinal fusion. Trans Orthop Res Soc 1999;24:270.

# 33.4 GROWTH FACTORS AND GENE THERAPY IN SPINAL FUSION

**JOHN LOUIS-UGBO ■ SCOTT D. BODEN**

## OSTEOINDUCTIVE GROWTH FACTORS

Bone healing involves a complex interaction of many local autocrine and systemic regulatory factors. These factors trigger undifferentiated mesenchymal cells to migrate, proliferate, and differentiate into bone-forming cells. The transplanted autogenous bone matrix and the hematoma formed after decortication of the spine provides a pool of these growth factors that mediate osteoinduction. The transforming growth factor (TGF)-β superfamily of polypeptide growth (including TGF-β1 through TGF-β5, bone morphogenetic proteins [BMPs] 2 through 9, and growth and differentiation factors [GDFs]) constitute the most important growth factors implicated in fracture healing. Other growth factors present in the callus during the fracture healing process include fibroblast growth factor, platelet-derived growth factor, and insulin-like growth factor (IGF). TGF-β and other growth factors are released by platelets and osteoprogenitor cells. These proteins are thought to stimulate cellular proliferation and differentiation of osteoblasts and to direct bone matrix formation.

## Functions of Growth Factors

TGF-β seems to have some synergistic and antagonistic effects with BMPs; however, it is unable to initiate the entire osteoinduction cascade by itself and form ectopic bone, a property uniquely exhibited by some of the BMPs. The BMPs have a myriad of functions ranging from extracellular and skeletal organogenesis to bone regeneration. Fibroblast growth factors are mitogenic and angiogenic factors that are important in neovascularization and wound healing. Platelet-derived growth factors function as local tissue growth regulators that initially were isolated from blood platelets, underscoring one of the important roles of the clot in fracture healing. IGFs are other examples of matrix-synthesizing growth factors that are important in bone healing (see Tables 33.2-2 and 33.2-3).

## Bone Morphogenetic Proteins

The BMPs comprise a family of at least 15 structurally related, low-molecular-weight noncollagenous glycoproteins. Wozney et al, using molecular cloning, identified the specific molecules, of which all but one (BMP-1) belong to an expanding TGF-β superfamily of GDFs. There are three subclasses of BMPs based on amino acid sequences found in osteoinductive extracts of bone:

- Subgroup 1 (human BMP-2, BMP-4, and *Drosophila* [fruit fly] decapentaplegic [dpp])
- Subgroup 2 (human BMP-5, BMP-6, BMP-7 [osteogenic protein-1])
- Subgroup 3 (BMP-8, and *Drosophila* 60A)

Human BMP-3 (osteogenin) is less related. Presently, single BMPs are available through recombinant gene technology, and mixtures of BMPs are available as purified bone extracts for basic science research and clinical trials. Heterodimeric BMP-2/BMP-7 has been shown to be more potent than homodimers in induction of osteoblast differentiation.

### Mechanism of Action of Bone Morphogenetic Proteins (Osteoinductive Properties)

The BMPs play an important role in embryonic endochondral and intramembranous bone formation, and they are thought to promote the normal healing process after fractures. BMPs are known to bind to specific receptors on a variety of different cell types, including mesenchymal stem cells, osteoblasts, and osteoclasts. These receptors subsequently activate second messenger systems within the cytoplasm, which affect the expression of BMP response genes in the nucleus. Within the cell, a set of small signal modulating molecules called *SMADs* further modulates the BMP signal (see Table 33.1-6). These secondary messengers compose a family of small signal transducing molecules within the intracellular domain that can be either negative or positive modulators of a BMP signal. Subsequently, BMP receptor stimulation leads, directly or indirectly, to cellular chemotaxis, proliferation, and differentiation. With lower concentrations, BMPs promote the differentiation of mesenchymal stem cells into chondrocytes, which lay down a cartilaginous matrix. This matrix then calcifies, is invaded by blood vessels, and remodels into mature bone, a process termed *endochondral bone formation*. At higher concentrations, BMPs can induce direct bone formation, recapitulating normal intramembranous bone formation.

### Delivery Systems for Bone Morphogenetic Proteins

There are currently three strategies for delivery of osteoinductive growth factors, as follows:

- Use of extracted and partially purified mixture of proteins that include BMPs from animal or human cortical bone, popularized by Urist et al
- Use of recombinant human BMPs (rhBMPs), which was

## TABLE 33.4-1 PROPERTIES OF AN IDEAL GROWTH FACTOR CARRIER

Ability to retain and release the BMP in a controlled fashion

Biocompatibility

Should not interfere with normal bone healing

Biomechanically strong (not squeezed easily at fusion site)

User friendly

Easy to manufacture

Should act as a three-dimensional space occupier

Act as scaffolding across which de novo bone formation can occur

Retain the BMP at the site of application to prevent extraneous bone formation

Resorption timing of the carrier also is important to match the anticipated speed of osteoinduction

Ability to detect osteoinduction via plain radiographs

enabled by the cloning and sequencing of many of the BMP genes

▪ Use of gene therapy, which involves delivery of the DNA encoding a growth factor rather than delivery of the protein itself

The properties of an ideal growth factor carrier are listed in Table 33.4-1.

### Purified Bone Morphogenetic Proteins in Spinal Fusions

Human BMP extracts prepared on a limited basis in the laboratory of Urist and a commercially available extract of bovine BMP mixture known as NeOsteo (Centerpulse Biologics, Austin, TX) have been used in the treatment of nonunions and spinal fusion. The bovine extract has shown successful osteoinduction in ectopic locations in rats and nonhuman primates. Also, it has been used as a bone graft substitute for segmental defect repair in dogs and posterolateral spinal fusion in rabbits and nonhuman primates. The growth factor has been used with hydroxyapatite, calcium carbonate, and demineralized bone matrix carriers. Preliminary human clinical trials currently are under way.

Boden et al showed the efficacy of highly purified bovine BMP in rabbit and nonhuman primate intertransverse process fusion models. They found a dose-dependent response in the rabbit model, which indicated that a concentration threshold must be overcome before BMP can induce bone formation effectively. In similar experiments with rhesus monkeys, effective spinal fusion was achieved with purified BMP in 18 weeks. These experiments highlighted the need for higher doses of BMP in primates compared with doses needed for rodents. Also, the healing time required for primates was significantly longer (18 to 24 weeks). Lovell et al, using polylactic acid polymer as carrier in a dog posterior intervertebral fusion model, reported on the improvement of spinal fusion success rate and fusion mass when partially purified BMP was used. The fusion rate was 71% in levels with BMP compared with 17% in control levels.

### Recombinant Bone Morphogenetic Proteins in Spinal Fusions

RhBMP-2 (Genetics Institute, Cambridge, MA, and Medtronic Sofamor Danek, Memphis, TN) has been used extensively for in vitro and in vivo safety and efficacy studies. Extensive data show that this growth factor is a morphogen, not a mitogen, and induces cells to differentiate and form endochondral bone in ectopic and heterotopic locations. Several preclinical studies have shown that rhBMP-2 is successful in repair of segmental long bone defects in rats, dogs, and sheep and in posterolateral spinal fusion in rabbits, dogs, and nonhuman primates. There is adequate evidence that rhBMP-2 and rhBMP-7 (Creative Biomolecules, Hopkinton, MA) when used in pharmacologic doses in various animal models are efficacious and superior to autogenous grafts in achieving spinal fusion. BMP-4, BMP-6, BMP-9, and, to a lesser extent BMP-5, also have been shown to induce new bone formation.

### Animal Studies

In a study on the efficacy of rhBMP-7 (OP-1; Stryker Biotech, Hopkinton, MA) in a mongrel dog posterior spinal fusion model, Cook et al observed that rhBMP-7 could induce stable fusion formation 6 weeks after implantation, and this often led to complete fusions by 12 weeks. This was significantly faster than autograft alone, which did not fuse until 24 weeks after implantation. Muschler et al also reported the effectiveness of rhBMP-2 with a biodegradable carrier in a beagle posterior spinal fusion model. They compared rhBMP-2 with a PLGA carrier, autograft bone alone, and polylactic glycolic acid (PLGA) carrier alone. At 12 weeks, they found the union score and biomechanical strength of the fusion mass was equivalent between rhBMP-2 + PLGA and autograft bone. Additionally, both were superior to PLGA alone. Schimandle et al evaluated rhBMP-2 in a rabbit intertransverse process fusion model. They found that rhBMP-2, delivered either with a collagen carrier or with autograft bone, was superior to autograft bone alone in producing spinal fusion. rhBMP-2 with autologous iliac crest bone resulted in 100% fusion compared with 42% fusion with autologous bone alone. rhBMP-2 also produced more mature bone formation that was biomechanically superior to that formed with autologous bone alone at 4 to 5 weeks.

**Morphology of Fusion Mass.** Holliger et al studied the difference in morphologic features of the fusion mass between rhBMP versus autograft material in rabbit intertransverse process fusion with computed tomography (CT). They showed that fusion masses derived from rhBMP-2 had higher volume and better attachment to the transverse process than with autologous bone alone. They also showed that the weak point of the fusion mass was distributed more randomly with rhBMP-2 than at the attachment site to the transverse process, which happened 11 of 12 times for autograft. Sandhu et al, in a dog posterior spinal fusion, found that the crucial element was the dose of BMP, and it was unrelated to whether there was decortication of the fusion model.

## Carrier Media

Several animal studies evaluating the efficacy of various carrier molecules have been done. Inorganic carriers of BMP that have shown efficacy in promoting spinal arthrodesis include true bone ceramic derived from sintered bovine bone and hydroxyapatite/tricalcium phosphate. Organic carriers include polylactic acid polymers, collagen and noncollagenous protein carriers, mineralized or demineralized bone matrix, and autograft. Fischgrund et al evaluated the use of rhBMP-2 with various types of carrier materials and the effect of rhBMP-2 as an adjunct to autogenous iliac crest bone graft in a dog lumbar intertransverse process fusion model. No significant difference between carriers for rhBMP-2 could be determined; however, PLGA acid carrier sites were associated with a greater incidence of voids within the fusion mass. rhBMP-2, when added to autograft, significantly increased the volume and the maturity of the resulting fusion mass. Sheehan et al also showed that a composite of rhBMP-2, autogenous bone, and collagen produced biomechanically stiffer and larger fusion masses than either autograft or collagen alone.

**Dose Response Studies.**    Sandhu et al evaluated the effect of rhBMP-2 in an adult beagle posterolateral fusion model. They found that 2300 µg of rhBMP in an open cell polylactic acid polymer was superior to autograft iliac crest bone graft in achieving a single-level lumbar intertransverse process fusion. The same investigators showed in a later study that the effect of increasing BMP dose produced less dramatic enhancement. In this experiment, rhBMP-2 was implanted in multiple doses (58, 115, 230, 460, and 920 µg). All specimens with BMP were fused solidly by 3 months. There was no significant difference in biomechanical, radiographic, or histologic characteristics of the quality of intertransverse process fusion from the 58-µg to 2300-µg doses, almost a 40-fold difference. In a similar study on the dose response in a nonhuman primate model of intertransverse process spinal fusion, Boden et al observed a dose-dependent increase in the amount and quality of bone throughout the ceramic carrier based on qualitative assessment. They used a 60% hydroxyapatite/40% tricalcium phosphate ceramic block with multiple doses of rhBMP-2 (0, 6, 9, or 12 mg per side). All monkeys treated with rhBMP-2 achieved fusion.

**Anterior Interbody Fusions.**    Anterior interbody fusion using rhBMP-2 also has been investigated. In a sheep anterior lumbar interbody fusion model, Sandhu et al showed 100% intervertebral osseous union using an implanted cylindrical and threaded titanium interbody fusion device containing rhBMP2. Only 33% of the control animals implanted with the fusion cage containing autograft alone achieved fusion. Boden et al studied two doses in an anterior lumbar interbody fusion in a nonhuman primate model. They showed that successful fusion could be done using laparoscopic techniques with titanium-threaded cages and collagen soaked in rhBMP-2. The bovine-derived absorbable collagen sponges were soaked in either 750 µg/mL or 1500 µg/mL of rhBMP-2. The fusions were evaluated with plain radiographs, CT scans, manual palpation, and histo-logic analysis. Solid spinal fusion occurred with both doses of rhBMP-2; however, the higher dose led to a more rapid fusion. This study was particularly important because higher species, such as nonhuman primates, historically have lower fusion rates.

Hecht et al reported on the efficacy of rhBMP-2-soaked collagen sponge with allograft dowel in rhesus macaque anterior lumbar interbody fusion at the lumbosacral junction (L7-S1). They used one freeze-dried smooth cortical dowel allograft cylinder filled with autograft bone (control) or filled with an absorbable collagen sponge soaked with rhBMP-2. The three monkeys with rhBMP-2 showed radiographic signs of fusion at 8 weeks. The control animals were slower to show new bone formation, and two of the three control animals did not have bone union develop. Zdeblick et al used the alpine goat model for multilevel anterior cervical discectomy and fusion to compare the use of a standard titanium intervertebral fusion device (BAK Sulzer Spinetech, Minneapolis, MN) with autogenous bone graft, autogenous bone graft with a hydroxyapatite-coated BAK device, and a BAK device filled with rhBMP-2. Successful arthrodesis was more obvious with rhBMP-2-filled cages (95%) than with the hydroxyapatite-coated cage (62%) or the standard cage (48%). Although biomechanical testing did not reveal a statistically significant difference in stiffness between the groups, there was a tendency for the spines in the animals that received rhBMP-2 to be stiffer.

**Minimally Invasive Techniques.**    Using a minimally invasive, video-assisted lumbar intertransverse process arthrodesis technique, Boden et al examined the feasibility, efficacy, and safety of using rhBMP-2 to achieve spinal fusion through two small portals. This method was performed initially in rabbits, then a rhesus monkey model was employed. The video-assisted arthrodesis combined with growth factor technology was a safe, feasible, and effective method of spinal fusion in the rabbit and rhesus monkey. It was thought that this minimally invasive procedure would decrease the morbidity of paraspinal muscle denervation and devascularization seen with open intertransverse process fusion techniques. The morbidity associated with graft site harvesting would be eliminated with the use of the osteoinductive bone graft substitute. Cunningham et al evaluated rhBMP-7 in anterior thoracoscopic fusions in sheep. Four months after surgery, they found that the BAK device with rhBMP-7 had the highest fusion rate and better bone formation than an empty BAK device. These studies support the prospect of less painful and less morbid spinal arthrodesis procedures with faster and stronger fusions.

**Overcoming Spinal Fusion Healing Inhibition.**    The powerful osteoinductive property of BMP may serve to overcome biologic impediments to fusion and facilitate the use of minimally invasive techniques of spinal fusion. In two studies, rhBMP-2 overcame the inhibitory effect of nicotine and a nonsteroidal antiinflammatory drug in a rabbit intertransverse process fusion model. Osteoinductive protein-1 (BMP-7; Stryker Biotech, Hopkinton, MA) was able to overcome the inhibitory effects of nicotine in a rabbit posterolateral spinal fusion model and to induce bone fusion reliably at 5 weeks. This finding suggests that BMPs might offer a method for overcoming the inhibitory effects of nicotine on spinal fusion.

# OTHER GROWTH FACTORS IN SPINAL FUSION

GDF-5 also is a member of the TGF-β superfamily that is required for proper skeletal patterning and development in the vertebrate limb. Spiro et al studied the osteoinductive activity of recombinant human GDF-5 (rhGDF-5) in combination with a mineralized collagen osteoconductive bone graft matrix (Healos; Orquest, CA) in a rabbit posterolateral lumbar fusion model. Healos alone, Healos plus rhGDF-5, or autograft harvested from the iliac crest were employed. Healos plus rhGDF-5 was found to form bone that was histologically and mechanically equivalent to that which was formed in response to autogenous bone alone. Although there are fewer published animal studies with rhGDF-5, the early results seem promising.

Kandziora et al studied the effect of a poly-(D,L-lactide) (PDLLA) carrier system combined with IGF-I and TGF-β1 in a sheep cervical spine interbody fusion model. When compared with autograft, IGF-I and TGF-β1 application by a poly-(D,L)-lactide-coated interbody cage significantly improved interbody bone matrix formation; however, the growth factors were not able to increase the incidence of solid bone fusion.

## Human Clinical Trials

Based on the highly promising results of the preclinical investigations, several pilot human trials have been initiated. Several preliminary investigations of rhBMP-2 for anterior and posterior spinal fusion also have begun. It is anticipated that data from these well-controlled feasibility trials should become available within the next few years. Boden et al have reported on the first pilot study examining the osteoinductive capacity of rhBMP-2 for a human spinal fusion application. In a limited randomized multicenter study involving 14 patients, threaded interbody fusion cages were filled with either rhBMP-2/collagen sponge or autogenous iliac crest bone graft and implanted for anterior lumbar interbody fusion. The rhBMP-2 patients, not requiring iliac crest harvest, had a shorter hospital stay compared with the autograft control patients (2 days versus 3.3 days). Of the rhBMP-2 patients, 10 of 11 were judged fused by 3 months after surgery, and all 11 were fused by 6 months. Of the three control patients, one was deemed a nonunion after 1 year. Among the rhBMP-2-induced fusions, CT scan reconstructed images consistently showed new bone growth through and anterior to the cages 6 and 12 months after surgery. Since that study, nearly 350 patients have been implanted with 99.5% fusion success rate as assessed by CT scans.

Kleeman et al performed a clinical prospective study to compare laparoscopic anterior lumbar interbody fusion using rhBMP-2 in titanium tapered cages with autogenous bone in threaded cortical bone dowels in 45 patients. Twenty-two patients underwent a laparoscopic anterior lumbar interbody fusion with an rhBMP-2-soaked collagen sponge within a tapered titanium cage, and 23 patients underwent a laparoscopic anterior lumbar interbody fusion with threaded cortical bone dowels packed with autograft. The rhBMP-2 group had a shorter operative time and length of hospital stay compared with the autograft group. Both groups reported improvement of back pain, leg pain, and overall satisfaction; however, the rhBMP-2 group improved to a higher level based on full restoration of function, the Oswestry outcome questionnaire, and the SF-36 back profile; the difference was statistically significant.

A randomized prospective clinical pilot trial was performed to determine if the dose and carrier for rhBMP-2 that was successful in rhesus monkeys could induce consistent radiographic posterolateral spinal fusions in humans. Patients enrolled in this study had single-level disc degeneration, grade I or less spondylolisthesis, mechanical low back pain with or without leg pain, and failed at least 6 months of nonoperative treatment. Twenty-five patients undergoing lumbar arthrodesis were randomized (1:2:2 ratio):

- Autograft/TSRH pedicle screw instrumentation (n = 5)
- rhBMP-2/TSRH (n = 11)
- rhBMP-2 only without internal fixation (n = 9)

The carrier was 60% hydroxyapatite/40% tricalcium phosphate granules (10 cm$^3$/side) with 20 mg of rhBMP-2/side. The radiographic fusion rate was 40% (2 of 5) in the autograft/TSRH group and 100% (20 of 20; $p = 0.05$) with rhBMP-2 with or without TSRH internal fixation. The authors concluded that rhBMP-2 with the biphasic calcium phosphate granules consistently induced radiographic posterolateral lumbar spinal fusion with or without internal fixation in patients with not greater than grade I spondylolisthesis. Also, there was a statistically greater and quicker improvement in patient-derived clinical outcome measures, including Oswestry and SF-36, in the rhBMP-2 groups.

NeOsteo (BMP protein extract) is being evaluated in posterolateral spinal fusion for degenerative spondylolisthesis; human pilot data have shown early promising results. Although the use of BMPs has shown promise in smaller animals, there is evidence to suggest that the high doses required for successful treatment of higher order animals, including humans, may be less practical for multilevel fusions through currently available means. The development of an ideal delivery system for BMP remains a clinical challenge.

Pilot studies done to determine the efficacy of rhBMP-7 in human spinal fusion procedures have been less encouraging. Laursen et al reported the use of OP-1 as an intracorporeal bone graft stimulator in unstable thoracolumbar burst fractures in five human subjects. OP-1 was found not to be efficacious, however, because all the cases failed to heal, and in one case, severe bone resorption occurred. Jeppsson et al evaluated OP-1 in cervical spine posterior fusion in four patients with rheumatoid disease. No bone formation occurred in three patients, and the study was stopped. Patel et al reported their initial experience with OP-1 for posterolateral spinal fusion in humans. In this study, 16 patients underwent decompression and fusion for spinal stenosis and degenerative spondylolisthesis, 12 patients received combined autograft and OP-1, and 4 patients received autograft alone. No adverse effects were seen, but the radiographic fusion rate was less than 70%. There were no problems with bone overgrowth or restenosis. At a 2-year follow-up assessment, results had been maintained, and restenosis had not occurred.

# GENE THERAPY IN SPINAL FUSION

Although recombinant and extracted BMP mixtures now seem capable of inducing bone growth in humans, administration of milligram doses of these proteins would be costly, and the delivery systems remain to be optimized. These issues have led several investigators to explore the use of gene therapy for the control of bone formation. Gene therapy allows for factors to be expressed in cells for longer periods and may direct bone formation more naturally by prolonged expression of more physiologic concentrations of growth factor rather than single boluses of a large dose.

The duration of protein production that is required and the anatomic location where the protein must be delivered determine the type of strategy employed for gene therapy. Several different gene therapy options are available, as follows:

- Gene therapy can be systemic or regional.
- The gene can be introduced directly to a specific anatomic site (in vivo technique), or specific cells can be harvested from the patient, expanded, and genetically manipulated in tissue culture, then reimplanted (ex vivo technique).
- The vehicle (vector) for gene delivery to the cell can be viral or nonviral (Table 33.4-2).

The delivery of the BMP transgenes to the host can be accomplished using two approaches:

- Ex vivo transduction of cells with the BMP gene, followed by the implantation of the transduced cells into the host animal
- Direct injection of a BMP vector, which inserts the BMP transgene directly into host cells

## Mechanisms of Action

In ex vivo gene transfer, cells are harvested from the patient, and DNA is transferred to cells in tissue culture. The genetically modified cells subsequently are administered to the patient. In addition to providing an osteoinductive gene to a desired site, the ex vivo approach has the additional advantage of supplying cells (e.g., bone marrow cells) that are capable of participating in osteoinduction. In vivo gene transfer involves the introduction of the specific gene directly into the body with the expectation that it will reach the target cell. To initiate gene expression, exogenous DNA must penetrate the cell, avoid lysosomal degradation, and enter the nucleus where the transcriptional machinery resides. When a virus is used as a vector, portions of the viral genome are deleted to prevent replication and create space for the insertion of the therapeutic DNA. DNA may be incorporated into the host cell's chromosomes, or it may remain extrachromosomal (episomal). Cellular uptake of DNA that is not associated with any delivery vehicle (naked DNA) is usually an inefficient process. Despite this inefficiency, naked DNA has been used successfully to promote osteogenesis.

## Applications in Spinal Fusion

Several direct and ex vivo BMP gene therapy studies have been used to fuse the spine successfully in animals. Riew et al showed that mesenchymal cells transduced with the BMP-2 gene can promote osteogenesis in the paraspinal region in the rabbit. They attempted to prolong the bone-inducing effect of BMP-2 using an adenoviral vector carry-

## TABLE 33.4-2  GENE THERAPY VECTORS

| Vectors | Description | Advantages | Disadvantages |
|---|---|---|---|
| Plasmids | Circular constructs of naked DNA | Unrestricted size of genes delivered; relative lack of toxicity | Inefficient gene transfer |
| Liposomes | Lipid vesicles (coupling of cationic liposomes with anionic DNA) | Delivers unrestricted size of genes | Relative inefficient gene transfer |
| Particle-mediated gene transfer | Gene delivery by bombardment of target cells with microprojectiles coated with DNA | Circumvents the cell membrane barrier; multiple genes with a large amount of DNA can be delivered | Transient gene expression; lack of stable gene expression |
| Retrovirus | Integrating vectors (i.e., the viral genome must be integrated into the target cell genome before expression is possible) | Reliable transfer and integration of genes to a wide array of different cells | Concern of insertional mutagenesis |
| Adenoviruses | Standard E1,E3 deleted gutless vectors—no adenovirus genes | Highest efficiency gene transfer | Transient gene transfer host immune response |
| Other viral vectors | Adeno-associated virus, herpes simplex virus, lentivirus AAV | | |

ing the human BMP-2 gene to transduce expanded marrow-derived mesenchymal stem cells in New Zealand White rabbits. Of the five study rabbits, only one (20%) showed radiographic evidence of new bone formation on the side implanted with Adv-BMP-2 5 weeks after surgery. No new bone was noted on the control Adv-β-gal side. No new bone formation was observed on either side in the other four study rabbits.

Wang et al transfected culture-expanded marrow cells with an adenoviral vector (Adv-BMP-2) to produce BMP-2 in a rat intertransverse spinal fusion model. The transfected cells were soaked onto a guanidine-extracted, deactivated, demineralized bone matrix carrier and implanted into the rat spine between the transverse processes of L4-5. At 4 weeks, all rats that had been implanted with Adv-BMP-2-producing marrow cells showed 100% fusion. All rats (100%) that had been implanted with recombinant BMP-2 alone also had complete arthrodesis by 4 weeks. All other groups did not show fusion at 8 weeks' time. Alden et al investigated the effect of percutaneous spinal fusion employing BMP-2 using adenovirus-mediated gene transfer techniques in an athymic (immunocompromised) rat model. Twelve animals divided into four groups were studied as follows:

- Adv-BMP-2 bilaterally
- Adv-BMP-2 on the right
- Adv-β-gal on the left
- Adv-β-gal bilaterally

CT scan and histology revealed new bone formation at each of the Adv-BMP-2-injected sites, but no changes were observed at the Adv-β-gal control sites. The investigators concluded that in vivo endochondral bone formation was possible using direct adenoviral construct injection into the paraspinal musculature. In both studies, cells were genetically modified to overexpress the protein, turning them into a biologic BMP-2 factory, which can be implanted into the site of spinal fusion. Riew et al achieved only 20% fusion, however, whereas Wang et al did not show any advantage in terms of fusion rates over recombinant protein. Although these studies show feasibility, they do not show a clear advantage of using gene transfer in place of recombinant BMP-2.

Lieberman et al, using the same BMP-2 gene transfer model as Wang, showed a histologic difference in the bone formed by genetically modified cells compared with bone formed by recombinant protein. The genetically modified cells appeared to form bone with finer trabecular architecture than that formed by recombinant BMP-2. This observation suggests that gene transfer and local expression of BMP-2 may lead to biologic effects that are different from the addition of exogenous protein.

Lim mineralization protein-1 (LMP-1) has been shown to be effective in inducing spinal fusion in vivo. LMP-1 cDNA, a novel intracellular protein, initiates membranous bone formation in vitro and in vivo when transfected into buffy coat white blood cells. Although LMP-1 is an intracellular protein, it is thought to act via secretion of soluble osteoinductive factors that subsequently induce expression of other BMPs and their receptors. Boden et al used a posterior spinal fusion model in nude rats and grafted guanidine-extracted demineralized bone matrix with bone marrow cells transfected with the LMP-1 cDNA. At 4 weeks, the sites with active LMP-1 cDNA had 100% fusion compared with 0% fusion at sites with the inactive reverse copy of LMP-1 cDNA. Radiographic and histologic examinations showed that virtually no bone induction was apparent in the absence of active LMP-1 cDNA. Viggeswarapu et al showed that LMP-1 is able to induce intertransverse process fusion when delivered by a replication incompetent type 5 adenovirus in immunocompetent rabbits. They did ex vivo transfection of LMP-1 cDNA into bone marrow or peripheral blood buffy coat cells. These cells were combined with a collagen and ceramic composite sponge and implanted into the posterolateral spine in rabbits. In their study, all 10 rabbits treated with cells expressing LMP-1 achieved fusion, as tested by manual palpation. None of the control rabbits treated with cells not expressing LMP-1 achieved fusion. CT scans showed that the presence of LMP-1 expressing cells increased the fusion mass density and that the bone formation was confined mostly to the carrier. Although these findings are preliminary, the potential benefit of regional gene therapy for spinal fusion applications is significant, and considerable work in this area is ongoing.

## SUGGESTED READING

Boden SD, Kang JD, Sandhu HS, Heller JG. 2002 Volvo Award for Low Back Pain Research. Use of rhBMP-2 to achieve posterolateral lumbar spine fusion in humans: a prospective and randomized clinical pilot trial. Spine 2002;27:2662–2673.

Boden SD, Martin GJ, Horton WC, et al. Laparoscopic anterior spinal arthrodesis with rhBMP-2 in a titanium interbody threaded cage. J Spinal Disord 1998;11:95–101.

Cunningham BW, Kotani Y, McNulty PS, et al. Video-assisted thoracoscopic surgery versus open thoracotomy for anterior thoracic spinal fusion: a comparative radiographic, biomechanical, and histologic analysis in a sheep model. Spine 1998;23:1333–1340.

Fischgrund JS, James SB, Chabot MC, et al. Augmentation of autograft using rhBMP-2 and different carrier media in the canine spine fusion model. J.Spinal Disord 1997;10:467–472.

Hecht B, Fischgrund J, Herkowitz H, et al. The use of recombinant human bone morphogenic protein 2 (rhBMP-2) to promote spinal fusion in a nonhuman primate anterior interbody fusion model. Spine 1999;24:629–636.

Holliger EH, Trawick RH, Boden SD, Hutton WC. Morphology of the lumbar intertransverse process fusion mass in the rabbit model: a comparison between two bone graft materials—rhBMP-2 and autograft. J Spinal Disord 1996;9:125–128.

# OUTCOMES ASSESSMENT

**BERNARD A. PFEIFER**

*Scientific method* requires the formulation of a hypothesis, testing a sample to prove or disprove its validity, and applying the principle tested to the entire population. Adherence to this process reduces bias and promotes valid interpretation of data. Testing of the hypothesis requires the appropriate experimental design and measurement apparatus. *Process improvement (quality control)* is a closed-loop system in which a problem is identified, a remedy is selected, data on the effectiveness of the remedy are collected, and the remedy is assessed and either modified or continued based on the data collected.

Both of these techniques can and should be applied to the clinical practice of medicine. The outcome initiatives were started in the late 1980s as a response to the rising cost of health care. Regional variation in rates of surgery, especially for the treatment of spinal problems, pointed out the need to assess the results of treatment and formulate a best method for appropriate patient care. Only with "hard" data can one choose from the multiple options available to select the best care for a given problem. In addition, insurers are assessing process quality through the use of health employer data and information set questionnaires and other outcome measures. New initiatives are under way to use quality incentives to stimulate better patient care through financial remuneration based on outcome measures of quality.

Still, the most appropriate use of patient-based outcomes assessment tools is simply to find the best treatment for the patient. Rothman used the SF-36 health status questionnaire to prove the high level of improvement that came with total hip arthroplasty and compared these outcomes with surgery for herniated disc, total knee arthroplasty, and scoliosis. Surgery for disc herniation showed the second best improvement, with total knee arthroplasty third. Patients operated on for scoliosis showed deterioration in health status.

Haher used a new Scoliosis Research Society instrument to show that an anterior approach to curve correction had better acceptance and patient-perceived result than posterior correction for equivalent curves; this was despite the "objective" outcome of solid fusion and percent correction seen by the operating surgeons. An additional study by D'Andrea compared the radiographic outcome of scoliosis patients with this patient-based outcomes questionnaire

and showed little correlation between the surgeon's success criterion and the patient's self-perception. These examples show the power of outcomes research.

Outcomes assessment is a less formal process. This evaluation uses an outcomes instrument for periodic reassessment of practice patterns, usually with comparison to a large group of similar patients. The outcomes assessment movement had a surge in the 1980s and 1990s with varied success.

Cardiac surgeons under the leadership of their academy have kept outcomes records on their surgical patients with an easily definable end point (i.e., survival); this has been a reaction to outside surveillance but has led to quality improvements for cardiac surgery patients. In spinal surgery, the North American Spine Society first presented its low back outcomes instrument in 1991. This instrument was an effort by a committee within the group to propose a questionnaire that would be accepted generally for use in low back patient analysis. The instrument was designed to measure pain and function, employment status, expectation, and success of meeting the expectation. The instrument development followed the principles outlined subsequently.

The American Academy of Orthopedic Surgeons (AAOS) incorporated this instrument into its MODEMS database, while at the same time a private group, the National Spinal Network, formulated its own instrument set. In the latter part of the 1990s, both groups came together in accepting the MODEMS data set as a standard. Although the National Spinal Network still is functioning, the AAOS MODEMS project has ceased to exist as a data-gathering and comparative group.

Several device manufacturers have their own study groups that perform outcomes assessment. The inherent bias in this approach may be overcome through the use of accepted instruments and independent analysis of the data.

Outcomes assessment can be quite arduous. The quality of the data set affects the accuracy of the conclusions drawn from it. Pitfalls include the office mechanics of data collection, expense of data entry, privacy, and concern regarding the end use of the data collected.

Most offices use a paper form that the patient completes, with subsequent key data entry into the computer. The general patient population must accept the instrument selected. Kiosks and computer data tablets have been tried but rely on the sophistication of the end user (patient) and have no way of verification of accuracy. Native language of the patient must be considered so as not to introduce a translation error.

One also has to consider patient flow. In an office where most of the patients are seen for consultation and only a small portion go on to surgery, a decision must be made to distribute the forms economically. If all patients receive and complete one, many will be discarded if the patients are seen for one consultation only. If forms are given to patients selected for a procedure, it may be late in the process (i.e., the patient may be tired), and the completion rate and accuracy may suffer. Optimal use would be incorporation of a smaller form within a general patient intake form with a longer one for patients selected for a procedure of interest. Having a single staff member responsible for the tracking is ideal; if the surgeon reviews the form at some point during the interview, this adds to the success of the project.

Pooling of data provides a benchmark against which to assess the current patient or group of patients. Consideration of the patient's privacy prevents dissemination of identifying data; yet if no identifying data are sent to the data repository, the same patient may be duplicated. This bias can occur when the same patient completes another data set in a second participating physician's office. Solutions to this problem include unique identifiers from combinations of patient-identifying data (e.g., part of birth date plus part of social security number) or by comparing the patient with a set of normative data at any given point in time.

One successful venture was the Maine Medical Assessment Foundation established by the Maine Medical Association. This group was federally funded and would send nurses to participant offices to contact patients directly and have them complete questionnaires and analyze the data obtained. The group showed the usefulness of surgery for herniated disc and spinal stenosis. Funding was insufficient to allow further study of spinal fusion, however, and the project has since disbanded.

Finally, physicians' concerns that the data will be used to their detriment has been a factor in the limited success of these projects thus far. Although studies have shown that the anonymous presentation of data to physicians has led to beneficial change in rates of procedures, there still seems to be a reticence to participate in pooled outcomes data unless it has been mandated.

# INSTRUMENT SELECTION: PATIENT-BASED OUTCOMES INSTRUMENTS

Patient-based outcomes instruments fall into two broad categories:

- General health status
- Region (or disease) specific

Examples of the former include the SF-36, designed by Ware, and the Musculoskeletal Functional Assessment, championed by Swiontkowski. Examples of the latter are the Oswestry Disability Index, the North American Spine Society (NASS) Instrument, the MODEMS instrument from the AAOS, and the Scoliosis Research Society instrument.

In taking any measurement, one has to use an appropriate, accurate, sensitive, and accepted device to assess the situation. For patient-based outcomes instruments, this process has been recognized as follows:

- An expert panel is assembled to select appropriate items.
- A pilot test is run, and the results are assessed to reduce the number of items.
- The test is given to groups of patients, and a retest is given a short time later to ensure reliability; Pearson coefficients >0.05 are preferred.
- The range of responses is analyzed to avoid clustering, and analyzing edge effects tests validity. Cronbach's $\alpha$ coefficient, a measure of item applicability in a scale, >0.86 is preferred.
- Sensitivity to change is assessed by analyzing pretreatment and posttreatment groups.

This type of testing is costly and arduous but required if one is to apply the instrument across a population of patients. In addition, cultural issues have to be assessed for applicability of the instrument to a diverse patient population or for international application. Finally, an assessment of normative results (i.e., results obtained from a group of "normal" individuals) may strengthen the usefulness of the instrument. A comprehensive review of these instruments was undertaken by NASS. Their Compendium of Outcomes Instruments is recommended for review before making a selection.

# SPECIFIC OUTCOMES INSTRUMENTS AND APPLICATIONS

## Pain Diagrams

Pain diagrams, as Palmer first reported in 1949, are one method of assessing patient condition. Since that time, numerous articles have appeared assessing the strengths and weaknesses of pain diagrams. The best more recent summary is by Ohnmiss. The diagram consists of anterior and posterior outlines of the body with patients asked to draw symbols indicating the location and the nature of their pain. Symbols usually are given for ache, numbness, pins and needles, stabbing, and burning. When Palmer first reported the diagram, a simple observational characterization of the response in organic and nonorganic terms was proposed. Uden expanded this classification into subgroups: organic, possibly organic, possibly inorganic, and inorganic. Intraobserver reliability was 85% for senior observers and 77% for junior observers. Ransford published a penalty point scoring system in which points were assigned for pain not in usual locations seen for root compression and other "commonly encountered causes of back and leg pain." High reliability has been reported with the use of this method. Margolis used a scoring method based on the method used in burn centers to evaluate extent of injury; a grid was placed over the drawing, and if a mark was placed in that region, a point was scored.

Ransford showed that the pain diagram agreement with the Minnesota Multi-Phasic Personality Inventory (MMPI) was 89% overall with a sensitivity of 93% and a specificity of 79%. Although Uden showed the pain diagram correctly predicted herniated disc on myelography, Rankine showed poor prediction of root compression seen on magnetic resonance imaging. Mckoy found a significant negative correlation between pain drawing scores and outcomes 6 months after surgery. The pain diagram has been found to have a significant correlation with MMPI hysteria scale and presence of Waddell criterion, both of which have a negative correlation with surgical success, so this result in not unexpected. In her summary publication correlation with discogram findings, Ohnmiss showed that the location of pain indicated on the diagram was related to the symptomatic level of the disc. In L3-4 disruption, pain was distributed in the anterior portion; L4-5 pain was distributed in anterior and posterior portions; and L5-S1 pain was distributed in the posterior portion. It seems that the best use of the pain diagram is in identifying patients with inorganic pain and patients with radiculopathy. There may be a correlation with the level of disc disruption.

## Visual Analogue Scale

The visual analogue scale is a straight line drawing usually labeled from 0 to 10 on which the patient is asked to rate his or her pain. Adding gradations to create a ruler has expanded this system, and images have been added to facilitate patient selection. It is a simple and effective method to allow the patient to rate the amount of pain and compare pretreatment and posttreatment levels. Million et al reported the test-retest reliability of this specific version of the visual analogue scale. They showed $r = 0.88$ for each of the individual scales and $r = 0.97$ for the total in a test administered by an examiner. The test has been correlated with isokinetic and nondynamometric tests.

## SF-36

The SF-36 is the result of 2 decades of evolution of an instrument designed to assess a patient's well-being. It was developed by Ware et al in 1984 for a Harris survey and later modified for a medical outcomes study. The *SF* stands for *Short Form* because participants did not complete earlier questionnaires that were deemed too long. The 36 questions are divided into eight domains or scales (Table 34-1).

## Minnesota Multi-Phasic Personality Inventory

The MMPI is a psychiatric test that should be administered by a qualified professional. As such, it does not perform as an outcomes instrument but as a test that has been studied and associated with prediction of surgical outcomes. It originally was described in 1942 by Starke and has been modified by Butcher. There are 10 scales generated from a questionnaire of 360 to 570 questions. Most important for the spine patient are the hysteria, hypochondriasis, and depression scales. Normative and other testing has been carried out for this instrument.

## Oswestry Low Back Pain Disability Questionnaire

The Oswestry Low Back Pain Disability Questionnaire is an 11-question instrument first published by Fairbank in 1980. It has been modified to a version 2.0, in which the question regarding pain intensity has been changed from that of medication usage to intensity. The score is a disability score, and a higher score implies more disability, which sounds counterintuitive. The instrument has been shown to have high test-retest reliability and has been validated against the Roland-Morris Questionnaire. The scoring is a simple addition of the responses, then doubling. Change greater than 15% is considered significant. The instrument's primary author has published a review of its use and functionality. The test has been criticized in that the result is counterintuitive; a higher numeric score indicates more disability and a patient that is faring poorly. Nonetheless, its simplicity, length, and acceptance have made it a valuable test.

## Roland Morris Disability Questionnaire

The Roland Morris Disability Questionnaire instrument is an outgrowth of the Sickness Impact Profile and first was reported in 1983. It is a 24-question yes/no format describing back pain; brevity and ease of understanding by the recipient are its hallmark. The Sickness Impact Profile on which it is based has been studied extensively; this instrument still is relatively untested.

## TABLE 34-1  SHORT-FORM 36

| Scale | Label | Phenomena Captured |
|-------|-------|--------------------|
| Physical functioning | PF | Physical function |
| Role–physical | RP | Physical disability |
| Bodily pain | BP | Physical disability and well-being |
| General health | GH | Physical and mental personal evaluation |
| Vitality | VT | Physical and mental well-being |
| Social functioning | SF | Physical and mental disability |
| Role–emotional | RE | Mental disability |
| Mental health | MH | Mental function and well-being |

<table>
<tr><td colspan="2">Please answer the following questions as to how your neck feels. This data will be used for research and tracking reasons only. Thank you for your time to complete this questionnaire.</td><td>Your Name _____<br><br>Date of Birth ___/___/_____     Today's Date ___/___/___</td></tr>
</table>

L U M B A R   I N T A K E   6 - 2 0 0 0

In the **past week** how often have **you suffered:** (Please circle one.)

| | None of the time | A little of the time | Some of the time | A good bit of the time | Most of the time | All of the time |
|---|---|---|---|---|---|---|
| 38. Back Pain? | 1 | 2 | 3 | 4 | 5 | 6 |
| 39. Leg pain? | 1 | 2 | 3 | 4 | 5 | 6 |
| 40. Numbness or tingling in leg and/or foot? | 1 | 2 | 3 | 4 | 5 | 6 |
| 41. Weakness in leg and/or foot? | 1 | 2 | 3 | 4 | 5 | 6 |

In the **past week,** how *bothersome* have these symptoms **been**? (Please circle one.)

| | Not at all bothersome | Slightly bothersome | Somewhat bothersome | Moderately bothersome | Very bothersome | Extremely bothersome |
|---|---|---|---|---|---|---|
| 42. Back Pain? | 1 | 2 | 3 | 4 | 5 | 6 |
| 43. Leg pain? | 1 | 2 | 3 | 4 | 5 | 6 |
| 44. Numbness or tingling in leg and/or foot? | 1 | 2 | 3 | 4 | 5 | 6 |
| 45. Weakness in leg and/or foot? | 1 | 2 | 3 | 4 | 5 | 6 |

In the **past week,** please tell us **how pain has affected your ability to perform** the following daily activities. (Circle the **ONE** statement that best describes your average ability.)

N=39–41,43–45=_____

| | I can dress myself without pain | I can dress myself without increasing pain | I can dress myself but pain increases | I can dress myself but with significant pain | I can dress myself but with very severe pain | I cannot dress myself due to pain |
|---|---|---|---|---|---|---|
| 46. Getting dressed (in the **past week**) | 1 | 2 | 3 | 4 | 5 | 6 |

| | I can lift heavy objects without pain | I can lift heavy objects but it is painful | Pain prevents me from lifting heavy objects off the floor, but I can lift heavy objects if they are on a table | Pain prevents me from lifting heavy objects, but I can lift light to medium objects if they are on a table | I can only lift light objects due to pain | I cannot lift anything due to pain |
|---|---|---|---|---|---|---|
| 46. Lifting (in the **past week**) | 1 | 2 | 3 | 4 | 5 | 6 |

**Figure 34-1** Part 1.

| | I can run or walk without pain | I can walk comfortably, but running is painful | Pain prevents me from walking more than 1 hour | Pain prevents me from walking more than 30 minutes | Pain prevents me from walking more than 10 minutes | I an unable to walk or can walk only a few steps at a time |
|---|---|---|---|---|---|---|
| 48. Walking and Running (in the <u>past week</u>). | 1 | 2 | 3 | 4 | 5 | 6 |

| | I can sit in any chair as long as I like | I can only sit in a special chair for as long as I like | Pain prevents me from sitting more than 1 hour | Pain prevents me from sitting more than 30 minutes | Pain prevents me from sitting more than 10 minutes | Pain prevents me from sitting at all |
|---|---|---|---|---|---|---|
| 49. Sitting (in the <u>past week</u>). | 1 | 2 | 3 | 4 | 5 | 6 |

| | I can stand in as long as I want | I can stand as long as I want but it gives me pain | Pain prevents me from standing more than 1 hour | Pain prevents me from standing for more than 30 minutes | Pain prevents me from standing for more than 10 minutes | Pain prevents me from standing at all |
|---|---|---|---|---|---|---|
| 50. Standing (in the <u>past week</u>). | 1 | 2 | 3 | 4 | 5 | 6 |

| | I sleep well | Pain occasionally interrupts my sleep | Pain interrupts my sleep half of the time | Pain often interrupts my sleep | Pain always interrupts my sleep | I never sleep well |
|---|---|---|---|---|---|---|
| 51. Sleeping (in the <u>past week</u>). | 1 | 2 | 3 | 4 | 5 | 6 |

| | My social and recreational life is unchanged | My social and recreational life is unchanged but it increases pain | My social and recreational life is unchanged but it severely increases pain | Pain has restricted my social and recreational life | Pain has severely restricted my social and recreational life | I have essentially no social and recreational life because of pain |
|---|---|---|---|---|---|---|
| 52. Social and Recreational life (in the <u>past week</u>). | 1 | 2 | 3 | 4 | 5 | 6 |

| | I can travel anywhere | I can travel anywhere but it gives me pain | Pain is bad but I can manage to travel over two hours | Pain restricts me to trips of less than one hour | Pain restricts me to trips of less than 30 minutes | Pain prevents me from traveling |
|---|---|---|---|---|---|---|
| 53. Traveling (in the <u>past week</u>). | 1 | 2 | 3 | 4 | 5 | 6 |

| | My sex life is unchanged | My sex life is unchanged but causes some pain | My sex life is nearly unchanged but it is very painful | My sex life is severely restricted by pain | My sex life is nearly absent because of pain | Pain prevents any sex life at all |
|---|---|---|---|---|---|---|
| 54. Sex life (in the <u>past week</u>). | 1 | 2 | 3 | 4 | 5 | 6 |

PD = 38,42,46–54 = _____

**Figure 34-1**  Part 2.

| As a result of my treatment, I expect.. | Not likely | Slightly likely | Somewhat likely | Very likely | Extremely likely |
|---|---|---|---|---|---|
| 36. Complete pain relief | 1 | 2 | 3 | 4 | 5 |
| 37. Moderate pain relief | 1 | 2 | 3 | 4 | 5 |
| 38. To be able to do more everyday household or yard activities | 1 | 2 | 3 | 4 | 5 |
| 39. To be able to sleep more comfortably | 1 | 2 | 3 | 4 | 5 |
| 40. To be able to go back to my usual job | 1 | 2 | 3 | 4 | 5 |
| 41. To be able to do more sports, go biking, or go for long walks | 1 | 2 | 3 | 4 | 5 |

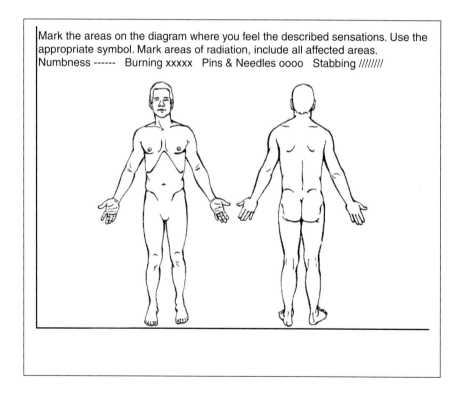

Mark the areas on the diagram where you feel the described sensations. Use the appropriate symbol. Mark areas of radiation, include all affected areas.
Numbness ------   Burning xxxxx   Pins & Needles oooo   Stabbing ////////

Please circle the number that best describes the amount of pain you had in the past week.

| | |
|---|---|
| Pain as bad as it can be | 10 |
| | 9 |
| excruciating | |
| | 8 |
| | 7 |
| severe | |
| | 6 |
| moderate | 5 |
| | 4 |
| mild | |
| | 3 |
| | 2 |
| slight | |
| | 1 |
| none | 0 |

**Figure 34-1**   Part 3. Example of an office-based low back outcomes instrument. The NASS pain disability score is calculated by averaging items 38, 42, and 46 through 54. The neurologic impairment score is calculated by averaging items 39 through 45. The expectation score is calculated by taking the average of the responses in that area (items 36 to 41). The pain diagram and visual analogue scale stand alone.

## North American Spine Society Low Back Pain Outcomes Instrument

The NASS Low Back Pain Outcomes Instrument was developed by a committee of the NASS and first formally reported in 1996. The committee added to the Oswestry base questions concerning amount of back pain to form a pain score. Six additional questions concerning amount of and bothersomeness of leg symptoms created a neurologic score. Both scores were an average of the responses to the individual questions that made up the scale (range 0 to 5). A lower score indicates a better functioning patient. Finally, there were questions regarding expectations for outcomes (for the intake form) and satisfaction with treatment (for the follow-up form). The instrument was psychometrically studied with good validity and reliability characteristics.

## Author's Instrument

I use an office-based instrument for the lumbar spine that incorporates some of the aforementioned instruments. Figure 34-1 shows this composite instrument.

## Other Instruments

### MODEMS Questionnaires

The AAOS began an ambitious project in 1992 to design a complete set of musculoskeletal outcomes instruments that could be used for any musculoskeletal outcomes research or assessment. For the spine, the instrument design phase of the project was coordinated with various subspecialty societies under the auspices of the Council of Spine Societies. The NASS low back pain outcome instrument was the basis for the MODEMS spine instrument. The low back module was kept intact with minor modifications. For the cervical spine, the instrument was reworded, changing "back" to "neck" and "leg" to "arm." Parallel scores (i.e., pain disability and neurologic impairment) were established. An attempt was made to add scales to measure myelopathy by questioning stiff and shaky leg symptoms. In addition, questions to assess comorbidity and an associated scale were constructed. Finally, the SF-36 was added, and a pain diagram substitution was created. The expectation scale and the expectation-met scale were retained from the NASS instrument. All scores were "normalized" to a 0-to-100 scale with higher numbers indicating better function or a patient in better condition. The questionnaires have undergone va-

### TABLE 34-2 NURICK CLASS

| | |
|---|---|
| Grade 0 | Root signs, no cord signs or symptoms |
| Grade 1 | Cord signs, no difficulty walking |
| Grade 2 | Slight difficulty walking, works full-time |
| Grade 3 | Gait difficulty does not allow work, can walk unassisted |
| Grade 4 | Able to walk only with assistance |
| Grade 5 | Chair bound or bedridden |

### TABLE 34-3 JAPANESE ORTHOPEDIC ASSOCIATION MYELOPATHY SCALE (MAXIMUM SCORE 5 17)

| | | |
|---|---|---|
| 1. | Upper extremity motor | |
| | Unable to feed self | 0 |
| | Unable to handle chopsticks, uses spoon | 1 |
| | Handle chopsticks with much difficulty | 2 |
| | Handle chopsticks with slight difficulty | 3 |
| | No deficit | 4    Max = 4 |
| 2. | Lower extremity motor function | |
| | Unable to walk | 0 |
| | Need walking aid on flat floor | 1 |
| | Needs hand rail on stairs | 2 |
| | Lack of stability and smooth reciprocation | 3 |
| | No impairment | 4    Max = 4 |
| 3. | Sensory deficit—upper extremity | |
| | Severe sensory loss or pain | 0 |
| | Mild sensory loss | 1 |
| | Normal | 2    Max = 2 |
| 4. | Sensory deficit—lower extremity | |
| | Same grading as per upper extremity | Max = 2 |
| 5. | Sensory deficit—trunk | |
| | Same grading as per upper extremity | Max = 2 |
| 6. | Bladder function | |
| | Urinary retention | 0 |
| | Severe difficulty | 1 |
| | Mild dysfunction | 2 |
| | Normal | 3    Max = 3 |

## TABLE 34-4 FRANKEL SCALE

| | |
|---|---|
| Frankel A | Sensory complete |
| Frankel B | Sensory incomplete |
| Frankel C | Motor useless |
| Frankel D | Motor useful |
| Frankel E | Normal |

lidity and reliability testing, and normative data have been obtained. In addition, a scoliosis questionnaire was devised that measured the patient's view of their attractiveness (cosmesis); this was added to the low back questionnaire.

The MODEMS instruments were tested as part of the overall MODEMS data-gathering project. The above-specified additions resulted in a lengthy questionnaire. The MODEMS questionnaires have not been widely accepted and have been criticized on the basis of length of instrument and arduous nature of data entry. In addition, they were part of a project to pool data in a central repository that suffered from poor participation. Nonetheless, it is a worthy effort, and one can use selected parts to create valuable scales that can provide helpful data. The normative data were obtained by administering the questionnaire to people selected by a research firm to represent a normal cross section of the population. This is the first instrument to have this feature and provides a benchmark against which the patient can be measured.

### Cervical Spine Research Society Questionnaire

BenDebba developed a questionnaire at Johns Hopkins that measures cervical outcomes. Good validity and reliability data were reported. The questionnaire is about as long as the MODEMS instrument without the SF-36 and the comorbidity questions. Excellent patient acceptance was reported. No scale has been created with the measure, but the questions stand independent of each other.

### Scoliosis Research Society Questionnaire

Haher devised a shorter questionnaire than the MODEMS to measure impact of deformity on patients with scoliosis. The validity and reliability testing of this instrument was coupled nicely with a study of anterior versus posterior approach to the correction of curve and indicated a preference for the former approach. The questionnaire has been modified by Asher but with minimal change. It seems to be most valuable in adolescent patients, but more recent reports showed its response to patient condition and that its ceiling and floor effects, internal consistency, reproducibility, and validity were equal to or better than the SF-36 domains with which it was compared.

## MEASURES OF PATIENT STATUS: NOT SELF-REPORTED

Several valuable indices incorporate patient report with physical examination parameters to assess the status of the patient. The Japanese Orthopedic Association myelopathy scale and Nurick classification are valuable for degenerative conditions. The Glasgow Coma Scale, the Frankel classification of quadriplegia, and the American Spinal Injury Association classification are examples of this type of assessment item for a patient after trauma to the spinal cord.

The Nurick scale attempts to quantify patient impairment from myelopathy based on ability to ambulate (Table 34-2). The Japanese Orthopedic Association first presented its myelopathy impairment scale in 1990 (Table 34-3). This scale takes into account and scores in graded fashion the patient's ability to walk, do fine motor tasks with the upper

## TABLE 34-5 AMERICAN SPINAL INJURY ASSOCIATION MOTOR SCORE

| Level | Muscle Group | Right | Left | |
|---|---|---|---|---|
| C5 | Elbow flexors | _____ | _____ | |
| C6 | Wrist extensors | _____ | _____ | |
| C7 | Elbow extensors | _____ | _____ | |
| C8 | Finger flexors | _____ | _____ | |
| T1 | Finger abductors | _____ | _____ | |
| L2 | Hip flexor | | _____ | _____ |
| L3 | Knee extensors | _____ | _____ | |
| L4 | Ankle dorsiflexor | _____ | _____ | |
| L5 | Toe extensor | | _____ | _____ |
| S1 | Plantar flexor | | _____ | _____ |
| | Max | 50 | 50 | Total 100 |
| Grades: | 0—Absent | | | |
| | 1—trace, flicker | | | |
| | 2—poor, moves gravity eliminated | | | |
| | 3—fair, moves against gravity | | | |
| | 4—good, moves against resistance | | | |
| | 5—normal | | | |

## TABLE 34-6 GLASGOW COMA SCALE

| | | | |
|---|---|---|---|
| 1. | Eye opening: | | Max = 4 |
| | Spontaneous | 4 | |
| | Responds to sound | 3 | |
| | Responds to Pain | 2 | |
| | Never | 1 | |
| 2. | Verbal response: | | Max = 5 |
| | Oriented | 5 | |
| | Confused conversation | 4 | |
| | Inappropriate words | 3 | |
| | Incomprehensible words | 2 | |
| | None | 1 | |
| 3. | Motor response | | Max = 6 |
| | Obeys commands | 6 | |
| | Localizes pain | 5 | |
| | Flexion withdrawal | 4 | |
| | Abnormal | 3 | |
| | Extension | 2 | |
| | None | 1 | |
| | | | Max = 15 |

extremities, feel sensation in trunk and extremities, and control bladder function. It has been modified for use in Western countries by substituting use of knife and fork for chopstick use. Numerous publications have cited the scale, but there has never been a scientific test of its sensitivity and specificity.

Frankel described a gradation of the patient's motor ability for use with spinal injury patients (Table 34-4). He divided this gradation into motor useful and motor useless. This scale is useful in tracking a patient's progress or regression during the course of therapy. The American Spinal Injury Association expanded on the Frankel classification. The same level of function for each individual motor group is retained, but key muscle groups are identified, and a point score is given for each side (Table 34-5). A separate notation of bladder and bowel function and the lowest sensory level present are noted. The classification provides a valuable way of tracking a patient's progress. Finally, in tracking the trauma patient, the Glasgow Coma Scale is a valuable adjunct because a patient with spinal injury often has a concomitant head injury that requires assessment (Table 34-6).

## SUGGESTED READING

Asher M, Min Lai S, Burton D, Manna B. Discrimination validity of the Scoliosis Research Society-22 patient questionnaire: relationship to idiopathic scoliosis curve pattern and curve size. Spine 2003;28:74–82.

BenDebba M, Heller J, Ducker TB, Eisinger JM. Cervical spine outcomes questionnaire: its development and psychometric properties. Spine 2002;27:2116–2123.

Bergner M, Bobbitt RA, Pollard WE, et al. The sickness impact profile: validation of a health status measure. Med Care 1976;14:57–67.

Butcher JN, Tellegen A. Common methodological problems in MMPI research. J Consult Clin Psychol 1978;46:620–628.

Chan CW, Goldman S, Ilstrup DM, et al. The pain drawing and Waddell's nonorganic physical signs in chronic low-back pain. Spine 1993;18:1717–1722.

Daltroy LH, Cats-Baril WL, Katz JN, et al. The North American Spine Society lumbar spine outcome assessment instrument, reliability and validity tests. Spine 1996;21:741–748.

D'Andrea LP, Betz RR, Lenke LG, et al. Do radiographic parameters correlate with clinical outcomes in adolescent idiopathic scoliosis? Spine 2000;25:1795–1802.

Dzioba RB, Doxey NC. A prospective investigation into the orthopedic and psychological predictors of outcome of first lumbar surgery following industrial injury. Spine 1984;9:264–268.

Fairbank J, Pynsent PB. The Oswestry index. Spine 2000;25:2940–2953.

Fairbank JCT, Couper J, Davies JB, O'Brien JP. The Oswestry low back pain disability questionnaire. Physiotherapy 1980;66:271–273.

Haher TR, Gorup JM, Shin TM, et al. Results of the Scoliosis Research Society instrument for evaluation of surgical outcome in adolescent idiopathic scoliosis: a multicenter study of 244 patients. Spine 1999;24:1435–1440.

# INDEX

*Note: Page numbers followed by "f" indicate figures; those followed by "t" indicate tables.*